YOU CAN'T SEE THEM, TASTE THEM, OR SMELL THEM—BUT CALORIES COUNT.

"My own diet"—what works best for each individual—is the most successful diet in the United States today. Forget fads. With the sound advice and calorie information found in *The Calorie Counter*, 6th Edition, you can make consistent small changes in the way you eat that will help you lose weight and keep it off.

- **Understand calories**
- **Understand portions**
- **Determine the calories you need daily**
- **Calculate the calories you burn through exercise and everyday activities**
- **Find out the truth about dieting myths**
- **Manage "mindless eating"**
- **Stop battling your weight**

THE CALORIE COUNTER, 6th Edition

The only weight-loss guide you will ever need.

D0037319

Books by Karen J. Nolan and Jo-Ann Heslin

The Calorie Counter (*Sixth Edition*)
The Complete Food Counter (*Fourth Edition*)
The Ultimate Carbohydrate Counter (*Third Edition*)
The Protein Counter (*Third Edition*)
The Diabetes Counter (*Fourth Edition*)
The Most Complete Food Counter (*Third Edition*)

**Books by Annette B. Natow, Jo-Ann Heslin
and Karen J. Nolan**

The Cholesterol Counter (*Seventh Edition*)
The Fat Counter (*Seventh Edition*)
The Healthy Wholefoods Counter

Books by Annette B. Natow and Jo-Ann Heslin

Eating Out Food Counter
The Healthy Heart Food Counter
The Vitamin and Mineral Food Counter

**Ebooks by Karen J. Nolan, Jo-Ann Heslin
and Annette B. Natow**

The Most Complete Food Counter (*Second Edition*)

Apps by Karen J. Nolan and Jo-Ann Heslin

Your Complete Food Counter

(http://itunes.apple.com/us/app/
your-complete-food-counter/id444558777?mt=8)

Published by POCKET BOOKS

THE
CALORIE
COUNTER

SIXTH EDITION

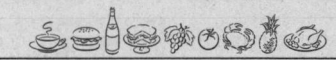

**Karen J. Nolan, Ph.D.
and Jo-Ann Heslin, M.A., R.D.**

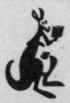

POCKET BOOKS
New York   London   Toronto   Sydney   New Delhi

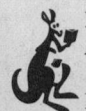
Pocket Books
A Division of Simon & Schuster, Inc.
1230 Avenue of the Americas
New York, NY 10020

This Pocket Books paperback edition January 2013

POCKET and colophon are registered trademarks of Simon & Schuster, Inc.

For information about special discounts for bulk purchases, please contact Simon & Schuster Special Sales at 1-866-506-1949 or business@simonandschuster.com.

The Simon & Schuster Speakers Bureau can bring authors to your live event. For more information or to book an event, contact the Simon & Schuster Speakers Bureau at 1-866-248-3049 or visit our website at www.simonspeakers.com.

Manufactured in the United States of America

10 9 8 7 6 5 4 3 2 1

ISBN 978-1-4516-2163-1

For

Our families, who support us through every project.

ACKNOWLEDGMENTS

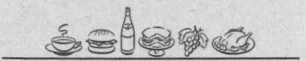

For all her continuous support and help, our agent, Nancy Trichter.

For her suggestions and editing skills, Sara Clemence.

For all her patience, comments and questions—our favorite reviewer, Jean Schwarsin.

Without the tireless cooperation of Stephen Llano and the production department at Pocket Books, *The Calorie Counter*, 6th Edition would never have been completed.

A special thank-you to our editor, Emilia Pisani.

We would also like to thank all of our readers for their suggestions and questions. Your input helps us provide you with the most useful information.

Man is to be compared to a clock, going all the time, rather than to an automobile engine, working only at intervals....

In order to have energy to spend ... we must first acquire it ... protein, fat and carbohydrate ... are the fuels which supply energy for the human machine.

Mary Swartz Rose, Ph.D.
Feeding the Family
The Macmillan Company, 1919

CONTENTS

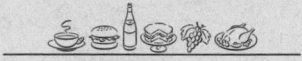

Introduction	1
Understanding Calories	5
Understanding Portions	8
Calories You Need	12
Real Men Can Count Calories	15
The Truth, and Nothing but the Truth	20
Calories You Use	25
Minimize Mindless Eating	32
Oops! What Now—Taking Charge in Tough Situations	36
Tracking Calories	42
Using Your Calorie Counter	46

PART ONE

Brand-Name, Nonbranded (Generic), and Take-out Foods

53

PART TWO

Restaurant Chains

511

INTRODUCTION

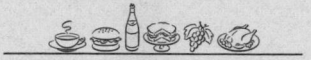

If losing weight were easy, no one would weigh too much.

If you're looking at this book, you are probably trying to lose weight. You aren't alone; *losing weight has become one of the most important health concerns in America*.

Everyone is scrambling to solve the problem of America's expanding waistlines. The federal government, public health organizations, professional organizations, educators, pharmaceutical companies, food manufacturers, and even restaurant chains all want to slow down the nation's weight gain epidemic. But new policies, programs, food formulations, and drug approvals occur slowly. Like most people we talk to every day, you are not willing to wait. *You want to lose weight now!*

So let's get started—

Calories are tiny energy powerhouses found in all the food you eat except water. You take in calories every time you eat.

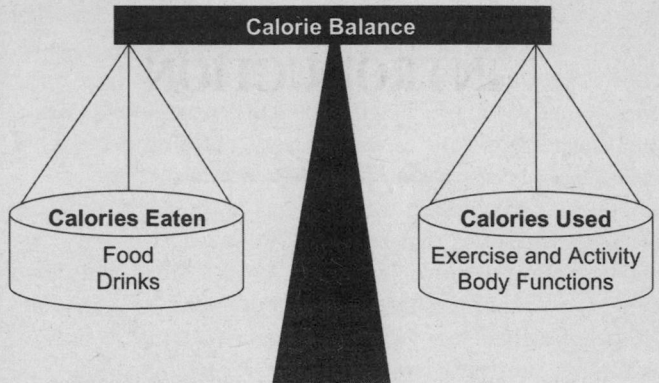

Determining the proper calorie intake is similar to balancing a scale. To maintain your weight, the calories you eat must be about equal to the calories your body uses to keep working, plus the calories you use in daily activities and in exercise. If you are:

Maintaining your weight—you are eating roughly the same number of calories that your body uses up. Your weight should remain about the same over time.

Gaining weight—you are eating more calories than your body uses up through activity. You will store these extra calories, and your weight will go up.

Losing weight—you are eating fewer calories than your body uses. You will be pulling calories that have been stored as fat, and your weight will go down.

Weight gain results from a combination of your genes and your environment.

There isn't much you can do about your genetic profile, which was fixed before you were born. Take a look at your relatives. Are they long and lean? Are they apple-shaped, holding most of their weight from the waist down? Are they short or tall? Your genetic profile will have a lot to do with your weight and body shape, but that does not mean you are doomed to be overweight. You *can* control your environment, especially your eating environment. And that's what we hope *The Calorie Counter* will help you do.

Food is everywhere we turn during the day. And most of us live lifestyles that require little physical activity; we make an effort to move. In the last 10 years, Americans have gained a total of more than 1 billion pounds—68% of adults are overweight. The extra weight we are carrying is putting a drain on our health-care system, increasing our risk for diabetes and heart disease, and shortening our lives.

Losing weight doesn't just happen. Deciding to lose weight is easy, but the follow-through can be a real challenge. You have to let go of bad habits (not easy!) and embrace new habits for eating and exercise. But we promise—it can be done!

Two important things you should know:

The most successful diet in the U.S. today is called "my own diet." Forget fads. With the sound advice and the calorie information found in this book, you can design your own diet—one that works.

Consistent small changes will add up to big results. When it comes to losing weight or *maintaining* your weight loss, making many small changes in the way you relate to food will result in more success than making a few big changes, which usually don't last.

Skeptical?

If you eat 100 fewer calories each day for a year, and change nothing else in your life, you will lose 10 pounds. All you would have to do is give up 1 slice of bread or 1 cookie or 1 small soda each day. A small change for a big result. Make a few more of those small changes, and the end result could be very impressive.

Our best eating advice, in a nutshell:

- Eat less, but enjoy what you eat
- Eat lots of fruits and vegetables
- Eat whole grains instead of refined carbs (like white bread)
- Eat less sugar (but you don't have to give it up)
- Eat more good fats like olive oil, fish, and nuts
- Eat lean proteins—fish, chicken without the skin, lean beef, pork, and lamb
- Enjoy a glass of wine, but not the whole bottle
- Move more and move often—find ways to be active throughout the day

---

10%

Losing 10% of your body weight—15 pounds for someone who weighs 150 pounds, 20 pounds for a person weighing 200 pounds, or 30 pounds if the scale says 300 pounds—is all that is needed to significantly improve your health.

Lose 10% of your current body weight and you will have:

Lower blood pressure
Improved cholesterol levels
Decreased risk for diabetes
Better sex

Reaching your ideal weight is great, but even just a 10% drop in body weight improves both your health and appearance.

UNDERSTANDING CALORIES

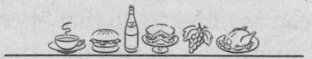

You can't see them, taste them, or smell them, but calories count!

Every time you eat, you take in calories. All foods, except water, have some. Calories are calories, whether they come from apples or chocolate fudge. Your body is a machine that uses food calories as fuel. When the amount of fuel you take in equals the amount of fuel you need to run your body, your weight remains constant. There is no extra fuel to store and no deficit to make up. Eat too many calories, and your body uses what it needs and stores the leftovers for future use. You see this storage on your thighs, hips, and waist. Eat too few calories and your body draws on its fuel reserves to meet demands. Your thighs, hips, and waist get slimmer as your fuel surplus is depleted.

You can think of the extra pounds you are carrying around as a warehouse of stored fuel. Remove calories from the warehouse and you lose weight. Add to the inventory in the warehouse and you gain.

Again and again, studies have shown that if you cut calories, you lose weight. A study published in early 2012 once again showed that the reason people gained weight is that they ate too many calories. It didn't matter what percentage of carb, fat, or protein a person ate as long as the overall amount of calories eaten daily were not excessive. It doesn't matter if calories come from bread, meat, salad dressing, or even vegetables. **When you eat too many calories, even from healthy foods, you gain weight.**

The key to long-term weight control is to burn as many calories as you eat. In order to do that effectively, you need to know how many calories you need and how many calories you burn in activity. Then you can see if the two balance each other.

And the Numbers Are . . .

On average, we eat 300 more calories a day than we ate 35 years ago. Today, the average man is 17 pounds heavier, and the average woman weighs 19 pounds more.

Women report eating 1,877 calories a day; men, 2,618 calories.

The catch: up to 75% of people underreport what they eat!

Beware Calories in a Glass (or Bottle . . . or Can . . .)

At most restaurants drink refills are free. You'll quickly get more soda and coffee without even asking. You get more, so you drink more. You're thinking, *It's free, so why shouldn't I drink it?* One reason—liquid calories could be helping you pack on extra pounds. It seems our bodies don't process calories from drinks the same way we process calories from food.

Alcohol drinks and clear liquids like soda, fruit drinks, energy drinks, and sweetened tea are potential diet disasters. Alcoholic drinks can be very calorie dense (see page 54), and they make you eat more. Studies show if you have a glass of wine with dinner, you'll eat more food—as much as 40% more calories.

Beverages also have a very low satisfaction level, which means they don't make you feel full. The more you are offered, the more you drink, often without considering the calories. Soda is the single largest source of calories in the American diet. The increased intake of calorie-containing clear drinks parallels our sharp rise in weight gain over the last 3 decades.

At the same time, the portion sizes of typical beverages have increased. We've gone from an 8-ounce bottle of Coke to unlimited soda refills served in a quart-sized glass. A small coffee now averages 10 ounces in contrast to the old 5-ounce cup. Add cream and sugar and your small coffee contains 100 calories. And few of us ever order "small." Multiply that by 3 or 4 cups a day and you start to see why it's hard to lose weight.

To keep calories down when you are thirsty:

- Choose low- or no-calorie drinks.

- Drink nonfat milk instead of whole milk.

- Dilute fruit drinks with mineral water.

- Dilute alcohol with low- or no-calorie mixers.

- Drink light beer, and not too many.

- Order hot cocoa with skim milk and no whipped topping.

- Order coffee minus the whipped toppings and other add-ons.

- Drink water: it's thirst quenching and calorie free.

Think About What You Drink

Researchers estimate that 20% of daily calories (close to 300 calories) comes from sugary drinks.

UNDERSTANDING PORTIONS

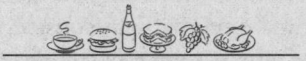

Smaller portions = a smaller you.

With the exception of a slice of bread, the portion sizes of commonly eaten foods have steadily grown over the last 20 years. Even the average restaurant dinner plate is 2 inches larger! We've gotten so used to these exaggerated amounts that we think of them as normal.

What Research Has Shown

Larger portions encourage people to overeat, even foods that they don't like or that don't taste good.

Serving large portions encourages people to eat up to 40% more calories at a meal.

After eating a large portion or a regular portion, people rated their feelings of fullness the same even though they ate more of the large portion.

Twenty years ago, the muffin or bagel you bought with your morning coffee weighed 2 ounces. Today, 4 to 6 ounces is more the norm. When burger shops first opened, an average soda was 8 ounces, regular French fries were 2.5 ounces, and the burger plus bun weighed less than 4 ounces. Today, a medium soda averages 20 ounces, and the French fries and burger have been supersized. They're 2 to 5 times larger than the original, adding up to a 1,000-calorie meal.

PORTION DISTORTION

Today's "normal" portion is actually a supersized serving.

FOOD ITEM	20 YEARS AGO CALORIES (PORTION)	TODAY CALORIES (PORTION)	CALORIE DIFFERENCE
Soda	150 (12 ounces)	400 (32 ounces)	+250
Muffin	210 (1.5 ounces)	500 (4 ounces)	+290
Pepperoni Pizza	500 (2 slices)	850 (2 slices)	+350
Chicken Caesar Salad	390 (1½ cups)	790 (3½ cups)	+400
Movie theater popcorn	270 (5 cups)	630 (11 cups)	+360
Chicken stir-fry	435 (2 cups)	865 (4½ cups)	+430

You may think larger portions are bargains without appreciating how many extra calories you're eating. According to a government survey, Americans typically eat 2½ times the standard serving of potatoes, 4 times the standard serving of pasta, and 2 times the standard serving of rice. A standard serving for all is ½ cup.

Seeing Is Believing

These visual cues will help you keep portion sizes reasonable, which automatically reduces calories.

computer mouse	=	*4-ounce portion of meat, chicken, seafood*
		or
		1 medium baked potato
yo-yo	=	*a mini bagel or 100 calories. How many yo-yos fit into your bagel, muffin, or pastry?*
tennis ball	=	*medium piece of fresh fruit*
Ping-Pong ball	=	*a 2-ounce serving of cheese*
		or
		2 tablespoons salad dressing, gravy, sour cream, peanut butter
music CD	=	*1 medium-sized pancake or small waffle*
quarter	=	*1 pat butter*

When you snack, pick single-serving packages. How many times have you opened a bag of chips just to have a few, and before you knew it the bag was empty? A 1-ounce, snack-size bag of chips allows you to enjoy a favorite treat without sabotaging your weight loss goals. Single-serving pudding, ice cream, pretzels, peanuts, cookies, and snack-size yogurt will help keep you from overindulging.

Many people don't realize that larger portions have more calories. They figure a soda is a soda, no matter how big—without calculating that a 32-ounce soda has 400 calories. Next time you order, think small—soda, coffee, movie theater popcorn, ice cream cones, and French fries. We even eat large portions of good-for-you fruits and vegetables.

Supersizing the Good Stuff

Typical fruits, a good-for-you food, have been supersized. It is hard to find small oranges, apples, bananas, and pears.

A small orange = 45 calories; a large one 86.

A small apple = 55 calories; a large one 110.

A small banana = 90 calories; a large one 121.

A small pear = 86 calories; a large one 133.

Buy and eat small whenever possible.

CALORIES YOU NEED

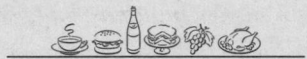

Most people don't know how many calories they need
each day, and most people don't know how many
calories they eat. Both are vital to weight control.

Most of us eat more than we admit and exercise less than we
should. The consequence is that we weigh more than we
would like to and blame it all on our metabolism—even if
we're not quite sure what that is.

Human metabolism is the sum of all the chemical reactions that occur in your body. Your body takes in foods,
burns some to generate power, uses some to produce new
material, and routes the rest into storage for future use. The
chemical reactions that occur either break down large com-
pounds into smaller units (the foods you eat, for example,
are broken down into smaller units of energy), or build com-
plex structures from smaller units (your muscles are made
up of fragments that come from the protein foods you eat,
like eggs). Human metabolism is the sum total of all the reactions needed to keep your body alive and moving. The energy required to make all this happen can be translated into
the calories you need each day.

Approximately 60% to 75% of your daily calories are
used just to keep you alive. Energy is needed to maintain
your body's temperature, allow your nerves to work, let

you breathe, keep your heart beating, allow your organs to function, nourish your body tissues, and repair and replace body fluids and parts. It's a big job, and it goes on 24 hours a day.

An interesting thing about this basic energy requirement is that different tissues in the body have different levels of activity. Fat tissue is less active and needs less energy. Muscle tissue, even at rest, is more active and uses up more energy. If you exercise and develop more muscle tissue, your body burns more calories every day just keeping your muscles healthy.

The rest of the calories you need each day are used to support activity. Obviously, you need fewer if you are relatively inactive and more if you are very active.

You Should Know—

The U.S. produces enough food to provide every person in the country with 3,900 calories a day.

Few of us need anywhere close to that amount.

Food producers are in fierce competition to get you to pick their products. Beware—all those extra calories can be tempting, and they pack on pounds.

To find out how many calories you need each day, you need to do two things. First, decide how much you want to weigh. Not your current weight; what is your target weight? Second, select an activity factor that fits your current activity level.

1. Your target weight is: _____.
2. Your activity factor is: _____.
   20 = Very active men
   15 = Moderately active men or very active women

    13 = Inactive men, moderately active women, and peo-
        ple over 55
    10 = Inactive women, repeat dieters, seriously over-
        weight people
 3. Target Weight × Activity Factor = Calories needed
    each day

For example, if your target weight is 130 and you are a
moderately active woman (factor 13), you need about 1,600
to 1,700 calories a day.

$$130 \text{ pounds} \times 13 = 1,690 \text{ calories}$$

Eating this number of calories each day would guarantee
weight loss, because you are getting only enough calories to
support your target weight, not your current heavier weight.
Couple this calorie intake with some added exercise and the
weight will come off even faster.

REAL MEN CAN COUNT CALORIES

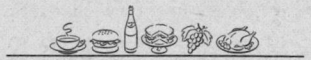

If a man cuts calories, he'll lose more weight
and he'll lose it faster than a woman will.

Announcing you are on a diet is not manly. Munching on salad, eating yogurt topped with granola, or sipping green tea does not conjure up a macho image. But over half of American men weigh too much, and many are trying to drop pounds.

According to the National Center for Health Statistics, 72% of American men are overweight, while only 64% of women are, based on their Body Mass Index (BMI). Having a BMI of more than 25 tips you into the overweight group. You may only be carrying around a few extra pounds, but as time goes on these "extra" pounds add up as you slide from the overweight category into the much too heavy, obese group. Clearly, losing weight is no longer for women only.

BMI is not a foolproof way to measure overweight. A person with a very muscular, dense body build and a low percentage of body fat could end up with the same BMI as someone who truly is overweight and has a high percentage of body fat. One way to sort out the difference is to measure waistlines. Experts say that people with a BMI of 25

YOUR BODY MASS INDEX (BMI)

HEIGHT	WEIGHT																					
	100	105	110	115	120	125	130	135	140	145	150	155	160	165	170	175	180	185	190	195	200	205
5'0"	20	21	22	22	23	24	25	26	27	28	29	30	31	32	33	34	35	36	37	38	39	40
5'1"	19	20	21	22	23	24	25	26	26	27	28	29	30	31	32	33	34	35	36	37	38	39
5'2"	18	19	20	21	22	23	24	25	26	27	28	28	29	30	31	32	33	34	35	36	37	37
5'3"	18	19	19	20	21	22	23	24	25	26	27	27	28	29	30	31	32	33	34	35	35	36
5'4"	17	18	19	20	21	21	22	23	24	25	26	27	28	28	29	30	31	32	33	33	34	35
5'5"	17	17	18	19	20	21	22	22	23	24	25	26	27	27	28	29	30	31	32	32	33	34
5'6"	16	17	18	19	19	20	21	22	23	23	24	25	26	27	27	28	29	30	31	31	32	33
5'7"	16	16	17	18	19	20	20	21	22	23	23	24	25	26	27	27	28	29	30	31	31	32
5'8"	15	16	17	17	18	19	20	21	21	22	23	24	24	25	26	27	27	28	29	30	30	31
5'9"	15	16	16	17	18	18	19	20	21	21	22	23	24	24	25	26	27	27	28	29	30	30
5'10"	14	15	16	17	17	18	19	19	20	21	22	22	23	24	24	25	26	27	27	28	29	30
5'11"	14	15	15	16	17	17	18	19	20	20	21	22	22	23	24	24	25	26	26	27	28	29
6'0"	14	14	15	16	16	17	18	18	19	20	20	21	22	22	23	24	24	25	26	26	27	28
6'1"	13	14	15	16	16	17	17	18	18	19	20	20	21	22	22	23	24	24	25	26	26	27
6'2"	13	13	14	15	15	16	17	17	18	19	19	20	21	21	22	23	23	24	24	25	26	26
6'3"	12	13	14	15	15	16	16	17	17	18	19	19	20	21	21	22	23	23	24	24	25	26
6'4"	12	13	13	14	15	15	16	16	17	18	18	19	19	20	21	21	22	23	23	24	24	25

to 35 and waistlines over 40 inches for men and more than 35 inches for women are considered overweight. They face increased health risks because they are carrying around too many pounds.

Use the BMI scale on page 16 to see where you stand. Find your height on the left of the chart. Find the weight closest to your weight across the top of the chart. Follow the weight column down and the height column across until they meet. Your BMI is the number at the intersection of your weight and height.

Your BMI is _____.

A study that included more than 50,000 men showed that 3 lifestyle factors predicted weight gain—less time exercising, more time watching TV, and eating between meals. Eating a soup bowl of ice cream while sitting in your recliner waving the remote at the TV will not make you trim.

In all fairness, most weight loss research has been done with women. But the few studies we have on men tell us very good news. Men are very successful at losing weight. They can eat more food and still lose weight, they lose weight faster, and when they trip up they are less likely to feel guilty and get derailed.

You Should Know—

> *The bigger a man's waistline, the lower his testosterone level, sex drive, sperm count, and likelihood of conceiving a child.*

Sadly, many men don't take weight loss seriously until they have a major health problem, like diabetes or a heart attack. What men need to realize is that making lifestyle changes before a catastrophe hits could prevent it from ever happening.

You may feel dieting is wimpy but striving for health and

fitness is manly. Aerobic exercise—walking, jogging, and bike riding—helps to lower pounds and reduce fat around your middle. Lowering body weight by as little as 10% can improve your health risks and increase your stamina on the basketball court and in the bedroom.

Watching calories is a simple and easy way for men to lose weight. You don't have to drastically change your eating pattern—your buddies will never be the wiser—you just need to adjust the amount and type of foods you eat. Swap fried chicken and fries for grilled chicken and a baked potato. Share a bucket of buffalo wings, but eat 3 instead of 6 and skip the blue cheese dip. Enjoy pizza, but stick with plain cheese. If you are daring, try the veggie-topped—just pass on the meat lover's or extra cheese.

You Should Know—

Men are more likely to overeat pizza, pasta, hamburgers, or casseroles.

Women get tripped up when it comes to sweets and snacks.

Simply downsizing portions will help most men lose weight.

Men, want to be in shape, ripped, trim?

- Drink alcohol, but in moderation.

- Go easy on calorie-containing drinks. They add up quickly. Water has zero calories.

- Rev up your metabolism—eat breakfast, lift weights.

- Don't sit around eating chips; go for a run, or at least a walk.

- Make smart food choices. Instead of a double burger with bacon and cheese, order a regular burger with lettuce and tomato.

- Cook at home, where you can control portions and cut calories. Notice all the men cooking on the food channels.

- Don't wait till you have been diagnosed with a problem to start losing weight.

- Count calories. It is a simple strategy for trimming down, and it works.

A Simple Trick—Don't Clear the Table

When leftover chicken wing bones were visible, guys watching a football game ate 27% less than those without the visual cue to signal how much they had eaten.

A tough guy can count calories and do it successfully—he just doesn't want to announce it to the world.

THE TRUTH, AND NOTHING BUT THE TRUTH

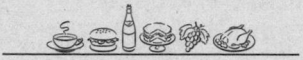

People who wear belts stop eating sooner than people who don't.

There are many misconceptions about what makes you gain weight and what doesn't. Here are a few that come up again and again. Let's set the record straight.

Sugar and fast food do not make you fat.

There is no specific food that causes weight gain. The only thing that makes you fat is eating too many calories. If you eat too much sugar and too many fast foods, you will gain weight. If you eat both in moderation, you won't. People who eat a lot of sugar or fast food also frequently eat larger portions, eat more often, and eat fewer good-for-you foods, like fruits, vegetables, and whole grains. Fat, sugar, and salt make foods taste more appealing and create a situation where it is easier to overeat. But the bottom line in weight gain is driven by portion size, not the specific foods eaten.

Smoking is not an effective weight-loss strategy.

As a matter of fact, research has shown that smoking encourages the accumulation of belly fat. Smokers, even lean ones, have thicker waists than nonsmokers.

Skipping meals does not help you cut calories.

People who eat many small amounts during the day are slimmer than those who eat few larger meals. Regular breakfast skippers are 450% more likely to be overweight. *Eat when you're hungry, stop when you're full* is a simple rule that is difficult to follow. But those who do follow it usually eat fewer calories than people who sit down to a big lunch or dinner simply because the clock says it's time to eat.

Nighttime calories are no more fattening than daytime calories.

Time of day doesn't matter; the calorie count does. You can eat all the calories you need for an entire day between midnight and 6:00 a.m., if you wish. As long as you don't eat any more during the rest of the day, you won't gain weight. The warning against late-night eating *does* have value if the calories eaten watching TV or coping with stress are on top of the calories you've already eaten during the day.

You Should Know—

It may be women's brains and not their stomachs that lead to overeating.

An imaging study showed that a woman's brain drives her to overeat when she is presented with her favorite foods or when she is under emotional stress.

The same is not true for men.

One package does not always equal one serving.

Read food labels carefully to see if a package—even a smaller one—contains more than 1 serving. Many foods and snacks are packaged as single serving, and that's exactly what you are getting—1 serving. But other "smaller" sized packages may hold more than 1 serving. For example, a small bag of chips may hold 2½ servings. A package of cookies may be 2 servings. Some large muffins give calories for half a muffin—who eats half a muffin, even a large one? Remember that if you eat the whole package, you'll be eating more calories than those listed for one serving.

Fat free and sugar free are not calorie free.

Buying fat-free or sugar-free foods seems virtuous and can seduce you into eating larger amounts. But beware: some brands of sugar-free cookies and fat-free crackers have the same number of calories as—and sometimes more than—the regular versions. Few foods are calorie free. If a fat-free salad dressing has half the calories of a regular version and you use twice as much, or if you eat a box of sugar-free cookies, there is no calorie benefit.

You won't burn fat faster if you exercise harder.

The intensity of your exercise makes no difference as long as you burn more calories than you eat. It doesn't matter how long it takes you to go a distance: the more ground you cover, the more calories you burn. For each pound you weigh, you burn 1 calorie per mile. So whether walking, hiking, jogging, or sprinting, a 100-pound person burns 100 calories a mile on a flat surface, a 200-pound person uses 200 calories, and so on. Keep in mind that the time you exercise is only a small part of the day. A daily active lifestyle may actually burn more calories than a single exercise session, so take the stairs, don't use the drive-thru, and play with the kids at the park.

Exercise Myths

Continued calorie burning after exercise lasts only 15 to 35 minutes, not hours, as once believed.

Exercise burns calories, not fat. But chipping away at excess flab doesn't require that you selectively burn fat—you just need to burn more calories than you eat and you'll get slimmer.

So, keep moving.

Water is a powerful calorie burner.

Seventy-five percent of people don't drink enough water. When you have too little water in your body, your metabolism slows down and you burn fewer calories. Exercising, running errands, and being out in the sun can all make you mildly dehydrated. Water, juice, seltzer, mineral water, milk, and even caffeine-containing coffee, tea, and soda all contribute to your fluid intake. If you don't urinate at least every 4 hours when you are awake, you probably need to be drinking more.

Your friends and family can make you fat.

Researchers have found that obesity can spread as a social epidemic. If people in your close social network are eating too much, exercising too little, and weigh too much, you are likely to adapt these habits and mimic their behavior. As you get heavier, you pass along these behaviors to others within your social network.

If you have a close friend who is obese, your risk for obesity increases by 57%. Among adult siblings, sisters had a greater effect on other sisters (67%) than sisters had on their brothers (44%). Men were more likely to gain weight if their male friends were heavy. In marriage, husbands and wives had an equal influence on each other. If one gained weight, there was about a 40% chance the other would too.

If overweight is contagious, thinness can be as well. Support groups like Alcoholics Anonymous (AA) have demonstrated that you can modify a person's social network and behavior for the better. Where AA succeeds and weight loss groups don't is the AA premise that there is a need for lifetime support. Maybe we need to devise public health programs that provide lifetime maintenance for those who lose weight so their social network promotes a more realistic, slimmer body image with positive eating and exercise messages.

Sleep Too Little, Weigh Too Much

Getting too little sleep triggers regions of the brain that increase hunger.

In our sleep-deprived lives, poor sleep habits can cause weight gain.

Plus, more hours awake mean more time to eat, and if you're tired, you're less likely to exercise—all adding up to extra pounds.

Aim for at least 7 hours a night.

People who sleep more weigh less.

CALORIES YOU USE

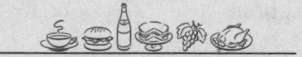

When it comes to weight loss, every
calorie you burn is a good one.

Activity burns calories. Activity also builds muscles, which
burn calories 70 times faster than fat does. Someone who has
been relatively inactive will see health benefits from using
up just 500 extra calories a week through activity. If you're
a true couch potato, this may be the level at which to start,
though real weight loss and fitness benefits start to kick in
when you use up 1,000 calories a week through activity.
Consider 2,000 calories as a great goal to strive for over time.

Everything you do counts, from planned activities to real-
life fitness: walking, gardening, golf, tennis, even house-
work. The more active you are, the more calories you burn.
And the really good news is that research has shown you
benefit from exercise whether the activity is continuous or
done in small bursts. Being active for as little as 10 minutes at
a time not only burns calories but also has a positive impact
on your health. The key is to *move* every day.

Don't Sit Your Life Away

Americans average 23 hours a week in front of the
TV. That adds up to almost 10 years over a lifetime!

Real-Life Fitness

- Pace while you're talking on the phone.

- Deliver memos and messages in person rather than by e-mail or phone.

- Go window shopping.

- Clean your house—washing floors, vacuuming carpets, washing windows, or scrubbing bathrooms equals vigorous exercise.

- Garden—weeding, hoeing, cutting the lawn, raking, or trimming bushes burns as many calories as playing a game of tennis.

- Turn your lunch break into an hour-long excursion.

- Carry a basket when shopping for a few items—it's like a free weight that keeps getting heavier and heavier; switch arms for a maximum workout.

- Sign up for a charity walk, bike, or run.

- Turn off the TV one night a week and plan something active.

- Make exercise a hobby—take golf, tennis, or skating lessons.

- Park your car at the farthest end of the parking lot.

- Take the stairs—you burn 10 calories for every flight you climb; over a lifetime that uses up thousands of calories.

- Dance—salsa, hip-hop, polka, tango, or line dance; square dancers can cover 5 miles in an evening.

- Grocery shop—one hour of pushing, lifting, and bending in the supermarket uses as many calories as a half hour on a treadmill.

- Spend rainy weekend afternoons walking around a museum; when the sun shines, go to the zoo.

- Wash the car.

- Go bowling instead of to the movies.

- Walk the dog.

- Push the baby in a stroller or take the kids to the playground.

- Be an active spectator—walk around the soccer field while the kids are playing.

- Play active games as a family—badminton, volleyball, stickball, croquet, basketball.

- Practice yoga.

Walk More, Weigh Less—Use a Pedometer

*Researchers have set guidelines for
how many steps per day
you need to walk to achieve weight control.*

Women—Steps Per Day

Age 18 to 40—12,000

Age 40 to 50—11,000

Age 50 to 60—10,000

Age 60 and older—8,000

Men—Steps Per Day

Age 18 to 50—12,000

Age 50 and older—11,000

*3,000 steps in 30 minutes =
a moderate-intensity workout.*

Daily activity helps you reach your target weight faster. Depending on your current level of activity, aim to use up 500 to 1,000 calories a week. Your ultimate goal is to double this amount as you become more fit. In the table "Using Up Calories," below, find the activity you've done and the weight column closest to your current weight. Multiply the calories burned in 1 minute by the number of minutes you were active.

For example, if you weigh 150 pounds and you weeded your flowerbed for 15 minutes, you used up almost 89 calories.

Gardening (weeding)
5.9 (calories burned in 1 minute) × 15 minutes = 88.5 calories

If your activity goal for the week is to burn 500 calories, you've already burned 89 with one simple chore.

Keep track of the calories you burn each day, and total the amount you burn in a week.

USING UP CALORIES

POUNDS	100	125	150	175	200
ACTIVITY	CALORIES USED PER MINUTE				
Archery	3.1	4.0	4.8	5.6	6.4
Auto repair	2.8	3.5	4.2	4.8	5.5
Badminton	3.6	4.6	5.4	6.4	7.3
Baseball	3.1	4.0	4.7	5.5	6.3
Basketball	4.9	6.2	9.9	11.5	13.2
Bicycling					
5 mph	1.9	2.4	2.9	3.4	3.9
10 mph	4.2	5.3	6.4	7.4	8.5
Bowling	2.7	3.4	4.1	4.5	5.5
Boxing	6.2	7.8	9.3	10.9	12.4
Calisthenics, light	3.4	4.3	5.2	6.1	7.0
Canoeing, 4 mph	4.4	5.5	6.7	7.8	8.9

POUNDS	100	125	150	175	200
ACTIVITY	**CALORIES USED PER MINUTE**				
Card playing	1.0	1.6	1.9	2.2	2.5
Carpentry	2.6	3.2	3.8	4.6	5.3
Chopping wood	4.8	6.0	7.2	8.4	9.6
Croquet	2.7	3.4	4.1	4.7	5.4
Dancing					
Active (square, salsa)	4.5	5.6	6.8	7.9	9.1
Aerobic dance	6.0	7.6	9.1	10.8	12.1
Moderate (waltz)	3.1	4.0	4.8	5.6	6.4
Fencing, moderate	3.3	4.1	5.0	5.8	6.7
Fishing	2.8	3.5	4.2	4.9	5.6
Football, touch	5.5	6.9	8.3	9.7	11.1
Gardening					
Lawn mowing, manual	3.0	3.8	4.6	5.2	5.9
Lawn mowing, power	2.7	3.4	4.1	4.7	5.4
Light gardening	2.4	3.0	3.6	4.2	4.8
Weeding	3.9	4.9	5.9	6.8	7.8
Golf					
Foursome (carry clubs)	2.7	3.4	4.1	4.5	5.4
Twosome (carry clubs)	3.6	4.6	5.4	6.4	7.3
Gymnastics	3.0	3.8	4.5	5.3	6.0
Handball	6.2	6.5	9.9	11.5	13.2
Hiking 3 mph	4.5	5.5	6.8	7.9	9.1
Hockey, field	5.0	7.6	9.1	10.8	12.1
Hockey, ice	6.6	8.3	10.0	11.7	13.4
Horseback riding					
Walk	1.9	2.4	2.9	3.4	3.9
Trot	2.7	3.4	4.1	4.8	5.4
Gallop	5.7	7.2	8.7	10.1	11.6
Horseshoes	2.5	3.1	3.8	4.4	5.2
House painting	2.3	2.9	3.5	4.0	4.6
Housework					
Dusting	1.8	2.3	2.6	3.1	3.5
Making beds	2.6	3.2	3.8	4.6	5.3
Ice Skating	4.2	5.2	6.4	7.4	8.5

POUNDS	100	125	150	175	200
ACTIVITY	**CALORIES USED PER MINUTE**				
Judo	8.5	10.6	12.8	14.9	17.1
Karate	8.5	10.6	12.8	14.9	17.1
Lacrosse	9.5	11.9	14.3	16.6	19.0
Motorcycling	2.4	3.0	3.6	4.2	4.8
Mountain climbing	6.5	8.2	9.8	11.5	13.1
Paddle ball	5.7	7.2	8.7	10.1	11.6
Pool (billiards)	1.5	1.9	2.2	2.6	3.0
Racquetball	6.5	8.1	9.8	11.4	13.0
Rollerblading, 9 mph	4.2	5.3	6.4	7.4	8.5
Rowing	3.4	4.2	5.0	5.9	6.7
Rowing machine	9.1	11.4	13.7	16.0	18.2
Running, steady rate					
5 mph	6.0	7.6	9.1	10.8	12.2
7 mph	9.7	12.1	14.6	17.1	19.5
Sailing, small boat	4.2	5.2	6.4	7.4	8.5
Scuba diving, moderate	9.4	11.8	14.1	16.5	18.8
Shoveling snow	5.2	6.5	7.8	8.9	10.2
Skiing, alpine downhill	6.4	8.0	9.6	11.2	12.8
Skiing, cross-country					
2.5 mph	5.0	6.2	7.5	8.8	10.0
4 mph	6.5	8.2	9.9	11.5	13.2
Soccer	5.9	7.4	8.9	10.3	11.8
Squash	6.7	8.4	10.1	11.8	13.5
Swimming					
Backstroke	2.5	3.1	3.8	4.4	5.1
Breaststroke	3.1	4.0	4.8	5.6	6.4
Front Crawl	4.0	5.0	6.0	7.0	8.0
Table tennis	3.4	4.3	5.2	6.3	7.2
Tennis					
Doubles	3.4	4.3	5.2	6.1	7.0
Singles	5.0	6.2	7.5	6.8	10.0
Typing	1.5	1.9	2.3	2.7	3.1
Volleyball	2.9	3.6	4.4	5.1	5.9

POUNDS	100	125	150	175	200
ACTIVITY	**CALORIES USED PER MINUTE**				
Walking					
1 mph	1.5	1.9	2.3	2.7	3.1
2 mph	2.1	2.6	3.2	3.7	4.3
4 mph	4.2	5.3	6.4	7.4	8.5
Washing floors	3.0	3.8	4.6	5.3	6.1
Washing windows	2.8	3.5	4.2	4.8	5.5
Waterskiing	5.0	6.2	7.5	8.8	10.0
Weight training					
Free weights	3.9	4.9	5.9	6.8	7.8
Nautilus	4.2	5.3	6.3	7.4	8.4
Universal	5.3	6.6	8.0	9.3	10.6

Calorie Cost of Love

A kiss = 6 to 12 calories, depending on the intensity.

Lovemaking = 125 to 300 calories,
depending on the level of passion.

MINIMIZE MINDLESS EATING

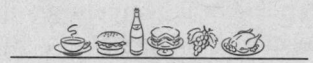

Each of us makes over 112 food decisions a day.

You're thinking, *That's not possible!* But it is. Each morning you decide to eat or not. Cereal or toast? Toast with butter? Or butter and jelly? One slice or two? Coffee, tea, or coke? Milk or sugar? One spoonful or two? Fruit or juice? Large or small glass? Seconds?

These choices are considered *low involvement* decisions, and often you're not even aware you're making them. They are mindless choices, but over time they can make a significant impact on what and how much you eat.

You Should Know—

Eating in response to external signals—food advertisements, food smells, TV commercials, candy dish on a coworker's desk, free food samples while shopping—is more likely to cause overeating than normal hunger signals. Most of us are rarely hungry.

Your home and office are full of hidden persuaders, but there are a number of things you can do to become a more mindful eater.

Put distance between you and food.

The greater the distance you have to travel to get food, the less you eat. Empty the candy dish on your desk. At home, leave all food in the kitchen cabinets. Don't stock a mini refrigerator in the family room. Putting distance between you and food gives you enough time to pause and say, "Do I really want that?" Keep less healthy foods out of your immediate line of sight, and move better-for-you food to eye level in the kitchen cabinets and refrigerator.

Use small plates, serving spoons, and bowls.

Large serving bowls encourage overeating. People take over 50% more food when given a large plate or when served from a large bowl. The next time you eat ice cream, use a dessert dish instead of a soup bowl. You generally eat whatever you serve yourself, so if you overserve, you overeat. Shapes also effect consumption. You drink less from tall, slim glasses and more out of short, fat ones. Try eating dinner off salad plates instead of large dinner plates.

Don't be seduced by the "health halo."

Lowfat, *reduced calorie*, *low carb*, *sugar free*, and *light* are all terms used to make you think a food is good for you. But too much of *any* food equals too many calories. People order more and eat more when they believe the choices are healthy. A restaurant-size dinner salad drenched in dressing is more than anyone needs to eat at one sitting. Even healthy foods need to be eaten in moderation.

Buying bulk adds bulk.

Warehouse stores encourage you to buy bigger sizes, which leads to eating more, and eating more frequently. People take larger helpings out of larger packages. Single servings and individual packs are smarter purchases. Or repack larger amounts into smaller sizes to discourage overeating.

Order small.

Regardless of the choice, go for the smallest option. At a restaurant order a lunch or half portion, or have an appetizer for your main course. Select the small or regular coffee, even if it's called "tall." Try a kid's meal. Eat medium-size apples, oranges, and baked potatoes. Order a one-scoop cone. Remember, *smaller sizes = a smaller you.*

Rework your eating environment so it works *for* you, not against you. Eat at the table in the kitchen or dining room, not in front of the TV. Once you are more aware of mindless eating, you can counteract mindless choices with mindful solutions. Simple strategies are more likely to succeed than willpower. Start small, easy, and doable—success, no matter how small, breeds success.

When Do You Eat Too Much?

Asked when they were most likely to overeat, 57% of people said at night, 25% said afternoon, and only 3% noted morning. Simply knowing this can help you cut calories and avoid temptation.

What Do the Experts Recommend?

A group of 23 food and nutrition experts (Jo-Ann Heslin, R.D., was invited to be part of the group) was asked to give ideas and suggestions for how Americans could achieve healthy eating and maintain a healthy weight. Here are their recommendations.

- Eating healthy meals and snacks deserves a large slice of our time-stressed lives.

- Give thought to what you eat. Most Americans are totally unaware of the choices they make every day.

- Retrain your taste buds to enjoy the flavor of healthy foods. Eat less sugar, sodium, and fat.

- Eat food for enjoyment and nourishment, not to soothe emotional issues. What are your food triggers?

- Downsize portions.

- Quit the clean plate club.

- Learn more about how many calories are in the foods you regularly eat.

- Learn more about food. It's fun and important to your health.

- Change slowly, and the changes are more likely to be permanent.

OOPS! WHAT NOW— TAKING CHARGE IN TOUGH SITUATIONS

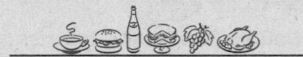

The road to success is always under construction.

You think you're unique. You're the only one who finds it hard to lose weight. Boy, are you wrong! The problems, questions and concerns you have about trying to lose weight are shared by most people in the same situation. To prove it, here the answers to the questions we hear most often.

Some of our suggestions may seem a little unorthodox, but we've learned that the key to success is flexibility. Not all problems can be solved perfectly. But every problem does have a compromise solution, one that allows you to go forward and lose weight.

Often after I eat and I'm full, I have an overwhelming urge to keep chewing. Why?

Eating is a pleasurable experience. You simply don't want to stop the fun. But you are able to recognize you're full, which is great. To satisfy the urge to keep chewing, try chewing a piece of gum or sipping on a large glass of flavored seltzer or mineral water and chopped ice. Ice gives you crunch without calories, and cold blunts taste. Both may help you subdue the urge to chew.

Whenever I fight with my husband, I bury my sorrow in bag of potato chips. Any suggestions?

Fights with people we love are tough to deal with, and many times we turn to food for comfort. Overeating is not the best response to an emotionally tough time, but if you find yourself in that spot, a simple switch to pretzels or popcorn will at least reduce your calorie intake.

If it's too late and you've already eaten the chips, let's do some math. A 6-ounce bag of potato chips has 900 calories. To use up the extra calories eaten, cut 200 calories a day from your eating plan for the next 3 days and add 10 to 20 minutes extra activity each day. This will compensate for the "Oops!"

When I can't sleep, I eat. How do I stop this?

In an ideal world, we would just tell you not to eat during the night. In real life, middle-of-the-night noshing is a tough habit to break. It's unlikely that you are eating because you're hungry. The habit is probably tied to some emotional issue you are coping with—a tough boss, difficult teenager, money worries, relationship problems. Separating eating and emotions is hard.

When you are tempted to raid the refrigerator after midnight, think high volume, low calories—popcorn, pretzel sticks, rice cakes, a large no-calorie drink with chopped ice, raw vegetables, a hunk of watermelon, a bowl of soup. If ice cream is your midnight munchie of choice, switch to Italian ice or ice pops, which have fewer calories than ice cream.

I have to keep candy and cookies in the house for the kids, which I wind up eating. How can I prevent this?

Let's stop kidding ourselves. Are you really buying the candy and cookies for the kids, or is it a great excuse to indulge? Buy some treats that are good for the whole family—sorbet, graham crackers, raisin bars, ice cream dixie cups. One of the best gifts you can give your children is to be a good role model. Healthy eating habits are contagious.

What do I do after I've eaten something I shouldn't?

Resist the "Now I've blown it!" syndrome. There will be days when you eat more than you've planned. There will be times when you can't be active. You will backslide. It's inevitable. Just don't let these glitches derail you. Have a backup plan for such occasions. A healthy lifestyle isn't based on one meal or one bout of activity. It's a consistent effort to make good choices and be active most of the time. When you trip up, just say "Oops!" Forgive yourself and get back on track.

I eat the most when I'm sad. How can I stop this?

Eating can be comforting. We often reach for food when we feel sad, lonely, frustrated, or overwhelmed. Eating pushes the emotion into the background—but not for long. When the feelings return, you eat more. This is a hard cycle to break, but you've already made a big step by realizing that you eat too much when you are sad.

What makes you happy? Visiting a friend? A long bubble bath? Exercising? Next time you feel sad, try a nonfood option for lifting your spirits. This is easier to suggest than to do, but now that you've identified a trigger for overeating you can change the behavior.

Exercise = Happiness

Regular exercise releases natural brain chemicals (endorphins) that lift your spirits and make you feel happier.

Instead of working on behavior changes, wouldn't it be simpler just to never eat chocolate cake again?

While you're attempting to reach your target weight, chocolate cake definitely falls into the once-in-a-blue-moon category, but no foods should ever be forbidden. Swearing an oath against eating future slices will most likely result in a chocolate cake binge in the not-too-distant future. If you don't binge, you'll be resentful, waiting for the day when you can eat chocolate cake again. You go off your diet, eat the chocolate cake and other foods you gave up while dieting, and before you know it, you've gained back all the weight you lost!

Let's rewrite this scenario. You love chocolate cake. You decide to have a small slice of chocolate cake every Saturday night. You also plan to take an extra-long bike ride every weekend to help burn up the extra calories. You trade an extra activity for a calorie-dense choice. Don't deprive yourself—just plan.

How do I stop family and friends from urging me to eat when I shouldn't?

Dieting dynamics are interesting. When you're successfully controlling your weight, people around often react in contradictory ways. Some become cheerleaders, celebrating each victory and reveling in your successes. Others try to test your resolve by tempting you with foods you're trying to limit.

Be firm; tell everyone how important it is for you to lose weight and that having support will make your job easier. Friends who try to derail your eating plan may be jealous of your success. Interact with them less often for the time being. Good friends help, they don't hinder.

There are nights when I just don't have the energy to cook a good meal. What then?

Assemble! The telephone and microwave are two indispensable kitchen tools. A take-out rotisserie chicken, bagged salad, microwave potatoes, and ice pops for dessert require no cooking, and it's a good-for-the-whole-family meal. Order in wisely—pizza with vegetables and no cheese; wonton soup with steamed shrimp and vegetables, plus a common-sense portion of brown rice. Don't fall into the trap of "If I don't cook dinner I won't eat well." Today, almost one-third of all meals eaten at home are warmed up, not cooked.

Do I have to eat breakfast to lose weight?

Breakfast eaters are thinner. Your body really needs refueling in the morning. Without breakfast you burn calories less efficiently, actually making it harder to lose weight. Maybe what you hate are traditional breakfast foods. Be inventive. Have a smoothie. Swap breakfast and lunch choices. Try dinner leftovers. A sandwich? Pizza? An English muffin pizza made with ¼ cup marinara sauce, 2 tablespoons of grated cheese and 2 tablespoons of sliced mushrooms has 225 calories.

I nibble when I cook. How can I stop?

You can nibble a few hundred extra calories making dinner. Try chewing gum. It is unlikely that you will nibble with gum in your mouth.

What can I eat when I take the kids for hamburgers?

There isn't a child alive who doesn't expect an occasional trip to the local hamburger spot with playgrounds, kid's meals and toys to collect. Though fast food spots are not the best choices for a dieter, there are choices you can make that don't derail your diet plan.

Order a regular hamburger, "undressed"—no cheese or special sauce. Top it with add-ons that won't add-up—tomato slices, lettuce, mustard, salsa, and pickle slices. Try grilled chicken sandwiches and a side salad or plain baked potato. Instead of a milk shake, order lowfat chocolate milk. Skip the unlimited soda refills unless you stick with diet soda. Order salad, dressing on the side, and use a commonsense portion. Even a "kid's meal" isn't a bad idea, because the portions are reasonable.

Sampling Counts

Sampling adds up. Each French fry = 11 calories.

You are painting yourself into the picture of a slimmer, fitter you. Occasionally you'll find yourself coloring outside the lines. When this happens, don't beat yourself up—just take action. One day of overeating or one day without activity does not make you a failure. Fasting, drastically cutting calories or adding an uncomfortable amount of exercise sets the stage for failure.

Appreciate that habits are hard to change but not impossible. You count! Make your weight-loss goals and activity plan a priority.

TRACKING CALORIES

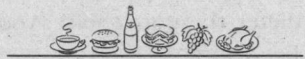

People cut calories by 10% when they simply write
down what they eat; 30% to 50% of those who
keep a food diary change their eating habits.

A large research study done at the Harvard School for Public Health confirmed that the most successful way to lose weight is to keep track of calories. It didn't matter if a person chose a lowfat, low carb, high carb, or high protein diet. If they counted calories, they lost weight. This proved, once and for all, calories count!

We know it's a chore to write down everything you eat and keep track of the calories, but it's worth it. The value of writing down what you eat makes you reflect on your choices, which makes you more aware of habits and gives you an opportunity to change behavior that is sabotaging your weight-loss efforts.

After a week of writing down calories, most people know how many calories are in 75% of what they usually eat. And, people who keep a food diary are more successful at losing weight, even during difficult times like holidays.

Your "Daily Food Diary," on page 45, will tell you a lot about how you eat, why you eat, and what you eat. Research has shown that men are more likely to omit items than women, both sexes are more likely to omit snack items, and meat items are more likely to be underestimated than other foods. No one will ever see what you write down, so be honest.

Why is the day of the week important? Some days, like weekends, you may eat more. Some people eat more on Friday, celebrating the end of a work week. Others eat more on Monday in response to the stress of a new week. If you find that some days trigger your overeating, it will be easier to change the pattern.

We appreciate that many people eat on a crazy schedule, so the day is broken into 3 periods. That will help you figure out when you do the most eating.

Morning (A.M.) is from midnight till noon. Many people eat in the middle of the night, so A.M. includes middle-of-the-night noshing, breakfast, coffee break, or morning snack.

Midday is from noon until dinner. It includes lunch and any afternoon or pre-dinner snack, like a drink after work.

Evening (P.M.) is dinnertime through midnight. It includes your evening meal and after-dinner, TV, and bedtime snacks.

After a few days, you'll begin to see patterns in your eating habits. Going too long without food or eating too frequently can both lead to eating too much. Ideally you want your calories to be spaced evenly throughout the day. But we know that isn't always possible.

By subtotaling your calories 3 times during the day, you can make adjustments for unexpected situations. For example, if a client comes in for lunch, you can skip your afternoon snack and eat a lighter dinner to compensate for the extra calories eaten at lunch.

Why does it matter if you eat alone or with company? Because we eat differently depending on the situation. Most people eat more with family and less with coworkers. Learning this about yourself can help you change habits that may be sabotaging your efforts to lose weight.

Finally, you'll want to note how many calories you burned through activity every day. Some days you may be more active than others, but if you start to fall into an inactive pattern, noting it will help you break the cycle quickly.

One meal or one day does not make a success or failure. But being totally honest with yourself can help keep you on the right track most of the time. Before you realize it, you'll be slimmer and fitter than ever.

Learning from the Losers

For almost 20 years the National Weight Control Registry has kept track of people who have lost at least 30 pounds and kept it off. These successful losers used the same general strategies to maintain long-term weight loss.

Eat a low calorie diet

Eat a lowfat diet and eat less saturated fat

Eat a moderate amount of carbohydrates

Go easy on fast food

Exercise regularly

It takes knowledge, motivation, action and time to create change.

DAILY FOOD DIARY

Your Target Calorie Amount _____

Day _____ Date _____

Food	Portion	Calories	Ate Alone	With Company
A.M.				
A.M. Calorie Total _____				
MIDDAY				
Midday Calorie Total _____				
P.M.				
P.M. Calorie Total _____				
Day's Calorie Total _____				

Activity	Minutes Active	Calories Burned
Total Calories Burned _____		

USING YOUR
CALORIE COUNTER

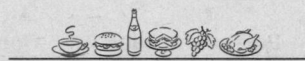

The Calorie Counter, 6th Edition, lists the calories and portion size for more than 20,000 foods. Now you can compare the values in your favorite foods and, when necessary, choose substitutes when you go out to shop or eat. This will save time and help you decide what to buy.

The counter section of the book is divided into two parts: Part One: Brand-Name, Nonbranded (Generic), and Take-out Foods (page 53); and Part Two: Restaurant Chains (page 511). Each part lists foods or restaurant chains alphabetically.

In Part One, for each category you will find nonbranded (generic) foods listed first, in alphabetical order, followed by an alphabetical listing of brand-name foods. The nonbranded listings will help you estimate calorie values when you don't see your favorite brand. They can also help you evaluate store brands. Large categories are divided into subcategories, such as canned, fresh, frozen, and ready-to-eat, to make it easier to find what you're looking for. Some categories have *see* and *see also* references, to help you find related items.

Because we eat out so often, more than 900 take-out foods are listed in Part One. These are found in the take-out subcategory in many categories throughout this section.

Look there for foods you take out or order in, since they are not nutrition labeled.

Most foods are listed alphabetically. In some cases, though, foods are grouped by category. For example, a tuna sandwich is found in the sandwich category. Other group categories include:

ALCOHOL DRINKS (Page 54)
Includes all alcoholic beverages and mixed drinks except beer, champagne, malt, and wine, which have their own separate categories.

ASIAN FOOD (Page 66)
Includes all types of Asian foods except egg rolls and sushi, which are found in the egg rolls and sushi categories.

DELI MEATS/COLD CUTS (Page 215)
Includes all sandwich meats except chicken, ham, and turkey, which have their own separate categories.

DINNER (Page 216)
Includes all prepared dinners listed by brand name except pasta dinners, which are found in the pasta dinners category.

NUTRITION SUPPLEMENTS (Page 329)
Includes all dieting aids, meal replacements, and drinks, except energy bars and energy drinks, which have their own separate categories.

SANDWICHES   (Page 411)
Includes popular sandwich, calzone,
and panini choices.

SNACKS   (Page 432)
Includes a variety of snack items, such
as pork rinds and cheese puffs.

SPANISH FOOD   (Page 455)
Includes all types of Spanish and
Mexican foods except salsa and
tortillas, which have their own
separate categories

In Part Two, Restaurant Chains (page 511), 112 national
and regional restaurant, coffee, doughnut, frozen yogurt, ice
cream, pizza, sandwich, soup, and sushi chains are listed.
Brand-name foods are required by federal law to have nutrition information on labels, but in most areas of the country
restaurants provide this information voluntarily.

With *The Calorie Counter* as your guide, you will never
again wonder how many calories are in the food you eat.

DEFINITIONS

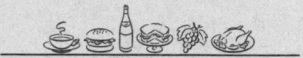

as prep (as prepared): refers to food that has been prepared according to package directions

lean and fat: describes meat with some fat on its edges that is not cut away before cooking, or poultry prepared with skin and fat as purchased

lean only: refers to lean meat that is trimmed of all visible fat, or poultry without skin

not prep (not prepared): refers to food that has not been cooked and may require the addition of other ingredients to prepare

shelf-stable: refers to prepared products found on the supermarket shelf that are not canned or frozen but are packaged and ready-to-eat or are ready to be heated and do not require refrigeration

take-out: describes prepared dishes that you purchase ready-to-eat; those included serve as a guide to the calories in the foods you purchase

ABBREVIATIONS

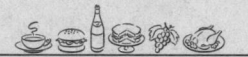

avg	=	average
diam	=	diameter
fl	=	fluid
frzn	=	frozen
g	=	gram
in	=	inch
lb	=	pound
lg	=	large
med	=	medium
mg	=	milligram
oz	=	ounce
pkg	=	package
pt	=	pint
prep	=	prepared
qt	=	quart
reg	=	regular
sec	=	second
serv	=	serving
sm	=	small
sq	=	square
tbsp	=	tablespoon
tsp	=	teaspoon
w/	=	with
w/o	=	without
<	=	less than

NOTES

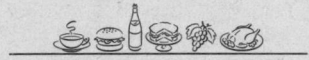

0 (zero) indicates there are no calories in that food.

Discrepancies in figures are due to rounding of values, product reformulation, and reevaluation. The current labeling law allows rounding. Some of the data listed is analysis data, obtained directly from manufacturers, not from labels; therefore, some values may differ slightly from labels because the values have not been rounded.

PART ONE

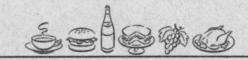

Brand-Name, Nonbranded (Generic), and Take-out Foods

> **Eating 100 calories less each day
> can help you lose 10 pounds in a year!
> It can be done with small changes—**
>
> - Use mustard, salsa, or fat-free mayonnaise in place of 1 tablespoon regular mayonnaise
> - Eat 1 slice of toast for breakfast instead of 2
> - Order a cup of soup instead of a bowl
> - Try a plain baked potato with pepper instead of sour cream
> - Eat cereal with nonfat milk instead of whole milk
> - Swap broiled for breaded and fried chicken fingers
> - Use tuna packed in water instead of oil
> - Swap a diet soda for regular soda
> - Enjoy a glass of wine instead of a martini
> - Have a chocolate kiss instead of a chocolate bar

FOOD	PORTION	CALS
ABALONE		
breaded & fried	1 serv (3 oz)	162
steamed	1 serv (3 oz)	127
ACAI JUICE		
Arthur's		
Acai Plus	1 bottle (11 oz)	230
Bossa Nova		
Acai Juice Blueberry	8 oz	89
Acai Juice Mango	8 oz	89
Acai Juice Original	8 oz	94
Acai Juice Passion Fruit	8 oz	89
Acai Juice Raspberry	8 oz	89
O.N.E.		
Amazon Acai	1 bottle (11 oz)	157
Ultra Lo-Gly		
Acai-Blue	1 bottle (10 oz)	45
Zola		
100% Juice	1 box (11 oz)	170
ACEROLA		
fresh	1 (5 g)	2
ACEROLA JUICE		
juice	1 cup	56
ADZUKI BEANS		
canned sweetened	½ cup	351
dried cooked w/o salt	½ cup	147
Arrowhead Mills		
Organic Dried not prep	¼ cup	130
AGAVE (see SYRUP)		
AKEE		
fresh	3.5 oz	223
ALCOHOL DRINKS (see also BEER AND ALE, CHAMPAGNE, MALT, WINE)		
7&7	1 serv	178
alabama slammer	1 serv	103
amaretto sour	1 serv	295
angel's kiss	1 serv	85
anisette	1 oz	111

FOOD	PORTION	CALS
antifreeze cocktail	1 serv	177
apricot brandy	1 oz	96
apricot sour	1 serv	164
aquavit	1 oz	65
b 52	1 serv	247
b&b	1 serv	75
bahama breeze	1 serv	70
bahama mama	1 serv	153
bailey's & amaretto	1 serv	184
banana colada	1 serv	376
bay breeze	1 serv	173
bend me over	1 serv	242
benedictine	1 oz	104
betsy ross	1 serv	206
black devil	1 serv	220
black russian	1 serv	184
bloody mary	1 serv	150
blue whale	1 serv	222
bourbon & soda	1 serv (4 oz)	105
bourbon sour	1 serv	166
brandy	2 oz	255
brandy alexander	1 serv	266
brandy sour	1 serv	164
bushwacker	1 serv	286
campari	2 oz	245
cherry heering	2 oz	245
coffee liqueur	1 serv (1.5 oz)	175
cognac	1 oz	67
cosmopolitan martini	1 serv	126
creme de almonde	1 oz	102
creme de banana	1 oz	99
creme de cassis	1 oz	82
creme de menthe	1 serv (1.5 oz)	186
curacao liqueur	1 oz	81
daiquiri	1 serv (2 oz)	112
daiquiri banana	1 serv	277
daiquiri frozen	1 serv	393
daiquiri frozen pineapple	1 serv	186
dark & stormy	1 serv	64
doctor pepper	1 serv	95

FOOD	PORTION	CALS
drambuie	2 oz	225
fuzzy navel	1 serv	247
gibson	1 serv (4 oz)	254
gin	1 serv (1.5 oz)	110
gin & tonic	1 serv (7.5 oz)	171
gin ricky	1 serv	114
grasshopper	1 serv	275
happy hawaiian	1 serv	434
harvey wallbanger	1 serv	198
head banger	1 serv	165
hot buttered rum	1 serv (8.8 oz)	316
hot toddy	1 serv	188
hurricane	1 serv	205
kamikaze	1 serv	136
long island iced tea	1 serv	292
lynchburg lemonade	1 serv	465
mai tai	1 serv	165
manhattan	1 serv	171
margarita	1 serv	173
margarita strawberry	1 serv	106
martini	1 serv (3 oz)	206
martini apple	1 serv	147
martini rum	1 serv	131
mellow yellow	1 serv	95
mexican grasshopper	1 serv	638
mint julep	1 serv	136
mississippi mud	1 serv	496
mudslide	1 serv	566
narragansett	1 serv	168
nutcracker	1 serv	730
old fashioned	1 serv	223
orange crush	1 serv	461
pain killer	1 serv	277
peppermint pattie	1 serv	344
pina colada	1 serv (4.5 oz)	245
planter's cocktail	1 serv	105
planter's punch	1 serv	233
presbyterian	1 serv	170
purple passion	1 serv	215
rob roy	1 serv	171

FOOD	PORTION	CALS
rum	1 serv (1.5 oz)	97
rum boogie	1 serv	134
rum cola	1 serv	209
rum highball	1 serv	170
rum punch	1 serv	448
rum screwdriver	1 serv	166
rum sour	1 serv	156
rum swizzle	1 serv	187
rusty nail	1 serv	159
sake	1 serv (1 oz)	39
salty dog	1 serv	210
scotch & soda	1 serv	104
sea breeze	1 serv	207
sex on the beach	1 serv	190
singapore sling	1 serv (4 oz)	115
slippery nipple	1 serv	142
sloe gin fizz	1 serv (2.5 oz)	132
snake bite	1 serv	362
southern comfort	1 serv (1.5 oz)	184
tequila	1 serv (1.5 oz)	117
tequila frozen screwdriver	1 serv	159
tequila gimlet	1 serv	150
tequila sour	1 serv	156
tequila stinger	1 serv	221
tequila sunrise	1 serv (6.8 oz)	232
tom collins	1 serv (7.5 oz)	121
vermouth cassis	1 serv	97
vodka	1 serv (1.5 oz)	97
vodka gimlet	1 serv	150
vodka sour	1 serv	138
vodka stinger	1 serv	378
whiskey	1 serv (1.5 oz)	105
whiskey sour	1 serv (3.5 oz)	162
white russian	1 serv	290
zombie	1 serv	235
Absolut		
Vodka	1 shot (1.5 oz)	98
Bacardi		
Gold Rum	1 shot (1.5 oz)	98

FOOD	PORTION	CALS
Capt. Morgan's		
Original Spiced Rum	1 shot (1.5 oz)	86
Crown Royal		
Canadian Whiskey	1 shot (1.5 oz)	96
Jack Daniel's		
Old No.7 Tennessee Whiskey	1 shot (1.5 oz)	98
Jose Cuervo		
Gold Tequila	1 shot (1.5 oz)	96
Seagram's		
Gin	1 shot (1.5 oz)	120
Smirnoff		
Vodka	1 shot (1.5 oz)	96

ALE (see BEER AND ALE)

ALFALFA

sprouts	½ cup	40

ALLIGATOR

cooked	3 oz	126

ALLSPICE

ground	1 tsp	5

ALMONDS

almond butter w/ salt	2 tbsp	203
almond butter w/o salt	2 tbsp	203
almond extract	1 tsp	38
almond paste	¼ cup	260
chocolate covered	6 pieces (0.6 oz)	102
dry roasted w/ salt	¼ cup	206
dry roasted w/o salt	¼ cup	206
honey roasted	¼ cup	214
jordan almonds	6 (0.7 oz)	99
oil roasted w/ salt	¼ cup	238
oil roasted w/o salt	¼ cup	238
praline	17 pieces (1.4 oz)	210
yogurt covered	6 pieces (0.8 oz)	122
American Almond		
Marzipan	2 tbsp	130
Arrowhead Mills		
Organic Almond Butter Creamy	2 tbsp	200

FOOD	PORTION	CALS
Back To Nature		
California Sea Salt Roasted	1 oz	160
Barney Butter		
Almond Butter Crunchy	2 tbsp (1.1 oz)	180
Almond Butter Smooth	2 tbsp (1.1 oz)	180
Diamond		
Slivered	¼ cup (1 oz)	170
Fisher		
Roasted & Salted	¼ cup (1 oz)	170
Frito Lay		
Roasted Salted	3 tbsp (1 oz)	190
Godiva		
Dark Chocolate Almonds	1 pkg (2 oz)	310
Justin's		
Almond Butter Classic	2 tbsp (1.1 oz)	200
Almond Butter Maple	2 tbsp (1.1 oz)	190
Love'n Bake		
Almond Paste	2 tbsp	140
Almond Schmear	2 tbsp	140
Roasted Butter	2 tbsp	180
Mrs. May's		
Almond Crunch	1 oz	156
Naturally More		
Almond Butter	2 tbsp	190
Nut Harvest		
Lightly Roasted	2 tbsp	180
Planters		
Chocolate Lovers Dark Chocolate	11 pieces (1.4 oz)	220
Flavor Grove Chili Lime	1 oz	170
Flavor Grove Sea Salt & Olive Oil	1 oz	170
NUT-rition Bone Health Mix	¼ cup (1.2 oz)	170
Slivered	1 pkg (2 oz)	330
Smoked	1 pkg (1.5 oz)	250
Sunkist		
Accents Italian Parmesan	1 tbsp	40
Accents Original Oven Roasted	1 tbsp	40
SunRidge Farms		
Dark Chocolate Cane Sweetened	11 (1.4 oz)	220

FOOD	PORTION	CALS
ALOE JUICE		
Alo		
Appeal Aloe Vera + Pomelo Pink Grapefruit & Lemon	8 oz	60
Awaken Aloe Vera + Wheatgrass	8 oz	50
Enliven Aloe Vera + 12 Fruits & Vegetables	8 oz	50
Enrich Aloe Vera + Pomegranate & Cranberry	8 oz	70
Exposed Aloe Vera Original	8 oz	60
TropiKing		
Aloe Vera Juice	8 oz	88
Aloe Vera Juice & Grape	8 oz	100
Aloe Vera Juice & Pineapple	8 oz	100
Aloe Vera Juice & Pomegranate	8 oz	120
AMARANTH		
grain uncooked	½ cup (3.4 oz)	365
leaves cooked	½ cup	14
Arrowhead Mills		
Organic Whole Grain not prep	¼ cup	180
ANCHOVY		
boneless	1 oz	60
canned in oil drained	1 can (2 oz)	94
fresh	1 (4 g)	8
fresh fillets	3 (0.4 oz)	21
Arroyabe		
In Olive Oil	1 oz	60
Polar		
Rolled Fillets w/ Capers In Olive Oil	7 pieces (0.6 oz)	40
ANGLERFISH		
raw	3.5 oz	72
ANISE		
seed	1 tsp	7
ANTELOPE		
roasted	4 oz	215
APPLE		
CANNED		
sliced sweetened	½ cup	68

FOOD	PORTION	CALS
Dole		
Squish'ems	1 pkg	80
Glory		
Fried Apples	½ cup	80
Jake & Amos		
Red Spiced Rings	1 (1 oz)	35
Polar		
Fuji	½ cup	50
DRIED		
chopped	½ cup	104
cooked w/o sugar	½ cup	73
rings	5	78
Bare Fruit		
Chips Cinnamon	1 pkg (0.6 oz)	43
Chukar Cherries		
Cherry Apple Slices	10 (1 oz)	110
Del Monte		
Dried Apples	¼ cup (1.4 oz)	110
Fruit Ripples		
Cinnamon Apple	1 pkg	50
Strawberry Apple	1 pkg	50
Mott's		
Snacks Freeze Dried	1 pkg (0.55 oz)	60
Mrs. May's		
Fruit Chips	1 pkg	35
Nature's Envy		
Apple Chips Original	1 pkg (0.8 oz)	80
Stoneridge Orchards		
Green Wedges	⅓ cup (1.4 oz)	140
Sun-Maid		
Apples	¼ cup (1.4 oz)	120
FRESH		
apple	1 sm	55
apple	1 med	72
apple	1 lg	110
candied	1 sm (4.9 oz)	179
candied	1 med (6.5 oz)	234
candied	1 lg (9.8 oz)	357
w/ skin sliced	1 cup	57
w/o skin sliced	1 cup	53

FOOD	PORTION	CALS
Chiquita		
Apple	1 (6.4 oz)	95
Apple Bites w/ Caramel	1 pkg (2.5 oz)	70
Apple Slices	1 pkg (2.2 oz)	30
Crunch Pak		
Foodles Apples w/ Raisins & Peanut Butter	1 pkg (5 oz)	260
Grab And Go Apples w/ Grapes	1 pkg	80
Grab And Go Apples w/ Peanut Butter	1 pkg	220
Party Tray Apple-tizer Grand Crunch & Munch	1/10 pkg	150
Snackers Apples w/ Caramel Dip & Cheese	1 pkg (4.7 oz)	230
Snackers Apples w/ Caramel Dip & Chocolate	1 pkg (4.7 oz)	260
Snackers Apples w/ Grapes & Caramel	1 pkg (4.7 oz)	140
Snackers Apples w/ Pretzels & Cheese	1 pkg (4.7 oz)	240
Snackers Apples w/ Raisins & Pretzels	1 pkg	210
Sweet Apples w/ Yogurt Dip	1/5 pkg	70
Dole		
Apple	1 med (5.4 oz)	80
Earthbound Farms		
Organic Slices	1 pkg (2 oz)	30
Eastern Select		
Gala	1 (5.5 oz)	80
Grapple		
Grape Flavored	1 med (6.4 oz)	95
Mrs. Prindable's		
Caramel Triple Chocolate	1/4 apple (1.7 oz)	120
Caramel Walnut	1/4 apple (2 oz)	160
Ready Pac		
Apples w/ Caramel Dip	1 pkg (6 oz)	200
Apples w/ Peanut Butter Dip	1 pkg (5.7 oz)	340
Sullivan		
McIntosh	1 (5.4 oz)	80
FROZEN		
sliced w/o sugar	1/2 cup	42
REFRIGERATED		
Country Crock		
Cinnamon Apples	1/2 cup (4.4 oz)	130
Dole		
Fruit Crisp Apple Cinnamon	1 pkg (4 oz)	160
Parfait Apples & Creme	1 pkg (4.3 oz)	130

FOOD	PORTION	CALS
TAKE-OUT		
baked no sugar added	1 (5.6 oz)	90
baked w/ sugar	1 (6 oz)	162
fried apple rings	1 serv (2.7 oz)	91
scalloped	½ cup (3.3 oz)	90
APPLE JUICE		
cider	1 cup	117
juice + vitamin C & calcium	1 cup	117
mulled cider	1 serv	265
unsweetened w/o vitamin C	1 cup	117
Apple & Eve		
100% Juice	8 oz	110
Back To Nature		
100% Juice	1 pkg (6 oz)	80
Fizz Ed.		
Green Apple	1 can (8.4 oz)	100
Kedem		
100% Juice	8 oz	100
Land O'Lakes		
Juice	1 cup (8 oz)	120
Mott's		
100% Natural	1 bottle (14 oz)	200
Nantucket Nectars		
100% Juice Pressed Apple	8 oz	120
Organic Cloudy Apple	8 oz	120
Ocean Spray		
Juice	8 oz	100
Old Orchard		
100% Juice Apple Cider	8 oz	130
R.W. Knudsen		
Organic 100% Juice	8 oz	120
Santa Cruz		
Organic	8 oz	120
Smart Juice		
Organic 100% Juice	8 oz	117
Snapple		
100% Juice Green Apple	8 oz	160
Juice Drink Apple	8 oz	110

FOOD	PORTION	CALS
Tastee		
Cider 100% Juice	8 oz	120
Tree Ripe		
Organic 100% Juice	6 oz	80
Tropicana		
Orchard Style	1 bottle (14 oz)	200
Trop50 Farmstand Apple	8 oz	50
Walnut Acres		
Organic Juice	8 oz	110
APPLESAUCE		
sweetened	½ cup	97
unsweetened	½ cup	52
Beth's Farm Kitchen		
Chunky	2 tbsp (1 oz)	50
GoGo Squeeze		
Apple	1 pkg (3.2 oz)	60
Apple Banana	1 pkg (3.2 oz)	60
Apple Cinnamon	1 pkg (3.2 oz)	50
Apple Peach	1 pkg (3.2 oz)	60
Mott's		
Healthy Harvest Granny Smith No Sugar Added	1 pkg (3.9 oz)	50
Organic Original	½ cup (4.5 oz)	110
Organic Unsweetened	½ cup (4.3 oz)	50
Single-Serve Cinnamon	1 pkg (4 oz)	100
Musselman's		
Unsweetened	1 pkg (4 oz)	50
Revolution Foods		
Organic Unsweetened	1 pkg (4 oz)	50
Santa Cruz		
Organic	½ cup (4.5 oz)	60
Organic Apple Apricot	1 pkg (4 oz)	60
Organic Apple Blueberry	1 pkg (4 oz)	60
Organic Apple Cherry	½ cup (4.5 oz)	60
APRICOT JUICE		
nectar	6 oz	106
Ceres		
100% Juice	8 oz	130
Santa Cruz		
Organic Nectar	8 oz	120

FOOD	PORTION	CALS
APRICOTS		
canned heavy syrup	½ cup	91
canned in juice	½ cup	59
canned in water	½ cup	33
canned light syrup	½ cup	80
dried halves	6	51
dried halves cooked w/o sugar	½ cup	106
fresh	1	17
fresh sliced	½ cup	40
frozen sweetened	½ cup	119
Del Monte		
Halves In Heavy Syrup	½ cup (4.5 oz)	100
Dole		
Fresh	3 (4 oz)	60
Elizabeth's Natural		
Turkish Dried	5 (1.8 oz)	90
Harvest Bay		
Dried	5 (1.4 oz)	60
Mariani		
Ultimate Dried	¼ cup (1.4 oz)	100
S&W		
Whole In Heavy Syrup	½ cup (4.5 oz)	120
Sunsweet		
Dried	¼ cup (1.4 oz)	130
ARROWHEAD		
corm boiled	1 med	9
ARROWROOT		
raw	1 root (1.2 oz)	21
raw root sliced	1 cup	78
Bob's Red Mill		
Starch	¼ cup	110
ARTICHOKE		
CANNED		
hearts in oil	1 serv (3 oz)	100
Cento		
Hearts Quartered Marinated	2 pieces	20
Gertie's Finest		
Tapenade	2 tbsp	29

FOOD	PORTION	CALS
Native Forest		
Organic Hearts Quartered	1 serv (4 oz)	35
Polar		
Hearts	2	18
Hearts Quartered Marinated	1 oz	25
Progresso		
Hearts	2	30
Hearts Marinated	2 (1.1 oz)	60
Reese		
Cocktail Artichokes Original	½ jar (5 oz)	50
Roland		
Hearts	½ cup (4.6 oz)	50
The Gracious Gourmet		
Artichoke Parmesan Tapenade	2 tbsp (1 oz)	30
FRESH		
cooked	1 med	60
hearts cooked	½ cup	42
Ocean Mist		
Lemon	1 (4.2 oz)	60
FROZEN		
cooked	1 cup	42
cooked w/o salt	1 pkg (9 oz)	108
C&W		
Hearts	12 pieces (3 oz)	40
TAKE-OUT		
stuffed	1 (8.8 oz)	397

ASIAN FOOD (*see also* CURRY, DINNER, EGG ROLLS, SAUCE, SOY SAUCE, SUSHI)

FOOD	PORTION	CALS
CANNED		
chow mein chicken w/o noodles	1 cup	194
La Choy		
Chow Mein Beef	1 cup	90
Chow Mein Chicken	1 cup (9.3 oz)	100
Sweet & Sour Noodles	1 cup	150
Teriyaki Chicken	1 cup (8.6 oz)	120
FRESH		
wonton wrapper	1 (0.3 oz)	23
Nasoya		
Won Ton Wraps	8 (2.1 oz)	160

FOOD	PORTION	CALS
FROZEN		
Amy's		
Asian Noodle Stir Fry	1 pkg	290
Indian Mattar Paneer	1 pkg (10 oz)	320
Indian Palak Paneer	1 pkg (9.9 oz)	270
Indian Paneer Tikka	1 pkg (9.4 oz)	320
Indian Vegetable Korma	1 pkg (9.4 oz)	310
Thai Stir Fry	1 pkg (9.4 oz)	310
Contessa		
Chow Mein Chicken w/ Sauce not prep	1¾ cups	320
Curry Chicken w/ Sauce not prep	1¾ cups	240
Fried Rice Chicken w/ Sauce not prep	1¾ cups	260
General Tsao Shrimp w/ Sauce not prep	1¾ cups	270
Kung Pao Shrimp w/ Sauce not prep	1¾ cups	200
Lo Mein Shrimp w/ Sauce not prep	1¾ cups	250
Stir-Fry Beef w/ Sauce not prep	1¾ cups	190
Stir-Fry Chicken w/ Sauce not prep	1¾ cups	160
Stir-Fry Shrimp w/ Sauce not prep	1¾ cups	120
Sweet & Sour Shrimp w/ Sauce not prep	1½ cups	180
Tandoori Chicken w/ Sauce not prep	1⅓ cups	200
Crazy Cuizine		
Korean Inspired	¼ pkg (5 oz)	240
Mandarin Orange Chicken	1 cup (5 oz)	260
Tangerine Beef	1 cup (5 oz)	360
Ethnic Gourmet		
Bhartha Eggplant	1 pkg (11 oz)	300
Dal Bahaar	1 pkg (11 oz)	360
Kaeng Kari Kai	1 pkg (10 oz)	390
Korma Chicken	1 pkg (10 oz)	340
Korma Vegetable	1 pkg (11 oz)	300
Kotopoulo Domato Ke Feta	1 pkg (10 oz)	340
Pad Thai Chicken	1 pkg (10 oz)	410
Pad Thai Shrimp	1 pkg (10 oz)	410
Tandoori Chicken w/ Spinach	1 pkg (10 oz)	170
French Meadow Bakery		
Vegetarian Dal Makhani	1 pkg (12 oz)	370
Glutino		
Gluten Free Chicken Pad Thai Peach	1 pkg (7 oz)	370
Healthy Choice		
Sweet & Sour Chicken	1 pkg (11.9 oz)	420

FOOD	PORTION	CALS
Helen's Kitchen		
Thai Yellow Curry w/ Tofu Steaks & Vegetables & Basmati Rice	1 pkg (9 oz)	280
Joy Of Cooking		
Beef & Broccoli	1 pkg (10.9 oz)	360
Chicken Fried Rice	1 pkg (10.9 oz)	460
General Tso's Chicken	1 pkg (10 oz)	400
Lo Mein Vegetable	1 cup (7.7 oz)	220
Naturals General Tso's Chicken	1 pkg (10 oz)	330
Naturals Mandarin Orange Chicken	1 pkg (10 oz)	340
Naturals Szechuan Peppercorn Beef	1 pkg (10 oz)	350
Naturals Teriyaki Mixed Vegetables	1 pkg (10 oz)	260
Sesame Orange Chicken	1 pkg (10.9 oz)	420
Soothing Lettuce Wraps	4 tbsp (2 oz)	90
Tempura Chicken Nuggets	¾ cup (3.5 oz)	230
Tropical Sweet & Sour Chicken	1 pkg (10.9 oz)	490
Lean Cuisine		
Cafe Cuisine Chow Fun Beef	1 pkg (9 oz)	320
Cafe Cuisine Sweet & Sour Chicken	1 pkg (10 oz)	300
Cafe Cuisine Thai-Style Chicken	1 pkg (9 oz)	260
Simple Favorites Chicken Chow Mein	1 pkg (9 oz)	240
Organic Classics		
Thai Chicken Curry	1 pkg (10 oz)	420
Purely Asian Brand		
Broccoli Beef	½ pkg (11 oz)	400
Mandarin Orange Chicken	½ pkg (12 oz)	450
Sweet & Sour Chicken	½ pkg (12 oz)	380
Tandoor Chef		
Chicken Tikka Masala	1 pkg (9.9 oz)	330
Tyson		
Meal Kit Chicken Fried Rice	2½ cups	440
MIX		
Nissin		
Chow Mein Chicken as prep	½ pkg (2 oz)	240
Chow Mein Thai Peanut as prep	½ pkg (2 oz)	270
SHELF-STABLE		
Dr. McDougall's		
Asian Entrée Pad Thai Noodle Gluten Free as prep	1 pkg (2 oz)	200
Asian Entrée Spicy Kung Pao Noodle as prep	1 pkg (2 oz)	220

FOOD	PORTION	CALS
Asian Entrée Teriyaki Noodle as prep	1 pkg (2 oz)	200
Asian Entrée Thai Peanut Noodles as prep	1 pkg (2 oz)	220
TAKE-OUT		
beef & broccoli	1 cup	221
beef w/ black bean sauce	1 serv (7 oz)	288
bo bia roll	1 (2.5 oz)	82
buddha's delight w/ cellophane noodles fat choi jai	1 serv (7.6 oz)	211
bun baked red bean	1 (1.1 oz)	102
cha siu bao steamed buns w/ chicken filling	1 (2.3 oz)	160
chicken masala	1 serv (8 oz)	430
chicken tandoori	1 serv (4 oz)	156
chicken tikka	1 serv (2.5 oz)	173
chinese garlic chicken	1 cup (5.7 oz)	290
chinese style fried egg noodles w/ seafood & lettuce	1 serv (14 oz)	694
chow mein beef w/o noodles	1 cup	271
chow mein chicken w/ noodles	1 cup (7.7 oz)	273
chow mein noodles	1 cup	237
chow mein pork w/o noodles	1 cup	284
chow mein shrimp w/ noodles	1 cup (7.7 oz)	262
chow mein shrimp w/o noodles	1 cup	154
chow mein vegetable w/o noodles	1 cup	224
dim sum deep fried beancurd w/ shrimp	1 (1.1 oz)	77
dim sum deep fried yam	1 (2.4 oz)	201
dim sum meat filled	3 pieces (4 oz)	124
dim sum pork hash	1 (1.1 oz)	59
dim sum shrimp	3 (4 oz)	307
dim sum steamed chives & prawns	1 (1.2 oz)	48
egg foo yung beef	1 patty (6 oz)	243
egg foo yung chicken	1 patty (3 oz)	121
egg foo yung pork	1 patty (3 oz)	125
egg foo yung shrimp	1 patty (3 oz)	153
filipino chicken adobo	1 serv (15 oz)	555
foochow fish ball	1 (1 oz)	36
fried rice	1 cup	333
fried rice beef	1 cup	346
fried rice chicken	1 cup	329
fried rice pork	1 cup	335
fried rice shrimp	1 cup	323

FOOD	PORTION	CALS
general tsao's chicken	1 cup (5 oz)	296
green beans szechuan style	1 cup	176
indian style fried egg noodles w/ eggs tomato sauce & lime	1 serv (15 oz)	721
korean spicy shredded chicken	1 serv (5 oz)	258
kung pao beef	1 cup	410
kung pao chicken	1 cup (5.7 oz)	434
kung pao pork	1 cup	460
kung pao shrimp	1 cup (5.7 oz)	345
lemon chicken w/o vegetables	1 serv (6.6 oz)	503
lo mein beef	1 cup	286
lo mein chicken	1 cup (7 oz)	280
lo mein meatless	1 cup	234
lo mein pork	1 cup	314
lo mein shrimp	1 cup	236
moo goo gai pan chicken	1 cup (7.6 oz)	272
moo shu pork w/o pancake	1 cup	512
pad thai w/ chicken	1 cup (7 oz)	358
pad thai w/ shrimp	1 cup (7 oz)	314
pakhoras	1 (2.5 oz)	163
paneer pakhora	1 (2.2 oz)	183
peking duck w/ pancakes & seafood sauce	1 serv (14 oz)	1871
pork w/ chinese cabbage	1 serv (4 oz)	120
sesame seed paste bun	1 (2.5 oz)	220
shrimp chips banh phong tom	6 med	214
shrimp w/ lobster sauce	1 cup	298
shu mai chicken & vegetable dumplings	6 (3.6 oz)	160
sukiyaki beef	1 cup	165
sukiyaki chicken	1 serv (18 oz)	436
sweet & sour chicken w/o rice	1 cup	670
sweet & sour pork w/ rice	1 cup	268
sweet & sour pork w/o rice	1 cup	231
sweet & sour shrimp	1 cup	480
szechuan chicken	1 cup (5.7 oz)	180
szechuan shrimp & vegetables	1 cup	159
tempura hawaiian fish tofu vegetable	2 cups	285
tempura vegetable	8 pieces	90
teriyaki beef	1 cup	454
teriyaki chicken	¾ cup	399
teriyaki chicken w/ rice	1 serv (11 oz)	430

FOOD	PORTION	CALS
teriyaki shrimp	1 cup	271
thai style pineapple rice w/ ham & pork floss	1 serv (7.7 oz)	408
wonton fried meat filled	1 (0.7 oz)	54
wonton meat & shrimp boiled	1 (0.5 oz)	19

ASPARAGUS

CANNED

spears	1	3
spears	1 cup	46
Del Monte		
Spears Extra Long	½ cup	20
Gertie's Finest		
White	1 oz	15
Green Giant		
Spears Extra Long	5 (4.4 oz)	20
McSweet		
Pickled Spears	6 (1 oz)	25
Native Forest		
White	1 serv (4 oz)	20
S&W		
Spears	½ cup (4.4 oz)	20
FRESH		
cooked	½ cup	20
spears cooked	4	13
spears raw	4	10
Alpine Fresh		
Fresh Green	5 spears (3.3 oz)	20
Dole		
Spears	5 med (2.8 oz)	15
Ocean Mist		
Spears	5 (3.3 oz)	25
FROZEN		
cooked	1 pkg (10 oz)	53
spears cooked	4	11
C&W		
Spears	7 (3 oz)	20
Joy Of Cooking		
Tender	½ cup (3.3 oz)	70
Seabrook Farms		
Spears	7 (2.9 oz)	20

FOOD	PORTION	CALS
ATEMOYA		
fresh	½ cup	94
AVOCADO		
california mashed	¼ cup	96
california peeled & pitted	1	289
florida mashed	¼ cup	69
florida peeled & pitted	1	365
Cabilfrut		
Hass fresh	⅕ med (1.1 oz)	55
Calavo		
Fresh	⅕ med (1 oz)	55
Chiquita		
Fresh	1 (7 oz)	322
Dole		
Fresh	⅕ med (1 oz)	50
Earthbound Farms		
Organic Fresh	⅕ med (1 oz)	55
Margaritaville		
Guacamole Zesty Island Garlic	1 oz	40
Simply Avo		
Hass Avocado Pulp	2 tbsp	50
Hass Halves	⅙ pkg (1.1 oz)	50
Wholly Guacamole		
Classic	2 tbsp (1 oz)	60
Organic	2 tbsp	50
Pico De Gallo Style	2 tbsp	40
TAKE-OUT		
guacamole	1 serv (2.2 oz)	105
BACON		
bacon grease	1 tbsp	116
beef breakfast strips cooked	3 strips	153
gammon lean & fat grilled	4.2 oz	274
pan fried	3 strips	109
turkey	2 (0.8 oz)	84
Boar's Head		
Fully Cooked Slices	3 (0.5 oz)	70
Butterball		
Turkey Bacon	1 slice (0.5 oz)	25

FOOD	PORTION	CALS
Dietz & Watson		
Gourmet	2 strips (0.5 oz)	70
Pancetta	⅙ pkg (0.5 oz)	50
Hormel		
Black Label Lower Sodium	2 slices (0.5 oz)	80
Microwave Ready	2 slices (0.5 oz)	80
Real Bits	1 tbsp (7 g)	25
Jimmy Dean		
Lower Sodium	1 slice (0.3 oz)	50
Original	1 slice (0.3 oz)	50
Thick Slice	1 slice (0.5 oz)	80
Organic Prairie		
Uncured Hardwood Smoked	2 strips (2 oz)	270
Uncured Turkey	2 strips (1 oz)	40
Oscar Mayer		
Bacon Bits	1 tbsp (7 g)	25
Fully Cooked	3 slices (0.5 oz)	70
Hardwood Smoked	2 slices (0.5 oz)	70
Lower Sodium	3 slices (0.5 oz)	70
Super Thick Applewood Smoked	0.6 oz	90
Turkey	0.5 oz	35
Turkey Lower Sodium	0.5 oz	35
Tyson		
Hickory Thick Cut	2 pieces (0.8 oz)	140
BACON SUBSTITUTES		
bacon bits meatless	1 tbsp	33
meatless	1 strip	16
Bob's Red Mill		
Bac'Ums	4 tsp	25
McCormick		
Bac'n Pieces	1 tbsp (7 g)	30
Worthington		
Stripples	2 strips (0.5 oz)	60
BAGEL		
cinnamon raisin	1 lg (4 in)	244
cinnamon raisin mini	1	71
egg	1 lg (4.5 in)	364
low carb	1 (4 oz)	216
oat bran	1 lg (4 in)	227

FOOD	PORTION	CALS
onion mini	1 (1.4 oz)	100
plain	1 sm (3 in)	190
plain	1 med (3.5 in)	289
plain	1 lg (4.5 in)	360
Enjoy Life		
Nut Gluten Free Classic Original	1 (3 oz)	270
Finagle A Bagel		
Cinnamon Raisin	1 (4 oz)	300
Everything	1 (4 oz)	310
Onion	1 (4 oz)	300
Plain	1 (4 oz)	290
Poppy Seed	1 (4 oz)	310
Sesame	1 (4 oz)	310
French Meadow Bakery		
100% Spelt	1 (3.4 oz)	270
Hemp	1 (3.4 oz)	280
Sprouted Cinnamon Raisin	1 (3.5 oz)	270
Natural Ovens		
Blueberry	1 (3 oz)	250
Brainy	1 (3 oz)	230
Whole Wheat	1 (3 oz)	230
New York Style		
Crisps Natural Whole Wheat	6	120
Crisps Plain	7	140
Pepperidge Farm		
100% Whole Wheat	1	250
100% Whole Wheat Mini	1 (1.4 oz)	100
Everything	1	260
Plain Mini	1	110
Thomas'		
100% Whole Wheat Mini	1 (1.5 oz)	110
Bagel Holes Plain	3 (1.6 oz)	120
Bagel Thins Everything	1 (1.6 oz)	110
Bagelbread Mini Squares 100% Whole Wheat	1 (2 oz)	150
Udi's		
Gluten Free Plain	1 (3.5 oz)	280
Gluten Free Whole Grain	1 (3.5 oz)	280

BAKING POWDER

baking powder	1 tsp	2
low sodium	1 tsp	5

FOOD	PORTION	CALS
Bob's Red Mill		
Baking Powder	1 tsp	5
Calumet		
Double Acting	⅛ tsp	0
Clabber Girl		
Baking Powder	⅛ tsp (0.6 g)	0
Davis		
Baking Powder	⅛ tsp (0.6 g)	0
Rumford		
Aluminum Free	⅛ tsp (0.6 g)	0
BAKING SODA		
baking soda	1 tsp	0
Arm & Hammer		
Baking Soda	¼ tsp	0
Bob's Red Mill		
Baking Soda	¼ tsp	0
BALSAM PEAR (BITTER GOURD)		
leafy tips cooked w/o salt	1 cup	20
leafy tips raw	1 cup	14
pods raw sliced	1 cup	16
pods sliced cooked w/ salt	1 cup	24
BAMBOO SHOOTS		
canned sliced	½ cup	12
fresh sliced cooked w/ salt	½ cup	7
raw sliced	½ cup	20
La Choy		
Bamboo Shoots	½ cup	10
Polar		
Sliced	½ cup	25
BANANA		
baked	1 (4.5 oz)	163
banana chips	1 oz	147
fresh	1 extra sm (<6 in)	72
fresh	1 sm (6 in)	90
fresh	1 med (7 in)	105
fresh	1 lg (8 in)	121
fresh mashed	½ cup	100
fresh sliced	1 cup	134

FOOD	PORTION	CALS
green fried	1 (3.1 oz)	152
green pickled	½ cup	240
green sliced fried	1 cup	323
powder	1 tbsp	21
red ripe	1 (7 in)	93
red ripe sliced	1 cup	134
whole dried	1 piece (1.2 oz)	130
Bob's Red Mill		
Chips	25 (1.4 oz)	210
Brothers-All-Natural		
Crisps	1 pkg (0.58 oz)	66
Chiquita		
Fresh	1 med (4.1 oz)	105
Crispy Green		
Crispy Bananas	1 pkg (0.5 oz)	55
Crunchies		
Freeze Dried Organic	¼ cup (0.3 oz)	32
Crunchy N'Yummy		
Organic Freeze Dried	1 pkg (1 oz)	110
Dole		
Fresh	1 med (4.4 oz)	110
Kopali		
Organic Dark Chocolate Covered	½ pkg (1 oz)	120
Nana Flakes		
100% Natural	1 tbsp (0.2 oz)	22
Tree Of Life		
Dried Sweetened	½ cup (1.6 oz)	240
TAKE-OUT		
batter dipped fried	1 sm (4 oz)	266
batter dipped fried sliced	1 cup	335
fried dwarf w/ cheese	1 (1.4 oz)	84
fritter	1 (2.3 oz)	197

BANANA JUICE

R.W. Knudsen		
Sensible Sippers Organic	1 box (4.23 oz)	35
Snapple		
Juice Drink Go Bananas	8 oz	110

FOOD	PORTION	CALS
BARBECUE SAUCE		
barbecue	2 tbsp	52
low sodium	2 tbsp	52
Annie's Homegrown		
Organic	2 tbsp (1.2 oz)	45
Bear-Man		
Black Bear Boogie	2 tbsp	40
Growlin' Grizzly	2 tbsp	60
Bone Suckin'		
Sauce	2 tbsp	40
Cattlemen's		
Classic	2 tbsp	60
Smokehouse	2 tbsp	60
Chef Hymie Grande		
Cascabel Express Barbecue Glaze	2 tbsp (1.2 oz)	30
Polapote Barbecue Glaze	2 tbsp (1.2 oz)	30
Dave's Gourmet		
Badlands BBQ	2 tbsp (1.1 oz)	40
David's Unforgettables		
Balsamic Spicy	2 tbsp (1 oz)	70
Jake & Amos		
Apple Butter Barbecue Sauce	2 tbsp (0.5 oz)	30
Naturally Fresh		
BBQ	2 tbsp	40
OrganicVille		
Original No Added Sugar	2 tbsp (1 oz)	50
Ribber City		
Kansas City	2 tbsp (1.1 oz)	40
Steel's		
No Sugar Added Gluten Free	2 tbsp (1.3 oz)	24
The Gracious Gourmet		
Spicy Barbeque Glaze	2 tbsp (1 oz)	35
Walden Farms		
Original Calorie Free	2 tbsp (1 oz)	0
World Harbors		
Bar-B	2 tbsp (1.2 oz)	70
Buccaneer Blends Fra Diavlo	2 tbsp (1.2 oz)	45
Buccaneer Blends Honey Mango	2 tbsp (1.3 oz)	60
Buccaneer Blends Sticky Rum	2 tbsp (1.2 oz)	50

FOOD	PORTION	CALS
BARLEY		
flour	1 cup	511
pearled cooked	1 cup (5.5 oz)	193
pearled uncooked	¼ cup	176
Arrowhead Mills		
Organic Pearled not prep	¼ cup	160
BARRACUDA		
broiled	4 oz	239
cooked flaked	1 cup	287
poached	4 oz	227
TAKE-OUT		
breaded & fried	4 oz	282
BARRAMUNDI		
Australis		
Barramundi	4 oz	90
Crispy Asian Sesame Panko	1 piece (4 oz)	240
Lemon Herb Butter	1 piece (6 oz)	170
BASIL		
fresh chopped	2 tbsp	1
ground	1 tsp	4
leaves fresh	5	1
BASS		
breaded baked	4 oz	205
pickled mero en escabeche	2 oz	156
striped baked	3 oz	105
striped bass farm raised	4 oz	110
BAY LEAF		
crumbled	1 tsp	2
BEANS (see also individual beans names)		
CANNED		
baked beans plain	½ cup	119
baked beans vegetarian	½ cup	119
baked beans w/ franks	½ cup	184
baked beans w/ pork	½ cup	134
baked beans w/ pork & tomato sauce	½ cup	119
refried beans	½ cup	134

FOOD	PORTION	CALS
Allens		
Original Baked	½ cup	150
Refried Black Beans No Fat Added	½ cup	120
Amy's		
Organic Refried	½ cup	140
Organic Refried Light In Sodium	½ cup (4.6 oz)	140
B&M		
Baked Original	½ cup (4.6 oz)	180
Barbeque Baked	½ cup (4.6 oz)	190
Country Style	½ cup (4.6 oz)	170
Vegetarian	½ cup (4.6 oz)	160
Bush's		
Boston Recipe	½ cup (4.6 oz)	150
Country Style	½ cup (4.6 oz)	160
Honey	½ cup	160
Maple Cured Bacon	½ cup (4.6 oz)	140
Original	½ cup (4.6 oz)	140
Vegetarian Fat Free	½ cup	130
Campbell's		
Pork & Beans	½ cup	140
Gebhardt		
Refried	½ cup	90
Refried Fat Free	½ cup	80
Refried Jalapeno	½ cup	100
Green Giant		
Three Bean Salad	½ cup	80
Hormel		
Kid's Kitchen Microwave Meals Beans & Wieners	1 pkg (7.7 oz)	310
Jake & Amos		
Four Bean Salad	2 tbsp	32
Old El Paso		
Refried Fat Free Spicy	½ cup	100
Pace		
Refried Salsa	½ cup	70
Read		
3 Bean Salad	⅓ cup	60
Rosarita		
Refried	½ cup	120
Refried Black Beans No Fat	½ cup	110

FOOD	PORTION	CALS
Refried Fat Free	½ cup	100
Refried Vegetarian	½ cup	120
Van Camp's		
Baked Beans Homestyle	½ cup	170
Beanee Weenee BBQ	1 can	260
Beanee Weenee Original	1 can	240
Beanee Weenee w/ Chili	1 can	240
Pork And Beans	½ cup	110
Wagon Master		
Pork & Beans	½ cup	130
FROZEN		
Lean Cuisine		
Simple Favorites Sante Fe Rice & Beans	1 pkg (10.4 oz)	290
TAKE-OUT		
baked beans	½ cup	191
barbecue beans	3.5 oz	120
frijoles a la charra w/ pork tomatoes & chili peppers	1 cup	341
refried beans	½ cup	43
three bean salad	1 cup	114

BEAN SPROUTS (see ALFALFA, SPROUTS)

BEAR

simmered	3 oz	220

BEAVER

roasted	4 oz	240

BEE POLLEN

bee pollen	1 tsp (5 g)	16
Tree Of Life		
Bee Pollen	1 tsp (7 g)	30

BEECHNUTS

dried	1 oz	163

BEEF (see also BEEF DISHES, JERKY, MEATBALLS, VEAL)

CANNED		
corned beef	1 oz	71
Hormel		
Corned Beef	1 serv (2 oz)	120
Dried Beef	1 oz	50

FOOD	PORTION	CALS
Libby's		
Corned Beef	2 oz	120
Potted Meat	¼ cup	120
Roast Beef w/ Gravy	⅔ cup	140
FRESH		
arm pot roast trim 0 fat braised	3.5 oz	297
arm pot roast trim ⅛ in fat braised	3.5 oz	302
beef crumbles 70% lean pan browned	3 oz	230
bottom round roast trim 0 fat braised	4 oz	253
bottom round roast trim 0 fat roasted	3.5 oz	187
bottom round roast trim ½ in fat braised	4 oz	337
bottom round roast trim ⅛ in fat braised	4 oz	280
bottom round roast trim ⅛ in fat roasted	4 oz	247
bottom sirloin butt roast trim 0 fat roasted	3.5 oz	182
brisket flat half trim ⅛ in fat braised	3.5 oz	298
brisket flat trim 0 fat braised	3.5 oz	221
brisket point half trim 0 fat braised	3.5 oz	358
brisket point half trim ¼ in fat braised	3.5 oz	404
brisket point half trim ⅛ in fat braised	3.5 oz	349
chuck boston cut roast trim 0 fat roasted	3.5 oz	207
chuck boston cut roast trim ¼ in fat roasted	3.5 oz	242
chuck bottom roast trim 0 fat braised	3.5 oz	334
chuck bottom roast trim ¼ in fat braised	3.5 oz	345
chuck fillet steak trim 0 fat broiled	4 oz	181
chuck top roast trim 0 fat broiled	4 oz	245
club steak trim ½ in fat broiled	4 oz	384
corned beef brisket cooked	3 oz	213
crosscut shank trim ¼ in fat stewed	1 serv (6.8 oz)	510
delmonico steak trim ¼ in fat broiled	4 oz	409
entrecote steak trim ½ in fat broiled	4 oz	413
eye round roast trim 0 fat roasted	4 oz	190
eye round roast trim ¼ in fat roasted	4 oz	283
filet mignon roast trim ⅛ in fat roasted	4 oz	367
filet mignon trim ¼ in fat roasted	4 oz	376
filet mignon trim 0 fat broiled	4 oz	247
filet mignon trim ⅛ in fat broiled	4 oz	303
ground 70% lean broiled	3.5 oz	273
ground 75% lean broiled	2.5 oz	195
ground 80% lean broiled	3 oz	234
ground 85% lean pan fried	3 oz	197

FOOD	PORTION	CALS
ground 90% lean pan fried	3 oz	173
ground 95% lean pan fried	3 oz	139
ground 97% lean irradiated	4 oz	160
ground lowfat w/ carrageenan raw	4 oz	160
london broil trim 0 fat broiled	3.5 oz	188
london broil trim ¼ in fat broiled	4 oz	260
new york strip steak trim 0 fat broiled	4 oz	219
oxtails cooked	6 pieces (6.3 oz)	472
porterhouse steak trim 0 fat broiled	1 lb	1252
porterhouse steak trim ¼ in fat broiled	1 lb	1492
porterhouse steak trim ⅛ in fat broiled	1 lb	1324
porterhouse steak trim ⅛ in fat broiled	4 oz	337
rib eye roast trim ¼ in fat roasted	3.5 oz	365
rib eye steak trim ⅛ in fat broiled	4 oz	221
rib roast trim ¼ in fat roasted	4 oz	406
rib steak trim ¼ in fat broiled	4 oz	388
round tip roast trim 0 fat roasted	4 oz	213
sandwich steaks thinly sliced	1 serv (2 oz)	173
shell steak trim ¼ in fat broiled	4 oz	366
shortribs lean & fat braised	1 serv (7.8 oz)	1060
skirt steak trim 0 fat broiled	4 oz	289
t-bone steak trim 0 fat broiled	4 oz	280
t-bone steak trim ¼ in fat broiled	1 lb	1388
t-bone steak trim ⅛ in fat broiled	1 lb	804
tip round roast trim ⅛ in fat roasted	4 oz	248
top loin steak boneless trim ⅛ in fat broiled	4 oz	299
top round roast trim 0 fat braised	4 oz	237
top round roast trim ¼ in fat braised	4 oz	281
top round roast trim ¼ in fat roasted	4 oz	265
top round steak trim ¼ in fat pan fried	4 oz	314
top sirloin steak trim ⅛ in fat broiled	4 oz	275
top sirloin steak trim ⅛ in fat pan fried	4 oz	355
tri-tip roast trim 0 fat roasted	3.5 oz	218
tri-tip steak trim 0 fat broiled	4 oz	300
Dietz & Watson		
Prime Rib Seasoned	3 oz	150
Laura's Lean		
Eye Of Round	4 oz	135
Flank Steak	4 oz	140
Ground Beef 92% Lean	4 oz	160

FOOD	PORTION	CALS
Ground Beef Patties	1 (4 oz)	160
Ground Round 96% Lean	4 oz	140
Ribeye Steak	4 oz	175
Sirloin Steak	4 oz	145
Sirloin Tip	4 oz	130
Strip Steak	4 oz	150
Tenderloin Filet	4 oz	145
Top Round	4 oz	135
Maverick Ranch		
Ground Beef 85% Lean not prep	4 oz	150
Ground Beef 96% Lean not prep	4 oz	130
NY Strip Steak not prep	4 oz	180
Ribeye Steak not prep	4 oz	215
Organic Prairie		
Grass Fed Ground	4 oz	240
Rumba		
Cheekmeat	4 oz	300
Crosscut Hind Shank	4 oz	190
Marrow Bones	4 oz	290
Oxtail	4 oz	260
Short Ribs	4 oz	400
READY-TO-EAT		
dried beef smoked chopped	1 oz	37
roast beef spread	¼ cup	127
Applegate Farms		
Organic Roast Beef	2 oz	80
Healthy Ones		
Deli Roast Beef	2 oz	70
Laura's Lean		
Beef Pot Roast Au Jus	3 oz	110
Oscar Mayer		
Slow Roasted Shaved	¼ pkg (1.8 oz)	60
Tyson		
Beef Strips Seasoned	1 serv (3 oz)	130
TAKE-OUT		
roast beef rare	2 oz	70

BEEF DISHES
CANNED

corned beef hash	3 oz	155

FOOD	PORTION	CALS
Hormel		
Beef Stew	1 pkg (7.5 oz)	150
Corned Beef Hash	1 cup (8.3 oz)	390
Corned Beef Hash 50% Reduced Fat	1 cup (8.3 oz)	290
Roast Beef Hash	1 cup (8.3 oz)	390
Roast Beef In Gravy	1 serv (5.8 oz)	130
Libby's		
Corned Beef Hash	1 cup	420
Hawaiian Corned Beef	2 oz	120
FROZEN		
Quaker Maid		
Sandwich Steaks Pure Beef	1 serv (1.8 oz)	120
Tyson		
Steak Country Fried	1 (3.2 oz)	310
MIX		
Hamburger Helper		
Beef Pasta as prep	1 cup	270
Cheddar Cheese Melt as prep	1 cup	310
Cheesy Baked Potato as prep	1 cup	310
Chili Cheese as prep	1 cup	340
Double Cheesy Quesadilla as prep	1 cup	350
Italian Sausage as prep	1 cup	290
Microwave Singles Cheesy Lasagna	1 pkg	210
Philly Cheesesteak as prep	1 cup	320
Salisbury as prep	1 cup	260
Tomato Basil Penne as prep	1 cup	300
REFRIGERATED		
Hormel		
Beef Tips & Gravy	1 serv (4 oz)	170
Laura's Lean		
Meatloaf w/ Tomato Sauce	1 serv (5 oz)	230
Shredded Beef w/ Barbecue Sauce	1 serv (5 oz)	245
Tyson		
Chuck Roast w/ Vegetables	1 serv (4 oz)	320
Seasoned Meatloaf	1 serv (5 oz)	320
Steak Tips In Bourbon Sauce	1 serv (5 oz)	180
TAKE-OUT		
beef bourguignonne	1 cup	339
beef satay + peanut sauce	2 skewers	253
bool kogi korean marinated beef ribs	4 oz	190

FOOD	PORTION	CALS
bracciola	1 roll (4.7 oz)	276
bubble & squeak	5 oz	186
bulgoghi korean grilled beef	1 serv (5.2 oz)	256
chipped beef on toast	1 slice (5 oz)	226
cornish pasty	1 (8 oz)	847
goulash w/ potatoes	1 cup	298
greek moussaka	1 serv (8.5 oz)	450
irish stew	1 cup (7 oz)	280
kebab indian	1 (5.4 oz)	553
kheema	6.7 oz	781
koftas	5	280
meatloaf	1 lg slice (5 oz)	294
pepper steak	1 cup	317
pot roast w/ gravy	1 serv (6 oz)	320
samosa	2 (4 oz)	652
shepherds pie	1 serv (7 oz)	282
sloppy joes	1 serv (9 oz)	398
steak & kidney pie w/ top crust	1 slice (5 oz)	400
stew w/ potatoes & vegetables	1 cup	199
stroganoff swiss steak w/ sauce	1 cup	394
toad in the hole	1 (4.7 oz)	383

BEEFALO

ground	3.5 oz	171
roasted	3.5 oz	188
t-bone steak	3.5 oz	111

BEER AND ALE

alcohol free beer	7 fl oz	50
ale brown	10 oz	77
ale pale	10 oz	88
beer cooler	1 (16 oz)	194
beer light	12 oz can	103
beer regular	12 oz can	153
black & tan	1 serv (12 oz)	146
black velvet	1 (10 oz)	160
boilermaker	1 serv	216
lager	10 oz	80
lager & black	1 (14 oz)	241
mead	1 serv	250
pilsener lager	7 oz	85

FOOD	PORTION	CALS
shandy	1 serv	125
stout	10 oz	102
trojan horse	1 (16 oz)	189
Amstel		
Light	1 bottle (12 oz)	95
Bard's		
Gluten Free	1 bottle (12 oz)	155
Beck's		
Pilsner	1 bottle (12 oz)	138
Bud		
Dry	1 bottle (12 oz)	130
Budweiser		
Beer	1 bottle (12 oz)	145
Bud Light	1 bottle (12 oz)	110
Coors		
Lite	1 bottle (12 oz)	104
Non-Alcohol	1 bottle (12 oz)	66
Original	1 bottle (12 oz)	149
Super Dry	1 bottle (12 oz)	149
Corona		
Extra	1 bottle (12 oz)	149
Guinness		
Draft In A Bottle	1 bottle (12 oz)	128
Extra Stout	1 bottle (12 oz)	174
Heineken		
Beer	1 bottle (12 oz)	150
Icehouse		
5.0	1 bottle (12 oz)	149
Keystone		
Light	1 bottle (12 oz)	103
Kilarney's		
Red Lager	1 bottle (12 oz)	197
Killian's		
Beer	1 bottle (12 oz)	163
LaBatt		
Blue	1 bottle (12 oz)	127
Lowenbrau		
Beer	1 bottle (12 oz)	160
Michelob		
Porter	1 bottle (12 oz)	196
Ultra	1 bottle (12 oz)	95

FOOD	PORTION	CALS
Miller		
Genuine Draft	1 bottle (12 oz)	143
Lite	1 bottle (12 oz)	96
MGD 64	1 bottle (12 oz)	64
O'Douls		
Non-Alcoholic	1 bottle (12 oz)	65
RedBridge		
Gluten Free	1 bottle (12 oz)	160
Sierra Nevada		
Porter	1 bottle (12 oz)	194
Smirnoff		
Ice	1 bottle (12 oz)	241
Weinhard's		
Amber Light	1 bottle (12 oz)	135
Blond Lager	1 bottle (12 oz)	161
Hefeweizen	1 bottle (12 oz)	151
Pale Ale	1 bottle (12 oz)	147
BEET JUICE		
juice	7 oz	72
BEETS		
CANNED		
harvard	½ cup	90
pickled	½ cup	74
sliced	½ cup	37
Freshlike		
Pickled Sliced	4 slices (1 oz)	20
Greenwood		
Harvard	1 serv (4.4 oz)	100
Pickled	1 oz	25
Jake & Amos		
Harvard	1 serv (4 oz)	90
Rise 'N Roll		
Pickled Baby Beets	3 (1 oz)	30
S&W		
Sliced	½ cup (4.3 oz)	35
Sliced Pickled	1 oz	15
FRESH		
greens cooked w/o salt	½ cup	19
sliced cooked	½ cup	37
whole cooked	2 med (3.5 oz)	44

FOOD	PORTION	CALS

BEVERAGES (see ALCOHOL DRINKS, BEER AND ALE, CHAMPAGNE, COFFEE, DRINK MIXERS, ENERGY DRINKS, FRUIT DRINKS, ICED TEA, MALT, MILK SHAKE, SMOOTHIES, SODA, TEA/HERBAL TEA, WATER, WINE, YOGURT DRINKS)

BISCUIT
FROZEN
Jimmy Dean

FOOD	PORTION	CALS
Snack Size Sausage On A Biscuit	2	400
MIX		
plain as prep	1 (2 oz)	190
Bisquick		
Heart Smart	⅓ cup	140
REFRIGERATED		
plain baked	1 (1 oz)	93
Immaculate Baking Co.		
Buttermilk	1 (2 oz)	170
Pillsbury		
Buttermilk	3 (2.2 oz)	150
Flaky Layers	3 (2.2 oz)	160
Grands! Butter Tastin'	1 (2 oz)	190
Grands! Buttermilk Reduced Fat	1 (2 oz)	170
Grands! Golden Wheat Reduced Fat	1 (2.1 oz)	180
Grands! Original	1 (2 oz)	190
Grands! Original Reduced Fat	1 (2 oz)	170
Perfect Portions Butter Tastin'	1 (1.9 oz)	190
TAKE-OUT		
buttermilk	1 lg (2.7 oz)	280
oatcakes	2 (4 oz)	115
plain	1 sm (1.2 oz)	127
tea biscuit	1 (3 oz)	210
w/ egg	1 (4.8 oz)	373
w/ egg & bacon	1 (5.3 oz)	458
w/ egg & ham	1 (6.7 oz)	442
w/ egg & sausage	1 (6.3 oz)	581
w/ egg & steak	1 (5.2 oz)	410
w/ egg cheese & bacon	1 (5.1 oz)	477
w/ ham	1 (4 oz)	386
w/ sausage	1 (4.4 oz)	485

BISON (see BUFFALO)

FOOD	PORTION	CALS
BLACK BEANS		
dried cooked w/o salt	1 cup (6 oz)	227
Allens		
Black Beans	½ cup	100
Goya		
Black Beans	½ cup (4.3 oz)	90
Tree Of Life		
Organic	½ cup (4.6 oz)	130
BLACKBERRIES		
canned in heavy syrup	½ cup	118
fresh	½ cup	31
unsweetened frzn	½ cup	48
Cascadian Farm		
Organic frzn	1 cup	80
Dole		
Fresh	1 cup (5.1 oz)	60
Marion frzn	1 cup (4.9 oz)	90
Oregon		
In Light Syrup	½ cup	120
BLACKBERRY JUICE		
canned	6 oz	65
BLACKEYE PEAS		
CANNED		
cowpeas	1 cup (8.4 oz)	185
w/ pork	1 cup (8.4 oz)	199
DRIED		
catjang cooked w/o salt	1 cup (6 oz)	200
cooked w/o salt	1 cup (5.8 oz)	160
FRESH		
cowpeas leafy tips chopped cooked w/o salt	1 cup (1.9 oz)	12
TAKE-OUT		
blackeye peas & pork	1 cup (6.3 oz)	236
frijol de ojo negro guisados	1 cup (9.1 oz)	289
hopping john	1 cup (7.9 oz)	419
BLINTZE		
Golden		
Cheese	1 (2.1 oz)	80

FOOD	PORTION	CALS
Ratner's		
Cheese	1 (2.2 oz)	100
Tofutti		
Mintz's Blintzes Dairy Free	1 (2 oz)	140
TAKE-OUT		
cheese	1 (2.7 oz)	160
BLUEBERRIES		
canned in heavy syrup	½ cup	113
fresh	1 pt	229
fresh	½ cup	41
frzn unsweetened	½ cup	40
C&W		
Ultimate	¾ cup	70
Chukar Cherries		
Puget Sound Dried	¼ cup	160
White Chocolate Covered	3 tbsp (1.4 oz)	223
De-Lite		
Dried Sweetened	1 oz	86
Dole		
Blueberries frzn	1 pkg (3 oz)	50
Blueberries frzn	1 cup (4.9 oz)	70
Emily's		
Dark Chocolate Covered	¼ cup (1.4 oz)	170
LiteHouse		
Glaze	3 tbsp	70
Marie's		
Glaze	2 tbsp	40
Ocean Spray		
Fresh	1 cup	85
Stoneridge Orchards		
Organic Dried Wild Whole	⅓ cup (1.4 oz)	130
Whole Dried	⅓ cup (1.4 oz)	130
Sunsweet		
Dried	¼ cup (1.4 oz)	140
Top Crop		
Fresh	1 cup (4.9 oz)	80
Tree Of Life		
Dried	¼ cup (1.5 oz)	150

FOOD	PORTION	CALS
BLUEBERRY JUICE		
Ocean Spray		
Diet	8 oz	5
Tart Is Smart		
Wild Blueberry Concentrate	0.5 oz	35
Walnut Acres		
Organic	8 oz	130
BLUEFIN		
fillet baked	4.1 oz	186
BLUEFISH		
fresh baked	3 oz	135
BOAR		
wild roasted	3 oz	136
Natural Frontier Foods		
Wild Boar Steaks	1 (4 oz)	170
BOK CHOY (*see* CABBAGE)		
BONITO		
dried	1 oz	50
fresh	3 oz	117
BORAGE		
fresh chopped	1 cup	19
BOTTLED WATER (*see* WATER)		
BOYSENBERRIES		
frzn unsweetened	½ cup	33
in heavy syrup	½ cup	113
BRAINS		
beef pan fried	3 oz	167
beef simmered	3 oz	123
lamb braised	3 oz	123
lamb fried	3 oz	232
pork braised	3 oz	117
veal braised	3 oz	116
veal fried	3 oz	181
BRAN		
corn	1 cup (2.7 oz)	170

FOOD	PORTION	CALS
oat	½ cup (1.6 oz)	116
oat cooked	½ cup (3.8 oz)	44
rice	½ cup (2.1 oz)	187
wheat	½ cup (2 oz)	63
Bob's Red Mill		
Rice Bran	2 tbsp	60
Mother's		
Oat Bran not prep	½ cup (1.4 oz)	150
Quaker		
Unprocessed	⅓ cup (0.6 oz)	35
Tree Of Life		
Oat Bran	½ cup (1.6 oz)	120
Organic Wheat Bran	¼ cup (1.1 oz)	190

BRAZIL NUTS
dried unblanched	1 oz	186

BREAD
CANNED

boston brown	1 slice (1.6 oz)	88
B&M		
Raisin Brown Bread	½ in slice (2 oz)	130
FROZEN		
Cedarlane		
Organic Mediterranean Stuffed Focaccia	1 piece (4 oz)	295
Kineret		
Challah Pull Apart	1 piece	140
Pepperidge Farm		
Garlic	1 slice (2.5 in)	170
Texas Toast Five Cheese	1 slice	150
Whole Grain Texas Toast	1 slice	150
Tandoor Chef		
Tandoori Naan	1 piece (3 oz)	182
MIX		
cornbread	1 piece (2 oz)	188
READY-TO-EAT		
anadama	1 piece (1.1 oz)	87
baguette whole wheat	2 oz	140
cassava	1 piece (3.5 oz)	299
challah	1 slice (1.4 oz)	115
cinnamon	1 slice (0.9 oz)	69
cracked wheat	1 slice (1.1 oz)	78

FOOD	PORTION	CALS
cuban bread	1 slice (1.1 oz)	83
french	1 slice (1.1 oz)	88
italian	1 loaf (1 lb)	1255
navajo fry	1 piece	281
oat bran	1 slice (1.1 oz)	71
oatmeal	1 slice (0.9 oz)	73
pan criollo	1 piece (0.9 oz)	69
pannetone	1 slice (0.9 oz)	86
pita	1 sm (1 oz)	77
pita	1 lg (2 oz)	165
pita whole wheat	1 sm (1 oz)	74
pita whole wheat	1 lg (2.2 oz)	170
pumpernickel	1 slice (0.9 oz)	65
raisin	1 slice (1.1 oz)	88
rye	1 slice (1.1 oz)	83
seven grain	1 slice (1.1 oz)	80
wheat berry	1 slice (0.9 oz)	65
wheat bran	1 slice (1.3 oz)	89
wheat germ	1 slice (1 oz)	73
white cubed	1 cup	93
whole wheat	1 slice (1 oz)	69
Alvarado Street Bakery		
Sprouted Soy Crunch	1 slice (1.2 oz)	90
Sprouted Whole Wheat	1 slice	90
Arnold		
100% Natural Soft Honey Wheat	2 slices (2 oz)	150
Grains & More Double Omega	1 slice	110
Jewish Rye	1 slice	90
Sandwich Thins Multi-Grain	1 (1.5 oz)	100
Sandwich Thins Whole Grain White	1 (1.5 oz)	100
Whole Grains 100% Whole Wheat Double Fiber	1 slice	100
Whole Grains 7 Grain	1 slice	110
Whole Grains 12 Grain	1 slice (1.5 oz)	110
Whole Grains 15 Grain	1 slice	110
Aunt Gussie's		
Gluten Free Focaccia Bread Kalamata Olive	1 piece (2.7 oz)	180
Gluten Free Focaccia Bread Rosemary	1 piece (2.7 oz)	180
Baker's Inn		
9 Grain	1 slice	100

FOOD	PORTION	CALS
Cracked Wheat	1 slice	100
Honey White Made w/ Whole Grain	1 slice	110
Honey Whole Wheat	1 slice	100
Potato Made w/ Whole Grain	1 slice	100
Comfort Care		
Cabin Hearth Whole Wheat	1 oz	170
Ecce Panis		
Classic Ciabatta	⅛ loaf (2 oz)	180
Flatout		
Fold It Flatbread 5 Grain Flax	1 (1.7 oz)	100
Fold It Flatbread Traditional Country	1 (1.8 oz)	140
Light Original	1 (2 oz)	90
Light Sundried Tomato	1 (1.9 oz)	90
Soft & No Crust Garden Spinach	1 (2 oz)	130
The Original	1 (2 oz)	130
Wrap Healthy Grain Harvest Wheat	1 (2 oz)	120
Wrap Healthy Grain Whole Grain White	1 (1.9 oz)	110
Wrap Mini Healthy Grain Harvest Wheat	1 (1 oz)	70
Freihofer's		
100% Whole Wheat	1 slice	90
French Meadow Bakery		
100% Rye Salt Free	1 slice (1.6 oz)	90
100% Spelt	2 slices (2.4 oz)	170
European Sourdough Rye	1 slice (1.7 oz)	90
Gluten Free Multigrain	1 slice (1.8 oz)	150
Hemp	2 slices (2.4 oz)	200
Kamut	2 slices (3 oz)	170
Men's Bread	2 slices (2.4 oz)	200
Our Daily Bread	2 slices (2.4 oz)	160
Sprouted Cinnamon Raisin	1 slice (1.5 oz)	100
Summer	1 slice (1.2 oz)	90
Gillian's Foods		
Gluten Free Cinnamon Raisin	1 slice (2 oz)	130
Kontos		
Pocket-Less Pita Whole Wheat	1 (2.8 oz)	210
La Tortilla Factory		
Smart & Delicious Soft Wrap Whole Grain White	1 (2.2 oz)	100
Smart & Delicious Soft Wraps Multi Grain	1 (2.2 oz)	100
Smart & Delicious Soft Wraps Tomato Basil	1 (2.2 oz)	100

FOOD	PORTION	CALS
Smart & Delicious Soft Wraps Traditional	1 (2.2 oz)	90
Smart & Delicious Soft Wraps Whole Grain	1 (2.2 oz)	170
Manna Organics		
Banana Walnut Hemp	1 slice (2 oz)	140
Carrot Raisin	1 slice (2 oz)	130
Fig Fennel Flax	1 slice (2 oz)	120
Millet Rice	1 slice (2 oz)	130
Whole Rye	1 slice (2 oz)	150
Martin's		
Potato 100% Whole Wheat	1 slice (1.3 oz)	70
Matthew's		
Golden White	1 slice (1.1 oz)	90
Honey 12 Grain	1 slice (1.1 oz)	80
Mrs Baird's		
Acti-Fiber Wheat	2 slices (2.2 oz)	160
Whole Grain Wheat Sugar Free	1 slice (1.1 oz)	70
Natural Ovens		
100% Sweet Whole	1 slice	90
Carb Conscious Original	1 slice	80
Healthy Beginnings Better White	1 slice	110
Healthy Beginnings Honey Wheat	1 slice	120
Hunger Filler Whole Grain	1 slice	100
Organic Plus Whole Grain & Flax	1 slice	120
Whole Grain Oat Nut Crunch	1 slice	100
Nature's Own		
100% Whole Wheat	1 slice	50
9 Grain	1 slice	120
Hearty Oatmeal	1 slice	100
Wheat Double Fiber	1 slice	50
Wheat Light	2 slices	80
Wheat N' Fiber	1 slice	60
Whole Wheat w/ Organic Flour	1 slice	100
Nature's Pride		
100% Whole Wheat	1 slice (1.5 oz)	110
100% Whole Wheat Double Fiber	1 slice (1.5 oz)	100
Country Buttermilk	1 slice (1.5 oz)	110
Healthy Multi-Grain	1 slice (1.5 oz)	110
Honey Wheat	1 slice (1 oz)	70
Nutty Oat	1 slice (1.5 oz)	110

FOOD	PORTION	CALS
Oroweat		
100% Whole Wheat	1 slice (1.3 oz)	100
Country Potato	1 slice (1.3 oz)	100
Country Whole Grain White	1 slice (1.3 oz)	90
Double Fiber	1 slice (1.3 oz)	70
Honey Fiber Whole Grain	1 slice (1.3 oz)	80
Russian Rye	1 slice (1 oz)	80
Seven Grain	1 slice (1.3 oz)	100
Whole Grain & Flax	1 slice (1.3 oz)	100
Pepperidge Farm		
100% Natural Whole Grain German Dark Wheat	1 slice	100
Breakfast Apple & Grains	1 slice	90
Canadian White	1 slice	100
Carb Style7 Grain	1 slice	60
Farmhouse Hearty White	1 slice	120
Farmhouse Honey Wheat	1 slice (1.5 oz)	120
Farmhouse Honey Wheatberry	1 slice	120
Farmhouse Whole Grain White	1 slice (1.5 oz)	110
Fruit & Grain Cranberry Orange	1 slice (1.4 oz)	90
Honey Flax Whole Grain	1 slice (1.5 oz)	100
Hot & Crusty Italian	1 slice (2 in thick)	150
Jewish Rye Whole Grain Seeded	1 slice	70
Light Style 7 Grain	1 slice	45
Light Style Oatmeal	3 slices	140
Party Pumpernickel	5 slices	130
Swirl 100% Whole Wheat Cinnamon Raisins	1 slice (1 oz)	80
Very Thin White	3 slices	120
Vitality Oats & Barley	1 slice (1.5 oz)	120
Whole Grain 100% Soft Whole Wheat Double Fiber	1 slice	100
Whole Grain Soft Honey Oat	1 slice (1.5 oz)	100
Roman Meal		
Muesli	1 slice (1.5 oz)	110
Original Whole Grain	2 slices (2 oz)	130
Rudi's Organic Bakery		
100% Whole Wheat	1 slice	100
14 Grain	1 slice	90
Artisan Country French	1 slice	100
Artisan Rosemary Olive Oil	1 slice	100

FOOD	PORTION	CALS
Low Carb Right Choice	1 slice	45
Spelt Ancient Grain	1 slice	120
Whole Grain Apple N Spice	1 slice	110
S. Rosen's		
Hawaiian	1 slice	110
Rye Black Bavarian	1 slice	100
Sara Lee		
Soft & Smooth 100% Whole Wheat	1 slice	70
Soft & Smooth Whole Grain White	2 slices	150
Sonoma		
Wraps Organic Multi Grain	1 (2.4 oz)	180
Wraps Organic Wheat	1 (2.4 oz)	190
Wraps Original White Whole Wheat	1 (2.4 oz)	200
Stroehmann		
Dutch Country Twelve Grain	1 slice	100
Potato	1 slice	100
Sun-Maid		
Raisin Cinnamon Swirl	1 slice (1.2 oz)	100
The Baker		
Yoga Bread	1 slice	70
Thomas'		
Breakfast Original	1 slice	90
Sahara Pita Pockets Mini Whole Wheat	1 (1 oz)	70
Swirl Cinnamon Raisin	1 slice	120
Tumaro's		
Deli Style Wraps Cracked Pepper	1 (2.1 oz)	100
Deli Style Wraps Everything	1 (2.1 oz)	80
Deli Style Wraps Pumpernickel	1 (2.1 oz)	80
Deli Style Wraps Rye	1 (2.1 oz)	80
Deli Style Wraps Sour Dough	1 (2.1 oz)	80
Wraps Chipotle Chili & Peppers	1 (2.3 oz)	170
Wraps Sun Dried Tomato & Basil	1 (2.3 oz)	170
Udi's		
Gluten Free Cinnamon Raisin	2 slices (2.1 oz)	160
Gluten Free Whole Grain	2 slices (2 oz)	140
Wonder		
100% Whole Wheat Soft	2 slices (1.6 oz)	110
Classic White	1 slice (1 oz)	70
Light White	1 slice (0.8 oz)	40
Smart White	1 slice (0.9 oz)	50

FOOD	PORTION	CALS
Texas Toast	1 slice (1.4 oz)	100
Whole Grain White	2 slices (2 oz)	140
REFRIGERATED		
Pillsbury		
Italian	⅛ pkg (1.6 oz)	110
TAKE-OUT		
banana	1 slice (2 oz)	196
chapati as prep w/ fat	1 (1.6 oz)	95
chapati as prep w/o fat	1 (2.5 oz)	141
cornbread	1 piece (2.3 oz)	183
cornstick	1 (1.4 oz)	118
focaccia onion	1 piece (4.6 oz)	282
focaccia rosemary	1 piece (3.5 oz)	251
focaccia tomato olive	1 piece (4.7 oz)	270
garlic bread	1 slice (1 oz)	96
irish soda bread	1 slice (3 oz)	247
italian garlic	1 loaf (11 oz)	990
naan	1 bread (3.5 oz)	286
papadum fried	1 (6 g)	30
paratha plain	1 (1.6 oz)	136
poori indian puffed bread	1 piece (1.3 oz)	112
zucchini	1 slice (1.4 oz)	150

BREADCRUMBS

FOOD	PORTION	CALS
dry seasoned	¼ cup	115
fresh	¼ cup	30
plain	¼ cup	107
Edward & Sons		
Organic Lightly Salted	⅓ cup	110
Organic Panko	⅓ cup	110
Gillian's Foods		
Plain Gluten Free	¼ cup (1.2 oz)	60
Kikkoman		
Panko	½ cup (1.1 oz)	110
Krasdale		
Seasoned	¼ cup	120
Progresso		
Garlic & Herb	¼ cup (1 oz)	110
Italian Style	¼ cup (1 oz)	118
Panko Lemon Pepper	¼ cup (1 oz)	120

FOOD	PORTION	CALS
Panko Plain	¼ cup (1 oz)	110
Plain	¼ cup (1 oz)	110
Southern Homestyle		
Corn Flake Crumbs	2 tbsp	40
Tortilla Crumbs	2 tbsp	40

BREADFRUIT
fresh	1 sm (13.5 oz)	396
fried	1 cup	379
raw	1 cup	227

BREADNUTTREE SEEDS
dried	1 oz	104

BREADSTICKS
plain	1 sm	21
plain	1 lg	41
Fattorie & Pandea		
Fornini w/ Sea Salt	5 (1.2 oz)	140
Ferrara		
Slim Thin Torinese Style	6 (0.5 oz)	60
Pepperidge Farm		
Garlic frzn	1	160
Pillsbury		
Cornbread Twists	1 (1.4 oz)	140
Original Soft	2 (1.8 oz)	140
Stella D'Oro		
Original	1 (0.3 oz)	40
Roasted Garlic	1	45
Sesame	1 (0.4 oz)	50
Sodium Free	1 (0.3 oz)	40

BREAKFAST BARS (*see* CEREAL BARS, ENERGY BARS)

BROCCOFLOWER
fresh flowerets cooked	1 cup (2.9 oz)	26
fresh raw	1 cup (2.2 oz)	20
head fresh raw	1 lg (18 oz)	158

BROCCOLI
FRESH
chinese broccoli (gai lan) cooked	1 cup (3 oz)	19
cooked w/o salt chopped	½ cup (2.7 oz)	27

FOOD	PORTION	CALS
cooked w/o salt spear 5 in	1 (1.3 oz)	13
raab cooked	½ cup (3 oz)	28
raw	1 bunch (1.3 lbs)	207
raw floweret	1 (0.4 oz)	3
raw flowers	1 cup (2.5 oz)	20
raw spear 5 in long	1 (1.1 oz)	11
BroccoSprouts		
Broccoli Sprouts	½ cup	16
Dole		
Broccoli	1 stalk (5.2 oz)	50
Broccoli Slaw	1 cup (3 oz)	25
Mann's		
Broccoli Wokly	1 serv (3 oz)	25
Broccolini	8 stalks (3 oz)	35
Ocean Mist		
Rapini Broccoli Rabe Chopped Raw	1 cup	9
Ready Pac		
Microwave Broccoli Rabe as prep	½ cup (3 oz)	30
FROZEN		
chopped cooked w/o salt	1 cup (6.5 oz)	52
spears cooked w/o salt	1 cup (6.5 oz)	52
Birds Eye		
Broccoli & Cheese Sauce	½ cup	90
Steamfresh Cuts	1 cup (3.1 oz)	30
Steamfresh Florets	1 cup (2.3 oz)	30
C&W		
Broccoli & Cheddar Cheese Sauce	1⅓ cups	70
Florets	1 cup	30
Cascadian Farm		
Organic Florets	⅔ cup	20
Dr. Praeger's		
Broccoli Bites	2 (2 oz)	110
Green Giant		
Cuts as prep	⅔ cup	25
Pasta Broccoli & Alfredo Sauce as prep	1 cup	210
Steamers Broccoli & Cheese Sauce as prep	½ cup	45
Seabrook Farms		
Broccoli Raab	1 cup (2.9 oz)	25
Skyy		
Broccoli Bites	3 (2.8 oz)	180

FOOD	PORTION	CALS
TAKE-OUT		
batter dipped & fried	3 pieces (1.4 oz)	58
w/ cheese sauce	1 cup (8 oz)	242
BROWNIE		
brownie	1 (2 oz)	227
butterscotch	1 (1.2 oz)	151
Arrowhead Mills		
Gluten Free as prep	1	160
Betty Crocker		
Dark Chocolate as prep	1	170
Fudge Low Fat as prep	1	140
Original Supreme as prep	1	160
Triple Chunk as prep	1	180
Walnut as prep	1	170
Warm Delights Hot Fudge	1 pkg (3 oz)	370
Bob's Red Mill		
Gluten Free as prep	1	140
Duncan Hines		
Chocolate Fudge frzn	½12 pkg (1.4 oz)	170
Dark Chocolate Chunk Mix as prep	½16 pkg	170
Milk Chocolate Mix as prep	½20 pkg	180
Peanut Butter Cup Mix as prep	½16 pkg	170
Turtle Mix as prep	½16 pkg	160
Walnut Mix as prep	½16 pkg	180
Erin Baker's		
Organic Bites	1 (1 oz)	100
Organic Bites Double Chocolate Chip	1 (1 oz)	90
Fiber One		
Chocolate Fudge	1 (0.89 oz)	90
Chocolate Peanut Butter	1 (0.89 oz)	90
Foods By George		
Gluten Free	⅑ pkg (1.5 oz)	180
Foxy's Bake Shop		
Milk Chocolate	½ (1.7 oz)	200
White Chocolate	½ (1.7 oz)	200
French Meadow Bakery		
Gluten Free Fudge	1 (2.82 oz)	350
Glenny's		
100 Calorie 75% Organic	1 (1.45 oz)	100

FOOD	PORTION	CALS
Hershey's		
Brownie	½ pkg (1.5 oz)	190
Uncle Wally's		
Smart Portion	1 (0.9 oz)	80
VitaBrownie		
Brownie	1 (2 oz)	100
Dark Chocolate Pomegranate	1 (2 oz)	100

BRUSSELS SPROUTS
CANNED

FOOD	PORTION	CALS
Jake & Amos		
Pickled Dill Brussels Sprouts	2 tbsp	10
FRESH		
cooked	6 pieces	45
Dole		
Brussels Sprouts	4 (2.9 oz)	30
Ocean Mist		
Brussels Sprouts	4 (2 oz)	40
Select Gourmet		
Fresh	½ cup	35
FROZEN		
cooked	1 cup	65
Birds Eye		
Steamfresh Baby	10 (2.9 oz)	45
Steamfresh Singles Baby	1 pkg (3.2 oz)	50
C&W		
Petite	10 (3 oz)	45
Green Giant		
Baby & Butter Sauce as prep	½ cup	60

BUCKWHEAT

FOOD	PORTION	CALS
groats roasted cooked	1 cup (6 oz)	155
groats roasted uncooked	½ cup	292
Bob's Red Mill		
Organic Kernels	¼ cup	142
Wolff's		
Kasha not prep	¼ cup (1.6 oz)	170

BUFFALO (*see also* HOT DOG, JERKY, SAUSAGE)

FOOD	PORTION	CALS
burger	3 oz	202
chuck braised	4 oz	205

FOOD	PORTION	CALS
top round steak broiled	3 oz	313
water buffalo roasted	3 oz	111
High Plains Bison		
Filet Mignon	4 oz	120
Ground	4 oz	190
Pot Roast	4 oz	150
Ribeye Steak	4 oz	215
Shredded In BBQ Sauce	1 serv (5 oz)	250
Steak Top Sirloin	4 oz	110
Tenderloin Tips	4 oz	120
Natural Frontier Foods		
Burgers	1 (5 oz)	170
Ground	4 oz	170
Steaks	1 (4 oz)	160
BULGUR		
cooked	½ cup	76
uncooked	½ cup	239
Bob's Red Mill		
From Soft White Wheat	¼ cup	150
Near East		
Whole Grain Wheat Pilaf as prep	1 cup	200
TAKE-OUT		
tabbouleh	1 cup	198
BURBOT (FISH)		
fresh baked	3 oz	98
BURDOCK ROOT		
cooked w/o salt	1 cup	110
cooked w/o salt	1 root (5.8 oz)	146
BUTTER		
clarified butter	1 tbsp (0.4 oz)	112
clarified butter	¼ cup (1.8 oz)	449
ghee cow's milk	1 tbsp	126
ghee vegetable oil	1 tbsp	126
honey butter	1 tbsp (0.6 oz)	85
honey butter	¼ cup (2.5 oz)	338
light butter whipped salted	1 tbsp (0.3 oz)	48
stick salted	1 tbsp (0.5 oz)	102
stick salted	¼ cup (2 oz)	407

FOOD	PORTION	CALS
stick salted	1 (4 oz)	810
stick unsalted	1 tbsp (0.5 oz)	102
stick unsalted	¼ cup (2 oz)	407
stick unsalted	1 (4 oz)	810
whipped salted	1 tbsp (0.3 oz)	67
whipped salted	¼ cup (1.3 oz)	271
Cabot		
Salted	1 tbsp	100
Country Crock		
Spreadable Butter w/ Canola Oil	1 tbsp (0.4 oz)	80
Deerfield		
Creamy	1 tbsp	100
Earth Balance		
Butter Blend Unsalted	1 tbsp	100
Gopi		
Pure Ghee	1 tsp (5 g)	35
Horizon Organic		
European	1 tbsp	100
Karoun		
Unsalted	1 tbsp (0.5 oz)	100
Land O'Lakes		
Butter Spread Cinnamon Sugar	1 tbsp (0.5 oz)	70
Honey	1 tbsp (0.5 oz)	90
Light Salted	1 tbsp (0.5 oz)	50
Light Whipped Salted	1 tbsp (0.4 oz)	45
Roasted Garlic w/ Oil	1 tbsp (0.5 oz)	90
Salted	1 tbsp (0.5 oz)	100
Spreadable w/ Canola Oil	1 tbsp (0.5 oz)	100
Whipped Salted	1 tbsp (0.2 oz)	50
Molly McButter		
Natural Butter	1 tsp (2 g)	5
Organic Valley		
European Style	1 tbsp	110
Plugra		
European Style Unsalted	1 tbsp (0.5 oz)	100
Straus		
Organic European Style Lightly Salted	1 tbsp (0.5 oz)	110
Organic European Style Sweet Butter	1 tbsp (0.5 oz)	110

BUTTER SUBSTITUTES

stick	1 stick	811

FOOD	PORTION	CALS
Butter Buds		
Granules	1 pkg (2 g)	5
Sunsweet		
Lighter Bake	1 tbsp	35
BUTTERBUR		
canned fuki chopped	1 cup	3
fresh fuki	1 cup	13
BUTTERNUTS		
dried	1 oz	174
BUTTERSCOTCH (see also CANDY)		
E. Guittard		
Baking Chips	33 (0.5 oz)	80
Hershey's		
Chips	1 tbsp (0.5 oz)	80
CABBAGE (see also COLESLAW)		
chinese bok choy shredded cooked w/o salt	1 cup	20
chinese pe-tsai shredded cooked w/o salt	1 cup	17
green raw shredded	1 cup	19
green shredded cooked w/o salt	1 cup	34
japanese pickled	½ cup	22
red raw shredded	1 cup	22
red shredded cooked w/o salt	1 cup	44
savoy shredded cooked w/o salt	1 cup	35
Aunt Nellie's		
Sweet & Sour Red	2 tbsp (1 oz)	20
Dole		
Shredded Red Fresh	1½ cups (3 oz)	25
Glory		
Country Cabbage	½ cup	25
Ready Pac		
Ready Fixin's Shredded Red	2 cups (3 oz)	25
TAKE-OUT		
coleslaw w/ pineapple & dressing	1 cup (4.6 oz)	194
creamed	1 cup	158
kimchee	1 cup	32
stuffed cabbage w/ rice & beef	1 (3.6 oz)	117
sweet & sour red cabbage	4 oz	61

FOOD	PORTION	CALS

CACAO
Kopali

| Organic Dark Chocolate Covered Cacao Nibs | ½ pkg (1 oz) | 140 |

Navitas Naturals

Butter	1 tbsp	120
Nibs	1 oz	130
Powder	1 oz	120

Sunfood

| Organic Cacao Beans | 1 oz | 171 |
| Organic Cacao Nibs | 1 oz | 171 |

CACTUS

fresh cooked w/ fat	1 pad (1 oz)	11
fresh cooked w/o fat	1 cup (5.2 oz)	22
pricklypear	1 (3.6 oz)	42
pricklypear fresh	1 cup (5.2 oz)	61

CAKE (see also CAKE MIX)

battenburg cake	1 slice (2 oz)	204
cream puff shell	1 (2.3 oz)	239
crumpet	1 (2.3 oz)	131
dutch honey cake	1 slice (0.8 oz)	70
eccles cake	1 slice (2 oz)	285
madeira cake	1 slice (1 oz)	98
sponge	1 piece (1.3 oz)	110
sponge cake dessert shell	1 (0.8 oz)	70
treacle tart	1 slice (2.5 oz)	258
turnover guava	1 (2.7 oz)	239

Amy's

| Organic Chocolate | 1 slice | 170 |
| Toaster Pops Apple | 1 (2.1 oz) | 150 |

Aunt Trudy's

| Organic Baklava Soy Nut | 1 (1.8 oz) | 190 |

Balocco

| Il Panettone | 1 serv (3.5 oz) | 380 |

Bellino

| Pandoro | 1 (2.8 oz) | 330 |

Betty Crocker

| Warm Delights Cinnamon Swirl | 1 (3.3 oz) | 390 |

Coppenrath

| Mousse Cake Chocolate | ⅛ cake (1.8 oz) | 140 |

FOOD	PORTION	CALS
Mousse Cake Coconut	⅛ cake (1.8 oz)	140
Mousse Duets Chocolate	1 (3.2 oz)	290
Mousse Duets Lemon Chiffon	1 (3.2 oz)	280
Do Goodie		
Gluten Free Banana Bread	1 slice (2 oz)	150
Gluten Free Cupcake Chocolate	1	290
Gluten Free Cupcake Vanilla	1	290
Earth Cafe		
Cheesecake Vegan Blueberry Thrill	1 slice (2 oz)	193
Cheesecake Vegan Coconut Carob	1 slice (2 oz)	206
Cheesecake Vegan Rockin' Raspberry	1 slice (2 oz)	194
El Monterey		
Cheesecake Bites Caramel	1 (2 oz)	180
Cheesecake Bites Raspberry	1 (2 oz)	200
Entenmann's		
Apple Puffs	1 (3 oz)	290
Blackout Iced	⅛ cake (2.2 oz)	210
Cheese Buns	1 (3 oz)	320
Chocolate Chip Iced	⅛ cake (2.5 oz)	330
Chocolate Fudge	⅛ cake (2.2 oz)	240
Cinnamon Swirl Buns	1 (3 oz)	320
Coffee Cake Cheese Filled Crumb	⅛ cake (2 oz)	210
Danish Twist Cheese	⅛ cake (1.9 oz)	220
Danish Twist Raspberry	⅛ cake (1.8 oz)	210
Devil's Food Marshmallow Iced	⅛ cake (2.2 oz)	260
Fudge Iced Golden Cake	⅛ cake (2.2 oz)	260
Lemon Crunch	⅛ cake (3 oz)	320
Lemon Loaf	⅙ cake (2 oz)	210
Louisiana Crunch	⅛ cake (2.7 oz)	310
Utlimate Super Cinnamons	½ bun (2.5 oz)	280
Vanilla Bean Iced	⅛ cake (2.2 oz)	290
Fiber One		
Toaster Pastry Blueberry	1 (1.8 oz)	180
Toaster Pastry Chocolate Fudge	1 (1.8 oz)	160
Foods By George		
Gluten Free Crumb Cake	⅑ cake (2.2 oz)	280
Gluten Free Pound Cake	⅙ cake (2.7 oz)	290
French Meadow Bakery		
Gluten Free Cupcake Chocolate	1 (2 oz)	220
Gluten Free Cupcake Yellow	1 (2 oz)	230
Vegan Carrot	¼ cake (2.6 oz)	130

FOOD	PORTION	CALS
Glenny's		
Blondie 100 Calorie 75% Organic	1 (1.45 oz)	100
Gourmet Pastries		
Baklava Walnut	1 piece (1.8 oz)	240
Guiltless Gourmet		
Dessert Bowl Bananas Foster Cake	1 pkg (2 oz)	200
Dessert Bowl Black Velvet Cake	1 pkg (2 oz)	200
Hostess		
100 Calorie Pack Mini Carrot Cake	1 pkg (1.2 oz)	100
100 Calorie Pack Mini Chocolate Cupcakes	1 pkg (1.3 oz)	100
100 Calorie Pack Mini Coffee Cake Cinnamon Streusel	1 pkg (1.2 oz)	100
100 Calorie Pack Mini Golden Cupcakes	1 pkg (1.2 oz)	100
Cup Cakes Chocolate	1 (1.8 oz)	170
Ho Hos	1	120
Twinkies	1 (1.5 oz)	150
Kineret		
Babka Chocolate	1 piece (1 oz)	100
Lance		
Honey Bun	1 (3 oz)	320
Mrs. Freshley's		
Golden Cupcakes Creme Filled	1 pkg (1.3 oz)	100
Mrs. Smith's		
Carrot	⅙ cake (2.9 oz)	300
Cobbler Blackberry	1 serv (4 oz)	260
Singles Heavenly 100 New York Cheesecake	1 (0.9 oz)	100
Neuman's		
Date Nut Bread	1 oz	90
Pepperidge Farm		
Chocolate Coconut 3 Layer	⅛ cake	240
Devil's Food 3 Layer	⅛ cake	220
Golden 3 Layer	⅛ cake	230
Lemon 3 Layer	⅛ cake	240
Turnover Apple	1	290
Turnover Peach	1	290
Pillsbury		
Caramel Rolls	1 (1.7 oz)	170
Cinnamon Rolls w/ Icing	1 (3.5 oz)	310
Toaster Strudel	1 (2 oz)	200
Toaster Strudel Blueberry	1 (2 oz)	190

FOOD	PORTION	CALS
Toaster Strudel Cream Cheese	1 (2 oz)	200
Toaster Strudel Raspberry	1 (2 oz)	190
Toaster Strudel Wildberry	1 (2 oz)	190
Turnovers Cherry	1 (2 oz)	180
Prosperity		
Limoncello	1 serv (3.5 oz)	300
The Fillo Factory		
Organic Apple Strudel	1 (4.4 oz)	290
Organic Apple Turnovers	1 (3 oz)	180
Tortuga		
Caribbean Rum Golden Original	1 piece (4 oz)	400
Weight Watchers		
Lemon Creme	1 (0.9 oz)	80
TAKE-OUT		
angelfood	1 slice (2 oz)	143
apple crisp	1 serv (8.6 oz)	384
apple turnover	1 (6.6 oz)	661
baklava	1 piece (2.7 oz)	334
basbousa namoura	1 piece (1 oz)	60
bean cake	1 cake (1.1 oz)	130
black forest chocolate cherry	1 piece (2.5 oz)	187
boston cream pie	1 slice (3.2 oz)	232
cannoli w/ cannoli cream	1	369
carrot w/ icing	1 slice (4.7 oz)	543
cheesecake	1 slice (4.5 oz)	410
cheesecake chocolate	1 slice (4.5 oz)	489
chinese moon cake	1 (4.8 oz)	458
cobbler pineapple	1 cup (7.6 oz)	414
coconut mochiko filipino cake	1 piece (2.7 oz)	252
coffeecake iced	1 piece (1.6 oz)	175
cream puff custard filled chocolate frosted	1 (3.9 oz)	293
eclair	1 (3.5 oz)	262
french apple tart	1 (3.5 oz)	302
fruitcake	1 slice (1.5 oz)	139
funnel cake	1 (3.2 oz)	276
gingerbread	1 piece (2.4 oz)	213
jelly roll	1 slice (1.8 oz)	146
jelly roll lemon filled	1 slice (3 oz)	210
napoleon	1 (3 oz)	348
napoleon	1 mini (1 oz)	123

FOOD	PORTION	CALS
panettone	1/12 cake (2.9 oz)	300
petit fours	2 (0.9 oz)	120
pineapple upside down	1 piece (4.2 oz)	387
pound	1 slice (1 oz)	120
pound fat free	1 slice (2 oz)	160
pumpkin bread w/ raisins	1 slice (2.1 oz)	178
red velvet cupcake w/ cream cheese frosting	1 sm	272
red velvet w/ cream cheese frosting	1/16 cake	520
sacher torte	1 slice (2.2 oz)	240
sacher torte chocolate + apricot jam	1 serv	430
strawberry shortcake	1 serv (4.1 oz)	211
strudel apple	1 piece (2.2 oz)	175
strudel cheese	1 piece (2.2 oz)	195
strudel cherry	1 piece (2.2 oz)	179
strudel pineapple	1 piece (2.2 oz)	159
sweet potato w/ glaze	1 piece (2.7 oz)	275
tiramisu	1 piece (5.1 oz)	409
tiramisu	1 cake (4.4 lbs)	5732
torte chocolate ganache	1 slice (3.5 oz)	400
trifle w/ cream	6 oz	291
white w/ coconut icing	1 slice (3.9 oz)	399
zucchini bread	1 slice (1.4 oz)	150

CAKE ICING

FOOD	PORTION	CALS
chocolate	1/4 cup	269
vanilla	1/4 cup	322
Betty Crocker		
HomeStyle Mix Fluffy White as prep	6 tbsp	100
Rich & Creamy Butter Cream	2 tbsp (1.3 oz)	140
Rich & Creamy Chocolate	2 tbsp (1.2 oz)	130
Rich & Creamy Creamy White	2 tbsp (1.2 oz)	140
Rich & Creamy Lemon	2 tbsp (1.2 oz)	140
Rich & Creamy Vanilla	2 tbsp (1.2 oz)	140
Whipped Fluffy White	2 tbsp (0.8 oz)	100
Duncan Hines		
Chocolate Butter Cream	2 tbsp (1.2 oz)	140
Chocolate Fudge	2 tbsp (1.2 oz)	130
Classic Vanilla	2 tbsp	140
Cream Cheese	2 tbsp (1.2 oz)	140
Milk Chocolate	2 tbsp	140

FOOD	PORTION	CALS
Manischewitz		
Dairy Free Chocolate	2 tbsp (1.2 oz)	138
Naturally Nora		
Frosting Mix Chocolate as prep	1/12 pkg	150
Frosting Mix Vanilla as prep	1/12 pkg	170
Pillsbury		
Chocolate Fudge Sugar Free	2 tbsp (1 oz)	100
Creamy Supreme Buttercream	2 tbsp (1.2 oz)	150
Creamy Supreme Classic White	2 tbsp (1.2 oz)	150
Creamy Supreme Coconut Pecan	2 tbsp (1.2 oz)	160
Creamy Supreme Milk Chocolate	2 tbsp (1.2 oz)	140
Creamy Supreme Vanilla	2 tbsp (1.2 oz)	150
Easy Frost Chocolate Fudge	2 tbsp (1.2 oz)	140
Easy Frost Cream Cheese	2 tbsp (1.2 oz)	150
Easy Frost Vanilla	2 tbsp (1.2 oz)	150
Funfetti Pink Vanilla	2 tbsp (1.2 oz)	140
Vanilla Sugar Free	2 tbsp (1 oz)	100
Whipped Supreme Cream Cheese	1 tbsp (0.8 oz)	100
Whipped Supreme Strawberry	2 tbsp (0.8 oz)	110
CAKE MIX		
Betty Crocker		
Gingerbread as prep	1 piece	220
Pineapple Upside Down as prep	1/6 cake	390
Pound Cake as prep	1/8 cake	260
SuperMoist Carrot as prep	1/12 cake	260
SuperMoist Chocolate as prep	1/12 cake	250
SuperMoist Devil's Food as prep	1/12 cake	260
SuperMoist Lemon as prep	1/12 cake	240
SuperMoist Milk Chocolate as prep	1/12 cake	240
SuperMoist Spice as prep	1/12 cake	270
SuperMoist Vanilla as prep	1/12 cake	230
SuperMoist White as prep	1/12 cake	220
SuperMoist Yellow as prep	1/12 cake	230
Bisquick		
Heart Smart	1/3 cup	140
Duncan Hines		
Angel Food as prep	1/12 cake	140
Cupcake Mix Classic Yellow as prep	1	130
Decadent Carrot as prep	1/12 cake	260
Golden Butter Recipe as prep	1/12 cake	270

FOOD	PORTION	CALS
Lemon Supreme as prep	1/12 cake	270
Red Velvet as prep	1/12 cake	270
Yellow Classic as prep	1/12 cake	270
Naturally Nora		
Cheerful Chocolate as prep	1/12 pkg	300
Sunny Yellow as prep	1/12 pkg	280
Surprising Stars as prep	1/12 pkg	300
Uncle Wally's		
Slice 'N Bake Cupcakes Chocolate	1 (2.1 oz)	240

CALZONE (see SANDWICHES)

CANADIAN BACON
grilled	2 slices (1.6 oz)	87
Applegate Farms		
Natural	2 slices (2 oz)	90
Celebrity		
98% Fat Free	3 slices (1.8 oz)	60
Dietz & Watson		
Canadian Style	2 oz	70
Oscar Mayer		
Fully Cooked	3 slices (1.9 oz)	60

CANADIAN BACON SUBSTITUTES
Yves		
Meatless Canadian Bacon	2 slices (2 oz)	80

CANDY
butterscotch	1 piece (6 g)	24
candied cherries	1 (4 g)	12
candied citron	1 oz	89
candied lemon peel	1 oz	90
candied orange peel	1 oz	90
candied pineapple slice	1 slice (2 oz)	179
candy corn	1 oz	105
caramels	1 piece (8 g)	31
caramels chocolate	1 piece (6 g)	22
carob bar	1 (3.1 oz)	453
dark chocolate	1 oz	150
fondant	1 piece (0.6 oz)	57
fondant chocolate coated	1 piece (0.4 oz)	40
fondant mint	1 oz	105

FOOD	PORTION	CALS
fruit pastilles	1 tube (1.4 oz)	101
fudge brown sugar w/ nuts	1 piece (0.5 oz)	56
fudge chocolate marshmallow	1 piece (0.7 oz)	84
fudge chocolate marshmallow w/ nuts	1 piece (0.8 oz)	96
fudge chocolate w/ nuts	1 piece (0.7 oz)	81
fudge peanut butter	1 piece (0.6 oz)	59
fudge vanilla w/ nuts	1 piece (0.5 oz)	62
gumdrops	10 lg (3.8 oz)	420
gumdrops	10 sm (0.4 oz)	135
hard candy	1 oz	106
jelly beans	10 lg (1 oz)	104
jelly beans	10 sm (0.4 oz)	40
lollipop	1 (6 g)	22
marzipan	1 oz	128
milk chocolate	1 bar (1.55 oz)	226
milk chocolate crisp	1 bar (1.45 oz)	203
milk chocolate w/ almonds	1 bar (1.45 oz)	215
nougat nut cream	0.5 oz	49
peanut bar	1 (1.4 oz)	209
peanut brittle	1 oz	128
peanuts chocolate covered	10 (1.4 oz)	208
peanuts chocolate covered	1 cup (5.2 oz)	773
praline	1 piece (1.4 oz)	177
pretzels chocolate covered	1 oz	130
pretzels chocolate covered	1 (0.4 oz)	50
sesame crunch	20 pieces (1.2 oz)	181
taffy	1 piece (0.5 oz)	56
toffee	1 piece (0.4 oz)	65
truffles	1 piece (0.4 oz)	59
3 Musketeers		
Bar	1 (2.1 oz)	260
Fun Size	3 bars (1.6 oz)	190
Minis	7 (1.4 oz)	170
Mint	1 bar (1.2 oz)	150
5th Avenue		
Bar	1 (2 oz)	260
Almond Joy		
Bar	1 (1.6 oz)	220
Andes		
Dark Chocolate Covered Cherries	2 (1 oz)	110

FOOD	PORTION	CALS
Thins Cherry Jubilee	8 pieces (1.3 oz)	200
Thins Creme De Menthe	8 pieces (1.3 oz)	200
Annabelle's		
Skinny Hunk Chewy Nougat	1 bar (1 oz)	100
Baby Ruth		
Fun Size	2 bars (1.3 oz)	170
Snack Bars	2 (1.3 oz)	170
Bartons		
Cashew Toppers	1 (1 oz)	140
Baskin-Robbins		
Soft Candy Mint Chocolate Chip	2 (0.3 oz)	40
Sugar Free Hard Candy Cookies 'N Cream	4 (0.6 oz)	40
Benecol		
Smart Chews Caramel	1 piece	20
Benedetto		
Cubetti Mini Caramel Crunch Protein 1st	5 pieces (1.7 oz)	178
Cupola Mini Mint Protein 1st	5 pieces (1.7 oz)	122
Betty Crocker		
Fruit Gushers Rockin' Blue Raspberry	1 pkg (0.9 oz)	90
Blow Pop		
Regular	1 (0.6 oz)	60
Brach's		
Candy Corn	19 (1.4 oz)	140
Mellowcreme Pumpkins	6 pieces (1.5 oz)	150
Breath Savers		
Peppermint	1 (1.8 g)	5
Bubble Chocolate		
Dark Chocolate	1 bar (1.41 oz)	200
Milk Chocolate	1 bar (1.41 oz)	220
Butterfinger		
Crisp Bar	1 (2.1 oz)	270
Original Bar	1 (2.1 oz)	270
Snackerz	1 pkg (1.3 oz)	170
Cadbury		
Caramello	1 (1.6 oz)	220
Dairy Milk	7 blocks (1.4 oz)	200
Milk Chocolate Fruit & Nut	10 blocks (1.4 oz)	200
Milk Chocolate Roast Almond	7 blocks (1.4 oz)	210
Royal Dark	7 blocks (1.4 oz)	170

FOOD	PORTION	CALS
Cella's		
Milk Chocolate Covered Cherries	2 (1 oz)	120
Charleston Chews		
Chocolate	1 bar (1.9 oz)	230
Vanilla	1 bar (1.9 oz)	230
Charms		
Fluffy Stuff Cotton Candy	1 pkg (0.6 oz)	70
Sour Balls	1 (5 g)	20
Squares	2 pieces	20
Chew-ets		
Peanut Chews Original Dark	3 pieces	170
Choward's		
Mints All Flavors	3 (5 g)	20
Chuao Chocolatier		
Choco Pod Banana	1 (0.4 oz)	50
Choco Pod Passion	1 (0.4 oz)	50
Coco		
Brain Truffles Orange	1 (0.5 oz)	56
Preggers Truffles Dark Chocolate	1 (0.5 oz)	56
Coffee Spoons		
Flavored	1 (0.6 oz)	90
Coombs Family Farms		
Maple Candy	6 pieces (1.5 oz)	160
Crispy Cat		
Roasted Peanut	1 bar (1 oz)	220
Dare		
RealFruit Gummies All Flavors	8 pieces (1.4 oz)	120
Dots		
Gumdrops Fruit	11 (1.4 oz)	130
Dove		
Dark Chocolate Cranberry Almond	⅓ pkg (1.2 oz)	170
Milk Chocolate Roasted Almond	⅓ bar (1.2 oz)	180
E. Guittard		
Bar Quevedo Bittersweet 65% Cacao	1 (2 oz)	290
Bar Sur Del Lago Bittersweet 65% Cacao	1 (2 oz)	290
Elmer Chocolates		
Assorted	5 (2 oz)	240
Emily's		
Espresso Beans Dark Chocolate Covered	26 (1.4 oz)	220

FOOD	PORTION	CALS
Enjoy Life		
Boom Choco Boom Dark Chocolate Dairy Nut Soy Free	1 bar (1.4 oz)	200
Equal Exchange		
Organic Chocolate Espresso Bean	1 bar (1.4 oz)	216
Organic Milk Chocolate	1 bar (1.4 oz)	230
Organic Very Dark Chocolate	1 bar (1.4 oz)	220
Ferrero		
Rocher	3 pieces (1.3 oz)	220
Rondnoir	3 pieces (1.4 oz)	220
Frooties		
Chewy Candy Fruit Flavored	12 pieces (1.3 oz)	104
Ghirardelli		
Luxe Milk Chocolate	4 sq (1.5 oz)	220
Squares Milk Chocolate w/ Caramel Filling	3 (1.6 oz)	220
Squares Mint Indulgence	3 (1.6 oz)	210
Squares 60% Cacao Dark Chocolate	4 (1.5 oz)	220
Squares 60% Cacao Dark Chocolate w/ Caramel	3 (1.6 oz)	220
Gimme		
Dark Chocolate Omega 3	1 pkg (1 oz)	130
Dark Chocolate Probiotics	1 pkg (1 oz)	130
Milk Chocolate Calcium	1 pkg (1 oz)	120
Godiva		
Assorted Milk Chocolate	4 pieces (1.4 oz)	190
Gems Truffles Milk Chocolate	4 (1.5 oz)	200
Truffles Assorted	2 pieces (1.4 oz)	210
Good & Plenty		
Licorice	33 (1.4 oz)	140
Guylian		
Twists Milk Chocolate Truffle	5 pieces (1.2 oz)	230
Twists Original Praline	4 pieces (1.2 oz)	200
Hammond's		
Root Beer Drops	3 (0.6 oz)	60
Heath		
Bar	1 (1.4 oz)	210
Hershey's		
Bar Milk Chocolate w/ Almonds	1 (1.4 oz)	210
Bar Special Dark	1 (1.4 oz)	180
Bliss Dark Chocolate Bar	1 (1.3 oz)	160

FOOD	PORTION	CALS
Bliss Milk Chocolate	6 (1.5 oz)	210
Bliss Milk Chocolate Meltaway	6 (1.5 oz)	220
Bliss Milk Chocolate Raspberry Meltaway	6 (1.5 oz)	220
Cacao Reserve 35% Cacao Milk Chocolate w/ Hazelnuts	3 sq (1.3 oz)	220
Kisses Cherry Cordial	9 (1.5 oz)	180
Kisses Hugs	9 (1.4 oz)	210
Kisses Milk Chocolate	9 (1.4 oz)	200
Kisses Special Dark	9 (1.4 oz)	180
Milk Chocolate Bar	1 (1.5 oz)	210
Milk Chocolate w/ Almonds Bar	1 (1.5 oz)	210
Miniatures Special Dark	5 (1.4 oz)	190
Nuggets Milk Chocolate	4 (1.4 oz)	200
Nuggets Milk Chocolate w/ Almonds	4 (1.3 oz)	200
Pieces All Flavors	51 (1.4 oz)	190
Pot Of Gold Assorted Milk & Dark Chocolate	4 (1.4 oz)	200
Ice Breakers		
Coolmint	1 (0.8 g)	0
Jay's		
Cotton Candy	1 pkg (2 oz)	220
Jelly Belly		
Jelly Beans Cocktail Classics	1 pkg (0.75 oz)	80
Peas & Carrots	49 (1.4 oz)	140
Jer's		
Balls Peanut Butter Chocolate	1 piece (0.5 oz)	80
Original IncrediBar Peanut Butter	1 (1.8 oz)	210
Jolly Rancher		
Gummies	9 (1.4 oz)	120
Original Assortment	3 (0.5 oz)	50
Junior		
Caramels	1 box (1.4 oz)	170
Mints	1 box (1.4 oz)	170
KitKat		
Bar	1 (1.5 oz)	210
Kopali		
Organic Dark Chocolate Covered Espresso Beans	½ pkg (1 oz)	120
Lance		
Chewz Strawberry	1 pkg (1.1 oz)	120
Peanut Bar	1 (2.3 oz)	340

FOOD	PORTION	CALS
Let's Do Organic		
Black Licorice Bars	1 (0.9 oz)	80
Black Licorice Chews	8 (1.4 oz)	130
Gummi Bears	1 pkg (0.9 oz)	80
Lindt		
Lindor Truffles 60% Extra Dark	3 pieces (1.3 oz)	210
Lindor Truffles Swiss Dark Chocolate	3 (1.4 oz)	240
Petits Desserts Assorted	4 (1.3 oz)	210
Love Candy		
Dark Chocolate	1 bar (1.5 oz)	190
Milk Chocolate	1 bar (1.5 oz)	200
Yogurt Supreme	1 bar (1.5 oz)	190
Mama's Goodies		
Butter Nut Crunch Almond	1 piece (1.33 oz)	220
Butter Nut Crunch Macadamia & Coconut	1 piece (1.33 oz)	220
Butter Nut Crunch Sesame Seed	1 piece (1.33 oz)	220
Mamba		
Fruit Flavor	6 (0.9 oz)	170
Sour	6 (0.9 oz)	100
Maple Grove Farms		
Maple	5 pieces (1.5 oz)	160
Mike & Ike		
All Flavors	1 pkg (2 oz)	200
Milk Duds		
Chocolate	13 (1.4 oz)	170
Milkfuls		
Candy	6 (1.4 oz)	170
Milky Way		
Fun Size	2 bars (1.2 oz)	150
Mounds		
Bar	1 (1.7 oz)	230
Mr.Goodbar		
Bar	1 (1.7 oz)	250
Necco		
Banana Splits	4 (1.4 oz)	150
Clark Junior Bar	1 (0.5 oz)	60
Conversation Hearts Tiny	40 (1.4 oz)	160
Double Dipped Peanuts	15 (1.4 oz)	200
Junior Assorted Wafers	1 roll (0.5 oz)	50
Mary Janes	5 (1.4 oz)	160

FOOD	PORTION	CALS
Mint Juleps	4 (1.4 oz)	150
Nonpareils	10 (1.4 oz)	190
Squirrel Nut Caramel	5 (1.6 oz)	170
Nestle		
Crunch Stix	1 (0.6 oz)	90
NibMor		
Organic Vegan Dark Chocolate	½ bar (1.1 oz)	120
Organic Vegan Dark Chocolate w/ Almonds	½ bar (1.1 oz)	130
Organic Vegan Dark Chocolate w/ Cacao Nibs	½ bar (1.1 oz)	120
Organic Vegan Dark Chocolate w/ Crispy Brown Rice	½ bar (1 oz)	110
Panda		
Licorice Cherry	1 bar (1.1 oz)	100
PayDay		
Peanut Caramel	1 (1.8 oz)	240
Pot Of Gold		
Nut Assortment	4 (1.4 oz)	210
Pecan Caramel Clusters	4 (1.4 oz)	200
Truffle Assortment	3 (1.5 oz)	200
Pure Fun		
Organic Vegan Barrels Of Fun Root Beer Float	2 (0.5 oz)	60
Organic Vegan Candy Canes	1 (0.5 oz)	62
Organic Vegan Chocolate Meltdowns All Flavors	3 (0.6 oz)	70
Organic Vegan Citrus Slices All Flavors	3 (0.6 oz)	60
Organic Vegan Cotton Candy All Flavors	¼ pkg (0.5 oz)	60
Organic Vegan Jaw Boulders All Flavors	2 (0.5 oz)	58
Organic Vegan Pure Pops All Flavors	3 (0.6 oz)	60
Raisinets		
Candy	¼ cup (1.6 oz)	190
Reese's		
Crispy Crunchy Bar	1 (1.7 oz)	250
FastBreak	1 (2 oz)	260
NutRageous	1 (1.8 oz)	260
Peanut Butter Cups Miniatures Dark Chocolate	5 (1.5 oz)	220
Pieces Peanut Butter	1 pkg (1.5 oz)	210
ReeseSticks		
Wafer Bar Chocolate & Peanut Butter	1 (1.5 oz)	210
Ricochet		
Coffee Shots Sugar Free	5 (3 g)	10

FOOD	PORTION	CALS
Riesen		
Candy	4 (1.3 oz)	170
Ritter Sport		
Bar Cappuccino	1 (3.5 oz)	574
Bar Chocolate & Cornflakes	1 (3.5 oz)	525
Bar Chocolate Butter Biscuit	1 (3.5 oz)	556
Bar Chocolate Marzipan	1 (3.5 oz)	484
Bar Dark Chocolate	1 (3.5 oz)	525
Bar Milk Chocolate	1 (3.5 oz)	533
Bar Mousse Au Chocolat	1 (3.5 oz)	544
Bar White Chocolate Whole Hazelnuts	1 (3.5 oz)	562
Rolo		
Chewy Caramels In Milk Chocolate	3 pkg (1.7 oz)	220
Russell Stover		
All Dark Assorted	2 pieces (1.2 oz)	150
Assorted Chocolates	2 pieces (1.1 oz)	160
Private Reserve Triple Chocolate Mousse	3 pieces (1.3 oz)	220
Private Reserve Vanilla Bean Brulee	3 pieces (1.3 oz)	180
See's		
Assorted Chocolates	2 (1.2 oz)	160
Nuts & Chews	3 (1.6 oz)	240
Soft Centers	2 (1.4 oz)	170
Sencha Naturals		
Green Tea Mints All Flavors	3	5
Shaman Chocolates		
Organic Extra Dark Chocolate 82% Cacao	½ bar (1 oz)	158
Organic Milk Chocolate w/ Macadamia Nuts & Hawaiian Pink Sea Salt	½ bar (1 oz)	91
Skinny Cow		
Heavenly Crisp Bar	1 (0.8 oz)	110
Skittles		
Original Fruit	1 pkg (2.2 oz)	250
Sour	1 pkg (1.8 oz)	200
Skor		
Toffee & Milk Chocolate	1 (1.4 oz)	200
Slim-Fast		
Protein Snack Chews Peanut Butter	1 pkg (0.9 oz)	100
Smile Chocolatiers		
Choclatea Ginger Tea Milk Chocolate 37% Cacao	½ bar (1.5 oz)	230

FOOD	PORTION	CALS
Choclatea Herbal Chai Tea Dark Chocolate 64% Cacao	½ bar (1.5 oz)	220
Choclatea Pistachio Green Tea White Chocolate	½ bar (1.5 oz)	240
Choclatea Pomegranate White Tea Very Dark Chocolate 72% Cacao	½ bar (1.5 oz)	220
Choclatea White Tea Very Dark Chocolate 72% Cacao	½ bar (1.5 oz)	220
Sour Patch		
Kids Soft & Chewy	1 pkg (1 oz)	100
Starbucks		
Truffles Caffe Mocha	3 (1.3 oz)	200
Sugar Babies		
Candy	30 pieces (1.5 oz)	180
Chocolate	19 pieces (1.4 oz)	180
Sugar Daddy		
Pop	1 lg (1.7 oz)	200
SunRidge Farms		
Rainbow Drops Milk Chocolate	¼ cup (1.4 oz)	170
Surf Sweets		
Gummy Bears	16 (1.4 oz)	130
Gummy Worms	4 (1.4 oz)	130
Jelly Beans	31 (1.4 oz)	140
Sour Worms	8 (1.4 oz)	130
Symphony		
Almonds & Toffee	1 (1.5 oz)	220
Take 5		
Original	1 pkg (1.5 oz)	200
Terra Nostra		
Organic Bar Creamy Milk Raisins & Pecans	4 sections (1.2 oz)	180
Organic Bar Vegan Intense Dark	4 sections (1.2 oz)	180
Organic Bar Vegan Ricemilk Choco	4 sections (1.2 oz)	190
Organic Bar Vegan Robust Dark Raisins & Pecans	4 sections (1.2 oz)	170
Thorntons		
Chocolates Summer Collection	1	65
Toblerone		
Bittersweet w/ Honey & Almond Nougat	⅓ bar (1.2 oz)	170
Milk Chocolate w/ Honey & Almond Nougat	⅓ bar (1.2 oz)	170
White w/ Honey & Almond Nougat	⅓ bar (1.2 oz)	180

FOOD	PORTION	CALS
Toffifay		
Candy	5 (1.4 oz)	200
Tootsie Roll		
Midgees	6	140
Pops	1 (0.6 oz)	60
Pops Caramel Apple	1 (0.6 oz)	60
Truffulls		
Chocolate Caramel Gluten Free	1 (1.13 oz)	120
Chocolate Mint Gluten Free	1 (1.13 oz)	120
Twix		
Fun Size	1 (0.6 oz)	80
Twizzlers		
Licorice	4 (1.6 oz)	150
Strawberry	4 (1.6 oz)	160
Werther's		
Caramel Milk Chocolate	6 (1.3 oz)	230
Original	3 (0.5 oz)	60
Original Sugar Free	5 (0.5 oz)	40
Whitman's		
Assorted Chocolates	4 pieces (1.5 oz)	210
Whoppers		
Malted Milk Balls	18 (1.4 oz)	190
Wolfgang		
Blueberries Dipped In Dark Chocolate	2 (0.7 oz)	80
Cranberries Dipped In Dark Chocolate	2 (1 oz)	130
Raspberries Dipped In Dark Chocolate	2 (1.1 oz)	130
Wonka Exceptionals		
Bar Chocolate Waterfall	4 sq (1.4 oz)	210
Bar Domed Dark Chocolate	4 sq (1.4 oz)	200
Fruit Jellies All Flavors	14 (1.5 oz)	130
Fruit Marvels All Flavors	10 (1.4 oz)	140
York		
Peppermint Patty	1 (1.4 oz)	140
Young & Smylie		
Licorice Black	11 (1.5 oz)	140
Licorice Strawberry	11 (1.5 oz)	150
Zagnut		
Peanut Butter & Coconut	3 (1.5 oz)	200
Zero		
Bar	1 (1.8 oz)	230

FOOD	PORTION	CALS
CANTALOUPE		
dried	3.5 pieces (1.4 oz)	140
fresh cubed	1 cup	57
fresh half	½	94
Chiquita		
Fresh Cup Up	1 cup (6.2 oz)	60
Dole		
Fresh	¼ med (4.7 oz)	45
CAPERS		
capers	1 tbsp	2
CARAWAY		
seed	1 tbsp	22
CARDAMOM		
ground	1 tsp	6
CARDOON		
fresh cooked w/o salt	1 serv (3.5 oz)	22
fresh shredded	1 cup (6.2 oz)	30
Ocean Mist		
Cardone Fresh Shredded	1 cup (6.2 oz)	36
CARIBOU		
roasted	3 oz	142
CARISSA		
fresh	1	12
CAROB		
carob mix	3 tsp	45
carob mix as prep w/ whole milk	9 oz	195
flour	1 cup	185
flour	1 tbsp	14
Bob's Red Mill		
Powder Toasted	2 tsp	25
Tree Of Life		
Chips Malt Sweetened	50 (0.5 oz)	70
CARP		
fresh cooked	3 oz	138
fresh cooked	1 fillet (6 oz)	276
fresh raw	3 oz	108

FOOD	PORTION	CALS
roe raw	1 oz	37
roe salted in olive oil	2 tbsp (1 oz)	40

CARROT JUICE
Canned	6 oz	73
Hollywood		
100% Juice	1 can (12 oz)	120
Lakewood		
Organic	6 oz	73
Odwalla		
100% Juice	8 oz	70

CARROTS
CANNED
slices	½ cup	17
slices low sodium	½ cup	17
Allens		
Tiny Sliced	½ cup (4.5 oz)	45
Del Monte		
Savory Sides Honey Glazed	½ cup	70
S&W		
Julienne	½ cup (4.3 oz)	35
FRESH		
baby raw	1 (0.5 oz)	6
raw	1 (2.5 oz)	31
raw shredded	½ cup	24
slices cooked	½ cup	35
Chiquita		
Carrot Bites w/ Ranch Dressing	1 pkg (2.5 oz)	50
Crunch Pak		
Baby Carrots w/ Ranch Dressing	⅕ pkg	50
Dole		
Mini Cut	11 (3 oz)	30
Earthbound Farms		
Organic Tops On	1 (2.7 oz)	35
Organic w/ Organic Ranch Dip	1 pkg (2.2 oz)	90
Ready Pac		
Baby Carrots	7 (3 oz)	40
FROZEN		
slices cooked	½ cup	26

FOOD	PORTION	CALS
Birds Eye		
Steam & Serve Carrots & Cranberries	1 cup	130
C&W		
Whole Baby	⅔ cup	35
Green Giant		
Honey Glazed	1 cup	90
Joy Of Cooking		
Bite Size	½ cup (3.3 oz)	70
CASABA		
cubed	1 cup (6 oz)	46
melon fresh	¼ (14 oz)	115
CASHEW JUICE		
O.N.E.		
Cashew Fruit	1 bottle (11 oz)	140
CASHEWS		
cashew butter w/o salt	1 tbsp	94
dry roasted w/ salt	18 nuts (1 oz)	160
dry roasted w/ salt	1 oz	163
oil roasted w/ salt	1 oz	163
oil roasted w/o salt	1 oz	163
Arrowhead Mills		
Organic Cashew Butter	2 tbsp	160
Back To Nature		
Jumbo Sea Salt Roasted	1 oz	160
Frito Lay		
Whole Salted	3 tbsp	180
Lance		
Cashews	1 pkg (1.5 oz)	270
Navitas Naturals		
Cashews	1 oz	160
Nut Harvest		
Whole Sea Salted	2 tbsp (1 oz)	170
Peeled Snacks		
Nut Picks Cashew Later	1 pkg (1 oz)	180
Planters		
Chocolate Lovers Milk Chocolate	10 pieces (1.5 oz)	230
Halves & Pieces	1 oz	160
Halves & Pieces Lightly Salted	1 oz	160
Whole Honey Roasted	1 oz	150

FOOD	PORTION	CALS
Sunfood		
Organic	1 oz	164
Tree Of Life		
Cashew Butter Creamy	2 tbsp	180
Yumnuts		
Chili Lime	¼ cup (1 oz)	170
Chocolate	¼ cup (1 oz)	160
Honey	¼ cup (1 oz)	170
Toasted Coconut	½ cup (1 oz)	170
CASSAVA		
diced cooked w/o fat	1 cup (4.6 oz)	213
root raw	1 (14.3 oz)	653
TAKE-OUT		
fritter crab meat stuffed	1 (4.4 oz)	341
CATFISH		
channel breaded & fried	3 oz	194
wolffish atlantic baked	3 oz	105
Simmons		
Farm Raised	4 oz	140
CAULIFLOWER		
flowerets fresh	1 (0.5 oz)	3
flowerets fresh cooked w/o salt	3 (2 oz)	12
fresh	1 cup	25
fresh cooked w/o salt	1 cup	29
fresh head small	1 (9.2 oz)	66
frzn cooked w/o salt	1 cup	34
green fresh	1 cup	20
green fresh small head	1 (11.4 oz)	101
pickled	¼ cup	14
pickled chow chow	¼ cup	74
Birds Eye		
Steamfresh Garlic Cauliflower	1 cup (2.4 oz)	40
Dole		
Fresh	1 cup (3.4 oz)	25
Jake & Amos		
Sweet Pickled Hot Cauliflower	1 tbsp	40
Mann's		
Cauliettes Fresh	1 serv (3 oz)	20

FOOD	PORTION	CALS
TAKE-OUT		
batter dipped fried	1 piece (0.9 oz)	55
batter dipped fried	1 cup	178
w/ cheese sauce	1 cup	249
CAVIAR		
black or red	2 tbsp	81
CELERY		
fresh	1 lg stalk (2.2 oz)	9
pickled	½ cup	10
raw diced	½ cup	8
seed	1 tsp	1
strips	1 cup	17
Dole		
Hearts	2 med (4 oz)	15
Earthbound Farms		
Organic Hearts	2 stalks (3.9 oz)	20
Ready Pac		
Sticks	5 (3 oz)	10
TAKE-OUT		
creamed	½ cup	87
stir fried	½ cup	30
stuffed w/ cheese	1 (5 inch)	38
CELERY JUICE		
juice	1 cup	42
CELERY ROOT		
fresh cooked w/o salt	1 cup (5.4 oz)	42
fresh cut up	1 cup (5.5 oz)	66
CELTUCE		
raw	3.5 oz	22
CEREAL		
bran flakes	¾ cup	90
corn flakes	1¼ cups	110
farina as prep w/ water	¾ cup	88
granola	½ cup	285
oatmeal instant as prep w/ water	1 cup (8.2 oz)	138
oatmeal regular & quick as prep w/ water	¾ cup (6.1 oz)	149
oatmeal regular & quick not prep	⅓ cup (0.9 oz)	104

FOOD	PORTION	CALS
puffed rice	1 cup	56
puffed wheat	1 cup	44
shredded mini wheats	1 cup	107
shredded wheat rectangular	1 biscuit (0.8 oz)	85
Alpen		
High Fibre	1 serv (1.6 oz)	154
No Sugar Added	1 serv (1.6 oz)	158
Alti Plano Gold		
Instant Quinoa Hot Cereal Spiced Apple Raisin	1 pkg	160
Instant Quinoa Organic Hot Cereal Oaxacan Chocolate	1 pkg	170
Amy's		
Bowls Organic Cream Of Rice	1 pkg (8.9 oz)	170
Bowls Organic Multigrain	1 pkg (8.9 oz)	190
Annie's Homegrown		
Bunny O's Honey	¾ cup (1 oz)	110
Bunny O's Organic	¾ cup (1 oz)	120
Arrowhead Mills		
Organic Amaranth Flakes	1 cup	140
Organic Kamut Flakes	1 cup	120
Organic Multigrain Flakes	1 cup	170
Organic Nature O's	1 cup	130
Organic Puffed Corn	1 cup	60
Organic Puffed Millet	1 cup	60
Organic Puffed Wheat	1 cup	60
Organic Rice Flakes Sweetened	1 cup	180
Organic Shredded Wheat	1 cup	190
Organic Spelt Flakes	1 cup	120
Back To Nature		
Granola Apple Blueberry	½ cup (1.8 oz)	200
Granola Chocolate Delight	½ cup (1.75 oz)	220
Granola Classic	½ cup (1.8 oz)	200
Granola Sunflower & Pumpkin Seed	½ cup (1.6 oz)	290
Granola To Go Ginger Roasted Almonds w/ Flax Seed	1 serv (1.5 oz)	190
Granola To Go Wild Blueberry Walnut w/ Flax Seed	1 serv (1.5 oz)	190
Bakery On Main		
Granola Apple Cinnamon Walnut	½ cup (2 oz)	240
Granola Fiber Power Cinnamon Raisin	½ cup (2 oz)	230

FOOD	PORTION	CALS
Granola Maple Raisin Almond	½ cup (2 oz)	240
Granola Super Fruit & Nut	½ cup (2 oz)	250
Barbara's Bakery		
Alpen No Sugar Added	⅔ cup	200
Organic Breakfast O's Fruit Juice Sweetened	1 cup	120
Organic Brown Rice Crisps Fruit Juice Sweetened	1 cup (1 oz)	120
Organic Corn Flakes Fruit Juice Sweetened	1 cup	110
Organic Ultima High Fiber	½ cup	90
Organic Ultima Pomegranate	½ cup	100
Organic Wild Puffs Fruity Punch	1 cup	110
Puffins Honey Rice Gluten Free	¾ cup (1 oz)	120
Puffins Multigrain Gluten Free	¾ cup (1 oz)	110
Puffins Originals	¾ cup (0.9 oz)	90
Shredded Oats Bite Size	1¼ cups (2 oz)	220
Shredded Wheat	2 biscuits (1.4 oz)	140
Basic 4		
Whole Grain	1 cup (1.9 oz)	200
Bear Naked		
Cranberry Raisin	⅔ cup (2 oz)	210
Fit Vanilla Almond Crunch	¼ cup (1.1 oz)	120
Granola Fruit And Nut	¼ cup (1.1 oz)	140
Granola Heavenly Chocolate	¼ cup (1.1 oz)	130
Peak Flax Oats And Honey w/ Blueberries	¼ cup (1.1 oz)	130
Better Balance		
Protein Cereal All Flavors Gluten Free	1 oz	100
Bob's Red Mill		
Farina Creamy Brown Rice not prep	¼ cup	150
Muesli Old Country	¼ cup	110
Natural Granola No Fat	½ cup	180
Organic Right Stuff Hot Cereal 6 Grain not prep	¼ cup	140
Rolled Oats Gluten Free not prep	½ cup	160
Boo Berry		
Cereal	3 cup (1.2 oz)	130
Bready Brek		
Original	1 serv (1 oz)	108
Cascadian Farm		
Organic Clifford Crunch	1 cup	100
Organic Granola Oats & Honey	⅔ cup (1.9 oz)	230

FOOD	PORTION	CALS
Chappaqua Crunch		
Original Granola	⅓ cup	115
Simply Granola w/ Raisins	⅓ cup	120
Simply Granola w/ Raspberries	⅓ cup	110
Cheerios		
Apple Cinnamon	¾ cup (1 oz)	120
Banana Nut	¾ cup (1 oz)	120
Chocolate	¾ cup (1 oz)	100
Honey Nut	¾ cup (1 oz)	110
MultiGrain	1 cup (1 oz)	110
Whole Grain Oat	1 cup (1 oz)	100
Yogurt Burst Strawberry	¾ cup (1 oz)	120
Chex		
Chocolate	¾ cup (1.1 oz)	130
Corn Gluten Free	1 cup (1.2 oz)	120
Multi-Bran	¾ cup (1.6 oz)	160
Rice Gluten Free	1 cup (0.9 oz)	100
Wheat	¾ cups (1.6 oz)	160
Chia Goodness		
Apple Almond Cinnamon	2 tbsp (1 oz)	130
Cranberry Ginger	2 tbsp (1 oz)	130
Original	2 tbsp (1 oz)	140
Cinnamon Toast Crunch		
Cinnamon Sugar	¾ cup (1.1 oz)	130
Cocoa Puffs		
Cereal	¾ cup (1 oz)	100
Cookie Crisp		
Cereal	¾ cup (0.9 oz)	100
Count Chocula		
Cereal	¾ cup (0.9 oz)	110
Country Choice Organic		
Multigrain Hot Cereal not prep	½ cup	130
Oats Old Fashioned not prep	½ cup	150
Oats Quick not prep	½ cup	150
Dorset Cereals		
Berries & Cherries	½ cup	150
Simply Delicious Muesli	½ cup	200
Super Cranberry Cherry & Almond	½ cup	200
Dr. McDougall's		
Organic Instant Oatmeal	1 pkg (1 oz)	120
Organic Maple 4 Grain	1 pkg (2.6 oz)	260

FOOD	PORTION	CALS
Earthbound Farms		
Organic Granola Maple Almond	½ cup	260
Enjoy Life		
Allergen Gluten Free Granola Cinnamon	½ cup	160
Erewhon		
Aztec Crunchy Corn & Amaranth	1 cup (1 oz)	110
Barley Plus not prep	¼ cups (1.6 oz)	170
Brown Rice Cream not prep	¼ cup (1.6 oz)	170
Cocoa Crispy Brown Rice	1 cup (1.8 oz)	200
Crispy Brown Rice No Salt Added	1 cup (1 oz)	110
Crispy Brown Rice Original	1 cup (1 oz)	110
Organic Instant Oatmeal Apple Cinnamon not prep	1 pkg (1.2 oz)	130
Organic Instant Oatmeal w/ Oat Bran	1 pkg (1.8 oz)	130
Rice Twice	¾ cup (1 oz)	120
Erin Baker's		
Granola Fruit & Nut	½ cup (1.6 oz)	190
Granola Oatmeal Raisin	½ cup (1.6 oz)	180
Granola Ultra Protein Power Crunch	½ cup (1.6 oz)	200
Farina		
Original as prep	1 cup	120
Feed		
Granola Apple A Day	¼ cup (1 oz)	130
Granola Bittersweet'ness	¼ cup (1 oz)	130
Granola Raisin Nut	¼ cup (1 oz)	130
Sweet Mango	¼ cup (1 oz)	120
Fiber One		
Caramel Delight	1 cup (1.8 oz)	180
Frosted Shredded Wheat	1 cup (2.1 oz)	200
Honey Clusters	1 cup (1.8 oz)	160
Original	½ cup (1 oz)	60
Raisin Bran Clusters	1 cup (2 oz)	170
Glucerna		
Crunchy Flakes'N Raisins	1 bowl (1.6 oz)	140
Crunchy Flakes'N Strawberries	1 bowl (1.5 oz)	150
Glutenfreeda		
Granola Apple Almond Honey	¼ cup (1 oz)	150
Oatmeal Instant as prep	1 pkg (1.8 oz)	190
Glutino		
Gluten Free Apple Cinnamon	½ cup	120
Gluten Free Honey Nut	½ cup	130

FOOD	PORTION	CALS
Golden Grahams		
Cereal	¾ cup (1.1 oz)	120
Health Valley		
Empower	1 cup	200
Granola Low Fat Tropical Fruit	⅔ cup	180
Heart Wise	1 cup	200
Organic Cherry Lemon Blast Ems	¾ cup	120
Organic Golden Flax	¾ cup	190
Organic Multigrain Apple Cinnamon Square Ems	1¼ cup	210
Organic Oat Bran O's	¾ cup	100
Rice Crunch-Ems	1 cup	110
Honest Foods		
Granola Planks Maple Almond Crunch	½ bar (2 oz)	250
Kaia Foods		
Organic Granola Buckwheat Cinnamon Raisin	½ cup (2 oz)	230
Organic Granola Buckwheat Cocoa Bliss	½ cup (2 oz)	220
Kashi		
7 Whole Grain Flakes	1 cup	180
7 Whole Grain Honey Puffs	1 cup	120
7 Whole Grain Nuggets	½ cup	210
7 Whole Grain Pilaf as prep	½ cup	170
GoLean	1 cup	140
GoLean Crunch!	1 cup	190
GoLean Crunch! Honey Almond Flax	1 cup	200
GoLean Instant Hot Cereal Creamy Truly Vanilla	1 pkg	150
GoLean Instant Hot Cereal Hearty Honey & Cinnamon	1 pkg	150
Good Friends	1 cup	170
Granola Mountain Medley	½ cup	220
Heart To Heart Instant Oatmeal Golden Brown Maple	1 pkg	160
Heart To Heart Instant Oatmeal Raisin Spice	1 pkg	150
Heart To Heart Oat Flakes & Blueberry Clusters	1¼ cups	200
Heart To Heart Toasted Oat	¾ cup	110
Honey Sunshine	¾ cup (1.1 oz)	100
Mighty Bites All Flavors	1 cup	110
Organic Promise Autumn Wheat	1 cup	190
Organic Promise Cinnamon Harvest	1 cup	190

FOOD	PORTION	CALS
Organic Promise Strawberry Fields	1 cup	120
Vive Probiotic Digestive Wellness	1¼ cups	170
Kellogg's		
Corn Pops	1 box (1 oz)	110
Raisin Bran	1 cup (2.1 oz)	190
Kix		
Corn Puffs	1¼ cups (1 oz)	110
Honey	1¼ cups (1.1 oz)	120
Kozy Shack		
Ready Grains Apple Cinnamon	1 pkg (7 oz)	210
Ready Grains Maple Brown Sugar	1 pkg (7 oz)	190
Ready Grains Original	1 pkg (7 oz)	180
Ready Grains Strawberry	1 pkg (7 oz)	210
Lucky Charms		
Swirled	¾ cup (1 oz)	110
Lundberg		
Purely Organic Hot'n Creamy Rice	⅓ cup	190
Malt-O-Meal		
Apple Zings	1 cup (1.2 oz)	130
Chocolate not prep	3 tbsp (1.2 oz)	130
Coco Roos	¾ cup (1 oz)	120
Crispy Rice	1¼ cups (1.2 oz)	130
Golden Puffs	¾ cup (1 oz)	110
Honey Nut Scooters	1 cup (1 oz)	110
Mateys Marshmallow	1 cup (1 oz)	120
Original Cream Hot Wheat not prep	3 tbsp (1.2 oz)	130
Original not prep	3 tbsp (1.2 oz)	130
Tootie Fruities	1 cup (1.1 oz)	130
McCann's		
Irish Oatmeal Instant Apples & Cinnamon not prep	1 pkg (1.2 oz)	130
Irish Oatmeal Instant Maple & Brown Sugar not prep	1 pkg (1.5 oz)	160
Irish Oatmeal Instant Regular not prep	1 pkg (1 oz)	100
Irish Oatmeal Quick Cooking not prep	½ cup (1.4 oz)	150
Irish Oatmeal Steel Cut not prep	¼ cup (1.4 oz)	150
Mom's Best Naturals		
Blue Pom Wheat-fuls	1 cup (1.9 oz)	210
Honey Grahams	¾ cup (1 oz)	130
Mallow Oats	1 cup (1 oz)	120
Raisin Bran	1 cup (2.1 oz)	230

FOOD	PORTION	CALS
Mother's		
Barley Hot Cereal not prep	⅓ cup (1.7 oz)	160
Peanut Butter Bumpers	1 cup (1.2 oz)	130
Rolled Oats not prep	½ cup (1.4 oz)	150
Toasted Oat Bran	¾ cup (1.1 oz)	120
Naked Granola		
Taste Of Seattle Nights	½ pkg (1.2 oz)	110
Natural Ovens		
Great Granola	½ cup	250
Nature's Path		
Organic Granola Flax Plus Pumpkin	¾ cup (1.9 oz)	260
Organic Granola Pomegran Plus	½ cup	140
Organic Smart Bran	⅔ cup	90
Nature's Plus		
Organic Oatmeal Hemp Plus	1 pkg	160
New Morning		
Cocoa Crispy Rice	¾ cup (1 oz)	120
Oatios Original	1 cup (1 oz)	110
Newman's Own		
Sweet Enough Honey Flax Flakes	¾ cup	100
Sweet Enough Honey Nut O's	¾ cup	110
Sweet Enough Wheat Puffs	¾ cup	100
Oatmeal Crisp		
Crunchy Almond	1 cup (2.1 oz)	240
Post		
100% Bran	½ cup (0.8 oz)	80
Bran Flakes	1 cup	100
Cocoa Pebbles	¾ cup (1 oz)	110
Golden Crisp	¾ cup (1 oz)	110
Grape-Nuts	½ cup (2 oz)	200
Grape-Nuts Trail Mix Crunch	1 cup (1.7 oz)	170
Grape-Nuts O's	1 cup (1 oz)	120
Great Grains Raisins Dates & Pecans	¾ cup (2 oz)	200
Honey Bunches Of Oats	1 cup (1.8 oz)	200
Honey Bunches Of Oats Peaches	1 cup	120
Honeycomb	1⅓ cups (1 oz)	120
LiveActive Mixed Berry Crunch	1 cup	190
LiveActive Nut Harvest Crunch	1 cup	220
Oreo O's	1 cup	110
Raisin Bran	1 cup (2 oz)	190

FOOD	PORTION	CALS
Selects Blueberry Morning	2 oz	220
Selects Cranberry Almond Crunch	¾ cup (1.8 oz)	200
Shredded Wheat Frosted	2 oz	180
Shredded Wheat'N Bran	2 oz	200
Shredded Wheat Original	2 biscuits (1.6 oz)	160
Shredded Wheat Spoon Size	1 cup (1.7 oz)	170
Toasties Corn Flakes	1 cup (1 oz)	100
Quaker		
Instant Oatmeal Apples & Cinnamon	1 pkg (1.2 oz)	130
Instant Oatmeal Cinnamon & Spice	1 pkg	170
Instant Oatmeal Cinnamon Roll	1 pkg	160
Instant Oatmeal Crunch Mixed Berry	1 pkg	190
Instant Oatmeal Express Baked Apple	1 pkg	200
Instant Oatmeal For Kids Dinosaur Eggs	1 pkg	190
Instant Oatmeal Lower Sugar Maple & Brown Sugar	1 pkg	120
Instant Oatmeal Maple Brown Sugar w/ Pecans	1 pkg	160
Instant Oatmeal Nutrition For Women Golden Brown Sugar	1 pkg	170
Instant Oatmeal Organic Regular	1 pkg	100
Instant Oatmeal Regular	1 pkg	100
Instant Oatmeal Simple Harvest Multigrain Maple Brown Sugar w/ Pecans	1 pkg (1.48 oz)	160
Instant Oatmeal Strawberries & Cream	1 pkg	130
Instant Oatmeal Supreme Apple Raisin	1 pkg	150
Instant Oatmeal Supreme Cinnamon Pecan	1 pkg	180
Instant Oatmeal Take Heart Golden Maple	1 pkg	160
Instant Oatmeal Weight Control Banana Bread	1 pkg	160
Oat Bran Hot Cereal not prep	½ cup	150
Oatmeal Squares	1 cup (2 oz)	210
Ralston		
Corn Flakes	1 cup (1 oz)	100
Raisin Bran	1 cup (2 oz)	190
Ready Brek		
Chocolate	1 serv (1 oz)	108
Rice Krispies		
Roasted Rice	1¼ cups (1.2 oz)	130
Roman Meal		
Cream Of Rye not prep	⅓ cup (1.4 oz)	130
Elements Cranberry Passion	1 cup (1.6 oz)	160
Hot Cereal not prep	⅓ cup (1.3 oz)	120

FOOD	PORTION	CALS
Silhouette Solution		
Oatmeal Cinnamon Apple	1 pkg (1.39 oz)	150
Skinner's		
Raisin Bran	1 cup (1.9 oz)	170
South Beach		
Crunch Strawberry Harvest	1 cup	170
Crunch Vanilla Almond	1 cup	180
Granola Clusters Cherry Almond	1 pkg (1 oz)	130
Granola Clusters Mixed Berry	1 pkg (1 oz)	130
Special K		
Cereal	1 box (0.8 oz)	90
Stark Sisters		
Granola Lo-Fat Raspberry Blueberry	½ cup	230
Granola Nutty Maple	½ cup	250
Granola Original Maple Almond	½ cup	240
Sunbelt		
Granola Low Fat Cinnamon & Raisins	½ cup	250
Total		
Cinnamon Crunch	1 cup (1.8 oz)	190
Raisin Bran	1 cup (1.9 oz)	160
Whole Grain	¾ cup (1 oz)	100
Trix		
Swirls	1 cup (1.1 oz)	120
Udi's		
Gluten Free Granola Au Naturel	¼ cup (1.1 oz)	120
Uncle Sam		
Mixed Berries	1 cup (1.9 oz)	190
Original	¾ cup (1.9 oz)	190
Weetabix		
Crunchy Bran	1 serv (1.4 oz)	122
Multigrain	1 serv (1.3 oz)	127
Oatibix Bites	1 serv (1.4 oz)	148
Oatibix Flakes	1 serv (1 oz)	114
Organic	2 biscuits (1.2 oz)	120
Organic Crispy Flakes	¾ cup	110
Wheatena		
Toasted Wheat	⅓ cup	160
Wheaties		
Cereal	¾ cup (1 oz)	100

FOOD	PORTION	CALS
YogActive		
Probiotic High Fibre Wheat Strawberry Raspberry	⅔ cup	160
Probiotic Kiwi	⅔ cup	120
Probiotic Strawberry	⅔ cup	130
Probiotic Strawberry Dark Chocolate	⅔ cup	130
Yogi		
Granola Crisps Baked Cinnamon Raisin	½ cup	120
Granola Crisps Fresh Strawberry Crunch	½ cup	120
Granola Crisps Mountain Blueberry Flax	½ cup	110
CEREAL BARS (*see also* ENERGY BARS, FRUIT AND NUT BARS)		
Alpen		
Fruit & Nut	1	109
Light Chocolate & Fudge	1	63
Raspberry & Yogurt	1	120
Annie's Homegrown		
Organic Peanut Butter	1 (1 oz)	120
Aristo		
Acai Blueberry Lime	1 (1.3 oz)	130
Pomegranate & Cranberry	1 (1.3 oz)	140
Attune		
Wellness Yogurt & Granola Lemon Creme	1 (1.4 oz)	180
Wellness Yogurt & Granola Strawberry Bliss	1 (1.4 oz)	180
Bakery On Main		
Granola Gluten Free Extreme Trail Mix	1 (1.3 oz)	140
Granola Gluten Free Peanut Butter Chocolate Chip	1 (1.2 oz)	140
Barbara's Bakery		
Fruit & Yogurt Cherry Apple	1	150
Nature's Choice Blueberry	1 (1.3 oz)	150
Organic Crunchy Granola Cinnamon Crisp	2 (1.5 oz)	190
Bear Naked		
Grain-ola Tropical Fruit	1 (2 oz)	220
Cascadian Farm		
Organic Chewy Granola Fruit & Nut	1 (1.2 oz)	140
Cheerios		
Honey Nut	1 (1.4 oz)	160
Cinnamon Toast Crunch		
Milk 'N Cereal	1 (1.6 oz)	180

FOOD	PORTION	CALS
Corazonas		
Oatmeal Squares Banana Walnut	1 (1.8 oz)	190
Oatmeal Squares Chocolate Chip	1 (1.8 oz)	190
Oatmeal Squares Cranberry Flax	1 (1.8 oz)	180
Country Choice Organic		
Oatmeal Squares Apple Cinnamon	1 (2 oz)	210
Oatmeal Squares Maple	1 (2 oz)	210
Earnest Eats		
Almond Trail Mix	1 (1.94 oz)	210
Choco Peanut Butter	1 (1.94 oz)	230
Cran Lemon Zest	1 (1.94 oz)	210
Enjoy Life		
Allergen Gluten Free Caramel Apple	1 (1 oz)	110
Fiber One		
Chocolate Caramel & Pretzel	1 (0.8 oz)	90
Oats & Caramel	1 (1.4 oz)	140
Oats & Chocolate	1 (1.4 oz)	140
Oats & Peanut Butter	1 (1.4 oz)	150
Fruition		
Blueberry	1 (1.7 oz)	160
Cran-Raspberry	1 (1.7 oz)	160
Lemon	1 (1.7 oz)	160
Fullbar		
Cocoa Chip	1 (1.59 oz)	160
Fit Chewy Brownie	1 (1.76 oz)	180
Fit Toffee Crunch	1 (1.76 oz)	180
Peanut Butter Crunch	1 (1.59 oz)	170
Glenny's		
Organic Muesli Chocolate Chip	1 (1.6 oz)	170
Organic Muesli Raisins & Dates	1 (1.6 oz)	170
Slim Carb Bars Brownie Cheesecake	1 (1.3 oz)	130
Slim-1 w/ Acai Very Berry Blast	1 (1.1 oz)	100
Slim-1 w/ GreenTea Double Fudge	1 (1.1 oz)	100
Glutino		
Gluten Free Breakfast Bar Apple	1 (1.4 oz)	120
Gluten Free Breakfast Bar Chocolate	1 (1.4 oz)	110
Gluten Free Organic Chocolate & Peanut	1 (1 oz)	110
Gluten Free Organic Wildberry	1 (1 oz)	100
Gnu		
Flavor & Fiber Banana Walnut	1 (1.6 oz)	140

FOOD	PORTION	CALS
Flavor & Fiber Chocolate Brownie Bar	1 (1.6 oz)	140
Flavor & Fiber Cinnamon Raisin	1 (1.6 oz)	130
Flavor & Fiber Expresso Chip	1 (1.6 oz)	140
Flavor & Fiber Lemon Ginger	1 (1.6 oz)	130
Flavor & Fiber Orange Cranberry	1 (1.6 oz)	130
Flavor & Fiber Peanut Butter	1 (1.6 oz)	140
Health Valley		
Cafe Creations Cinnamon Danish	1 (1.4 oz)	130
Date Almond Low Fat	1 (1.5 oz)	150
Granola Chocolate Chip Low Fat	1 (1.5 oz)	160
Granola Moist & Chewy Dutch Apple	1 (1 oz)	100
Granola Trail Mix Cranberries Nuts & Yogurt Chips	1 (1.2 oz)	140
Organic Fig Cobbler	1 (1.4 oz)	130
Organic Raspberry Tarts	1 (1.4 oz)	150
Organic Strawberry Cobbler	1 (1.3 oz)	130
Peanut Butter & Grape	1 (1.3 oz)	130
Hershey's		
Sweet & Salty Granola Bar Reese's w/ Chocolate	1 (1.2 oz)	160
Sweet & Salty Granola Bar w/ Pretzels	1 (1.2 oz)	140
Honest Foods		
Cran Lemon Zest	1 (2.2 oz)	240
Farmer's Trail Mix	1 (2.2 oz)	240
Jungle Grub		
Berry Bamboozle w/ Vanilla Icing Gluten Free	1 (0.9 oz)	100
Chocolate Chip Cookie Dough w/ Chocolate Coating Gluten Free	1 (0.9 oz)	100
Peanut Butter Groove w/ Vanilla Icing Gluten Free	1 (0.9 oz)	100
Kardea		
Lemon Ginger	1 (1.34 oz)	140
Kashi		
TLC Chewy Granola Dark Mocha Almond	1 (1.2 oz)	130
TLC Chewy Granola Honey Almond Flax	1 (1.2 oz)	140
TLC Soft Baked Apple Spice	1 (1.2 oz)	110
TLC Soft Baked Blackberry Graham	1 (1.2 oz)	110
TLC Soft Baked Ripe Strawberry	1 (1.2 oz)	110
Kellogg's		
FiberPlus Antioxidants Berry Yogurt Crunch	1 box (1.4 oz)	130

FOOD	PORTION	CALS
FiberPlus Antioxidants Chocolate Chip	1 (1.2 oz)	120
FiberPlus Antioxidants Chocolatey Peanut Butter	1 (1.2 oz)	130
FiberPlus Antioxidants Dark Chocolate Almond	1 (1.2 oz)	130
KeriBar		
Vegan Apple Peanut Butter	1 (1.4 oz)	140
Vegan Cherry Almond	1 (1.4 oz)	140
Vegan Strawberry Chocolate Chip	1 (1.4 oz)	130
Kind		
Peanut Butter Dark Chocolate + Protein	1 (1.4 oz)	180
Kudos		
Granola Chocolate Chip	1 (1 oz)	120
Lean Body		
Hi-Protein Granola Peanuts'N Chocolate	1 (2.8 oz)	340
Natural Ovens		
Great Granola Mixed Fruit	1 (1.4 oz)	150
Nature Valley		
Chewy Trail Mix Fruit & Nut	1 (1.2 oz)	140
Crunchy Granola Peanut Butter	2 (1.5 oz)	190
Oats 'N Honey	2 (1.5 oz)	190
Protein Chewy Peanut Almond & Dark Chocolate	1 (1.4 oz)	190
Protein Chewy Peanut Butter Dark Chocolate	1 (1.4 oz)	190
Sweet & Salty Granola Almond	1 (1.2 oz)	160
Nutri-Grain		
Apple Cinnamon	1 (1.3 oz)	120
Planters		
Nut-rition Antioxidant Almonds Blueberries & Dark Chocolate	1 (1.2 oz)	160
Nut-rition Bone Health Honey Roasted Peanuts Cashews & Almonds	1 (1.2 oz)	160
Nut-rition Energy Honey Roasted Peanuts Almonds & Chocolate	1 (1.2 oz)	170
Nut-rition Heart Healthy Cranberry Almond Peanut	1 (1.2 oz)	160
Post		
Honey Bunches Of Oats Banana Nut	1 (1.2 oz)	140
Honey Bunches Of Oats Oatmeal Raisin	1 (1.2 oz)	130
ProBar		
Cran-Lemon Twister	1 (3 oz)	360

FOOD	PORTION	CALS
Kettle Corn	1 (3 oz)	390
Koka Moka	1 (3 oz)	360
Old School PB&J	1 (3 oz)	370
Superfood Slam	1 (3 oz)	380
Quaker		
Breakfast Bar Apple Crisp	1 (1.3 oz)	130
Breakfast Bar Iced Raspberry	1 (1.3 oz)	130
Breakfast Bites Iced Raspberry	1 pkg (1.3 oz)	130
Breakfast Bites Strawberry	1 pkg (1.3 oz)	130
Chewy Chocolate Chip	1 (0.8 oz)	100
Chewy Cookies & Cream	1 (0.8 oz)	90
Chewy 90 Calorie Cinnamon Sugar	1 (1 oz)	90
Chewy 90 Calorie Honey Nut	1 (0.8 oz)	90
Chewy Dipps Peanut Butter	1 (1 oz)	150
Chewy Granola w/ Protein Peanut Butter & Chocolate	1 (1 oz)	110
Chewy Low Fat S'mores	1 (1 oz)	110
Crunchy Granola Oats & Berries Oatmeal Raisin	1 (1 oz)	130
Oatmeal To Go	1 (2.1 oz)	220
Oatmeal To Go Raspberry Streusel	1 (2.1 oz)	220
Q-Smart Cranberry Vanilla Almond	1 (1 oz)	120
Trail Mix Cranberry Raisin & Almond	1 (1.2 oz)	150
Reese's		
SnackBarz Peanut Butter	1 (0.9 oz)	120
Revolution Foods		
Jammy Sammy Apple Cinnamon & Oatmeal	1 (1 oz)	100
Organic Jammy Sammy PB & Grape	1 (1 oz)	110
Organic Jammy Sammy PB & Strawberry	1 (1 oz)	110
Roman Meal		
Whole Grain & Fruit	1 (2 oz)	190
Silhouette Solution		
Blueberry Pomegranate	1 (1.3 oz)	130
Peanut Passion	1 (1.3 oz)	130
South Beach		
Fiber Fit Granola Mocha	1 (1.2 oz)	120
Fiber Fit Granola S'Mores	1 (1.2 oz)	120
Sweet & Savory		
Cocoa Pistachio	1 (3 oz)	390

FOOD	PORTION	CALS
Tasty		
Carrot Cake	1 (1.2 oz)	110
Pumpkin Pie	1 (1.2 oz)	120
Weetabix		
Oaty Chocolate	1	67
Weetos	1	88
Wings Of Nature		
Organic Almond Raisin	1 (1.4 oz)	170
Organic Cafe Mocha Coffee	1 (1.2 oz)	153
Organic Cranberry Crunch	1 (1.4 oz)	170
Organic Espresso Coffee	1 (1.4 oz)	180
Yotta		
Apple Cinnamon	1 (1.2 oz)	120
Cherry	1 (1.2 oz)	120
Orange	1 (1.2 oz)	120
Zone Perfect		
Cookie Dough Chocolate Chip	1 (1.58 oz)	180
Cookie Dough Oatmeal Raisin	1 (1.58 oz)	170
Cookie Dough Peanut Butter	1 (1.58 oz)	190
Sweet & Salty Cashew Pretzel	1 (1.58 oz)	200
Sweet & Salty Trail Mix	1 (1.58 oz)	200

CHAMPAGNE

champagne	1 serv (3.5 oz)	84
mimosa	1 serv	117
punch	1 serv (4 oz)	73
sekt german champagne	1 serv (3.5 oz)	84

CHAYOTE

fresh cooked	1 cup	38
raw	1 (7 oz)	49
raw cut up	1 cup	32
Dole		
Fresh cooked	½ cup (2.8 oz)	17

CHEESE (see also CHEESE DISHES, CHEESE SUBSTITUTES, COTTAGE CHEESE, CREAM CHEESE, CREAM CHEESE SUBSTITUTES, NEUFCHATEL)

american	1 oz	93
american cheese spread	1 oz	82
beaufort	1 oz	115
bel paese	1 oz	112
blue	1 oz	100

FOOD	PORTION	CALS
blue crumbled	1 cup (4.7 oz)	477
bocconcini smoked	1 oz	90
brick	1 oz	105
brie	1 oz	95
cacio di roma sheep's milk cheese	1 oz	130
caerphilly	1.4 oz	150
camembert	1 oz	85
cantal	1 oz	105
caraway	1 oz	107
chabichou	1 oz	95
chaource	1 oz	83
cheddar	1 oz	114
cheddar low sodium	1 oz	113
cheddar lowfat	1 oz	49
cheddar reduced fat	1.4 oz	104
cheddar shredded	1 cup	455
cheshire	1 oz	110
cheshire reduced fat	1.4 oz	108
colby	1 oz	112
colby low sodium	1 oz	113
colby lowfat	1 oz	49
comte	1 oz	114
coulommiers	1 oz	88
crottin	1 oz	105
derby	1.4 oz	161
edam reduced fat	1.4 oz	92
emmentaler	1 oz	115
feta	1 oz	75
fontina	1 oz	110
frais	1.6 oz	51
gjetost	1 oz	132
gloucester double	1.4 oz	162
goat fresh	1 oz	23
goat hard	1 oz	128
gorgonzola	1 oz	107
gouda	1 oz	101
grana padano parmesan shaved	1 tbsp	20
gruyere	1 oz	117
lancashire	1.4 oz	149
leicester	1.4 oz	160

FOOD	PORTION	CALS
limburger	1 oz	93
lymeswold	1.4 oz	170
maroilles	1 oz	97
monterey	1 oz	106
morbier	1 oz	99
mozzarella	1 oz	80
mozzarella fresh	1 oz	80
mozzarella part skim	1 oz	72
muenster	1 oz	104
parmesan grated	1 tbsp	23
parmesan hard	1 oz	111
picodon	1 oz	99
pimento	1 oz	106
pont l'eveque	1 oz	86
port du salut	1 oz	100
provolone	1 oz	100
pyrenees	1 oz	101
quark 20% fat	1 oz	33
quark 40% fat	1 oz	48
quark made w/ skim milk	1 oz	22
queso anejo	1 oz	106
queso asadero	1 oz	101
queso chihuahua	1 oz	106
queso fresco	1 oz	41
queso manchego	1 oz	107
queso panela	1 oz	74
raclette	1 oz	102
reblochon	1 oz	88
ricotta part skim	½ cup (4.4 oz)	171
ricotta whole milk	½ cup (4.4 oz)	216
romadur 40% fat	1 oz	83
romano	1 oz	110
roquefort	1 oz	105
rouy	1 oz	95
saint marcellin	1 oz	94
saint nectaire	1 oz	97
saint paulin	1 oz	85
sainte maure	1 oz	99
selles sur cher	1 oz	93
stilton blue	1.4 oz	164

FOOD	PORTION	CALS
stilton white	1.4 oz	145
swiss	1 oz	107
swiss processed	1 oz	95
tilsit	1 oz	96
tome	1 oz	92
triple creme	1 oz	113
vacherin	1 oz	92
wensleydale	1.4 oz	151
whey cheese	1 oz	126
yogurt cheese	1 oz	80
Alpine Lace		
Reduced Fat Provolone	1 slice (0.8 oz)	70
Reduced Fat Swiss	1 slice (0.8 oz)	70
Reduced Fat White American	1 slice (0.8 oz)	70
Reduced Sodium Muenster	1 slice (0.8 oz)	90
Applegate Farms		
Organic Cheddar Milk	1 slice (0.7 oz)	85
Organic Muenster Kase	1 slice (0.8 oz)	85
Yogurt Cheese w/ Probiotics	1 slice (0.7 oz)	80
Athenos		
Blue Crumbled	¼ pkg (1.1 oz)	110
Feta Black Peppercorn	1 oz	80
Feta Crumbled Garlic & Herb	⅕ pkg (1.2 oz)	90
Gorgonzola Crumbled	2 tbsp (1.1 oz)	110
Mozzarella Fresh	1 in cube (1 oz)	80
Boar's Head		
Imported Swiss	1 oz	110
Cabot		
Cheddar Extra Sharp	1 oz	110
Cheddar Horseradish	1 oz	110
Cheddar Light 50% Reduced Fat	1 oz	70
Cheddar Light 50% Reduced Fat Omega-3	1 oz	70
Cheddar Light 75% Reduced Fat	1 oz	60
Cheddar Shake	2 tsp	25
Cheddar Tomato Basil	1 oz	110
Monterey Jack	1 oz	110
Pepper Jack 50% Reduced Fat	1 oz	70
Swiss Slices	1 (1 oz)	110
Connoisseur		
Asiago Spread	1 tbsp	90

FOOD	PORTION	CALS
Brie Spread	2 tbsp	90
Gorgonzola Spread	1 tbsp	90
Wheel Asiago Pesto	2 tbsp	90
Wheel Swiss Bacon	2 tbsp	90
Cracker Barrel		
Fontina	1 slice (0.7 oz)	80
Sharp Cheddar 2% Milk	1 oz	90
Dietz & Watson		
Aalsbruk Edam	1 oz	90
American Yellow	1 slice (1 oz)	110
Cheddar Sharp	1 oz	110
Danish Blue	1 oz	100
Danish Havarti	1 oz	110
Gorgonzola	1 oz	100
Muenster	1 slice (0.7 oz)	75
DiGiorno		
Shredded Three Cheese Parmesan Romano & Asiago	¼ cup (1 oz)	110
Dragone		
Mozzarella Whole Milk	1 oz	90
Parmesan Wedge	1 oz	100
Ricotta Part Skim	¼ cup (2.2 oz)	90
Easy Cheese		
American	2 tbsp (1.1 oz)	90
Cheddar	2 tbsp (1.1 oz)	90
Finlandia		
Baby Muenster	1 oz	100
Double Gloucester Deli Slices	1 slice (0.8 oz)	83
Gouda Deli Slices	1 slice (0.8 oz)	79
Havarti Deli Slices	1 slice (0.8 oz)	86
Muenster Deli Slices	1 slice (0.8 oz)	86
Swiss Deli Slices	1 slice (0.8 oz)	86
Swiss Light Deli Slices	1 slice (0.8 oz)	57
Viola	2 tbsp (1 oz)	87
Fresh Made		
Farmers Cheese Nonfat	2 tbsp	15
Friendship		
Farmer	2 tbsp (1 oz)	50
Farmer No Salt Added	2 tbsp (1 oz)	50

FOOD	PORTION	CALS
Frigo		
Mozzarella Part Skim	1 oz	80
Parmesan Shredded	¼ cup (1 oz)	100
Ricotta Whole Milk	¼ cup (2.2 oz)	110
Romano Shredded	¼ cup (1 oz)	100
Grana Padano		
PDO Cheese	1 oz	120
Hans All Natural		
Spread Cheddar & Jalapeno	2 tbsp (1 oz)	90
Spread Swiss Cheese & Almonds	2 tbsp (1 oz)	90
Haolam		
Cheddar Sliced	1 slice (1 oz)	114
Horizon Organic		
American	1 slice (0.7 oz)	60
Cheddar	1 oz	110
Monterey Jack	1 oz	100
Shred Mexican	¼ cup	110
Shred Parmesan	1 tbsp	20
Slice Provolone	1 slice (0.7 oz)	70
Sticks Colby	1 (1 oz)	110
String Mozzarella	1 stick (1 oz)	80
J.L. Kraft		
Spreadable Feta & Spinach	2 tbsp	80
Karoun		
Ackawi	1 oz	110
Ani	1 in cube (1 oz)	110
Labne Kefir	2 tbsp (1 oz)	80
Paneer	1 oz	90
Kraft		
Cheddar Sharp Shredded 2% Milk	¼ cup	80
Crumbles Three Cheese	¼ cup (1 oz)	110
LiveActive 2% Milk Marbled Colby & Monterey Jack	1 stick (1 oz)	90
LiveActive Cheddar Cheese Sticks	1 (1 oz)	120
LiveActive Colby & Monterey Jack Cubes	7 (1 oz)	110
LiveActive Mozzarella Sticks	1 (1 oz)	80
Shredded Mexican Style Cheddar & Monterey Jack	¼ cup	110
Singles 2% Milk Pepperjack	1 slice (0.7 oz)	45
Swiss Extra Thin Slices	1 (0.6 oz)	60

FOOD	PORTION	CALS
Land O'Lakes		
American	1 slice (0.7 oz)	70
Chedarella	1 oz	110
Cheddar	1 oz	110
Snack 'N Cheese To Go Cheddar Mild	1 serv (0.7 oz)	80
Snack 'N Cheese To Go Cheddar Mild Reduced Fat	1 serv (0.5 oz)	60
Snack 'N Cheese To Go Co-Jack	1 serv (0.7 oz)	80
Snack 'N Cheese To Go Co-Jack Reduced Fat	1 serv (0.7 oz)	60
Swiss	1 oz	110
Laughing Cow		
Blue Light	1 wedge (0.7 oz)	35
Creamy Swiss Light	1 wedge (0.7 oz)	35
Creamy Swiss Original	1 wedge (0.7 oz)	50
French Onion Light	1 wedge (0.7 oz)	35
Garlic & Herb Light	1 wedge (0.7 oz)	35
Mozzarella Sun-Dried Tomato & Basil Light	1 wedge (0.7 oz)	35
Queso Fresco & Chipotle Light	1 wedge (0.7 oz)	35
Lifeway		
Farmer	2 tbsp (1.1 oz)	40
Farmer Lite	2 tbsp (1.1 oz)	25
Sweet Kiss Spread Peach	1 oz	50
Sweet Kiss Spread Raisins	1 oz	45
Molly McButter		
Natural Cheese	1 tsp (2 g)	5
Organic Valley		
Blue Crumbles	1 oz	100
Cheddar Mild	1 oz	110
Feta	1 oz	60
Monterey Jack Shredded	¼ cup	80
Muenster	1 slice (0.7 oz)	80
Provolone	1 slice (0.7 oz)	70
Swiss	1 oz	110
Pizza Zing		
Spicy Hot Cheese Shake	2 tsp	15
Rosenborg		
Danish Camembert	1 oz	80
Rouge Et Noir		
Breakfast	1 oz	90
Brie Garlic	1 oz	90

FOOD	PORTION	CALS
Brie Pesto	1 oz	90
Brie Tomato Basil	1 oz	90
Brie Triple Creme	1 oz	110
Camembert	1 oz	90
Le Petit Bleu	1 oz	110
Le Petit Chevre	1 oz	90
Marin French Blue	1 oz	110
Marin French Gold	1 oz	110
Schlosskranz	1 oz	85
Saladena		
Goat Crumbles	¼ cup	80
Sap Sago		
Fat Free Cheese Grated	1 tsp	10
Sargento		
4 Cheese Italian Shredded	¼ cup	80
4 Cheese Mexican Reduced Fat Shredded	¼ cup (1 oz)	80
American Burger	1 slice (0.7 oz)	70
Bistro Blends Shredded Italian Pasta Cheese	¼ cup (1 oz)	90
Blue Crumbled	¼ cup (1 oz)	100
Cheddar Chipotle Shredded	¼ cup	100
Cheddar Chipotle Sticks	1 (0.7 oz)	80
Cheddar Mild Cubes	7 (1 oz)	120
Cheddar Mild Shredded Reduced Sodium	¼ cup (1 oz)	110
Cheddar White Vermont Sharp	1 slice (0.7 oz)	80
Cheddar White Vermont Sharp Shredded	¼ cup (1 oz)	110
Cheese Dips Cheddar & Buttery Pretzels	1 pkg (3.8 oz)	360
Cheese Dips Cheddar & Tortilla Chips	1 pkg (3 oz)	320
Colby-Jack Sticks Reduced Sodium	1 (0.7 oz)	80
Jarlsberg	1 slice (0.8 oz)	80
Monterey Jack Shredded	¼ cup (1 oz)	110
Mozzarella Reduced Fat Shredded	¼ cup (1 oz)	80
Mozzarella Shredded	¼ cup (1 oz)	80
Muenster	1 slice (0.7 oz)	80
Nacho & Taco Shredded	¼ cup (1 oz)	110
Parmesan Grated	2 tsp (5 g)	25
Parmesan Shredded	2 tsp	20
Pepper Jack Reduced Sodium	1 slice (0.7 oz)	70
Provolone	1 slice (0.7 oz)	70
Provolone Reduced Sodium	1 slice (0.7 oz)	70
Ricotta Fat Free	¼ cup	50

FOOD	PORTION	CALS
Ricotta Light	¼ cup	60
Ricotta Whole Milk	¼ cup	90
String Light	1 piece (0.7 oz)	50
String Reduced Sodium	1 (0.7 oz)	60
Swiss Reduced Fat	1 slice (0.7 oz)	60
Swiss Shredded	¼ cup (1 oz)	110
Swiss Thick Slice	1 slice (1 oz)	110
Swiss Thin Sliced	1 slice (0.6 oz)	70
Smart Balance		
Creamy Cheddar Slices	1 (0.7 oz)	40
Fat Free Lactose Free Slices	1 (0.7 oz)	40
Sorrento		
Mozzarella Fresh	1 oz	90
Stella		
3 Cheese Italian Shredded	¼ cup	100
Asiago Wedge	1 oz	110
Gorgonzola Wedge	1 oz	100
Kasseri Wedge	1 oz	110
The Greek Gods		
Kefir Cheese	2 tbsp (1 oz)	80
Treasure Cave		
Blue Cheese Crumbled	¼ cup (1 oz)	100
Feta Crumbled	¼ cup (1 oz)	80
Gorgonzola Crumbled	¼ cup (1 oz)	100
Weight Watchers		
String Light	1 stick (0.8 oz)	50
Wholesome Valley		
Organic American	1 slice (0.7 oz)	50
Yanni		
Grilling Cheese Original	1 oz	80

CHEESE DISHES
Alexia

Cheddar Bites	3 (1.2 oz)	110
Mozzarella Stix	2 pieces (1.3 oz)	120
Banquet		
Mozzarella Nuggets	7	270
Farm Rich		
Cheese Sticks	2 (2 oz)	170
Mozzarella Sticks Marinara Stuffed	2 (2.3 oz)	160
Mozzarella Bites	4 (1.8 oz)	150

FOOD	PORTION	CALS
Stouffer's		
Welsh Rarebit	¼ pkg (2.5 oz)	140
The Fillo Factory		
Tyropita Cheese Fillo Appetizers	3 (3 oz)	230
TAKE-OUT		
fondue	½ cup (3.8 oz)	247
fried mozzarella sticks	3 (4.6 oz)	503
souffle	1 serv (7 oz)	504
welsh rarebit	1 slice	228

CHEESE SUBSTITUTES

FOOD	PORTION	CALS
mozzarella	1 oz	70
soya cheese	1.4 oz	128
Daiya		
Cheddar Style Shreds	¼ cup (1 oz)	90
Mozzarella Style Shreds	¼ cup (1 oz)	90
Playfood		
Cheesey Cheese	1 oz	60
Rice		
American Flavor	1 slice (0.7 oz)	50
American Flavor Vegan	1 slice (0.7 oz)	45
Shreds Mozzarella Flavor	⅓ cup (1 oz)	70
Sheese		
Blue Style	1 oz	100
Cheddar Style Medium	1 oz	100
Creamy Mexican	2 tbsp	80
Creamy Original	2 tbsp	80
Super Stix		
Mozzarella Flavor	1 (1 oz)	70
Tofutti		
Better Ricotta Milk Free	¼ cup (2.2 oz)	100
Soy American	1 slice (0.7 oz)	80
Soy Mozzarella	1 slice (0.7 oz)	80
Vegan Gourmet		
Cheese Alternative Cheddar	1 oz	50
Cheese Alternative Monterey Jack	1 oz	70
Cheese Alternative Mozzarella	1 oz	70
Cheese Alternative Nacho	1 oz	45
Veggie		
American Flavor	1 slice (0.6 oz)	40
Grated Parmesan Flavor	2 tsp	15

FOOD	PORTION	CALS
Pepper Jack Flavor	1 oz	60
Shreds Cheddar Flavor	1 oz	70
Veggy		
Mozzarella Flavor	1 slice (0.7 oz)	40

CHERIMOYA
fresh	1	515

CHERRIES
CANNED

FOOD	PORTION	CALS
maraschino	1 (4 g)	7
maraschino	¼ cup (1.4 oz)	66
sour in heavy syrup	½ cup	116
sour in light syrup	½ cup	94
sour water packed	½ cup	44
sweet juice pack	½ cup	68
sweet pitted in heavy syrup	½ cup	105
sweet water pack	½ cup	57
Chukar Cherries		
Cherry Jubilee Dessert Sauce	1 tbsp	40
Del Monte		
Sweet Dark Pitted In Heavy Syrup	½ cup (4.2 oz)	100
Jake & Amos		
Brandied Sweet	½ cup (4.4 oz)	90
S&W		
Sliced	½ cup (4.7 oz)	140
The Gracious Gourmet		
Spiced Sour Cherry Spread	1 tbsp (0.5 oz)	15
DRIED		
bing unsulfured	¼ cup	130
montmorency tart pitted	⅓ cup	160
rainier unsulfured	⅓ cup	140
tart	½ cup	200
yogurt covered	¼ cup	170
Bob's Red Mill		
Tart	⅓ cup	140
Chukar Cherries		
Bing	3 tbsp	130
Bing Chocolate Covered	3 tbsp (1.4 oz)	180
Cabernet Dark Chocolate Covered	2 tbsp (1.5 oz)	180
Columbia River Tart	⅓ cup	120

FOOD	PORTION	CALS
Rainier	3 tbsp	130
Totally Tart	⅓ cup	140
De-Lite		
Tart	1 oz	95
Emily's		
Dark Chocolate Covered	11 (1.4 oz)	180
Peeled Snacks		
Fruit Picks Cherry-Go-Round	1 pkg (1.5 oz)	130
Raisinets		
Dark & Milk Chocolate	¼ cup (1.6 oz)	200
Stoneridge Orchards		
Bing	⅓ cup (1.4 oz)	130
Organic Montmorency Whole	⅓ cup (1.4 oz)	135
Sunsweet		
Cherries	¼ cup (1.4 oz)	100
FRESH		
Sour	1 cup	52
sour pitted	1 cup	78
sweet	20	86
Chiquita		
Cherries	1 cup (4.8 oz)	87
Dole		
Cherries	1 cup (4.9 oz)	90
Domex Superfresh Growers		
Rainier	21 (5 oz)	90
FROZEN		
sour unsweetened	½ cup	36
sweet sweetened	½ cup	115
Dole		
Dark Sweet	1 cup (4.9 oz)	90
CHERRY JUICE		
tart cherry concentrate	1 cup	140
Cheribundi		
Skinny Cherry	8 oz	90
Tart Cherry	8 oz	130
Whey Cherry	8 oz	160
Froose		
Cheerful Cherry	1 box (4.2 oz)	80
HP		
Tart Montmorency Concentrate	1 oz	80

FOOD	PORTION	CALS
Old Orchard		
Very Cherre 100% Tart Cherry Juice	8 oz	130
Santa Cruz		
Organic 100% Juice Red Tart	8 oz	120
Smart Juice		
Organic 100% Juice Tart Cherry	8 oz	140
Tart Is Smart		
Tart Cherry Concentrate	1 oz	80
CHERVIL		
seed	1 tsp	1
CHESTNUTS		
chinese steamed	3 (1 oz)	43
creme de marrons	1 oz	73
japanese roasted	1 oz	57
ready-to-eat vacuum packed	5 (1 oz)	40
roasted	3 (1 oz)	70
Gefen		
Whole Roasted & Peeled	¼ cup (1.4 oz)	52
Matiz		
Organic	7–8	86
CHEWING GUM		
bubble gum	1 block	20
stick	1 piece	7
sugarless	1 piece	5
Bubble Yum		
Original	1 piece (8 g)	25
Sugarless	1 piece (5 g)	10
Choward's		
Scented Gum	3 pieces	10
Dubble Bubble		
Gumball	1 piece	10
Extra		
Sugar Free All Flavors	1 piece	5
Flare		
Warming Cinnamon	1 piece	5
Orbit		
Sugarfree Citrusmint	1 piece	<5
White Melon Breeze	2 pieces	5

FOOD	PORTION	CALS
Stride		
All Flavors	1 piece (1.9 g)	<5
Spark	1 piece (1.9 g)	5
Trident		
Extra Care	1 piece	<5
White Peppermint	2 pieces (3 g)	5
Vitamingum		
Fresh Sugar Free All Flavors	1 piece (3 g)	5
Sport Bubblegum	1 piece (6 g)	15
Winterfresh		
Gum	1 stick	10
CHIA SEEDS		
dried	1 oz	134
Health Warrior		
Chia Bar Peanut Butter Chocolate	1 (0.9 oz)	100
Chia Seeds	1 tbsp (0.5 oz)	60
TruRoots		
Chia	1 tbsp (0.4 oz)	55

CHICKEN (*see also* CHICKEN DISHES, CHICKEN SUBSTITUTES, DINNER, HOT DOG, MEATBALLS)

FOOD	PORTION	CALS
CANNED		
chicken spread	1 serv (2 oz)	88
meat drained	1 can (5 oz)	230
w/ broth	½ can (2.5 oz)	117
Hormel		
Chunk White & Dark	2 oz	70
Premium Chunk Breast	2 oz	60
Swanson		
Chunk Breast In Water	2 oz	50
Tyson		
Premium Chunk	½ can (2 oz)	60
Premium Chunk Breast	½ can (2 oz)	60
FRESH		
back w/ skin roasted bones removed	1 (3.7 oz)	318
back w/o skin roasted bones removed	1 (2.8 oz)	191
breast roasted diced	1 cup (5 oz)	231
breast w/ skin battered fried bones removed	½ breast (4.9 oz)	364
breast w/ skin floured fried bones removed	1 (3.4 oz)	218
breast w/ skin roasted bones removed	½ breast (3.4 oz)	193

FOOD	PORTION	CALS
breast w/ skin stewed bones removed	½ breast (3.9 oz)	202
breast w/o skin fried bones removed	½ breast (3 oz)	161
breast w/o skin roasted bones removed	½ breast (3 oz)	142
breast w/o skin stewed bones removed	1 (3.3 oz)	143
broiler/fryer w/ skin roasted bones removed	½ (10.5 oz)	715
capon meat & skin roasted bones removed	½ (1.4 lbs)	1459
cornish hen w/ skin roasted	½ (4.5 oz)	335
cornish hen w/ skin roasted	1 (9 oz)	668
cornish hen w/o skin roasted	½ (4 oz)	147
cornish hen w/o skin roasted	1 (7.7 oz)	295
dark meat w/o skin roasted diced	1 cup (5 oz)	287
drumstick w/ skin battered floured & fried bones removed	1 (1.7 oz)	120
drumstick w/ skin battered fried bones removed	1 (2.5 oz)	193
drumstick w/ skin roasted bones removed	1 (1.8 oz)	112
drumstick w/ skin stewed bones removed	1 (2 oz)	116
drumstick w/o skin fried bones removed	1 (1.5 oz)	82
drumstick w/o skin roasted bones removed	1 (1.5 oz)	76
drumstick w/o skin stewed bones removed	1 (1.6 oz)	78
feet cooked	1 (1.2 oz)	73
ground crumbled fried	3 oz	161
ground patty cooked	1 lg (2.8 oz)	190
ground patty cooked	1 med (2.1 oz)	142
ground patty cooked	1 sm (1.7 oz)	114
meat & skin stewed bones removed	¼ chicken (4.6 oz)	372
neck w/ skin battered fried	1 (1.8 oz)	172
neck w/ skin fried	1 (1.3 oz)	120
neck w/ skin simmered	1 (1.3 oz)	94
roaster meat & skin roasted bones removed	¼ chicken (8.4 oz)	535
skin battered fried from ½ chicken	6.7 oz	749
skin floured fried from ½ chicken	2 oz	281
skin roasted from ½ chicken	2 oz	254
skin stewed from ½ chicken	2.5 oz	261
tail cooked	1 (1 oz)	84
thigh w/ skin battered & fried bones removed	1 (3 oz)	238
thigh w/ skin floured fried bones removed	1 (2.2 oz)	162
thigh w/ skin roasted bones removed	1 (2.2 oz)	153
thigh w/ skin stewed bones removed	1 (2.4 oz)	158
thigh w/o skin fried bones removed	1 (1.8 oz)	113

FOOD	PORTION	CALS
thigh w/o skin roasted bones removed	1 (1.8 oz)	109
thigh w/o skin stewed bones removed	1 (1.9 oz)	107
wing w/ skin battered fried bones removed	1 (1.7 oz)	159
wing w/ skin floured fried bones removed	1 (1.1 oz)	103
wing w/ skin roasted bones removed	1 (1.4 oz)	100
wing w/o skin fried bones removed	1 (0.7 oz)	42
wing w/o skin roasted bones removed	1 (0.7 oz)	43
wing w/o skin stewed bones removed	1 (0.8 oz)	43
Coleman		
Organic Breast Boneless Skinless	4 oz	120
Organic Drumsticks	4 oz	180
Foster Farms		
Back & Necks	4 oz	340
Breast Skinless Boneless	4 oz	120
Drumsticks not prep	1 (2.8 oz)	130
Ground not prep	4 oz	210
Party Wings	5 (3.8 oz)	230
Thighs	1 (4.6 oz)	270
Perdue		
Boneless Skinless Breasts cooked	3 oz	110
Breast Boneless Herb & Pepper	1 piece (4.8 oz)	140
Breast Boneless Roasted Garlic w/ White Wine	1 piece (4.8 oz)	110
Breast Boneless Skinless cooked	3 oz	100
Breast Perfect Portions Boneless Skinless	1 (4.8 oz)	130
Ground cooked	3 oz	170
Ground Breast cooked	3 oz	80
Oven Ready Cornish Hen Seasoned	4 oz	160
Oven Ready Roaster Bone-In Breast	4 oz	140
Oven Ready Roaster Seasoned	4 oz	210
Oven Stuffer Drumstick	1 (3.6 oz)	190
Patties cooked	1 (3 oz)	170
Thigh Filets Boneless Skinless	4 oz	150
Thighs Tender & Tasty Boneless Skinless cooked	3 oz	150
Whole Chicken Tender & Tasty cooked	3 oz	150
Whole Dark Meat cooked	3 oz	210
Whole White Meat cooked	3 oz	170
Wingettes cooked	3 oz	170
Wings cooked	3 oz	170

FOOD	PORTION	CALS
Rocky		
The Range Chicken Whole	4 oz	240
Rosie		
Organic Breast Boneless Skinless	4 oz	120
Tyson		
Breasts Boneless Skinless	4 oz	110
Cornish Hen	1 serv (4 oz)	200
Drumsticks	4 oz	150
Thigh Cutlets Boneless Skinless	4 oz	130
Whole Cut Up	4 oz	220
Wings	4 oz	220
FROZEN		
breast roll roasted	2 oz	75
fajita strips	1 (0.3 oz)	13
patty cooked	1 (3.5 oz)	287
Banquet		
Wings Hot & Spicy	¼ pkg (3 oz)	260
Barber		
Buffalo Fingers	1 (3.3 oz)	160
Nuggets 4 Cheese Stuffed	3 (3 oz)	230
Nuggets Cheddar & Bacon Stuffed	3 (3 oz)	240
Potato Chip Sticks	2 pieces (4.5 oz)	350
Bell & Evans		
Breaded Breast Nuggets	1 serv (4 oz)	220
Breasts Grilled	1 (2.75 oz)	90
Breasts Grilled Buffalo Style	1 (3 oz)	110
Burgers	1 (4 oz)	160
Chicken Tenders Gluten Free	1 serv (4 oz)	180
Wings Honey Barbeque	3 (4.6 oz)	160
Coleman		
Breast Nuggets Gluten Free	6 (2.7 oz)	130
Breast Strips	6 (2.7 oz)	130
Health Is Wealth		
Nuggets	4 (3 oz)	130
Organic Prairie		
Breast Boneless Skinless	4 oz	150
Ground	4 oz	200
Perdue		
Breast Chunks Breaded BBQ Glazed	3 oz	190
Breast Chunks Breaded General Tso's Glazed	3 oz	190

FOOD	PORTION	CALS
Breast Chunks Breaded Honey BBQ Glazed	3 oz	180
Breast Chunks Breaded Honey Dijon Glazed	3 oz	200
Simply Smart Grilled Chicken Strips	3 oz	110
Simply Smart Lightly Breaded Chicken Strips	3 oz	140
Simply Smart Roasted Chicken Chunks	3 oz	120
Tyson		
Any'tizers Barbeque Style Wings	3 (3.2 oz)	200
Any'tizers Homestyle Chicken Fries	7 (3.2 oz)	230
Any'tizers Popcorn Chicken	6 (2.8 oz)	220
Breast Pattie	1 (2.6 oz)	180
Cordon Bleu	1 piece (5.9 oz)	380
Diced Strips	1 serv (3 oz)	90
Kiev	1 piece (5.9 oz)	480
Weaver		
Breast Nuggets	4 (2.8 oz)	190
Breast Strips	2 (2.7 oz)	190
Patties Breast	1 (2.9 oz)	200
Popcorn Chicken	12 pieces (2.9 oz)	200
Wings Buffalo Style	3 (2.9 oz)	160
READY-TO-EAT		
Applegate Farms		
Organic Roasted	2 oz	60
Butterball		
Breast Oven Roasted Thin Sliced	4 slices (2 oz)	50
Breast Strips Oven Roasted	½ pkg (3 oz)	90
Carl Buddig		
Chicken Sliced	2 oz	85
Dietz & Watson		
Breast Southern Fried	3 slices (1.9 oz)	70
Foster Farms		
Breast Strips Grilled	3 oz	110
Cutlets Breaded	3 oz	180
Healthy Ones		
Oven Roasted 97% Fat Free	4 slices (2 oz)	60
Hormel		
Natural Choice Carved Breast Grilled	½ pkg (2 oz)	60
Oscar Mayer		
Breast Oven Roasted Thin Sliced	⅓ pkg (2 oz)	60
Breast Strips Breaded	½ pkg (3 oz)	170
Breast Strips Grilled	½ pkg (3 oz)	110

FOOD	PORTION	CALS
Perdue		
Breast Bites Popcorn Breaded	12 (3 oz)	190
Breast Strips Breaded Original	2 (2.6 oz)	160
Cutlets Breaded Original Nuggets Original	1 (3 oz)	200
Nuggets w/ Whole Grain Breading	4 (2.8 oz)	160
Short Cuts Carved Chicken Breast Original Roasted	½ cup (2.5 oz)	90
Short Cuts Chicken Breast Grilled	½ cup (2.5 oz)	90
Sara Lee		
Breast Oven Roasted	4 slices (2 oz)	45
Tyson		
Chicken Strips Fajita	1 serv (3 oz)	110
Honey Roasted Breast	2 slices (1.6 oz)	50
Hot Wings Buffalo Style	4	220
Roasted Whole Chicken Lemon Pepper	1 serv (3 oz)	120
Salad Kit Chunk Chicken	1 pkg (3.4 oz)	210
TAKE-OUT		
chicken tenders	4 (2.2 oz)	180

CHICKEN DISHES
FROZEN
Banquet

FOOD	PORTION	CALS
Boneless Popcorn Chicken	11 pieces	180
Wings Honey BBQ	¼ pkg (3 oz)	270
Barber		
Broccoli & Cheese Reduced Fat	1 piece (5.5 oz)	250
Cordon Bleu	1 piece (6 oz)	370
Cordon Bleu Reduced Fat	1 piece (5.5 oz)	260
Creme Brie & Apple	1 piece (6 oz)	350
Kiev	1 piece (6 oz)	430
Mashed Potato Stuffed	1 piece (6 oz)	340
Skinless Breast Stuffed	1 piece (6 oz)	280
Crazy Cuizine		
Teriyaki Chicken	1 cup (5 oz)	240
MIX		
Chicken Helper		
Asian Chicken Fried Rice as prep	1 cup	250
Classic Creamy Chicken & Noodles as prep	1 cup	280
Jambalaya as prep	1 cup	280

FOOD	PORTION	CALS
REFRIGERATED		
Tyson		
Chicken Breast Medallions In White Wine & Garlic Sauce	1 serv (5 oz)	140
Ventera		
Rollatini w/ Rice Stuffing & Marsala Wine Sauce	1 serv + sauce (6 oz)	230
TAKE-OUT		
arroz con pollo	1 serv (16 oz)	579
barbecued pulled chicken	1 serv (9 oz)	312
boneless breast w/ apple stuffing	1 serv (5 oz)	260
breast & wing breaded & fried	2 pieces (5.7 oz)	494
buffalo wing + sauce	2 (1.7 oz)	147
cacciatore breast + sauce	1 serv (5.9 oz)	323
cacciatore drumstick + sauce	1 serv (3.2 oz)	172
cacciatore thigh + sauce	1 serv (3.8 oz)	204
cacciatore wing + sauce	1 serv (2.1 oz)	113
chicharrones de pollo	3 (2.6 oz)	289
chicken & dumplings	1 cup (8.6 oz)	368
chicken & noodles in cream sauce	1 cup (8 oz)	323
chicken a la king	1 cup (8.5 oz)	465
chicken breast parmigiana	1 serv (5.8 oz)	278
chicken cordon bleu + sauce	1 roll (8 oz)	504
chicken creole w/o rice	1 cup (8.6 oz)	187
chicken kiev breast meat	1 serv (9 oz)	653
chicken meatloaf	1 lg slice (5 oz)	243
chicken paprikash	1½ cups	296
chicken pie w/ top crust	1 slice (5.6 oz)	472
chicken salad white meat	1 serv (4 oz)	300
chicken satay + peanut sauce	2 skewers	239
creamed chicken	1 cup (8.5 oz)	388
croquette	1 (2.2 oz)	159
curry	1 cup (8.3 oz)	288
curry breast half + sauce	1 (7 oz)	244
curry drumstick + sauce	1 (3.7 oz)	129
curry thigh + sauce	1 (4.4 oz)	154
curry wing + sauce	1 (2.4 oz)	84
drumstick & thigh breaded & fried	2 pieces (5.2 oz)	431
fricassee	1 cup (8.6 oz)	322
groundnut stew hkatenkwan	1 serv (15.7 oz)	576
jamaican jerk wings	4 wings (9.9 oz)	709

FOOD	PORTION	CALS
jambalaya w/ sausage & rice	1 cup (8.6 oz)	393
kobete turkish chicken w/ pastry	1 serv	513
rotisserie seasoned breast w/ skin	1 serv (3.5 oz)	184
rotisserie seasoned breast w/o skin	1 serv (3.5 oz)	148
rotisserie seasoned thigh w/ skin	1 serv (3.5 oz)	233
rotisserie seasoned thigh w/o skin	1 serv (3.5 oz)	196
sancocho de pollo dominican chicken stew	1 serv	702
stew	1 cup (8.8 oz)	176
tandoori chicken breast	1 serv	260
tandoori chicken leg & thigh	1 serv	300
tetrazzini	1 cup (8.6 oz)	369

CHICKEN SUBSTITUTES
Chicken Free Chicken
Country Smoked	2 oz	80

Gardein
Buffalo Wings	1 serv (3.5 oz)	120
Chick'n Filets	1 (3.5 oz)	120
Chick'n Scallopini	1 piece (2.5 oz)	90
Crispy Fingers	2 (3.2 oz)	160
Crispy Tenders	1 (1.8 oz)	90
Tuscan Breasts	1 (5.3 oz)	150

Gardenburger
Chik'n Grill	1 (2.5 oz)	100

Health Is Wealth
Chicken-Free Nuggets	3 pieces (2.9 oz)	120

Loma Linda
Fried Chik'n w/ Gravy	2 pieces (2.8 oz)	150

Morningstar Farms
Chik'n Roasted Herb	1 pattie (2.2 oz)	110
Meal Starters Chik'n Strips	12 pieces (3 oz)	140

Veat
Chick'n Free Nuggets	1 serv (2.5 oz)	140
Vegetarian Breast	1 (1.8 oz)	90

Veggie Patch
Chick'n Nuggets	4 (2.7 oz)	170

Vjana
Chickin Fillets	1 (3.5 oz)	270
Chickin Nuggets	3 (2.6 oz)	200

FOOD	PORTION	CALS
Worthington		
FriChik Original	2 pieces (3.2 oz)	140
Meatless Chicken Style	1 slice (2 oz)	90
Yves		
Meatless Smoked Chicken Slices	4 (2.2 oz)	100

CHICKPEAS
CANNED
chickpeas	1 cup	285
Allens		
Garbanzo Beans	½ cup	120
Green Giant		
Garbanzo Beans	½ cup	100
Progresso		
Chick Peas	½ cup (4.6 oz)	120
DRIED		
cooked	1 cup	269
Arrowhead Mills		
Organic Dried Chickpeas not prep	¼ cup	160
FROZEN		
Tandoor Chef		
Channa Masala	½ pkg (5 oz)	190

CHICORY
endive fresh chopped	½ cup	4
greens raw chopped	½ cup	21
root raw	1 (2.1 oz)	44
roots raw cut up	½ cup (1.6 oz)	33
witloof head raw	1 (1.9 oz)	9
witloof raw	½ cup (1.6 oz)	8

CHILI
powder	1 tbsp	24
Ahh!Gourmet		
Wriggly Sambal Chili Sauce Paste	4 tbsp	170
Allergaroo		
Gluten Free Chili Mac	1 pkg (8 oz)	240
Amy's		
136 Organic Black Bean Medium	1 cup	200
Whole Meals Chili & Cornbread	1 pkg	340
Comfort Care		
Vegetarian White	1 cup (8 oz)	150

FOOD	PORTION	CALS
Dennison's		
Con Carne	1 cup	350
Fat Free w/ Beans	1 cup	210
Turkey	1 cup	210
Vegetarian	1 cup	190
Dynasty		
Thai Chili Garlic Paste	1 tsp (5 g)	0
Frontera		
Chili Mix Chipotle Black Bean	½ cup (4.2 oz)	60
Chili Starter Green Chile White Bean	½ cup (4.4 oz)	80
Health Valley		
Chunky Spicy Vegetarian No Salt Added	1 cup	150
Vegetarian Spicy	1 cup	150
Heinz		
Chili Sauce	1 tbsp (0.6 oz)	20
High Plains Bison		
Campfire Chili	1 cup (8 oz)	190
Hormel		
Chili Mac	1 pkg (9.9 oz)	270
Chili No Beans	1 pkg (7.3 oz)	190
Chili No Beans Less Sodium	1 serv (8.3 oz)	220
Chili w/ Beans	1 serv (8.7 oz)	260
Chili w/ Beans Less Sodium	1 serv (8.7 oz)	260
Turkey Chili w/ Beans	1 serv (8.7 oz)	210
Vegetarian Chili w/ Beans	1 serv (8.7 oz)	190
Master Chili		
Chipotle Chicken No Bean	1 serv (8.3 oz)	230
Roasted Tomato w/ Bean	1 serv (8.7 oz)	210
McIlhenny		
Original Recipe	½ cup	50
Meals To Live		
White Chicken Chili Relleno w/ Ranchero Sauce	1 pkg (9 oz)	210
Mimi's Gourmet		
Organic Vegan Gluten Free 3 Bean w/ Rice	1 pkg (11.5 oz)	270
Organic Vegan Gluten Free Black Bean & Corn	1 pkg (10.5 oz)	250
Organic Vegan Gluten Free White Bean	1 pkg (10.5 oz)	230
Spice Hunter		
Powder Blend Salt Free	¼ tsp	0
Thai Kitchen		
Roasted Red Chili Paste	1 tbsp (0.5 oz)	50

FOOD	PORTION	CALS
Truitt Brothers		
Beef Natural Shredded	1 cup (9.4 oz)	240
Vegetarian	1 cup (9.4 oz)	220
Worthington		
Vegetarian	1 cup	280
TAKE-OUT		
chiles rellenos cheese filled	1 (5 oz)	365
chili con carne w/ beans	1 cup	264
chili con carne w/ beans & chicken	1 cup (8.9 oz)	218
con carne w/ beans & rice	1 cup	298
vegetarian con carne	1 cup	272

CHILI PEPPER (*see* PEPPERS)

CHINESE FOOD (*see* ASIAN FOOD)

CHINESE PRESERVING MELON

cooked	½ cup	11

CHIPS (*see also* SNACKS)

apple chips	10 (0.8 oz)	101
banana	1 oz	147
carrot	28 (1 oz)	95
corn	1 oz	147
plantain	1 oz	158
potato salted	1 oz	155
potato sticks	½ cup (0.6 oz)	94
potato sticks	1 pkg (1 oz)	148
potato unsalted	1 oz	152
potato unsalted reduced fat	1 oz	138
shrimp	4 sm (0.4 oz)	56
shrimp	4 med (0.9 oz)	141
shrimp	4 lg (1.4 oz)	219
soy	1 oz	107
sweet potato	1 oz	141
taro	10 (0.8 oz)	115
tortilla lowfat baked	1 oz	118
tortilla lowfat unsalted	1 oz	118
tortilla white corn	1 oz	139
tortilla yellow corn	1 oz	139
Bachman		
Corn Jumbo Chipitos	16 (1 oz)	150

FOOD	PORTION	CALS
Potato Golden Ridges	22 (1 oz)	160
Tortilla Black Bean	1 oz	140
Tortilla Restaurant Style	11 (1 oz)	140
Tortilla Toasted Sweet Potato	11 (1 oz)	130
Beanfields		
Bean & Rice Naturally Unsalted	⅙ pkg (1 oz)	140
Bean & Rice Pico De Gallo	⅙ pkg (1 oz)	140
Bean & Rice Sea Salt	⅙ pkg (1 oz)	140
Bean & Rice Sea Salt & Pepper	⅙ pkg (1 oz)	140
Beanitos		
Pinto Bean & Flax	10 (1 oz)	150
Better Balance		
Protein Chips Gluten Free All Flavors	1 oz	110
Betty Crocker		
Potato Kettle Cooked Lightly Salted	1 oz	120
Boulder Canyon		
Potato 50% Reduced Salt	14 (1 oz)	150
Potato Sour Cream & Chive	14 (1 oz)	150
Potato Spinach & Artichoke	14 (1 oz)	150
Brothers-All-Natural		
Potato Crisps Fresh Onion & Fresh Garlic	1 pkg	45
Potato Crisps Original w/ Sea Salt	1 pkg	45
Buffalo Nickel Wingers		
Potato Level 1: No Bull Barbecue	25 (1 oz)	120
Potato Level 3: Nacho Chiliehanga	25 (1 oz)	120
Potato Level 5: Fiery Buffalo Bleu	25 (1 oz)	120
Burger King		
Potato Flame Broiled	16 (1 oz)	150
Potato Ketchup & Fries	16 (1 oz)	150
Butterfield		
Potato Sticks Shoestring	1 pkg (1.7 oz)	250
Corazonas		
Potato Lightly Salted	1 oz	130
Potato Parmesan Peppercorn	1 oz	140
Potato Spicy Rio Habanero	1 oz	130
Tortilla Lightly Salted	14 (1 oz)	140
Tortilla Squeeze Of Lime	14 (1 oz)	140
Deep River Snacks		
Potato Baked Fries Sweet Maui Onion	1 oz	135
Potato Kettle Cooked Asian Sweet & Spicy	1 oz	150

FOOD	PORTION	CALS
Potato Kettle Cooked Original Salted	1 oz	150
Potato Kettle Cooked Rosemary & Olive Oil	1 oz	150
Potato Kettle Cooked Salt & Vinegar	1 oz	150
Potato Zesty Jalapeno	1 oz	150
Doritos		
Tortilla Flamas	11 (1 oz)	140
Tortilla Nacho Cheese	11 (1 oz)	150
Tortilla Spicy Nacho	12 (1 oz)	140
Tortilla Toasted Corn	13 (1 oz)	140
Flat Earth		
Baked Fruit Crisps Apple Cinnamon Grove	14 (1 oz)	130
Baked Fruit Crisps Peach Mango Paradise	14 (1 oz)	130
Baked Fruit Crisps Wild Berry Patch	14 (1 oz)	130
Baked Veggie Crisps Farmland Cheddar	14 (1 oz)	130
Baked Veggie Crisps Garlic & Herb Field	14 (1 oz)	130
Baked Veggie Crisps Tangy Tomato Ranch	14 (1 oz)	130
FoodShouldTasteGood		
Tortilla Buffalo	10 (1 oz)	130
Tortilla Chocolate Gluten Free	1 pkg (1 oz)	140
Tortilla Multigrain Gluten Free	1 pkg (1 oz)	140
Tortilla Sweet Potato Gluten Free	10 (1 oz)	130
French's		
Potato Sticks Barbecue	¾ cup	160
Potato Sticks Original	¾ cup	190
Fritos		
Corn Lightly Salted	1 oz	160
Corn Original	32 (1 oz)	160
Corn Scoops	10 (1 oz)	160
Frontera		
Tortilla Blue Corn	⅑ pkg (1 oz)	130
Tortilla Thick & Crunchy	⅑ pkg (1 oz)	130
Glenny's		
Organic Soy Barbeque	1 oz	110
Organic Soy Creamy Ranch	1 oz	110
Soy Crisps Apple Cinnamon	½ pkg (0.6 oz)	70
Soy Crisps Caramel	½ pkg (1.3 oz)	70
Soy Crisps Low Fat Lightly Salted	½ pkg (0.6 oz)	70
Soy Crisps No Salt	½ pkg (0.6 oz)	70
Soy Crisps Salt & Pepper	½ pkg (0.6 oz)	70
Soy Crisps White Cheddar	½ pkg (0.6 oz)	70

FOOD	PORTION	CALS
Spud Delites Sea Salt	1 pkg (1.1 oz)	100
Veggie Fries	½ pkg (0.6 oz)	70
Zen Health Tortilla Crisps Original	1 oz	110
Guiltless Gourmet		
Tortilla Blue Corn	18 (1 oz)	120
Tortilla Chili Lime	18 (1 oz)	120
Tortilla Chipotle	18 (1 oz)	123
Tortilla Yellow Corn	18 (1 oz)	120
Tortilla Yellow Corn Unsalted	18 (1 oz)	120
Hippie Chips		
Baked Potato Chive-Talkin' Sour Cream	1 pkg (0.7 oz)	90
Baked Potato Haight AshBerry Jalapeno	1 pkg (0.7 oz)	90
Baked Potato Memphis Blues Barbecue	1 pkg (0.7 oz)	90
Baked Potato Sea Of Love Salt	1 pkg (1 oz)	125
Baked Potato Woodstock Ranch	1 pkg (0.7 oz)	90
Jay's		
Potato	1 oz	150
Late July		
Organic Multigrain Dude Ranch	13 (1 oz)	120
Organic Multigrain Mild Green Mojo	13 (1 oz)	110
Lay's		
Potato Balsamic Sweet Onion	15 (1 oz)	160
Potato Chipotle Ranch	15 (1 oz)	160
Potato Classic	15 (1 oz)	160
Potato Garden Tomato & Basil	15 (1 oz)	160
Potato Kettle Cooked Crinkle Cut Spice Rubbed BBQ	15 (1 oz)	140
Potato Kettle Cooked Original	16 (1 oz)	160
Potato Kettle Cooked Spicy Cayenne & Cheese	16 (1 oz)	150
Potato Lightly Salted	15 (1 oz)	160
Potato Original Baked	15 (1 oz)	120
Potato Stax Sour Cream & Onion	12 (1 oz)	150
Potato Sweet Southern Heat Barbecue	15 (1 oz)	160
Potato Wavy Original	11 (1 oz)	160
Little Wings		
Multi Grain Hot Buffalo Wing w/ Bleu Cheese Drizzle	1 pkg (0.5 oz)	60
Lundberg		
Rice Chips Original Sea Salt	1 oz	140
Rice Chips Sesame Seaweed	1 oz	140
Rice Chips Wasabi	1 oz	140

FOOD	PORTION	CALS
Madhouse Munchies		
Potato Sea Salt	16	150
Potato Sea Salt & Vinegar	16	150
Tortilla White	9	140
Margaritaville		
Tortilla Sea Salt	1 oz	140
Maui Style		
Potato	14 (1 oz)	150
Shrimp Chips	1 oz	150
Mediterranean Snacks		
Baked Lentil Cucumber Dill	22 (1 oz)	110
Baked Lentil Roasted Pepper	22 (1 oz)	110
Baked Lentil Sea Salt	22 (1 oz)	110
Multi Grain Original	16 (1 oz)	130
Veggie Medley Original	28 (1 oz)	130
Mexi-Snax		
Tortilla Multi-Grain Blue	15 (1 oz)	140
Tortilla Pico De Gallo	15 (1 oz)	140
Tortilla Salted	15 (1 oz)	140
Tortilla Tamari	15 (1 oz)	130
Michael Season's		
Popped Black Bean Nacho	17 (1 oz)	120
Popped Black Bean Red Pepper	17 (1 oz)	120
Popped Black Bean Sea Salt	17 (1 oz)	120
Potato Crisps Thin Baked Low Fat	14	120
Potato Kettle Style Reduced Fat	18	130
Potato Reduced Fat	20	140
Potato Reduced Fat Unsalted	20	140
Poore Brothers		
Original	14 (1 oz)	140
Salt & Vinegar	15 (1 oz)	150
Sweet Maui Onion	14 (1 oz)	140
Popchips		
Potato Barbeque	19 (1 oz)	120
Potato Cheddar	20 (1 oz)	120
Potato Original	22 (1 oz)	120
Potato Parmesan Garlic	20 (1 oz)	120
Potato Salt & Pepper	11 (0.4 oz)	50
Potato Sea Salt & Vinegar	20 (1 oz)	120
Potato Sour Cream & Onion	20 (1 oz)	120

FOOD	PORTION	CALS
Pringles		
Jalapeno	15 (1 oz)	150
Loaded Baked Potato	15 (1 oz)	150
Minis Cheddar Cheese	1 pkg	120
Minis Original	1 pkg	120
Original	14 (1 oz)	160
Pizza	15 (1 oz)	150
Select Cinnamon Sweet Potato	28 (1 oz)	150
Select Parmesan Garlic	28 (1 oz)	140
Snack Stacks Original	1 pkg	140
Revolution Foods		
Organic Popalongs Whole Grains Cheesy Cheese	16 (0.7 oz)	90
Organic Popalongs Whole Grains Original	16 (0.7 oz)	100
Organic Popalongs Whole Grains Simply Cinnamon	16 (0.7 oz)	100
Rhythm		
Crispy Kale Bombay Curry	½ pkg (1 oz)	101
Crispy Kale Kool Ranch	½ pkg (1 oz)	100
Crispy Kale Zesty Nacho	½ pkg (1 oz)	106
Robert's American Gourmet		
Soy Crisps Country Barbecue	1 oz	130
Ruffles		
Baked Original Potato	9 (1 oz)	120
Original Potato	12 (1 oz)	160
Reduced Fat Potato	13 (1 oz)	140
Reduced Fat Sea Salted Potato	1 oz	140
Salba Smart		
Organic Blue Corn Omega-3 Enriched	1 oz	104
Santitas		
Tortilla Triangles White Corn	9 (1 oz)	140
Tortilla Triangles Yellow Corn	9 (1 oz)	140
Seneca		
Crispy Apple Apple Pie Ala Mode	12 (1 oz)	140
Crispy Apple Caramel	12 (1 oz)	140
Crispy Apple Cinnamon	14 (1 oz)	150
Crispy Apple Original	12 (1 oz)	140
Crispy Apple Sour Apple	12 (1 oz)	150
Sensible Portions		
Garden Veggie Sea Salt	1 pkg (0.5 oz)	70

FOOD	PORTION	CALS
Simply 7		
Hummus Chips Sea Salt	30 (1 oz)	130
Lentil Chips Sea Salt	31 (1 oz)	140
Snikiddy		
Fries Potato Bold Buffalo Gluten Free	1 oz	130
Fries Potato Classic Ketchup Gluten Free	1 oz	130
Fries Potato Original Gluten Free	1 oz	130
Fries Potato Southwest Cheddar Gluten Free	1 oz	130
Snyder's Of Hanover		
Kosher Dill	1 oz	140
MultiGrain Sunflower	1 oz	140
MultiGrain Sunflower Southwestern Cheddar	1 oz	140
MultiGrain Tortilla Lightly Salted	1 oz	130
MultiGrain Tortilla Strips Flaxseed Gold	1 oz	140
Organic Veggie Crisps	1 oz	140
Potato Original	1 oz	150
Sweet Potato Baked	1 oz	110
Tortilla Gluten Free MultiGrain	10 (1 oz)	150
Tortilla White Corn	1 oz	140
Stacy's		
Bagel Chips Everything	12 (1 oz)	130
Pita Chips Cinnamon Sugar	1 oz	140
Soy Thin Chips Sticky Bun	18 (1 oz)	130
SunChips		
Multigrain French Onion	15 (1 oz)	140
Multigrain Original	16 (1 oz)	140
T.G.I. Friday's		
Potato Cheese Pizza	16 (1 oz)	160
Tater Skins		
Cheddar Bacon	16 (1 oz)	150
Original	16 (1 oz)	150
Terra		
Exotic Vegetable Original	14 (1 oz)	150
Exotic Vegetable Zesty Tomato	14 (1 oz)	150
Kettles Potato Sea Salt & Pepper	15 (1 oz)	140
Parsnip Chips	12 (1 oz)	150
Potato Au Natural	18 (1 oz)	150
Potato Blues	1 oz	130
Potato Frites Sea Salt & Vinegar	1 oz	150
Potato Golds Original	1 oz	130

FOOD	PORTION	CALS
Potato Potpourri	1 oz	140
Potato Red Bliss	1 oz	140
Stix Original Exotic Vegetable	1 oz	150
Sweet Potato	17 (1 oz)	160
Sweets & Beets	16 (1 oz)	150
Taro	1 oz	140
The Whole Earth		
Tortilla Really Seedy Multigrain	9 (1 oz)	140
Thunder		
Potato Buffalo Wing w/ Blue Cheese	22 (1 oz)	150
Tostitos		
Tortilla Baked Scoops	14 (1 oz)	120
Tortilla Bite Size Rounds	24 (1 oz)	140
Tortilla Multigrain	8 (1 oz)	150
Tortilla Scoops	12 (1 oz)	140
Umpqua Indian Foods		
Nana Crisps	⅕ pkg (1 oz)	120
Veggie	¼ pkg (1 oz)	120
Utz		
Pita Natural w/ Sea Salt	1 oz	120
Potato	20 (1 oz)	150
Potato Baked	1 oz	110
Potato BBQ	20 (1 oz)	150
Potato Grandma Kettle	1 oz	140
Potato Homestyle Kettle	1 oz	140
Potato Kettle Classics	20 (1 oz)	150
Potato Mystic Kettle	1 oz	150
Potato Mystic Kettle Reduced Fat	1 oz	130
Potato Natural Lightly Salted Kettle	1 oz	140
Potato No Salt Added	20 (1 oz)	150
Potato Onion & Garlic	1 oz	150
Potato Ripple	20 (1 oz)	150
Sweet Potato Kettle Classics	20 (1 oz)	150
Tortilla Baked	10	120
Tortilla Organic Yellow Corn	1 oz	140
Vegetable Natural Exotic Medley	1 oz	160
Want'ems		
Wonton Asian BBQ	16 (1 oz)	140
Wonton Original	16 (1 oz)	140

FOOD	PORTION	CALS
Yogachips		
Organic Apple Chips Peach	1 pkg (0.35 oz)	35
Zapp's		
Potato Cajun Dill	1 oz	150
Potato No Salt	1 oz	150
Potato Original	1 oz	150
Potato Sizzlin Steak	1 oz	150
Sweet Potato Lightly Salted	1 oz	150
CHITTERLINGS		
pork cooked	3 oz	258
CHIVES		
freeze-dried	1 tbsp	1
fresh chopped	1 tsp	0
fresh chopped	1 tbsp	1

CHOCOLATE (see also CANDY, CHOCOLATE SPREAD, CHOCOLATE SYRUP, COCOA, HOT CHOCOLATE, ICE CREAM TOPPINGS, MILK DRINKS)

FOOD	PORTION	CALS
BAKING		
baking	1 oz	145
grated unsweetened	¼ cup	165
liquid unsweetened	1 oz	134
mexican baking	1 sq (0.7 oz)	85
squares unsweetened	1 sq (1 oz)	145
Baker's		
Semi-Sweet	0.5 oz	70
Unsweetened	0.5 oz	70
White	0.5 oz	80
Hershey's		
Unsweetened Block	1 (0.5 oz)	70
CHIPS		
milk chocolate	1 cup (6 oz)	862
semisweet	1 cup (6 oz)	804
semisweet	60 pieces (1 oz)	136
E. Guittard		
Cappuccino	30 (0.5 oz)	80
Milk Chocolate	12 (0.5 oz)	80
Semisweet	30 (0.5 oz)	70
Ghirardelli		
Semi-Sweet	32 (0.5 oz)	70

FOOD	PORTION	CALS
Hershey's		
Milk Chocolate	1 tbsp (0.5 oz)	70
Premier White	1 tbsp (0.5 oz)	80
Semi-Sweet	1 tbsp (0.5 oz)	70
Special Dark	1 tbsp (0.5 oz)	70
Sugar Free	1 tbsp (0.5 oz)	70
MIX		
drink mix powder	2–3 heaping tsp	75
drink mix powder as prep w/ whole milk	9 oz	226
Nesquik		
Chocolate Powder	2 tbsp (0.6 oz)	60
Chocolate Powder No Sugar Added	2 tbsp (0.4 oz)	35
Sunfood		
Organic Powder	2 tbsp (1 oz)	120

CHOCOLATE MILK *(see MILK DRINKS)*

CHOCOLATE SPREAD

Love'n Bake		
Chocolate Schmear	2 tbsp	140

CHOCOLATE SYRUP

chocolate fudge	1 tbsp (0.7 oz)	73
chocolate fudge	1 cup (11.9 oz)	1176
syrup	1 cup	653
syrup	2 tbsp	82
syrup as prep w/ whole milk	1 cup (9.9 oz)	254
Hershey's		
Lite	2 tbsp (1.2 oz)	45
Sugar Free	2 tbsp (1.1 oz)	15
Sundae Syrup Double Chocolate	2 tbsp (1.3 oz)	100
Syrup	2 tbsp (1.4 oz)	100
Nesquik		
Calcium Fortified	2 tbsp (1.3 oz)	100
Santa Cruz		
Organic	2 tbsp	110
Steel's		
No Sugar Added Fat Free	2 tbsp (1 oz)	50
U-Bet		
Original	2 tbsp (1.4 oz)	128

FOOD	PORTION	CALS
CHUTNEY		
apple	1.2 oz	68
coconut	2 oz	87
fresh mint	2 oz	18
mango	¼ cup (2 oz)	227
tomato	1 oz	90
Beth's Farm Kitchen		
Blazing Tomato	2 tbsp (1 oz)	25
Chukar Cherries		
Curried Cherry	1 tbsp	30
Patak's		
Major Grey	1 tbsp	60
Mango Hot	1 tbsp	60
Mango Sweet	1 tbsp	60
Robert Rothchild Farm		
Hot Peach & Apple	2 tbsp	45
School House Kitchen		
Bardshar	1 oz	80
The Gracious Gourmet		
Mango Pineapple	2 tbsp (1 oz)	45
Wild Thymes Farm		
Apricot Cranberry Walnut	1 tbsp	16
Plum Currant Ginger	1 tsp	20
CILANTRO		
fresh	1 tsp (2 g)	<1
fresh	¼ cup	1
fresh sprigs	5 (5 g)	1
CINNAMON		
cinnamon sugar	1 tsp	16
ground	1 tsp	6
sticks	0.5 oz	39
McCormick		
Grinder Cinnamon Sugar	1 tsp (3.5 g)	10
CISCO		
raw	3 oz	84
smoked	1 oz	50

FOOD	PORTION	CALS
CLAMS		
CANNED		
liquid only	1 cup	6
liquid only	3 oz	2
meat only	1 cup	236
meat only	3 oz	126
Chicken Of The Sea		
Chopped	¼ cup	30
Whole Baby	¼ cup	30
Polar		
Baby	¼ cup	30
FRESH		
cooked	20 sm	133
cooked	3 oz	126
raw	3 oz	63
raw	20 sm (6.3 oz)	133
raw	9 lg (6.3 oz)	133
FROZEN		
Mrs. Paul's		
Fried	18 (3 oz)	270
SeaPak		
Oven Crunchy Strips	1 serv (3 oz)	250
TAKE-OUT		
breaded & fried	20 sm	379
CLEMENTINES		
Cuties		
Fresh	2 (6 oz)	80
Disney Garden		
Clementines	1	35
CLOVES		
ground	1 tsp	7
COCOA (see also HOT CHOCOLATE)		
cocoa butter	1 tbsp	120
powder unsweetened	1 tbsp	12
CocoaVia		
Beverage Mix Dark Chocolate	1 pkg (0.28 oz)	30
Hershey's		
Cocoa	1 tbsp (5 g)	10

FOOD	PORTION	CALS
Honest CocoaNova		
Cherry Cacao	8 oz	50
COCONUT		
dried sweetened shredded	¼ cup	116
dried toasted	1 oz	168
dried unsweetened	1 oz	187
fresh from 1 coconut	14 oz	1405
fresh shredded	¼ cup	71
Baker's		
Angel Flake Sweetened	0.5 oz	70
Bob's Red Mill		
Shredded	3 tbsp	120
Let's Do Organic		
Organic Reduced Fat Shredded	1 can (0.5 oz)	70
Shredded	3 tbsp (0.5 oz)	110
Mounds		
Sweetened Flakes	2 tbsp (0.5 oz)	70
Prosperity		
Organic Coconut Flax Butter Garlic & Onion	1 tbsp	140
COCONUT JUICE		
coconut water fresh	½ cup	23
creamed sweetened canned	½ cup	264
milk canned	½ cup	276
Coco King		
Roasted w/ Pulp	1 can (11.75 oz)	130
w/ Pulp	1 can (11.85 oz)	130
CocoZona		
Coconut Water	1 bottle (14.5 oz)	70
Goya		
Coconut Water	1 can (11.8 oz)	120
Let's Do Organic		
Creamed	1 oz	220
Milk	¼ cup	100
O.N.E.		
Natural Coconut Water	1 box (11 oz)	60
Thai Kitchen		
Coconut Milk	⅓ cup (2.8 oz)	140
Lite Coconut Milk	2 oz	45
Zico		
Coconut Water All Flavors	1 pkg (11 oz)	60

FOOD	PORTION	CALS
COD		
atlantic canned	3 oz	89
atlantic canned	1 can (11 oz)	327
atlantic dried	3 oz	246
atlantic fresh cooked	1 fillet (6.3 oz)	189
atlantic fresh cooked	3 oz	89
atlantic fresh raw	3 oz	70
pacific fresh baked	3 oz	95
roe canned	1 oz	34
roe tarama	3.5 oz	547
Mrs. Paul's		
Filets Lightly Breaded	1 (4 oz)	220
TAKE-OUT		
roe baked w/ butter & lemon juice	1 oz	36
COFFEE (*see also* COFFEE BEVERAGES, COFFEE SUBSTITUTES)		
INSTANT		
decaffeinated as prep	8 oz	2
decaffeinated powder	1 rounded tsp	4
regular powder	1 rounded tsp	4
REGULAR		
brewed	8 oz	2
roasted beans	1 oz	64
Spava		
Calm Decaffeinated	1 cup	0
COFFEE BEVERAGES		
Click		
Espresso Protein Drink as prep	2 scoops (1.1 oz)	120
Emmi		
Caffe Latte Cappuccino	1 pkg (7.7 oz)	140
Caffe Latte Vanilla	1 pkg (7.7 oz)	140
General Foods		
International Coffees Vanilla Bean Latte	1 serv	60
Health Is Wealth		
Nutriccino Vitamin Infused All Flavors	1 bottle (9.5 oz)	190
Vitamin Coffee Ener-G Infused Vanilla Latte	1 bottle (9.5 oz)	190
Iced 'Spresso		
Ultra Light American Vanilla	1 bottle (9.5 oz)	90
Ultra Light Espresso Latte	1 bottle (9.5 oz)	70
N.O. Brew		
Iced Coffee not prep	1 serv (2.6 oz)	10

FOOD	PORTION	CALS
O.N.E.		
Coffee Fruit	1 bottle (11 oz)	107
POMx		
Iced Cafe Au Lait	1 bottle (10.5 oz)	170
Iced Cafe Vanilla	1 bottle (10.5 oz)	180
Seattle's Best Coffee		
Iced Latte	1 can (9.5 oz)	130
Iced Latte Vanilla	1 can (9.5 oz)	130
Iced Mocha	1 can (9.5 oz)	130
Wolfgang Puck		
Culinary Iced All Flavors	1 bottle (8.5 oz)	120
TAKE-OUT		
cafe amaretto w/ alcohol	1 serv	192
cafe au lait	1 cup (8 oz)	77
cafe brulot	1 cup	48
cafe brulot w/ alcohol	1 serv	130
cappuccino	1 cup (8 oz)	77
coffee con leche	1 cup (6 oz)	104
cuban coffee w/ rum & creme de cacao	1 (9 oz)	112
dutch coffee w/ gin	1 (7 oz)	181
espresso	1 cup (4 oz)	2
french coffee w/ orange liqueur & kahlua	1 (8 oz)	232
irish coffee	1 serv (8 oz)	209
italian coffee w/ strega	1 (7 oz)	163
latte w/ skim milk	1 serv (13 oz)	88
latte w/ whole milk	1 serv (14 oz)	143
mocha	1 serv (17 oz)	403
puerto rican coffee w/ rum & kahlua	1 (8 oz)	166
turkish	1 cup (4 oz)	50

COFFEE SUBSTITUTES
Pixie

Mate Latte Chai	½ cup (4 oz)	80
Mate Latte Dark Roast	½ cup (4 oz)	70
Mate Latte Mocha	½ cup (4 oz)	70
Mate Latte Original	½ cup (4 oz)	70

COFFEE WHITENERS
Baileys

Caramel	1 tbsp (0.5 oz)	40
French Vanilla	1 tbsp (0.5 oz)	40

FOOD	PORTION	CALS
Hazelnut	1 tbsp (0.5 oz)	35
Original Irish Cream	1 tbsp (0.5 oz)	40
Farmland		
Nondairy Creamer	2 tbsp	40
International Delight		
Amaretto	1 tbsp (0.5 oz)	40
Caramel Macchiato	1 tbsp (0.5 oz)	40
Caribbean Cinnamon Creme	1 tbsp (0.5 oz)	45
Dark Chocolate Cream	1 tbsp (0.5 oz)	35
English Almond Toffee	1 tbsp (0.5 oz)	45
French Vanilla	1 tbsp (0.5 oz)	45
French Vanilla Fat Free	1 tbsp (0.5 oz)	30
French Vanilla Sugar Free	1 tbsp (0.5 oz)	20
Irish Creme	1 tbsp (0.5 oz)	40
Vanilla Caramel Cream	1 tbsp (0.5 oz)	35
Vanilla Latte	1 tbsp (0.5 oz)	40
Silk		
French Vanilla	1 tbsp (0.5 oz)	20
Original	1 tbsp (0.5 oz)	15
WildWood		
Soymilk Creamer Plain	1 tbsp	15

COLESLAW
Dole

Classic Coleslaw	1½ cups (3 oz)	20
Kit Creamy Coleslaw as prep	1½ cups (3.5 oz)	100
Fresh Express		
3 Color Deli	1½ cups	20
Kit w/ Sweet & Creamy Dressing as prep	1 cup	120
Old Fashioned	2 cups	25
Mann's		
Broccoli Cole Slaw w/o Dressing	1 serv (3 oz)	25
Ready Pac		
Coleslaw	1½ cups (3 oz)	20
Coleslaw Mix as prep	1 cup (3.5 oz)	130
TAKE-OUT		
coleslaw w/ dressing	¾ cup	147
vinegar & oil coleslaw	3.5 oz	150

COLLARDS

fresh cooked	½ cup	17

FOOD	PORTION	CALS
frzn chopped cooked	½ cup	31
raw chopped	½ cup	6
Allens		
Seasoned Southern Style	½ cup (4.1 oz)	35
Glory		
Green Fresh	2 cups	25
Seasoned canned	½ cup	35
Sensibly Seasoned canned	½ cup	20
Seabrook Farms		
Chopped Greens frzn	½ cup (3.1 oz)	30

COOKIES
MIX
chocolate chip	1 (0.56 oz)	79
oatmeal	1 (0.6 oz)	74
oatmeal raisin	1 (0.6 oz)	74
Betty Crocker		
Caramelita Bars as prep	1	190
Chocolate Chip as prep	2	170
Oatmeal as prep	2	160
Peanut Butter as prep	2	150
Reese's Dessert Bar Mix No Bake as prep	1	180
Sugar as prep	2	160
Sunkist Lemon Bars as prep	1	140
Turtle Cookie Bars as prep	1	180
Duncan Hines		
Chocolate Chip as prep	2 (1.1 oz)	180

READY-TO-EAT
animal crackers	1 (2.5 g)	11
animal crackers	11 (1 oz)	126
animal crackers	1 box (2.4 oz)	299
australian anzac biscuit	1	98
butter	1 (5 g)	23
chocolate chip	1 box (1.9 oz)	233
chocolate chip	1 (0.4 oz)	48
chocolate chip low sugar low sodium	1 (0.24 oz)	31
chocolate chip lowfat	1 (0.25 oz)	45
chocolate chip soft-type	1 (0.5 oz)	69
chocolate w/ creme filling	1 (0.35 oz)	47
chocolate w/ creme filling chocolate coated	1 (0.60 oz)	82

FOOD	PORTION	CALS
chocolate w/ creme filling sugar free low sodium	1 (0.35 oz)	46
chocolate w/ extra creme filling	1 (0.46 oz)	65
chocolate wafer	1 (0.2 oz)	26
cream cheese	1 (1.1 oz)	141
digestive biscuits plain	2	141
fig bars	1 (0.56 oz)	56
fortune	1 (0.28 oz)	30
fudge	1 (0.73 oz)	73
gingersnaps	1 (0.24 oz)	29
graham	1 sq (0.24 oz)	30
graham chocolate covered	1 (0.49 oz)	68
graham honey	1 (0.24 oz)	30
hermits	1 (1 oz)	117
jumbles coconut	1 (1 oz)	121
ladyfingers	1 (0.38 oz)	40
macaroons	1 (0.8 oz)	97
madeleines	1 (0.8 oz)	86
marshmallow chocolate coated	1 (0.46 oz)	55
marshmallow pie chocolate coated	1 (1.4 oz)	165
molasses	1 (0.5 oz)	65
neapolitan tri-color cookie	1 (0.6 oz)	79
oatmeal	1 (0.6 oz)	81
oatmeal soft-type	1 (0.5 oz)	61
oatmeal raisin	1 (0.6 oz)	81
oatmeal raisin low sugar no sodium	1 (0.24 oz)	31
oatmeal raisin soft-type	1 (0.5 oz)	61
peanut butter sandwich	1 (0.5 oz)	67
peanut butter sandwich sugar free low sodium	1 (0.35 oz)	54
peanut butter soft-type	1 (0.5 oz)	69
pinenut cookies	1 (1.1 oz)	134
raisin soft-type	1 (0.5 oz)	60
reginette queen's biscuit	1 (0.8 oz)	86
shortbread	1 (0.28 oz)	40
shortbread pecan	1 (0.49 oz)	79
spritz	1 (0.4 oz)	42
sugar	1 (0.52 oz)	72
sugar low sugar sodium free	1 (0.24 oz)	30
sugar wafers w/ creme filling	1 (0.12 oz)	18

FOOD	PORTION	CALS
sugar wafers w/ creme filling sugar free sodium free	1 (0.14 oz)	20
toll house original	1 (0.8 oz)	105
vanilla sandwich	1 (0.35 oz)	48
vanilla wafers	1 (0.21 oz)	28
zeppole	1 (0.8 oz)	78
6 Hour Energy		
Almond Cranberry Chocolate Chunk	½ (1.25 oz)	100
ABC		
Vegan Colossal Chocolate Chip	1 (2.1 oz)	240
Vegan Double Chocolate Decadence	1 (2.1 oz)	240
Vegan Luscious Lemon Poppyseed	1 (2.1 oz)	240
Vegan Mac The Chip	1 (2.1 oz)	250
Vegan Peanut Butter Chocolate Chip	1 (2.1 oz)	240
Vegan Phenomenal Pumpkin Spice	1 (2.1 oz)	220
Almond Joy		
Cookies	2 (1 oz)	140
Almondina		
BranTreats w/ Cinnamon	4 (1 oz)	127
Gingerspice	4 (1 oz)	137
Sesame	4 (1 oz)	138
The Original	4 (1 oz)	133
The Original Chocolate Dipped	2	130
Anna's		
Almond Cinnamon	6 (1 oz)	140
Cappuccino	6 (1 oz)	140
Chocolate Mint	6 (1 oz)	140
Orange	6 (1 oz)	140
Vanilla Chocolate Chip	6 (1 oz)	140
Annie's Homegrown		
Bunny Ginger Gluten Free	29 (1 oz)	130
Bunny Gluten Free	27 (1 oz)	120
Bunny Grahams Chocolate	27 (1 oz)	130
Bunny Grahams Honey	28 (1 oz)	140
Archway		
Coconut Macaroon	2 (1.3 oz)	160
Frosty Lemon	1 (0.9 oz)	110
Fruit Filled Raspberry	1 (0.8 oz)	90
Arico		
Gluten Free Casein Free Almond Cranberry	1 bar (1.4 oz)	140

FOOD	PORTION	CALS
Gluten Free Casein Free Double Chocolate	1 (0.9 oz)	100
Gluten Free Casein Free Lemon Ginger	1 (0.9 oz)	90
Gluten Free Casein Free Peanut Butter	1 bar (1.4 oz)	160
Arrowroot		
Biscuit	1 (5 g)	20
Aunt Gussie's		
Biscotti Almond	1 (0.8 oz)	110
Biscotti Almond Sugar Free	2 (1 oz)	150
Biscotti Cinnamon Raisin No Sugar Added	1 (0.8 oz)	110
Biscotti Italian w/ Olive Oil	2 (1.2 oz)	160
Coconut Crisp	2 (1.1 oz)	170
Latte Sugar Free	1 (0.9 oz)	110
Lemon Sugar Free	3 (1.2 oz)	160
Mexican Wedding Cakes	3 (1.2 oz)	160
Snickerdoodle	2 (1.1 oz)	180
Vanilla Spritz Sugar Free Gluten Free	2 (0.9 oz)	110
Back To Nature		
Granola Cranberry Pecan	1 (1.1 oz)	130
Granola Honey Nut	1 (1.1 oz)	140
Bahlsen		
Delice	6 (1.1 oz)	150
Deloba	5 (1.2 oz)	170
Hannover Waffeln	6 (1.1 oz)	180
Hit Cocoa Creme Filling	2 (1 oz)	150
Hit Creme Filling	2 (1 oz)	140
Waffeletten	4 (1 oz)	160
Barbara's Bakery		
Fig Bars Traditional	1	60
Fig Bars Wheat Free	1	60
Organic 100 Calorie Mini Ginger	1 pkg (0.9 oz)	100
Snackimals Chocolate Chip	10 (1 oz)	120
Snackimals Wheat Free Oatmeal	10	120
Barnum's		
Animal Crackers	10 (1 oz)	120
Barry's Bakery		
French Twists Wild Raspberry	2 (0.5 oz)	60
Bear Naked		
Granola Soft Baked Fruit & Nut	1 (1 oz)	130
Breaktime		
Ginger	4 (1 oz)	130
Oatmeal	4 (1 oz)	130

FOOD	PORTION	CALS
Brent & Sam's		
Chocolate Chip	2 (0.8 oz)	110
Brown & Haley		
Almond Roca	6 (1 oz)	110
Brown Butter Cookie		
Brown Butter Sea Salt	1 (0.7 oz)	94
Buzz Strong's		
Real Coffee	1 (1.2 oz)	150
Cameo		
Sandwich Creme	2 (1 oz)	130
Caveman Cookies		
Alpine	2 (1 oz)	150
Original	2 (1 oz)	130
Tropical	2 (1 oz)	140
Chips Ahoy!		
Chocolate Chip	1 pkg (1.4 oz)	190
Mini	1 pkg (1.2 oz)	170
Reduced Fat	1 pkg (1.1 oz)	140
Comfort Care		
Cabin Hearth Chocolate Chip	1 (2 oz)	250
Cabin Hearth Oatmeal Peach	1 (2 oz)	200
Cabin Hearth Oatmeal Raisin	1 (2 oz)	200
Country Choice Organic		
Fit Kids Snackin' Grahams Chocolate	18 (1 oz)	110
Oatmeal Chocolate Chip	1 (0.8 oz)	100
Oatmeal Raisin	1 (0.8 oz)	100
Dare		
Lemon Creme	1 (0.7 oz)	100
Maple Leaf Creme	1 (0.6 oz)	80
Delacre		
Royal Moments Milk Chocolate Biscuits	2 (0.9 oz)	130
DiCamillo		
Biscotti DiPrato	5 (1 oz)	130
Divvies		
Chocolate Chip Vegan	1	130
Oatmeal Raisin Vegan	1	120
Do Goodie		
Gluten Free Chocolate Chip	1	140
Gluten Free Oatmeal Raisin	1	120

FOOD	PORTION	CALS
Earthbound Farms		
Organic Ginger Snaps	2	120
Emily's		
Fortune Dark Chocolate Covered	2 (1.4 oz)	140
Graham Cracker Milk Chocolate Covered	1 (1 oz)	150
Enjoy Life		
Allergen Gluten Free Gingerbread Spice	2 (1 oz)	100
Allergen Gluten Free No Oats Oatmeal	2 (1 oz)	120
Allergen Gluten Free Snickerdoodle	2 (1 oz)	130
Snack Bar Sunbutter Crunch	1 (1 oz)	140
Entenmann's		
Original Chocolate Chip	3 (1 oz)	140
Erin Baker's		
Breakfast Banana Toasted Flax	1 (3 oz)	300
Breakfast Banana Walnut	1 (3 oz)	300
Breakfast Caramel Apple	1 (3 oz)	280
Breakfast Double Chocolate Chunk	1 (3 oz)	300
Breakfast Mini Fruit & Nut	1 (1 oz)	100
Breakfast Oatmeal Raisin	1 (3 oz)	290
Breakfast Vegan Chocolate Chip	1 (3 oz)	310
Organic Breakfast Mini Peanut Butter	1 (1 oz)	110
Fauchon		
Assorted Chocolate	4 (2 oz)	330
Foods By George		
Gluten Free Biscotti	1 (0.8 oz)	90
French Meadow Bakery		
Coconutty Macaroons	2 (1.1 oz)	150
Gluten Free Chocolate Chip	1 (2.1 oz)	320
Rhubarb Bar	1 (2.7 oz)	250
Vegan Peanut Butter Bliss	2 (1.2 oz)	150
Gak's Snacks		
Organic Brownie Chip	1 (1 oz)	130
Organic Chocolate Chip	1 (1 oz)	140
Organic Oatmeal	1 (1 oz)	120
Gamesa		
Animalitos	14 (1 oz)	110
Emperador Vanilla Creme Sandwich	2 (0.9 oz)	120
Hawaianas Coconut	3 (1 oz)	130
Sugar Wafers Chocolate	3 (1.2 oz)	160

FOOD	PORTION	CALS
Ginger Snaps		
Cookies	4 (1 oz)	120
Girl Scout		
Do-si-dos	2 (0.8 oz)	110
Dulce De Leche	4 (1 oz)	160
Peanut Butter Sandwich	3 (1.2 oz)	160
Samoas	2 (1 oz)	140
Savannah Smiles	5 (1 oz)	140
Shout Outs!	4 (0.9 oz)	130
Tagalongs	2 (0.9 oz)	140
Thank U Berry Munch	2 (0.9 oz)	120
Thin Mints	4 (1.1 oz)	160
Trefoils	5 (1.2 oz)	160
Gluten-Free Pantry		
Gluten Free Buckwheat Raisin	1 (1 oz)	140
Gluten Free Chocolate Chunk	1 (1 oz)	140
Glutenfreeda		
Kookies Sugar	1	142
Glutino		
Gluten Free Wafers Chocolate	4	160
Gluten Free Wafers Lemon	3	150
Gottena		
Exquisit	5	170
Gourmet Pastries		
Kourabiethes Butter Almond	1 (1.1 oz)	150
Phoenicia Honey & Spice	1 (1.3 oz)	140
Grandma's		
Chocolate Brownie	1 (1.4 oz)	190
Peanut Butter	1 (1.2 oz)	170
Vanilla Creme Sandwich	5 (1.4 oz)	190
Health Valley		
Mini Mint Chocolate Chip	4 (1 oz)	120
Oatmeal Raisin	1 (0.8 oz)	90
Raisin Oatmeal Low Fat	3	110
White Chocolate Chunk	1 (1 oz)	140
Home Free		
Organic Chocolate Chip	1 (1 oz)	140
Organic Oatmeal	1 (1 oz)	120
Honey Maid		
Grahams Honey	1 (1.1 oz)	130
Grahams Honey Low Fat	1 (1.1 oz)	120

FOOD	PORTION	CALS
Jovial		
Checkerboard Organic	2 (0.9)	120
Chocolate Cream Filled Organic	2 (1.1 oz)	160
Crispy Cocoa Organic	3 (1 oz)	140
Fig Fruit Filled Organic	2 (1.1 oz)	130
Ginger Spice Organic	2 (1.1 oz)	150
Vanilla Cream Filled Organic	2 (1.1 oz)	160
Jules Destrooper		
Butter Crisp	2 (0.9 oz)	120
Kashi		
TLC Happy Trail Mix	1 (1 oz)	130
TLC Oatmeal Dark Chocolate	1 (1 oz)	130
TLC Oatmeal Raisin Flax	1 (1 oz)	130
Kay's Naturals		
Protein + Cookie Bites All Flavors Gluten Free	1 oz	110
Kedem		
Tea Biscuits Chocolate	2 (0.3 oz)	32
Tea Biscuits Vanilla	2 (0.3 oz)	32
Keebler		
100 Calorie RightBites Fudge Shoppe Fudge Grahams	1 pkg (0.7 oz)	100
100 Calorie RightBites Sandies Shortbread	1 pkg (0.7 oz)	100
Animal Crackers Frosted	8	150
Chips Deluxe Chocolate Lovers	1	90
Chips Deluxe Coconut	2	150
Chips Deluxe Fudge Stripes	1	100
Chips Deluxe Original	1 pkg (2 oz)	300
Chocolate Dip & Cookie Sticks	1 pkg (1 oz)	130
Danish Wedding	4	130
Dipping Delights Cheesecake	1	90
E.L. Fudge Original	1	90
Fudge Shoppe Fudge Stripes	3	150
Fudge Shoppe Grasshoppers	4	140
Fudge Shoppe Mint Creme Filled	2	160
Graham Honey	8 (1 oz)	110
Graham Original	8 (1 oz)	130
Oatmeal Country Style	2	130
Sandies Drops Butter Pecan	4	140
Sandies Fudge Drops	4 (1 oz)	140
Sandies Pecan Shortbread Reduced Fat	1	80

FOOD	PORTION	CALS
Scooby-Doo Graham Sticks	9	130
S'mores Snack	1 pkg (0.8 oz)	110
Soft Batch Chocolate Chip	1	80
Vanilla Wafers	8	140
Vienna Fingers	2 (1.1 oz)	150
Vienna Fingers Reduced Fat	2 (1.1 oz)	140
Khaya		
Krunchi Orange & Chocolate	5 (1.53 oz)	240
Shortbread Grapeseed	13 (1.15 oz)	193
Shortbread Orange Rooibos	13 (1.15 oz)	259
La Choy		
Fortune	4 (1 oz)	110
Lance		
Oatmeal Creme	1 (2.5 oz)	300
Van-O-Lunch	1 pkg (1.6 oz)	230
Late July		
Organic Mini Sandwich Milk Chocolate	10 (1 oz)	130
Organic Mini Sandwich White Chocolate	10 (1 oz)	140
Lean Body		
Cookie Bar Hi-Protein S'Mores	1 (3.2 oz)	360
Liz Lovely		
Vegan Cowboy	½ cookie (1.3 oz)	190
Vegan Cowgirl	½ cookie (1.5 oz)	210
Vegan Ginger Snapdragons	½ cookie (1.5 oz)	190
Loacker		
Quadratini Dark Chocolate	9 (1.1 oz)	160
Lorna Doone		
Shortbread	4 (1 oz)	140
LU		
Le Chocolatier	3 (1 oz)	150
Le Fondant	4 (1.1 oz)	170
Le Petit Beurre	4 (1.2 oz)	140
Petit Ecolier Dark Chocolate	2 (0.9 oz)	130
Petit Ecolier Milk Chocolate	2 (0.9 oz)	130
Pim's Orange	2 (0.9 oz)	100
Shortbread	2 (1 oz)	140
Lucy's		
Chocolate Chip Gluten Free Vegan	3	130
Cinnamon Thin Gluten Free Vegan	3	130
Oatmeal Gluten Free Vegan	3	120
Sugar Gluten Free Vegan	3	130

FOOD	PORTION	CALS
Luna		
Berry Pomegranate	1 (1.4 oz)	140
Peanut Butter Chocolate	1 (1.4 oz)	150
M&M's		
Milk Chocolate	1 pkg (1.15 oz)	150
Mallomars		
Cookies	2 (0.9 oz)	120
Market Day		
Chocolate Chip Peanut Free	1 (1 oz)	150
Mauna Loa		
Macadamia Nut Chocolate Chip	4 (1 oz)	150
Miss Meringue		
Meringue Chocolate	1 pkg (1 oz)	100
Montana Monster Munchies		
Original	½ (1.4 oz)	177
Raisin	½ (1.4 oz)	172
MoonPie		
Mini All Flavors	1 pkg (1.2 oz)	130
Mrs. Fields		
Cookie Dough Snacks Brownie Chocolate Chip	7 (1 oz)	120
Cookie Dough Snacks Chocolate Chip	7 (1 oz)	120
Murray's		
Sugar Free Chocolate Chip	3 (1.1 oz)	160
Sugar Free Chocolate Sandwich	3 (1 oz)	130
Sugar Free Fudge Dipped Grahams	4 (1 oz)	150
Sugar Free Ginger Snap	7 (1.1 oz)	130
Sugar Free Oatmeal	3 (1.1 oz)	140
Sugar Free Shortbread	8 (1 oz)	130
Nabisco		
100 Calorie Pack Alpha-Bits Mini	1 pkg	100
100 Calorie Pack Barnum's Animal Choco	1 pkg	100
100 Calorie Pack Lorna Doone	1 pkg	100
100 Calorie Pack Teddy Grahams Mini Cinnamon	1 pkg	100
Grahams Original	8 (1.1 oz)	130
Nairn's		
Oat Fruit & Cinnamon	2 (0.7 oz)	85
Oat Stem Ginger	2 (0.7 oz)	87
Nana's		
No Gluten Berry Vanilla	1 bar (1.2 oz)	130

FOOD	PORTION	CALS
No Gluten Chocolate	1 (3.5 oz)	360
No Gluten Ginger	1 (3.5 oz)	360
No Gluten Nana Banana	1 bar (1.2 oz)	130
No Wheat Oatmeal Raisin	1 (3.5 oz)	280
Vegan Chocolate Chip	1 (4 oz)	320
Vegan Peanut Butter	1 (4 oz)	360
Vegan Sunflower	1 (3.5 oz)	380
Napolitanke		
Lemon Orange	4 (0.7 oz)	108
Mocca	4 (0.7 oz)	101
Natural Ovens		
Oatmeal Raisin	1 (1.3 oz)	120
New Morning		
Honey Grahams	2 (1 oz)	130
New York Style		
Biscotti Almond	3 (1 oz)	130
Newtons		
Fig	2 (1.1 oz)	110
Fig 100% Whole Grain	2 (1.3 oz)	130
Fig Fat Free	2 (1 oz)	90
Fruit Thins Cranberry Citrus Oat	3 (1 oz)	140
Raspberry	2 (1 oz)	100
Nilla Wafers		
Cookies	1 oz	140
Reduced Fat	1 oz	110
Nonni's		
Biscotti Limone	1 (0.8 oz)	110
Biscotti Original	1 (0.7 oz)	90
Biscotti Triple Cioccolati	1 (1.3 oz)	170
NutraBalance		
High Fibre	1 (0.7 oz)	90
Nutter Butter		
Bites	1 pkg (1.2 oz)	170
Sandwich Cookie	1 (1 oz)	130
Oreo		
Cakesters Mini Golden 100 Calorie Pack	1 pkg (0.8 oz)	100
Double Stuff	1 (1 oz)	140
Golden Chocolate Creme	3 (1.2 oz)	170
Reduced Fat	3 (1.2 oz)	150
Sandwich Cookie	2 (1.2 oz)	160

FOOD	PORTION	CALS
Orion		
Choco Pie	1 (1 oz)	120
Pepperidge Farm		
Bordeaux	4 (1 oz)	130
Chantilly Raspberry	2	120
Chesapeake Dark Chocolate Pecan	1 (0.9 oz)	130
Chessmen	3 (0.9 oz)	120
Dark Chocolate Mint Chocolate Chunk	1	140
Gingerman	4	130
Lemon	4 (1.1 oz)	160
Medallion Milk Chocolate	5	160
Milano	2 (1 oz)	140
Milano French Vanilla	2	130
Milano Mint Chocolate Covered	4	130
Milano Sugar Free	3	170
Nantucket Chocolate Dipped	1	150
Nantucket Dark Chocolate Chunk	1	140
Pirouettes Cappuccino	2	120
Pirouettes Chocolate Mint	2	120
Sausalito Milk Chocolate Macadamia Nut	1	140
Shortbread	2	140
Soft Baked Milk Chocolate	1	150
Soft Baked Mystic Sugar	1 (1.1 oz)	140
Soft Baked Santa Cruz Oatmeal Raisin	1 (1.1 oz)	130
Tahiti	2	170
Pirouette		
Sandwich Vanilla Creamed	3 (1.1 oz)	133
Polar		
Fortune	2	56
Q.bel		
Wafer Rolls Dark Chocolate	1 pkg (0.9 oz)	120
Wafer Rolls Milk Chocolate	1 pkg (0.9 oz)	130
Quaker		
Breakfast Cookie Oatmeal Raisin	1	180
Ruger		
Wafers Vanilla	3 (1 oz)	160
Simply Shari's		
Gluten Free Almond Shortbread	2 (1 oz)	120
Gluten Free Chocolate Chip	2 (1 oz)	120
Gluten Free Fudge Brownies	2 (1 oz)	130
Gluten Free Shortbread	2 (1 oz)	130

FOOD	PORTION	CALS
SnackWell's		
Cookie Cakes Chocolate Mint	1 (0.6 oz)	50
Devil's Food Fat Free	1 (0.5 oz)	50
Sugar Free Lemon Creme	2 (1.1 oz)	130
Sugar Free Shortbread	2 (1 oz)	130
Snikiddy		
Cherry Oaties	1 pkg (0.8 oz)	110
South Beach		
Fiber Fit Double Chocolate Chunk	1 pkg (0.8 oz)	100
Fiber Fit Oatmeal Chocolate Chunk	1 pkg (0.8 oz)	100
Wafer Sticke Dark Chocolate Hazelnut Creme	1 pkg	100
Wafer Sticke Dark Chocolate Peanut Butter	1 pkg	100
Starbucks		
Almond Roca Buttercrunch Toffee	6 (1 oz)	110
Biscotti Chocolate Hazelnut	1 (0.9 oz)	100
Madeleines Petite French Cakes	3 (1.8 oz)	230
White Chocolate & Raspberry	2 (0.9 oz)	120
Stella D'Oro		
100 Calorie Pack Breakfast Treats Original	1 pkg (0.8 oz)	100
Almond Delight	1 (1 oz)	150
Angelica Goodies	1 (0.7 oz)	90
Anginetti	4 (1.1 oz)	130
Biscotti Almond	1 (0.7 oz)	90
Biscotti French Vanilla	1 (0.7 oz)	90
Breakfast Treats Chocolate	1 (0.9 oz)	110
Breakfast Treats Original	1 (0.7 oz)	90
Coffee Treats Almond Toast	2 (0.9 oz)	100
Coffee Treats Angel Wings	3 (1 oz)	160
Coffee Treats Anisette Sponge	2 (0.9 oz)	90
Coffee Treats Anisette Toast	3 (1.2 oz)	130
Coffee Treats Roman Egg Biscuits	1 (1.1 oz)	130
Egg Jumbo	3 (1.2 oz)	120
Lady Stella	3 (1 oz)	130
Margherite	2 (1 oz)	130
Swiss Fudge	3 (1.2 oz)	170
Teddy Grahams		
Chocolate Honey	24 (1.1 oz)	130
Temptations		
Chocolate Alps	1 bar (1.6 oz)	170
Chocolate Mocha	1 bar (1.6 oz)	170
No Gluten Chocolate Rush	1 bar (1.6 oz)	170

FOOD	PORTION	CALS
Titan		
High Protein Chocolate Chip	1 (1.4 oz)	150
High Protein Oatmeal Raisin	1 (1.4 oz)	150
High Protein Peanut Butter	1 (1.4 oz)	150
Voortman		
Chinese Almond	1 (0.9 oz)	130
Coconut Delight	1 (0.6 oz)	90
Dutch Creme	1 (0.8 oz)	110
Fudge Swirl	1 (0.6 oz)	80
Gingerboy	1 (0.7 oz)	100
Maple Leaf	1 (0.6 oz)	90
Molasses	1 (1 oz)	110
Peanut Delight	1 (0.9 oz)	130
Shortbread	1 (0.6 oz)	90
Sugar Free Chocolate Chip	1 (0.7 oz)	80
Sugar Free Lemon Wafers	3 (1 oz)	130
Sugar Free Oatmeal	1 (0.7 oz)	70
Sugar Free Vanilla Creme	2 (0.7 oz)	100
Sugar Free Wafers Peanut Butter	4 (1 oz)	150
Sugar Free Wafers Vanilla	3 (1 oz)	130
Turnover Blueberry	1 (0.9 oz)	110
Turnover Cherry	1 (0.9 oz)	110
Turnover Strawberry	1 (0.9 oz)	110
Wafer Chocolate Covered	1 (0.7 oz)	100
Wafer Vanilla	3 (1 oz)	140
Wafers Mini Chocolate	5 (1 oz)	130
Walkers		
Shortbread Chocolate Chip	2 (1 oz)	140
Shortbread Rounds	2 (1.2 oz)	180
Whippet		
Original	2 (1.2 oz)	150
World Of Grains		
Apple Cinnamon	1 pkg	130
Cranberry	1 pkg	130
Multigrain	1 pkg	130
WOW		
Chocolale Brownie	1 (1.4 oz)	161
Chocolate Chip Gluten Free	1 (1.4 oz)	170
Lemon Burst Gluten Free	1 (1.4 oz)	180
Peanut Butter	1 (1.4 oz)	170

FOOD	PORTION	CALS
Zwieback		
Toast	1 (8 g)	35
REFRIGERATED		
chocolate chip	1 (0.42 oz)	59
chocolate chip dough	1 oz	126
oatmeal	1 (0.4 oz)	56
oatmeal raisin	1 (0.4 oz)	56
peanut butter	1 (0.4 oz)	60
peanut butter dough	1 oz	130
sugar	1 (0.42 oz)	58
sugar dough	1 oz	124
Pillsbury		
Chocolate Chip	2 (1.3 oz)	170
Gingerbread	2 (1.1 oz)	170
Oatmeal Chocolate Chip	2 (1.3 oz)	170
Peanut Butter	2 (1 oz)	130
S'Mores	2 (1.3 oz)	160
Sugar	2 (1.3 oz)	170
TAKE-OUT		
biscotti w/ nuts chocolate dipped	1 (1.3 oz)	117
black & white	1 lg (3 oz)	302
finikia	1 (1.2 oz)	171
koulourakia butter cookie twist	1 (0.9 oz)	113
linzer tart	1 (2.4 oz)	280
CORIANDER		
leaf dried	1 tsp	2
leaf fresh	¼ cup	1
seed	1 tsp	5
CORN		
CANNED		
cream style	½ cup	93
w/ red & green peppers	½ cup	86
white	½ cup	66
yellow	½ cup	66
Del Monte		
Cream Style Sweet Corn	½ cup (4.4 oz)	70
Savory Sides In Butter Sauce	½ cup	90
Savory Sides Santa Fe	½ cup	70
Whole Kernel	½ cup (4.4 oz)	60

FOOD	PORTION	CALS
Green Giant		
Mexicorn	½ cup (3.3 oz)	90
Super Sweet Yellow & White	⅓ cup (2.6 oz)	60
Whole Kernel	½ cup (4.3 oz)	90
Jake & Amos		
Pickled Dill Baby Corn	2 tbsp	5
Orchids		
Whole Young Spears	½ cup (4.6 oz)	25
DRIED		
Crunchies		
Freeze Dried Corn Snack	⅓ cup (1 oz)	130
Freeze Dried Sweet Buttered	½ cup (1 oz)	100
Sunrich Naturals		
Toasted Corn Cool Ranch	1 pkg (1 oz)	100
FRESH		
white cooked	½ cup	89
white raw	½ cup	66
yellow cooked	1 ear (2.7 oz)	83
yellow cooked	½ cup	89
yellow raw	1 ear (3 oz)	77
yellow raw	½ cup	66
FROZEN		
cooked	½ cup	67
on the cob cooked	1 ear (2.2 oz)	59
Birds Eye		
Steamfresh Singles Super Sweet	1 pkg (3.2 oz)	80
Steamfresh Southwestern	⅔ cup (2.9 oz)	90
Steamfresh Sweet Mini Corn On The Cob	1 (3 oz)	90
C&W		
Cheddar Bacon	½ cup	130
Early Harvest Supersweet Petite	⅔ cup	70
Salsa Corn	1 cup	90
Glory		
Savory Accents Fried Corn	½ cup	110
Green Giant		
Cream Style	½ cup	110
Nibblers On-The-Cob	1 (2.1 oz)	70
Health Is Wealth		
Creamed	½ pkg (4.5 oz)	110
Stouffer's		
Souffle	½ pkg (6 oz)	150

FOOD	PORTION	CALS
TAKE-OUT		
fritters	1 (1 oz)	62
on the cob w/ butter cooked	1 ear	155
scalloped	1 cup	257

CORN CHIPS (see CHIPS)

CORNISH HEN (see CHICKEN)

CORNMEAL

cornmeal mush as prep w/ water	1 cup	223
cornmeal yellow	½ cup (2.2 oz)	236
whole grain blue	½ cup (1.9 oz)	201
yellow self-rising	½ cup (3 oz)	296
Indian Head		
Stone Ground	¼ cup	100
Martha White		
White Enriched	3 tbsp (1.2 oz)	120
White Self Rising	3 tbsp (1.1 oz)	100
Yellow Self Rising	3 tbsp (1.1 oz)	110
Quaker		
Instant Original not prep	1 pkg (1 oz)	100
Quick Grits not prep	¼ cup (1.3 oz)	130
TAKE-OUT		
corn pone	1 piece (2.1 oz)	128
fritter puerto rican style	1 (1.4 oz)	109
harina de maize con coco	½ cup	383
harina de maize con leche	1 cup	295
hush puppies	1 (0.8 oz)	74
johnnycake	1 piece (1.7 oz)	134

CORNSTARCH

cornstarch	1 tbsp (0.3 oz)	34
cornstarch	¼ cup (1.1 oz)	122
Argo		
Cornstarch	1 tbsp (0.3 oz)	30
Bob's Red Mill		
Cornstarch	1 tbsp	30
Clabber Girl		
Cornstarch Calcium Fortified	1 tbsp (0.4 oz)	35
Rumford		
Cornstarch Calcium Fortified	1 tbsp (0.4 oz)	35

FOOD	PORTION	CALS
COTTAGE CHEESE		
creamed large curd	½ cup (4 oz)	110
creamed small curd	½ cup (3.7 oz)	103
dry curd	½ cup (2.5 oz)	52
lowfat 1%	½ cup (4 oz)	81
lowfat 1% lactose reduced	½ cup (4 oz)	84
Axelrod		
Lowfat 1%	½ cup (4 oz)	90
Breakstone's		
2% Low Fat Small Curd	½ cup (4.4 oz)	100
4% Fat Small Curd	½ cup (4.4 oz)	120
LiveActive Mixed Berries	1 pkg (4 oz)	120
Cabot		
Cottage Cheese	½ cup	100
No Fat	½ cup	70
Friendship		
1% Lowfat	½ cup	90
1% Lowfat No Salt Added	½ cup	90
1% Lowfat Whipped	½ cup	90
2% Digestive Health	½ cup	90
2% Pot Style	½ cup	90
4% California Style	½ cup	110
Nonfat	½ cup	80
Horizon Organic		
Lowfat	½ cup	100
Regular	½ cup	120
Knudsen		
LiveActive Pineapple	1 pkg (4 oz)	110
Lactaid		
Lowfat	½ cup (4 oz)	80
Land O'Lakes		
1% Lowfat	½ cup (4 oz)	90
2% Lowfat	½ cup (3.7 oz)	100
Cottage Cheese	½ cup (3.7 oz)	110
Fat Free	½ cup (4 oz)	80
Nancy's		
Organic Lowfat	½ cup	80
Organic Valley		
Low Fat	½ cup	100

FOOD	PORTION	CALS
COTTONSEED		
kernels roasted	1 tbsp	51
COUSCOUS		
cooked	1 cup (5.5 oz)	176
dry	1 cup (6.1 oz)	650
Bob's Red Mill		
Pearl not prep	⅓ cup (2 oz)	210
Pearl Tricolor not prep	⅓ cup (2 oz)	210
Pearl Whole Wheat not prep	⅓ cup (2 oz)	190
Marrakesh Express		
Mango Salsa as prep	1 cup	190
Mushroom as prep	1 cup	190
Plain as prep	1 cup	270
Near East		
Mediterranean Curry as prep	1 cup	220
Original Plain as prep	1 cup	190
Parmesan as prep	1 cup	220
Toasted Pine Nut as prep	1 cup	230
Wild Mushroom & Herb as prep	1 cup	230
CRAB		
CANNED		
blue	½ cup	67
blue drained	1 can (6.5 oz)	124
Ace Of Diamonds		
Fancy w/ Leg Meat	¼ cup (2 oz)	40
Chicken Of The Sea		
Fancy	⅓ can (2 oz)	40
Jumbo Lump	⅓ can (2 oz)	35
Polar		
Claw Meat	¼ cup (2 oz)	37
Jumbo Lump Meat	¼ cup (2 oz)	39
Wild Planet		
Dungeness	2 oz	62
FRESH		
alaska king meat only steamed	3 oz	82
blue cooked flaked	1 cup (4 oz)	120
dungeness steamed	3 oz	94
queen steamed	3 oz	98

FOOD	PORTION	CALS
Dockside Classics		
Crabcakes	1 (2.5 oz)	150
FROZEN		
Mama Belle's		
Crab Cakes Maryland Style	1 (2 oz)	100
Mrs. Paul's		
Deviled Crab Cakes	1 (3 oz)	220
SeaPak		
Maryland Style Crab Cakes + Sauce	1 (4 oz)	240
TAKE-OUT		
alaska king leg steamed	1 leg (4.7 oz)	130
baked	1 (3.8 oz)	160
cakes	2 (4.2 oz)	186
crab imperial	1 crab (6.8 oz)	289
crab salad	1 serv (5.5 oz)	285
crab thermidor	1 serv (6.4 oz)	456
deviled	1 serv (4.5 oz)	254
dungeness steamed	1 crab (4.5 oz)	140
empanada de jueyes	1 (4.4 oz)	341
fried crab puffs	4 (3.2 oz)	323
kenagi korean crab cooked	1 serv (3 oz)	71
salmorejo de jueyes (in tomato sauce)	1 serv (4.5 oz)	215
soft-shell breaded & fried	1 med (2.3 oz)	216
taco de jueyes	1 (4.2 oz)	266
CRACKER CRUMBS		
cracker meal	1 cup	440
graham cracker crumbs	1 cup	355
Honey Maid		
Graham Cracker Crumbs	2½ tbsp (0.6 oz)	70
Keebler		
Graham	¼ cup	93
CRACKERS		
melba toast round	1	12
oyster cracker	¼ cup	48
saltines	1	13
water biscuits	3	92
zwieback	1 oz	107
34 Degrees		
Crispbread Sesame	19 (1.1 oz)	140
Whole Grain	9 (0.5 oz)	35

FOOD	PORTION	CALS
Annie's Homegrown		
Cheddar Bunnies Original	50 (1 oz)	140
Aunt Gussie's		
Cracker Flats Spelt Cinnamon Raisin	1 (1 oz)	100
Cracker Flats Spelt Everything	1 (0.8 oz)	60
Back To Nature		
Poppy Thyme	17 (1 oz)	130
Rice Thin Sesame Ginger	16	120
Sesame Tarragon	17 (1 oz)	130
Barbara's Bakery		
Rite Rounds Lite Original	5 (0.5 oz)	60
Wheatines Original	4	60
Better Cheddars		
Original	1.1 oz	160
Blue Diamond		
Nut-Thins Almond Country Ranch	16 (1 oz)	130
Bran Crispbread		
GG Scandinavian	1 (0.4 oz)	12
Bremner Wafers		
Cracked Wheat	7 (0.5 oz)	70
Original	7 (0.5 oz)	70
Soup & Chili Crackers	50 (0.5 oz)	60
Breton		
Garden Vegetable	4 (0.7 oz)	100
Minis Cheddar Cheese	20 (0.7 oz)	100
Brown Rice Snaps		
Cheddar	6	60
Original Tamari Seaweed	9	60
Unsalted Plain	8	60
Cheese Nips		
Cheddar	1 pkg (1.2 oz)	170
Cheez-It		
Crackers	13 (1 oz)	150
Chicken Biskit		
Original	1.1 oz	160
Daelia's		
Biscuits For Cheese Almond w/ Raisins	4 (1 oz)	133
Biscuits For Cheese Hazelnut w/ Figs	4 (1 oz)	133
Dare		
Crackers	3 (0.5 oz)	70

FOOD	PORTION	CALS
Original	4 (0.7 oz)	90
Reduced Fat & Salt	5 (0.7 oz)	80
Dr. Kracker		
Flatbread Klassic Seed	1 (1 oz)	120
Flatbread Pumpkin Seed Cheddar	1 (1 oz)	120
Flatbread Seeded Spelt	1 (1 oz)	120
Flatbread Seedlander	1 (1 oz)	120
Flatbread Spelt Sunflower Cheddar	1 (1 oz)	120
Krispy Grahams	5 (1 oz)	110
Flatout		
Edge On Baked Flatbread Four Cheese	15 (1 oz)	130
Edge On Baked Flatbread Garlic Herb	15 (1 oz)	120
Glutino		
Gluten Free	4 (0.5 oz)	70
Gluten Free Rusks	2 (0.7 oz)	80
GrainsFirst		
Autumn Harvest	7 (1.1 oz)	140
Grissol		
Crispy Baguettes Garden Herb	8 (1 oz)	110
Health Valley		
Organic Bruschetta Vegetable	4	70
Organic Cracked Pepper	4	70
Organic Cracker Stix Garlic Herb	8	70
Organic Whole Wheat	4	70
Kashi		
Heart To Heart Whole Grain	7 (1 oz)	120
TLC Natural Ranch	15 (1 oz)	130
TLC Original 7 Grain	15 (1 oz)	130
TLC Party Mediterranean Bruschetta	4	120
TLC Snack Fire Roasted Vegetable	5	130
TLC Toasted Asiago	15 (1.1 oz)	130
Keebler		
Club Multi-Grain	4	70
Club Original	4 (0.5 oz)	70
Club Reduced Fat	5	70
Club Snack Sticks	12	130
Puffed Original	24	140
Sandwich Cheese & Peanut Butter	1 pkg (1.4 oz)	200
Sandwich Toast & Peanut Butter	1 pkg (1.4 oz)	200
Sandwich Wheat & Cheddar	1 pkg (1.3 oz)	190

FOOD	PORTION	CALS
Toasteds Harvest Wheat	16	130
Toasteds Sesame	5	80
Toasteds Wheat	5	80
Town House Bistro	2	80
Town House FlipSides Original	5	70
Town House Original	5 (0.5 oz)	80
Town House Reduced Fat	6	60
Town House Reduced Sodium	5	80
Town House Toppers	3	70
Wheatables 33% Less Fat	19	140
Wheatables Original	17	140
Zesta Saltine Fat Free	5	60
Zesta Saltine Original	5	60
Kellogg's		
All Bran Garlic Herb	18 (1 oz)	120
Special K Cracker Chips Southwest Ranch	27 (1 oz)	110
Kim's Magic Pop		
Onion	1 (5 g)	15
Kitchen Table Bakers		
Aged Parmesan	3	80
Everything	3	80
Garlic	3	80
Jalapeno	3	80
Lance		
Captain Wafers	4	70
Nekot	1 pkg (1.7 oz)	240
Nipchee	1 pkg (1.4 oz)	190
Peanut Butter On Wheat	1 pkg (1.4 oz)	200
Toastchee	1 pkg (1.5 oz)	220
Toastchee Reduced Fat	1 pkg (1.4 oz)	180
Larzaroni		
Bruschette w/ Olives	9 (1.1 oz)	140
Mary's Gone Crackers		
Wheat Free Gluten Free Black Pepper	13 (1 oz)	140
Wheat Free Gluten Free Onion	13 (1 oz)	140
Wheat Free Gluten Free Original Seed	13 (1 oz)	140
Mediterranean Crackers		
Feta & Oregano	3 (0.6 oz)	91
Mediterranean Snacks		
Lentil Cracked Pepper Gluten Free	18 (1 oz)	110
Lentil Sea Salt Gluten Free	18 (1 oz)	110

FOOD	PORTION	CALS
Nabisco		
Garden Harvest Apple Cinnamon	16 (1 oz)	120
Garden Harvest Banana	16 (1 oz)	120
Garden Harvest Tomato Basil	16 (1 oz)	120
Garden Harvest Vegetable Medley	16 (1 oz)	120
Vegetable Thins	21 (1 oz)	150
Nairn's		
Oatcake Fine	2 (0.5 oz)	70
Oatcake Rough	2 (0.8 oz)	91
New York Style		
Crispini Seeds & Spice	6	120
Panetini Original	2	80
Panetini Three Cheese	2	80
Pita Chips Garlic	7	130
Pita Chips Natural Whole Wheat	7	120
Nonni's		
Panetini Roasted Garlic	5 (1 oz)	120
Panetini Sun Dried Tomato Basil	5 (1 oz)	120
Orkney		
Oatcakes Thin	4 (1.8 oz)	227
Pepperidge Farm		
100 Calorie Pack Goldfish Cheddar	1 pkg	100
100 Calorie Pack Goldfish Pretzel	1 pkg	100
Goldfish Cinnamon Graham	1 pkg	210
Goldfish Pizza	55	140
Goldfish Reduced Sodium Cheddar	60	140
Goldfish w/ Whole Grain Cheddar	55 (1.1 oz)	140
Snack Sticks Pumpernickel	15	120
Water Crackers	4	60
Wheat Crisps Spicy Salsa	16	140
Premium		
Saltines Fat Free	5 (0.5 oz)	60
Saltines Low Sodium	5 (0.5 oz)	80
Saltines Multigrain	5 (0.5 oz)	60
Saltines Original	5 (0.5 oz)	60
Ritz		
Bites Cheese	13 (1 oz)	150
Hint Of Salt	0.5 oz	80
Original	0.5 oz	80
Reduced Fat	5 (0.5 oz)	70

FOOD	PORTION	CALS
Roasted Vegetable	5 (0.5 oz)	80
Sociables		
Original	0.5 oz	70
SunRidge Farms		
Japanese Rice	¼ cup (1 oz)	110
Suzie's		
Flatbreads Garlic Salt	1 oz	70
Triscuit		
Fire Roasted Tomato	1 oz	120
Garden Herb	1 oz	120
Hint Of Salt	1 oz	130
Original	1 oz	120
Reduced Fat	1 oz	120
Rosemary & Olive Oil	1 oz	120
Thin Crisps Original	1 oz	130
Thin Crisps Quattro Formaggio	1.1 oz	140
True North		
Peanut Crunches	¼ cup (1 oz)	150
Pistachio Crisps	12 (1 oz)	140
Utz		
Cheese Peanut Butter	6	200
Vegetable Thins		
Original	21 (1.1 oz)	150
Vinta		
Original	3 (0.7 oz)	100
Wasa		
Hearty	1 (0.5 oz)	45
Light Rye	2 (0.6 oz)	60
Multi Grain	1 (0.5 oz)	45
Sourdough	1 (0.4 oz)	35
Whole Grain	1 (0.4 oz)	40
Whole Wheat	1 (0.5 oz)	50
Water Crackers		
Original	6 (0.5 oz)	60
Wellaby's		
Cheese Ups Classic Cheese Gluten Free	1 cup (1 oz)	122
Cheese Ups Parmesan	1 cup (1 oz)	122
Feta Oregano & Olive Oil Gluten Free	8 (1.1 oz)	130
Original Cheese Mini Gluten Free	8 (1.1 oz)	130

FOOD	PORTION	CALS
Westminster		
Oyster	1 pkg (0.5 oz)	66
Wheat Thins		
100% Whole Grain	1 oz	140
Low Sodium	1.1 oz	150
Original	16 (1.1 oz)	140
Reduced Fat	1 oz	130
Wheatsworth		
Crackers	5 (0.5 oz)	80
CRANBERRIES		
cranberry orange relish	¼ cup	118
dried	½ cup	85
fresh chopped	1 cup	13
fresh whole	1 cup	11
sauce	1 slice (2 oz)	86
sauce	¼ cup	109
Chukar Cherries		
North Cove Dried	¼ cup	100
Craisins		
Blueberry	⅓ cup	140
Cherry	⅓ cup	130
Dried Cranberries	⅓ cup	130
Orange	⅓ cup	130
De-Lite		
Dried Sweetened	1 oz	92
Dole		
Fresh Whole	1 cup (3.3 oz)	45
Earthbound Farms		
Organic Dried	⅓ cup	130
Emily's		
Milk Chocolate Covered	¼ cup (1.4 oz)	180
Fool		
Cranberry Spread	1 tbsp	30
Fruitaceuticals		
OmegaCrans Dried	¼ cup	91
Mariani		
Dried Sweetened	⅓ cup	130
Ocean Spray		
Fresh	2 oz	30

FOOD	PORTION	CALS
Jellied Sauce	¼ cup (2.5 oz)	110
Whole Berry Sauce	¼ cup (2.5 oz)	110
S&W		
Sauce Jellied	¼ cup (2.5 oz)	100
Sauce Whole Berry	¼ cup (2.5 oz)	100
Sarabeth's		
Relish	1 tbsp (0.7 oz)	45
Stoneridge Orchards		
Dried	⅓ cup (¼ oz)	140
Sun-Maid		
Dried Cape Cod	⅓ cup (1.4 oz)	130
Sunsweet		
Dried	⅓ cup (1.4 oz)	140
Tree Of Life		
Organic Jellied	¼ cup (2.5 oz)	100
Truitt Brothers		
Sauce Orchard Medley	⅓ cup (2.7 oz)	90
Wild Thymes Farm		
Cranberry Fig Sauce	1 tsp	19
Original Cranberry Sauce	1 tbsp	21

CRANBERRY BEANS

canned	½ cup	108
dried cooked w/o salt	½ cup	120
Goya		
Roman Beans Dried not prep	¼ cup (1.4 oz)	80

CRANBERRY JUICE

cranberry juice cocktail low calorie w/ vitamin C	8 oz	46
cranberry juice cocktail w/ vitamin C	8 oz	137
unsweetened	8 oz	116
Apple & Eve		
100% Juice	8 oz	130
Lakewood		
Organic	6 oz	50
Organic Light	6 oz	45
Nantucket Nectars		
Cranberry Cocktail	8 oz	130
Northland		
100% Juice No Sugar Added	8 oz	130

FOOD	PORTION	CALS
Ocean Spray		
100% Juice Cranberry Blend	8 oz	140
Cocktail	8 oz	120
Cocktail Light	8 oz	40
Diet	8 oz	5
White Cocktail Light	8 oz	40
White Cranberry	8 oz	110
White Cranberry Strawberry	8 oz	110
Old Orchard		
Cranberry Naturals Classic Cranberry	8 oz	80
Santa Cruz		
Organic Nectar	8 oz	110
SSips		
Cocktail	1 box (7 oz)	110
CRAYFISH		
cooked	3 oz	97
raw	8	24
raw	3 oz	76
CREAM (see also WHIPPED TOPPINGS)		
clotted cream	2 tbsp (1 oz)	164
creme fraiche	2 tbsp (1 oz)	100
half & half	¼ cup (2.1 oz)	79
half & half	1 pkg (0.5 oz)	20
half & half	1 tbsp (0.5 oz)	20
half & half fat free	4 oz	67
heavy whipping	½ cup (4.2 oz)	411
heavy whipping	1 tbsp (0.5 oz)	52
heavy whipping whipped	½ cup (2.1 oz)	207
light coffee	½ cup (4.2 oz)	234
light coffee	1 tbsp (0.5 oz)	29
light coffee	1 pkg (0.4 oz)	22
whipped pressurized can	½ cup (1 oz)	77
whipped pressurized can	4 tbsp (0.4 oz)	31
Cabot		
Whipped	2 tbsp	15
Horizon Organic		
Half & Half	2 tbsp	35
Heavy Whipping	1 tbsp	50
Lactaid		
Half & Half	2 tbsp (1 oz)	40

FOOD	PORTION	CALS
Land O'Lakes		
Aerosol Whipped Light Cream	2 tbsp (0.2 oz)	20
Half & Half	2 tbsp (1.1 oz)	35
Half & Half Fat Free	2 tbsp (1.1 oz)	20
Heavy Whipping	1 tbsp (0.5 oz)	50
Organic Valley		
Half & Half	2 tbsp (1 oz)	40
Straus		
Organic Half And Half	2 tbsp (1 oz)	35
CREAM CHEESE		
cream cheese	1 oz	99
cream cheese	1 pkg (3 oz)	297
Connoisseur		
Wheel Mango Peach	2 tbsp	110
Wheel Wild Blueberry	2 tbsp	100
Earth Balance		
Brick	2 tbsp	80
Tub	2 tbsp	80
Horizon Organic		
Reduced Fat	2 tbsp	70
Lifeway		
Whipped	2 tbsp	80
Nancy's		
Organic	2 tbsp	95
Organic Valley		
Cream Cheese	1 oz	100
Soft	2 tbsp	90
Philadelphia		
⅓ Less Fat	2 tbsp (1.1 oz)	70
Original	1 in cube (1 oz)	100
Whipped	2 tbsp	60
CREAM CHEESE SUBSTITUTES		
Tofutti		
Better Than Cream Cheese All Flavors	2 tbsp (1 oz)	60
Vegan Gourmet		
Alternative Cream Cheese	2 tbsp (1 oz)	90
CREAM OF TARTAR		
cream of tartar	1 tsp	8

FOOD	PORTION	CALS
CREPES		
basic crepe unfilled	1 (7 in)	112
Ekizian		
Chickpea Crepe	1 (7 in) (1.5 oz)	212
Tandoor Chef		
Masala Dosa	1 (3 oz)	162
CROAKER		
atlantic breaded & fried	3 oz	188
atlantic raw	3 oz	89
CROCODILE		
cooked	3 oz	78
CROISSANT		
apple	1 (2 oz)	145
butter	1 lg (2.4 oz)	272
butter mini	1 (1 oz)	114
cheese	1 (1.5 oz)	174
chocolate	1 (2 oz)	237
TAKE-OUT		
w/ egg & cheese	1 (4.5 oz)	368
w/ egg & sausage	1 (5 oz)	497
w/ egg cheese & bacon	1 (4.1 oz)	385
w/ egg cheese & ham	1 (5.1 oz)	402
w/ egg cheese & sausage	1 (5.6 oz)	539
w/ ham & cheese	1 (4 oz)	338
CROUTONS		
plain	1 cup (1 oz)	122
seasoned	1 cup (1.4 oz)	186
Chatham Village		
Cheese & Garlic	2 tbsp (7 g)	40
Edward & Sons		
Organic Lightly Salted	2 tbsp	30
Fresh Gourmet		
Butter & Garlic	7 (7 g)	35
Cheese & Garlic	12 (0.5 oz)	70
Classic Caesar	6 (7 g)	35
Cornbread Sweet Butter	½ cup (1 oz)	110
Country Ranch	6 (7 g)	35
Fat Free Garlic Caesar	12 (7 g)	30

FOOD	PORTION	CALS
Italian Seasoned	6 (7 g)	35
Organic Seasoned	5 (7 g)	30
Pepperidge Farm		
Whole Grain Seasoned	6	30
Zesty Italian	6	30

CUCUMBER

fresh peeled	1 med (7 oz)	24
fresh sliced	1 cup	14
fresh w/ peel sliced	½ cup	8
TAKE-OUT		
cucumber & onion salad w/ vinegar	1 cup	52
cucumber raita	1 serv (3.3 oz)	40
cucumber salad w/ oil & vinegar	1 cup	183
cucumber salad w/ sour cream dressing	1 cup	68
kimchee	½ cup (1.8 oz)	36
tzatziki	½ cup (3.4 oz)	72

CUMIN

seed	1 tsp (2 g)	8
seed	1 tbsp (6 g)	22

CURRANT JUICE

black currant nectar	7 oz	110
red currant nectar	7 oz	108
Fructal		
Black Currant	1 bottle (6.75 oz)	102
GoodBelly		
Black Currant Probiotic Drink	8 oz	120

CURRANTS

black fresh	½ cup	36
zante dried	½ cup	204
Sun-Maid		
Zante	¼ cup (1.4 oz)	120

CURRY

curry powder	1 tsp	7
curry sauce mix as prep	1 cup	120
curry sauce mix as prep w/ milk	1 cup	270
paste	1 tube (6 oz)	465
Ethnic Gourmet		
Gujarati Vegetable Curry	1 pkg (10 oz)	380

FOOD	PORTION	CALS
Malay Chicken Curry	1 pkg (10 oz)	410
Simmer Sauce Bombay Curry	4 oz	70
Fortun's		
Finishing Sauce Mulligatawny Curry	¼ cup (2 oz)	60
French Meadow Bakery		
Fragrant Chicken Curry	1 pkg (12 oz)	280
Helen's Kitchen		
Indian Curry w/ Tofu Steaks & Rice	1 pkg (9 oz)	300
Kikkoman		
Sauce Thai Red Curry	¼ cup (2.2 oz)	90
Sauce Thai Yellow Curry	¼ cup (2.2 oz)	90
Knorr		
Curry Sauce Indian Madras	1 oz	30
Curry Sauce Thai	1 oz	35
Patak's		
Curry Paste Biryani	2 tbsp	180
Garam Masala Paste	2 tsp	130
Tandoori Paste	2 tbsp	30
Vegetable Curry w/ Rice Rich Creamy Coconut	1 pkg	400
Vegetable Curry w/ Rice Rich Tomato & Onion	1 pkg (10.5 oz)	290
Vegetable Curry w/ Rice Tangy Lemon & Cilantro	1 pkg	300
Vindaloo Paste	2 tbsp	160
So-Yah!		
Creamy Coconut Curry	1 pkg (10 oz)	190
Red Vindaloo Curry	1 pkg (10 oz)	150
Spice Hunter		
Curry Seasoning Salt Free	¼ tsp	0
Tandoor Chef		
Chicken Curry	1 pkg (9.9 oz)	330
Kofta Curry	½ pkg (5 oz)	100
TastyBite		
Green Curry Vegetables & Jasmine Rice	1 pkg (12 oz)	320
Yellow Curry Vegetables & Jasmine Rice	1 pkg (12 oz)	380
Thai Kitchen		
Green Curry Paste	1 tbsp (0.5 oz)	15
Red Curry Paste	1 tbsp (0.5 oz)	15
TAKE-OUT		
beef curry	1 cup	432
beef kurma	1 serv (10 oz)	611

FOOD	PORTION	CALS
chicken curry ½ breast	1 serv	160
chicken curry boneless	1 serv (6.2 oz)	219
chicken curry leg & thigh	1 serv	180
chickpea curry	1 serv (8.3 oz)	305
eggplant curry	1 serv (8 oz)	241
lamb curry	1 cup	257
mixed vegetable curry	1 serv (7.7 oz)	398
pea & potato curry	1 serv (7 oz)	284
pork vandaloo curry	1 serv	620
potato curry	1 serv (5.5 oz)	791
sambhar dhal curry	1 serv (10 oz)	177
shrimp curry	1 cup (8.3 oz)	276

CUSK

fillet baked	3 oz	106

CUSTARD

MIX

egg custard as prep w/ 2% milk	1 serv (3.5 oz)	112
egg custard as prep w/ whole milk	1 serv (3.5 oz)	122
flan as prep w/ 2% milk	1 serv (3.5 oz)	103
flan as prep w/ whole milk	1 serv (3.5 oz)	113

READY-TO-EAT

Kozy Shack

Custard	1 pkg (4 oz)	130

Signature

Flan Coffee	1 pkg (4.5 oz)	340
Flan Vanilla	1 pkg (4.5 oz)	350

TAKE-OUT

baked	½ cup (5 oz)	147
flan	½ cup (5.4 oz)	222
flan de calabaza	1 serv (3.5 oz)	225
flan de coco	½ cup (4.3 oz)	345
flan de pina	1 serv (4.2 oz)	186
flan de pini	½ cup (4.6 oz)	202
puerto rican corn custard	½ cup (4.9 oz)	553
tocino del cielo heaven's delight	1 cup	856
zabaione	½ cup (2 oz)	135

CUTTLEFISH

steamed	3 oz	134

FOOD	PORTION	CALS
DANDELION GREENS		
fresh cooked	½ cup	17
raw chopped	½ cup	13
DANISH PASTRY		
READY-TO-EAT		
Entenmann's		
Pecan Danish Ring	⅛ ring (1.9 oz)	240
TAKE-OUT		
cheese	1 (2.5 oz)	266
cinnamon	1 (5 oz)	572
fruit	1 (5 oz)	527
lemon	1 (2.5 oz)	263
raisin nut	1 (2.3 oz)	280
DATES		
deglet noor chopped	¼ cup (1.3 oz)	104
deglet noor dried	1 (7 g)	20
jujube dried	1 oz	75
jujube fresh	1 oz	30
jujube preserved in sugar	1 oz	91
medjool	1 (0.8 oz)	66
Bard Valley Growers		
Medjool	1	63
Bob's Red Mill		
Dried Crumbles	⅓ cup	130
Dole		
California Chopped	¼ cup (1.4 oz)	120
Earthbound Farms		
Organic Dried	6 (1.4 oz)	120
SunDate		
Fancy Medjool	3 (1.4 oz)	120
Sun-Maid		
Pitted	¼ cup (1.4 oz)	110
Tree Of Life		
Deglet Noor Pitted	5 (1.5 oz)	120
Organic Medjool	5 (1.5 oz)	120

DEER (*see* JERKY, VENISON)

FOOD	PORTION	CALS
DELI MEATS/COLD CUTS (*see also* BEEF, CHICKEN, HAM, MEAT SUBSTITUTES, TURKEY)		
barbecue loaf pork & beef	1 slice (0.8 oz)	40
beerwurst beef	2 oz	155
berliner pork & beef	1 slice (0.8 oz)	53
blood sausage	1 slice (0.9 oz)	95
bologna beef	1 slice (1 oz)	88
bologna beef & pork lowfat	1 slice (1 oz)	64
bologna beef lowfat	1 slice (1 oz)	57
bologna beef reduced sodium	1 slice (1 oz)	88
bologna beef & pork	1 slice (1 oz)	87
braunschweiger pork	1 slice (1 oz)	92
corned beef brisket	2 oz	90
dutch brand loaf pork & beef	1 slice (1.3 oz)	104
headcheese pork	1 slice (1.6 oz)	71
honey loaf pork & beef	1 slice (1 oz)	35
lebanon bologna beef	2 slices (1 oz)	105
mortadella beef & pork	1 slice (0.5 oz)	47
olive loaf pork	2 slices (2 oz)	134
pastrami beef	1 slice (1 oz)	41
peppered loaf pork & beef	1 slice (1 oz)	41
pepperoni pork & beef	15 slices (1 oz)	135
picnic loaf pork & beef	1 slice (1 oz)	65
salami cooked beef & pork	1 slice (0.8 oz)	58
salami hard pork	3 slices (0.9 oz)	14
salami hard pork & beef less sodium	1 slice (1 oz)	113
sandwich spread pork & beef	¼ cup	141
summer sausage thuringer cervelat	2 oz	203
Applegate Farms		
Organic Genoa Salami Sliced	1 oz	100
Butterball		
Turkey Bologna	1 slice (1 oz)	60
Turkey Ham	1 slice (1 oz)	35
Carl Buddig		
Beef	2 oz	90
Corned Beef	2 oz	90
Dietz & Watson		
Bologna Beef	3 slices (1.9 oz)	170
Mortadella	2 oz	150
Sopressata	1 oz	90

FOOD	PORTION	CALS
Foster Farms		
Bologna Chicken	1 slice (1 oz)	60
Healthy Ones		
Pastrami 97% Fat Free	4 slices (2 oz)	60
High Plains Bison		
Pastrami	3 oz	80
Oscar Mayer		
Salami Beef	3 slices (1.8 oz)	150
DILL		
seed	1 tsp	6
sprigs fresh	5 (0.3 oz)	0
weed dry	1 tbsp	8

DINNER (*see also* ASIAN FOOD, CURRY, PASTA DINNERS, POT PIE, SPANISH FOOD)

FOOD	PORTION	CALS
A La Carte		
Stuffed Zucchini w/ Barley Risotto Chicken Stuffing in Tomato Sauce	1 serv (5 oz)	140
Amy's		
Country Dinner Vegetable Salisbury Steak	1 pkg (10.9 oz)	380
Banquet		
Boneless Pork Ribs	1 pkg	370
Chicken Fingers	1 pkg	460
Corn Dog Meal	1 pkg	470
Crock Pot Classics Chicken & Dumplings	⅔ cup	200
Crock Pot Classics Hearty Beef & Vegetables	⅔ cup	140
Crock Pot Classics Meatballs In Stroganoff Sauce	⅔ cup	300
Fish Sticks	1 pkg	360
Fried Beef Steak	1 pkg	390
Meatloaf	1 pkg	300
Original Fried Chicken	1 pkg	380
Salisbury Steak	1 pkg	300
Swedish Meatballs	1 pkg	430
Turkey	1 pkg	200
Betty Crocker		
Complete Meals Chicken & Buttermilk Biscuits	⅕ pkg (5.4 oz)	280
Complete Meals Stroganoff	⅕ pkg (5 oz)	200

FOOD	PORTION	CALS
Birds Eye		
Steamfresh Meals For Two Asian Chicken Vegetable Medley	½ pkg (11.9 oz)	290
Steamfresh Meals For Two Grilled Chicken Marinara	½ pkg (11.9 oz)	360
Steamfresh Meals For Two Sweet & Spicy Chicken	½ pkg (11.9 oz)	370
Voila! Pasta Primavera w/ Chicken	1⅔ cups	250
Voila! Shrimp Scampi	1¾ cups	190
Voila! Southwestern Chicken	2 cups	250
C&W		
Stir Fry Feast Pot Sticker + Sauce	2 cups	200
Stir Fry Feast Ultimate + Sauce	1½ cups	190
Campbell's		
Supper Bakes Cheesy Chicken w/ Pasta	⅙ pkg	170
Supper Bakes Garlic Chicken w/ Pasta	⅙ pkg	220
Supper Bakes Savory Pork Chops w/ Herb Stuffing	⅙ box	160
Supper Bakes Traditional Roast Chicken w/ Stuffing	⅙ pkg	160
Candle Cafe		
Ginger Miso Stir Fry	1 pkg (9 oz)	200
Seitan Piccata w/ Lemon Caper Sauce	1 pkg (9 oz)	210
Contessa		
Beef Goulash not prep	1¾ cups	210
Chicken Alfredo not prep	1¾ cups	330
Chicken Cacciatore not prep	1¾ cups	230
French Meadow Bakery		
Garlic Ginger Chicken	1 pkg (12 oz)	310
Gardein		
Burgundy Trio	1 pkg	230
Thai Trio	1 pkg	250
Glory		
Savory Singles Chicken & Dumplings	1 pkg	290
Savory Singles Chicken Smoked Sausage & Rice Casserole	1 pkg	440
Savory Singles Ham & Sausage Jambalaya	1 pkg	400
Savory Singles Turkey & Gravy w/ Cornbread Stuffing	1 pkg	440

FOOD	PORTION	CALS
Gluten Free Cafe		
Lemon Basil Chicken	1 pkg (9.2 oz)	340
Glutino		
Gluten Free Chicken Pomodoro w/ Brown Rice & Vegetables	1 pkg (9.1 oz)	190
Gluten Free Chicken Ranchero w/ Brown Rice	1 pkg (9.1 oz)	180
Green Giant		
Create A Meal Stir Fry Sweet & Sour as prep	1 cup	280
Skillet Meal Chicken Teriyaki as prep	1½ cups	240
Healthy Choice		
Bacon & Smokey Cheddar Chicken	1 pkg (8.6 oz)	240
Beef Tips Portabello	1 pkg (11.2 oz)	270
Country Breaded Chicken	1 pkg (10.6 oz)	340
Fire Roasted Tomato Chicken	1 pkg (11.6 oz)	310
Fresh Mixers Creamy Roasted Garlic Chicken	1 pkg (7.4 oz)	310
Fresh Mixers Steak Portobello	1 pkg (7.5 oz)	290
Fresh Mixers Sweet Hickory BBQ Chicken	1 pkg (7.9 oz)	370
Grilled Chicken Monterey	1 pkg (10.9 oz)	320
Lemon Pepper Fish	1 pkg (10.6 oz)	300
Lunch Steamers Garlic Herb Shrimp	1 pkg (8.5 oz)	260
Lunch Steamers Lemon Herb Chicken	1 pkg (8.7 oz)	210
Lunch Steamers Rosemary Chicken & Sweet Potatoes	1 pkg (8.9 oz)	170
Pineapple Chicken	1 pkg (9 oz)	380
Portabella Spinach Parmesan	1 pkg (9.3 oz)	270
Salisbury Steak	1 pkg (8 oz)	170
Spicy Caribbean Chicken	1 pkg (8.5 oz)	310
Turkey Breast & Cranberries	1 pkg (10.7 oz)	250
Hormel		
Compleats Microwave Meals Beef Steak & Peppers w/ Noodles	1 pkg (9.9 oz)	210
Compleats Microwave Meals Chicken Breast & Dressing	1 pkg (9.9 oz)	270
Compleats Microwave Meals Chicken Breast & Gravy w/ Mashed Potatoes	1 pkg (9.9 oz)	200
Compleats Microwave Meals Homestyle Beef w/ Potatoes & Gravy	1 pkg (9.9 oz)	220
Compleats Microwave Meals Meatloaf w/ Potatoes & Gravy	1 pkg (9.9 oz)	310

FOOD	PORTION	CALS
Compleats Microwave Meals Salisbury Steak w/ Slice Potato & Gravy	1 pkg (9.9 oz)	280
Compleats Microwave Meals Santa Fe Chicken w/ Rice & Beans	1 pkg (9.9 oz)	280
Compleats Microwave Meals Swedish Meatballs	1 pkg (9.9 oz)	350
Compleats Microwave Meals Sweet & Sour Chicken w/ Rice	1 pkg (9.9 oz)	290
Compleats Microwave Meals Teriyaki Chicken w/ Rice	1 pkg (9.9 oz)	270
Compleats Microwave Meals Tuna Casserole	1 pkg (9.9 oz)	240
Compleats Microwave Meals Turkey & Dressing w/ Gravy	1 pkg (9.9 oz)	290
Compleats Microwave Meals Turkey & Hearty Vegetables	1 pkg (9.9 oz)	180
Joy Of Cooking		
Braised Beef Tips & Egg Noodles	1 cup (7.7 oz)	220
Roasted Herb Chicken	1 cup (7.7 oz)	170
Kashi		
Black Bean Mango	1 pkg (10 oz)	340
Lemon Rosemary Chicken	1 pkg (10 oz)	330
Lime Cilantro Shrimp	1 pkg (10 oz)	250
Southwest Style Chicken	1 pkg (10 oz)	240
Sweet & Sour Chicken	1 pkg (10 oz)	320
Lean Cuisine		
Cafe Cuisine Chicken & Vegetables	1 pkg (10.5 oz)	220
Cafe Cuisine Chicken Marsala	1 pkg (8.1 oz)	250
Cafe Cuisine Lemon Pepper Fish	1 pkg (9 oz)	290
Cafe Cuisine Orange Chicken	1 pkg (9 oz)	300
Cafe Cuisine Roasted Garlic Chicken	1 pkg (8.8 oz)	170
Cafe Cuisine Steak Tips Portabello	1 pkg (7.5 oz)	150
Casual Cuisine Flatbread Melts Steakhouse Ranch	1 pkg (6.25 oz)	350
Comfort Classics Baked Chicken	1 pkg (8.6 oz)	240
Comfort Cuisine Beef Pot Roast	1 pkg (9 oz)	210
Comfort Cuisine Meatloaf w/ Gravy & Whipped Potatoes	1 pkg (9.4 oz)	250
Comfort Cuisine Roasted Turkey Breast w/ Dressing	1 pkg (9.75 oz)	290

FOOD	PORTION	CALS
Comfort Cuisine Salisbury Steak w/ Mac & Cheese	1 pkg (9.5 oz)	260
Dinnertime Selects Balsamic Glazed Chicken	1 pkg (12 oz)	330
Dinnertime Selects Chicken Florentine	1 pkg (13.25 oz)	410
Dinnertime Selects Chicken Portabello	1 pkg (12 oz)	390
Dinnertime Selects Salisbury Steak	1 pkg (12.5 oz)	270
Market Creations Chicken Poblano	1 pkg (10.5 oz)	300
Market Creations Shrimp Scampi	1 pkg (10.5 oz)	250
Market Creations Sweet & Spicy Ginger Chicken	1 pkg (10.5 oz)	280
Simple Favorites Quesadilla BBQ Chicken	1 pkg (5 oz)	280
Simple Favorites Stuffed Cabbage	1 pkg (9.5 oz)	210
Simple Favorites Swedish Meatballs	1 pkg (9.1 oz)	290
Spa Cuisine Chicken Mediterranean	1 pkg (10.5 oz)	240
Spa Cuisine Chicken In Peanut Sauce	1 pkg (9 oz)	280
Spa Cuisine Chicken Pecan	1 pkg (9 oz)	310
Spa Cuisine Lemon Chicken	1 pkg (9 oz)	290
Spa Cuisine Lemongrass Chicken	1 pkg (9.4 oz)	250
Spa Cuisine Rosemary Chicken	1 pkg (8.25 oz)	210
Spa Cuisine Salmon w/ Basil	1 pkg (9.5 oz)	210
Marie Callender's		
Chicken Fried Beef	1 meal	540
Chicken Teriyaki	1 meal	430
Golden Battered Filet Dinner	1 meal	450
Herb Roasted Chicken	1 meal	460
Meat Loaf w/ Gravy	1 meal	480
Old Fashioned Beef Pot Roast	1 meal	330
Salisbury Steak	1 meal	400
Slow Roasted Beef	1 meal	370
Sweet & Sour Chicken	1 meal	600
Turkey w/ Stuffing	1 meal	400
Meal Mart		
Stuffed Cabbage Beef Hungarian Style	¼ pkg (2.5 oz)	210
Meals To Live		
Grilled White Chicken w/ Brown Rice & Vegetables Gluten Free	1 pkg (9 oz)	260
Grilled White Chicken w/ Red Roasted Potatoes & Green Beans	1 pkg (8 oz)	200
Shrimp Jambalaya Gluten Free	1 pkg (9 oz)	220

FOOD	PORTION	CALS
Sliced Turkey w/ Balsamic Sauce & Butternut Squash Gluten Free	1 pkg (7 oz)	230
Stacked Eggplant w/ Seasoned White Chicken	1 pkg (9 oz)	200
White Chicken Fajita w/ Santa Fe Rice Gluten Free	1 pkg (9 oz)	240
Mon Cuisine		
Vegan Moroccan Couscous	1 pkg (10 oz)	280
Vegan Veal Schnitzel In Sauce	1 pkg (10 oz)	300
Vegetarian Stuffed Cabbage In Tomato Sauce	1 pkg (10 oz)	220
Moosewood		
Organic Vegetarian Moroccan Stew	1 pkg (10 oz)	150
Organic Bistro		
Alaskan Salmon Cakes	1 pkg (10 oz)	410
Chicken Citron	1 pkg (13.5 oz)	490
Ginger Chicken	1 pkg (13.25 oz)	490
Jamaican Shrimp Cakes	1 pkg (12 oz)	380
Savory Turkey	1 pkg (12 oz)	430
Spiced Chicken Morocco	1 pkg (12.2 oz)	390
Wild Salmon	1 pkg (13.1 oz)	500
Organic Classics		
Chicken Marsala w/ Mashed Potatoes	1 pkg (9.5 oz)	330
Jamaican Style Jerk Chicken w/ Wehani Rice	1 pkg (9.5 oz)	270
Lemon Chicken w/ Wehani Rice	1 pkg (9.5 oz)	320
Simply Sensible		
Beef Pot Roast & Gravy w/ Mashed Potatoes	½ pkg (8.5 oz)	220
Beef Tips & Gravy w/ Brown Rice	1 cup (7 oz)	200
Zing Chicken & Brown Rice	1 cup (7 oz)	230
South Beach		
Chicken Santa Fe Style Rice & Beans	1 pkg (8.9 oz)	340
Meatloaf w/ Gravy	1 pkg (8.9 oz)	210
Roasted Turkey	1 pkg (9.4 oz)	240
Stouffer's		
Beef Stew	1 pkg (11 oz)	280
Beef Stroganoff	1 pkg (9.75 oz)	380
Chicken A La King	1 pkg (11.5 oz)	360
Corner Bistro Bourbon Steak Tips	1 pkg (12 oz)	520
Corner Bistro Sesame Chicken	1 pkg (12.63 oz)	510
Country Fried Beef Steak	1 pkg (16 oz)	610
Creamed Chipped Beef	½ pkg (5.5 oz)	140
Fish Filet	1 pkg (9 oz)	400

FOOD	PORTION	CALS
Fried Chicken Breast	1 pkg (8.88 oz)	360
Green Pepper Steak	1 pkg (10.5 oz)	240
Grilled Chicken Teriyaki	1 pkg (9.38 oz)	300
Grilled Lemon Pepper Chicken	1 pkg (9 oz)	240
Pork Cutlet	1 pkg (10 oz)	370
Roast Pork	1 pkg (9.5 oz)	320
Roast Turkey Breast	1 pkg (16 oz)	390
Salisbury Steak	1 pkg (16 oz)	470
Stuffed Pepper	1 pkg (10 oz)	220
Swedish Meatballs	1 pkg (11.5 oz)	560
Sukhis		
Tikka Masala Chicken	1 serv (5 oz)	170
Swanson		
Chicken & Dumplings	1 cup	230
Chicken A La King	1 can	270
Taste Above		
Meatless Zesty BBQ w/ Veggie Beef & Rice	1 pkg (10 oz)	280
TastyBite		
Beans Marsala & Basmati Rice	1 pkg (12 oz)	426
Spinach Dal & Basmati Rice	1 pkg (12 oz)	372
Stir Fry Vegetables & Jasmine Rice	1 pkg (12 oz)	450
Vegetable Supreme & Basmati Rice	1 pkg (12 oz)	317
The Fillo Factory		
Fillo Pie Spinach & Cheese	⅕ pie (4.8 oz)	270
Weight Watchers		
Smart Ones Sesame Chicken	1 pkg (11.7 oz)	360
Yves		
Meatless Santa Fe Beef	1 pkg (10.5 oz)	360
Zatarain's		
Blackened Chicken w/ Yellow Rice	1 pkg (10.5 oz)	470
Jambalaya w/ Sausage	1 pkg (12 oz)	500
Red Beans & Rice w/ Sausage	1 pkg (12 oz)	510
Rice Bowl Big Easy	1 pkg (10 oz)	430
Sausage & Chicken Gumbo w/ Rice	1 pkg (12 oz)	300

DIP

FOOD	PORTION	CALS
shrimp cream cheese	¼ cup (2 oz)	152
spinach sour cream	¼ cup	155
Cabot		
French Onion	2 tbsp	50
Ranch	2 tbsp	50

FOOD	PORTION	CALS
Cedarlane		
Organic Five Layer Mexican	2 tbsp	60
Emerald Valley		
Organic Black Bean	1 tbsp (1 oz)	45
Fritos		
Bean	2 tbsp (1.2 oz)	35
Chili Cheese	2 tbsp (1.2 oz)	45
Guiltless Gourmet		
Black Bean Mild	2 tbsp (1.1 oz)	40
Health Is Wealth		
Vegetarian Spinach & Artichoke	3 tbsp (1 oz)	30
Kraft		
Green Onion	2 tbsp	60
Lay's		
Country Ranch Mix as prep w/ sour cream	2 tbsp (1.1 oz)	70
French Onion	2 tbsp (1.2 oz)	60
LiteHouse		
Avocado	2 tbsp	140
Caramel Low Fat	1 tbsp	110
Caramel Original	2 tbsp	110
Dilly	2 tbsp	150
Fruit Dip Chocolate Yogurt	2 tbsp	110
Fruit Dip Vanilla Yogurt	2 tbsp	60
Lite Ranch Veggie	2 tbsp	70
Organic Ranch	2 tbsp	130
Marie's		
French Onion Roasted	2 tbsp	100
Guacamole	2 tbsp	40
Honey Vanilla Cream Fruit Dip	2 tbsp	60
Spinach Parmesan	2 tbsp	90
Naturally Fresh		
Caramel	2 tbsp	100
Chocolate	2 tbsp	70
Cream Cheese Strawberry	2 tbsp	90
Ranch Lite	2 tbsp	80
Ranch Vegetable	2 tbsp	120
Road's End Organics		
Nacho Cheese Gluten Free	2 tbsp	20
Robert Rothchild Farm		
Artichoke	2 tbsp	60

FOOD	PORTION	CALS
Salpica		
Chipotle Hummus Bean	2 tbsp (1 oz)	40
Cowgirl White Bean	2 tbsp (1 oz)	25
Salsa Con Queso	2 tbsp (1 oz)	20
Snyder's Of Hanover		
Three Bean	2 tbsp	25
Tostitos		
Creamy Spinach	2 tbsp (1.1 oz)	50
Dip Creations Mix Freshly Made Guacamole as prep w/ avocados	2 tbsp (1.1 oz)	50
Zesty Bean & Cheese Medium	2 tbsp (1.2 oz)	45
Utz		
Jalapeno Cheddar	2 tbsp	260
Sour Cream & Onion	2 tbsp	60
Walden Farms		
Blue Cheese Calorie Free	2 tbsp (1 oz)	0
Ranch No Calorie	2 tbsp (1 oz)	0
Want'ems		
Sweet Chili Fusion	2 tbsp (1.1 oz)	50
Thai Mango Fusion	2 tbsp (1.1 oz)	40
Wild Thymes Farm		
Indian Vindaloo Curry	1 tbsp	12
Indonesian Peanut Sauce	1 tbsp	32
DOCK		
fresh cooked	3½ oz	20
raw chopped	½ cup	15
DOUGHNUTS		
chocolate glazed	1 med (1.5 oz)	175
chocolate w/ chocolate icing	1 med (2 oz)	218
creme filled	1 (3 oz)	307
custard filled	1 (2.3 oz)	235
french cruller glazed	1 med (1.4 oz)	169
jelly filled	1 (3 oz)	289
old fashioned plain	1 med (2 oz)	226
plain chocolate frosted	1 med (1.5 oz)	194
plain glazed	1 med (1.6 oz)	192
whole wheat sugared	1 med (1.6 oz)	162
Entenmann's		
Crumb	1 (1.9 oz)	230

FOOD	PORTION	CALS
Glazed	1 (2 oz)	250
Mini Rich Frosted Chocolate	1 (1.1 oz)	170
Old Fashion Plain	1 (1.7 oz)	230
Pop'Ems Cinnamon	4 (2 oz)	250
Pop'Ems Glazed Crullers	2 (1.6 oz)	210
Pop'Ems Holes Rich Frosted	4 (2.1 oz)	320
Rich Frosted	1 (1.9 oz)	240
TAKE-OUT		
andagi okinawan doughnut	1 (0.7 oz)	84
malasada portuguese ball	1 (1.1 oz)	118
DRINK MIXERS		
whiskey sour mix not prep	1 pkg (0.6 oz)	64
whiskey sour mix	2 oz	55
Angostura		
Bloody Mary	4 oz	20
Daiquiri	2 oz	72
Daiquiri Strawberry	8 oz	120
Grenadine	1 tsp	10
Margarita	4 oz	80
Pina Colada	4 oz	60
Arizona		
Pina Colada Virgin Cocktail	8 oz	90
Dave's Gourmet		
Bloody Mary Original	2 oz	25
Fever-Tree		
Bitter Lemon	1 bottle (6.8 oz)	75
Go Cocktails!		
On-The-Go Sugar Free Appletini	1 pkg (1.9 g)	5
On-The-Go Sugar Free Cosmo	1 pkg (2.2 g)	5
On-The-Go Sugar Free Lemon Drop	1 pkg (2.5 g)	5
On-The-Go Sugar Free Margarita	1 pkg (2.78 g)	5
Margaritaville		
Margarita Mix Mango	4 oz	120
Margarita Mix Original Lime	4 oz	110
McIlhenny		
Bloody Mary Mix as prep	1 cup	70
Modmix		
Mojito	2 oz	50
Organic Citrus Margarita	2 oz	70

FOOD	PORTION	CALS
Organic French Martini	2 oz	50
Organic Lavender Lemon Drop	2 oz	55
Organic Pomegranate Cosmopolitan	2 oz	55
Organic Wasabi Bloody Mary	2 oz	20
Monin		
Grenadine	1 oz	90
Mojito Mix	1 oz	84
White Sangria Mix	1 oz	91
Old Orchard		
Daiquiri Mixer Strawberry frzn as prep	8 oz	120
Margarita Mixer frzn as prep	8 oz	120
Pina Colada Mixer frzn as prep	8 oz	120
Prometheus Springs		
Capsaicin Spiced Elixir Citrus Cayenne	8 oz	70
Capsaicin Spiced Elixir Lychee Wasabi	8 oz	80
Capsaicin Spiced Elixir Mango Chili	8 oz	70
Capsaicin Spiced Elixir Spicy Pear	8 oz	70
DRUM		
freshwater baked	3 oz	130
freshwater fillet baked	5.4 oz	236
DUCK		
boneless roasted	½ duck (7.8 oz)	444
boneless w/o skin roasted	3.5 oz	201
boneless w/o skin roasted diced	1 cup (4.9 oz)	281
chinese pressed	1 cup (4.9 oz)	267
chinese pressed	3 oz	162
pekin breast boneless w/ skin roasted	1 (4.2 oz)	242
pekin breast w/o skin broiled	3 oz	133
pekin leg w/ skin w/o bone roasted	1 (3.2 oz)	200
pekin leg w/o skin & bone roasted	1 (2.6 oz)	134
w/ skin & bone roasted	1 serv (6 oz)	583
w/ skin & bone roasted	½ duck (13 oz)	1287
wing roasted bone removed	1 (1.1 oz)	101
Grimaud Farms		
Muscovy Duck Confit	1 serv (3 oz)	170
Muscovy Duck Whole	1 serv (3.7 oz)	200
TAKE-OUT		
breast battered & fried bone removed	½ (3.2 oz)	199
leg battered & fried bone removed	1 (2.5 oz)	155

FOOD	PORTION	CALS
DUMPLING		
Crazy Cuizine		
Potstickers Chicken w/ Sauce	8 (5 oz)	220
Potstickers Pork w/o Sauce	8 (5 oz)	240
Fujisan		
Chicken Shumai Dumplings	3 (3 oz)	130
Health Is Wealth		
Potstickers Vegan	2 (1.6 oz)	90
Healthy Choice		
Sweet Asian Potstickers Entree	1 pkg (9.9 oz)	340
Joyce Chen		
Chinese Style Potstickers Chicken & Vegetable	6	170
Chinese Style Potstickers Pork & Vegetable	6	170
Kahiki		
Potstickers Chicken	5 (3.3 oz)	230
Samosas Coconut Curry Chicken	4 (2.8 oz)	170
Lean Cuisine		
Market Creations Pot Stickers Chicken	1 pkg (10 oz)	270
Simple Favorites Asian Pot Stickers	1 pkg (9 oz)	260
Panni		
Spaetzle Authentic German not prep	2 oz	200
Pepperidge Farm		
Apple	1	250
Peach	1	320
Traveling Chef		
Potstickers Chicken + Dipping Sauce	5 pieces + 1 tbsp sauce	285
TAKE-OUT		
apple	1 (6.7 oz)	661
bread dumpling	1 lg	330
cherry	1 (2.7 oz)	238
cornmeal	1 (2.8 oz)	134
fried pork	1 (3.5 oz)	338
fried puerto rican style	1 med (1.1 oz)	117
gyoza potstickers vegetable	8 (4.9 oz)	210
peach	1 (2.7 oz)	253
piroshki meat filled	1 (3.4 oz)	348
steamed meat	1 (1.3 oz)	41
DURIAN		
fresh	3.5 oz	141

FOOD	PORTION	CALS

EDAMAME (see SOYBEANS)

EEL

FOOD	PORTION	CALS
fresh cooked	1 fillet (5.6 oz)	375
fresh cooked	3 oz	200
raw	3 oz	156
smoked	3.5 oz	330

EGG (see also EGG DISHES, EGG SUBSTITUTES)

CHICKEN

FOOD	PORTION	CALS
fresh small	1 (1.3 oz)	54
fresh medium	1 (1.5 oz)	63
fresh large	1 (1.8 oz)	72
hard or soft cooked	1	77
pickled	1	72
poached	1	73
scrambled plain	1 (2 oz)	61
sunny side up	2	155
white raw	1 (1.1 oz)	17
yolk raw	1 (0.5 oz)	55

Davidson's

FOOD	PORTION	CALS
Pasteurized Shell Eggs	1 lg	75

Egg Innovations

FOOD	PORTION	CALS
100% Organic Cage Free Large	1 (1.8 oz)	70

Egg-Land's Best

FOOD	PORTION	CALS
Extra Large	1 (2 oz)	80
Hard-Cooked Peeled	1 med (1.5 oz)	60
Large	1 (1.8 oz)	70

Good Earth Organics

FOOD	PORTION	CALS
Organic Instant Whites	1 pkg (0.5 oz)	50

Horizon Organic

FOOD	PORTION	CALS
Jumbo	1 (2.2 oz)	90

Jake & Amos

FOOD	PORTION	CALS
Pickled Red Beet Eggs	2 (5.3 oz)	200

Land O'Lakes

FOOD	PORTION	CALS
Farm Fresh Brown Extra Large	1 (1.8 oz)	70

Organic Valley

FOOD	PORTION	CALS
Egg Whites Pasteurized	¼ cup	25
Large Omega-3	1	70

Pete & Gerry's

FOOD	PORTION	CALS
Organic Large	1 (1.8 oz)	70

FOOD	PORTION	CALS
Safest Choice		
Pasteurized Fresh	1 lg (1.8 oz)	70
Tree Of Life		
White Large Natural Omega-3	1 (1.8 oz)	70
OTHER POULTRY		
duck 100 year old	1 (1 oz)	49
duck cooked	1 (2.5 oz)	129
duck preserved hard core	1 (1.8 oz)	80
duck preserved soft core	1 (1.8 oz)	80
duck salted	1 (1 oz)	54
goose cooked	1 (5 oz)	265
quail canned	1 (0.3 oz)	14
quail cooked	1 (0.5 oz)	24
turkey raw	1 (2.8 oz)	135
EGG DISHES		
Aunt Jemima		
Eggs & Sausage	1 pkg (6.2 oz)	320
Omelet Ham & Cheese	1 pkg (5.2 oz)	240
Scramble Ham & Egg	1 pkg (6.8 oz)	260
Cedarlane		
Zone Omelette Cheese	1 pkg (10.4 oz)	350
Jimmy Dean		
Breakfast Bowls D-Lights Sausage	1 pkg	230
Breakfast Bowls Eggs Potato & Ham	1 pkg	390
Breakfast Bowls Eggs Potato Sausage & Cheddar Cheese	1 pkg	490
Breakfast Skillets Bacon as prep	1 serv (4.5 oz)	370
Breakfast Skillets Ham as prep	1 serv (4.5 oz)	270
Breakfast Skillets Smoked Sausage as prep	1 serv (4.5 oz)	380
Omelets Ham & Cheese	1 (4.2 oz)	280
Omelets Sausage & Cheese	1 (4.3 oz)	270
Meals To Live		
Spinach Omelet w/ Turkey Sausage Gluten Free	1 pkg (7.5 oz)	190
Weight Watchers		
Smart Ones Smart Morning Wrap Egg Sausage & Cheese	2 (4 oz)	240
TAKE-OUT		
deviled	1 half	62
eggs benedict	2	825
omelet cheese	3 eggs	387

FOOD	PORTION	CALS
omelet mushroom	3 eggs	251
omelet mushroom & onion	3 eggs	294
omelet plain	3 eggs	338
omelet spanish	3 eggs	496
omelet spinach	3 eggs	279
omelet western	3 eggs	355
salad	½ cup	353
scotch egg	1 (4.2 oz)	301
tortilla de amarillo omelet w/ plantain	3 eggs	536

EGG ROLLS

egg roll wrapper fresh	1 (1.1 oz)	93
Blue Horizon Organic		
Spring Rolls Chinese Shrimp	3 (2.1 oz)	130
Spring Rolls Indian	3 (2.1 oz)	110
Spring Rolls Thai	3 (2.1 oz)	110
Spring Rolls Thai Shrimp	3 (2.1 oz)	130
Health Is Wealth		
Spinach	1 (3 oz)	170
Thai Spring Roll	2 (1.6 oz)	90
Kahiki		
Chicken	1 (3 oz)	160
Chipotle Lime Chicken	1 (3 oz)	170
Lemongrass Chicken Stix	3 (2.6 oz)	100
Pork & Shrimp	1 (3 oz)	140
Vegetable	1 (3 oz)	90
Lean Cuisine		
Casual Cuisine Spring Rolls Fajita Chicken	½ pkg	200
Casual Cuisine Spring Rolls Garlic Chicken	½ pkg	200
Simple Favorites Eggroll Vegetable	1 pkg (9 oz)	320
TAKE-OUT		
chicken	1 (3 oz)	140
lobster	1 (4.8 oz)	270
lumpia vegetable & shrimp	2 (3 oz)	120
meat & shrimp	1 (4.8 oz)	320
pork & shrimp	1 (5 oz)	300
shrimp	1 (2.2 oz)	156
spicy pork	1 (3 oz)	200
spring roll deep fried	1 (0.8 oz)	70
vegetable	1 (3 oz)	170

FOOD	PORTION	CALS
EGG SUBSTITUTES		
Bob's Red Mill		
Egg White Dried	2 tsp	15
Vegetarian Egg Replacer	1 tbsp	30
Egg Beaters		
Original	¼ cup (2.1 oz)	30
EggPro		
Powder	1 tbsp	15
Horizon Organic		
Liquid Egg	¼ cup	35
Quick Eggs		
Fat Free Cholesterol Free	¼ cup	30
EGGNOG		
eggnog	1 cup	342
eggnog	1 qt	1368
eggnog flavor mix as prep w/ milk	9 oz	260
Farmland		
Egg Nog	½ cup	180
Horizon Organic		
Lowfat	½ cup	140
Lactaid		
Eggnog	½ cup (4 oz)	170
Organic Valley		
Ultra Pasteurized	½ cup	180
Straus		
Organic	4 oz	160
TAKE-OUT		
eggnog	1 cup	306
EGGNOG SUBSTITUTES		
Silk		
Nog	½ cup (4 oz)	90
EGGPLANT		
cubed cooked w/ oil	1 cup	133
pickled	½ cup	33
slices grilled	1 (2 oz)	36
Cedarlane		
Eggplant Mediterranean	1 pkg (10 oz)	230
Celentano		
Eggplant Parmigiana	1 serv (7 oz)	330

FOOD	PORTION	CALS
Peloponnese		
Baba Ganoush	2 tbsp	40
Stonewall Kitchen		
Eggplant Spread	1 tbsp	25
TastyBite		
Punjab Eggplant	½ pkg (5 oz)	144
The Gracious Gourmet		
Tapenade Roasted Eggplant	2 tbsp (1 oz)	35
TAKE-OUT		
baba ghannouj	¼ cup	55
caponata	2 tbsp (1 oz)	30
iman bayildi eggplant w/ onion & tomato	1 serv (15.6 oz)	345
indian eggplant runi	1 serv	180
moussaka	1 serv (9 oz)	372
papoutsaki little shoes	1 serv (15.5 oz)	245
tempura	1 serv (1.5 oz)	118
ELDERBERRIES		
fresh	1 cup	105
ELDERBERRY JUICE		
elderberry	7 oz	76
ELK		
eye of round roasted	3.5 oz	151
ground cooked	3.5 oz	143
Natural Frontier Foods		
Filet	1 (4 oz)	140
EMU		
cooked	3 oz	130
ENERGY BARS (*see also* CEREAL BARS, FRUIT AND NUT BARS, NUTRITION SUPPLEMENTS)		
Activex		
Organic All Flavors	1 (1.6 oz)	200
Attune		
Wellness Chocolate Crisp	1 (0.7 oz)	100
Wellness Cool Mint Chocolate	1 (0.7 oz)	100
Balance		
100 Calories Peanut Butter Crisp	1 (1 oz)	100
100 Calories Vanilla Crisp	1 (1 oz)	100
Carbwell Chocolate Fudge	1 (1.8 oz)	190

FOOD	PORTION	CALS
Gold Chocolate Peanut Butter	1 (1.8 oz)	210
Gold S'mores Crunch	1 (1.8 oz)	210
Organic Apricot Mango Crisp	1 (1.6 oz)	180
Organic Cranberry Pomegranate Crisp	1 (1.6 oz)	180
Original Almond Brownie	1 (1.8 oz)	200
Original Mocha Crisp	1 (1.8 oz)	200
Pure Banana Cashew	1 (1.6 oz)	180
Pure Cherry Pecan	1 (1.6 oz)	190
Boomi Bar		
Almond Protein Plus	1	270
Cashew Almond Delicacy	1	260
Cranberry Apple	1	210
Merry Macadamia	1	220
Pistachio Pineapple	1	200
Bora Bora		
Organic Island Brazil Nut Almond	1 (1.4 oz)	200
Organic Peanut Peanut	1 (1.4 oz)	230
Organic Sesame Raisin	1 (1.4 oz)	170
Clif		
Apricot	1 (2.4 oz)	230
Black Cherry Almond	1 (2.4 oz)	250
Builders Chocolate	1 (2.4 oz)	270
Builders Lemon	1 (2.4 oz)	270
Chocolate Almond Fudge	1 (2.4 oz)	250
Chocolate Chip Peanut Crunch	1 (2.4 oz)	260
Crunchy Peanut Butter	1 (2.4 oz)	250
Mojo Chocolate Peanut	1 (1.6 oz)	210
Mojo Honey Roasted Peanuts	1 (1.6 oz)	200
Mojo Mountain Mix	1 (1.6 oz)	180
Mojo Peanut Butter & Jelly	1 (1.6 oz)	220
Nectar Cherry Pomegranate	1 (1.6 oz)	150
Nectar Dark Chocolate Walnut	1 (1.6 oz)	160
Oatmeal Raisin Walnut	1 (2.4 oz)	240
Spiced Pumpkin Pie	1 (2.4 oz)	240
Vanilla Almond	1 (2.4 oz)	270
ZBar Blueberry	1 (1.3 oz)	120
ZBar Honey Graham	1 (1.3 oz)	130
ZBar Spooky S'mores	1 (1.3 oz)	130
Glenny's		
Fruit & Nut Mixed Nut	1	230

FOOD	PORTION	CALS
Glucerna		
All Flavors	1 (0.7 oz)	80
Granola Gourmet		
Chocolate Espresso	1 (1.23 oz)	150
Ultimate Berry	1 (1.2 oz)	150
Ultimate Cran-Orange	1 (1.2 oz)	140
Ultimate Fudge Brownie	1 (1.3 oz)	150
Ultimate Mocha Fudge	1 (1.2 oz)	150
Green SuperFood		
Whole Food	1 (2.1 oz)	220
Whole Food Chocolate	1 (2.1 oz)	230
Halo		
Honey Graham	1 (1.3 oz)	150
Nutty Marshmallow	1 (1.3 oz)	150
Rocky Road	1 (1.3 oz)	160
S'Mores	1 (1.3 oz)	150
JojoBar		
Chocolate Cashew	1 (1.8 oz)	220
Peanut Butter & Jelly	1 (1.8 oz)	220
Kashi		
GoLean Chocolate Almond Toffee	1 (2.7 oz)	290
GoLean Cookies 'N Cream	1 (2.7 oz)	290
GoLean Crunchy Chocolate Peanut	1 (1.8 oz)	180
GoLean Malted Chocolate Chip	1 (2.7 oz)	290
GoLean Oatmeal Raisin Cookie	1 (2.7 oz)	280
GoLean Peanut Butter & Chocolate	1 (2.7 oz)	290
GoLean Roll Caramel Peanut	1 (1.9 oz)	200
GoLean Roll Fudge Sundae	1 (1.9 oz)	190
TLC Chewy Granola Cherry Dark Chocolate	1 (1.2 oz)	120
TLC Crunchy Granola Honey Toasted 7 Grain	1 (1.4 oz)	180
TLC Crunchy Granola Pumpkin Spice	1 (1.4 oz)	180
TLC Crunchy Granola Roasted Almond	1 (1.4 oz)	180
LaraBar		
Jocalat Chocolate	1 (1.7 oz)	190
Lean Body		
Gold Caramel Cookie Twist	1 (2.9 oz)	330
Living Harvest		
Organic Hemp Protein Forbidden Fruit	1 (1.6 oz)	170
Luna		
Berry Almond	1 (1.7 oz)	170

FOOD	PORTION	CALS
Chai Tea	1 (1.7 oz)	190
Dulce De Leche	1 (1.7 oz)	170
Mini Caramel Nut Brownie	1 (0.7 oz)	70
Mini S'mores	1 (0.7 oz)	80
Sunrise Apple Cinnamon	1 (1.7 oz)	180
Sunrise Strawberry Crunch	1 (1.7 oz)	170
Toasted Nuts 'N Cranberry	1 (1.7 oz)	170
Mrs. May's		
Trio Blueberry	1 (1.2 oz)	170
Trio Tropical	1 (1.2 oz)	170
Muscle Milk		
Light Chocolate Peanut Caramel	1 (1.59 oz)	170
Nature's Path		
Optimum Pomegran Cherry	1 (2 oz)	230
Nogii		
No Gluten High Protein Peanut Butter & Chocolate	1 (2 oz)	230
Nutiva		
Organic Flax & Raisin	1 (1.4 oz)	200
Organic Flaxseed Flax Chocolate	1 (1.4 oz)	200
Organic Original Hempseed	1 (1.4 oz)	210
Odwalla		
Berries GoMega	1	220
Carrot	1	220
Choco-walla	1	240
Cranberry C Monster	1	220
Super Protein	1	230
Superfood	1	230
POM		
Pomegranate Dipped In Chocolate	1 (1.8 oz)	210
POMx		
Coconut Dipped In Yogurt	1 (1.8 oz)	230
Pomegranate Dipped In Yogurt	1 (1.8 oz)	210
Prana Bar		
Apricot Goji	1 (1.7 oz)	220
Coconut Acai	1 (1.7 oz)	220
Pear Ginseng	1 (1.7 oz)	220
Premier		
Protein Bar Double Chocolate Crunch	1 (2.5 oz)	270
Protein Bar Yogurt Peanut Crunch	1 (2.5 oz)	290

FOOD	PORTION	CALS
PureFit		
Almond Crunch	1 (2 oz)	230
Peanut Butter Crunch	1 (2 oz)	240
Sencha Naturals		
Green Tea Bar Lively Lemongrass	1 (2 oz)	220
Green Tea Bar Original	1 (2 oz)	220
Simply Nutrilite		
Sweet & Salty	1 (1.6 oz)	170
Snickers		
Marathon Chewy Chocolatey Peanut	1 (1.94 oz)	210
South Beach		
Energy Mix	1 pkg (1 oz)	160
SoyJoy		
Soy & Fruit Banana	1 (1.1 oz)	130
Soy & Fruit Blueberry	1 (1.1 oz)	140
Soy & Fruit Mango Coconut	1 (1.1 oz)	140
SunRidge Farms		
Energy Nuggets	2 (1.4 oz)	200
Think5		
Red Berry	1 (2.5 oz)	240
Red Berry Chocolate Covered	1 (2.8 oz)	290
ThinkPink		
Blueberry Dark Chocolate	1 (2.1 oz)	240
Lemon Burst	1 (2.1 oz)	230
Peanut Butter Caramel	1 (2.1 oz)	230
White Chocolate Raspberry	1 (2.1 oz)	240
Titan		
High Protein Chocolate Peanut Butter Crunch	1 (2.8 oz)	320
High Protein Cookies And Cream	1 (2.8 oz)	330

ENERGY DRINKS

FOOD	PORTION	CALS
180		
Blue w/ Acai	1 can (8.2 oz)	120
Blue w/ Acai Low Calorie	1 can (8.2 oz)	15
Orange Citrus Blast	1 can (8.2 oz)	120
Orange Citrus Blast Sugar Free	1 can (8.2 oz)	5
Red w/ Gogi	1 can (8.2 oz)	130
1In3Trinity		
Energy Drink	1 can (8.4 oz)	10

FOOD	PORTION	CALS
Arizona		
Energy Low Carb	1 can (8 oz)	10
Rx Energy Fast Shot Natural Green Tea	1 bottle (2 oz)	10
Sports Orange	8 oz	50
B52		
Zero Sugar Citrus Berry	8 oz	10
Bai		
Antioxidant Infusion Jamaica Blueberry	8 oz	70
Antioxidant Infusion Kenya Peach	8 oz	70
Antioxidant Infusion Mango Kauai	8 oz	70
Bawls		
Guarana	8 oz	90
Guaranexx Sugar Free	1 bottle (10 oz)	0
Bing		
Energy Drink	1 can (12 oz)	40
Bloom		
All Flavors	1 can (10.5 oz)	100
Boost		
Beauty	1 bottle (12 oz)	220
Youth	1 bottle (12 oz)	200
Boozer		
Hangover Remedy	1 can (8.4 oz)	110
Brain Toniq		
Functional Drink	1 can (8.4 oz)	80
C1.5		
Extreme	1 can (8.4 oz)	120
Celsius		
Ginger Ale	1 bottle (12 oz)	10
Orange	1 bottle (12 oz)	10
Cintron		
Citrus Mango	8 oz	110
Citrus Mango Sugar Free	8 oz	0
Clif		
Quench Fruit Punch	8 oz	45
Quench Orange	8 oz	45
Coca-Cola		
Zero	8 oz	1
Coolah		
Original	8 oz	120

FOOD	PORTION	CALS
Cytomax		
Performance Drink Cool Citrus	1 pkg (1.4 oz)	140
DNA Energy		
Low Carb Citrus	8 oz	0
Dr. Tim's		
ISO-5	1 bottle (11.2 oz)	60
Jungle Juice	1 bottle (4 oz)	20
Emu		
Energy Drink	1 bottle (8.4 oz)	170
EQ Thirst Equalizer		
All Flavors	8 oz	60
EX		
Aqua Vitamins Lemon Lime	1 bottle (16.9 oz)	110
Chillout	1 can (8.4 oz)	80
Pure Energy	1 can (8.4 oz)	70
Slim Energy	1 can (8.4 oz)	20
Facedrink		
The Social Drink	1 bottle (2.5 oz)	3
Fever		
Stimulation Beverage All Flavors	8 oz	130
Fitness Edge		
Tropical Orange	1 bottle (12 oz)	170
Function		
Alternative Energy	8 oz	60
Brainiac Carambola Punch	8 oz	60
Urban Detox Citrus Prickly Pear	8 oz	60
Youth Trip Acai Grape	8 oz	60
Fuze		
Refresh Banana Coconut	8 oz	90
Refresh Peach Mango	8 oz	90
Refresh Strawberry Banana	8 oz	100
Slenderize Cranberry Raspberry	8 oz	5
Slenderize Low Carb Tropical Punch	8 oz	5
Slenderize Tangerine Grapefruit	8 oz	10
Vitalize Blackberry Grape	8 oz	100
Vitalize Orange Mango	8 oz	100
Gatorade		
All Flavors	8 oz	50
Ginger Boost		
Ginger Orange	8 oz	110

FOOD	PORTION	CALS
Gleukos		
Performance All Flavors	8 oz	70
Go Girl		
Bliss	1 can (11.5 oz)	35
Glo	1 can (12 oz)	35
Sugar Free	1 can (12 oz)	<5
Guayaki		
Organic Raspberry Revolution	8 oz	50
Organic Unsweetened	8 oz	15
Healthy Shot		
Double Protein Peach	1 bottle (2.5 oz)	100
High Protein All Flavors	1 bottle (2.5 oz)	110
Hiro		
Thermo	1 can (8.33 oz)	10
Vitality	1 can (8.33 oz)	10
Honeydrop		
Alive Blood Orange & Honey	8 oz	40
Strong Blueberries & Honey	8 oz	40
IChill		
Relaxation Shot Blissful Berry	1 bottle (2 oz)	0
Kidstrong		
All Flavors	8 oz	30
King 888		
Original	8 oz	110
Sugar Free	8 oz	0
Liv Naturals		
All Flavors	8 oz	70
Marquis Platinum		
Vitality Drink	1 can	30
Me		
Curious Blueberry Lime	1 can	70
Vivacious Tangerine Pineapple	1 can	70
Mix1		
All Flavors	1 bottle (11 oz)	200
Mr. Re		
Restorative	1 can (11 oz)	80
Nawgan		
Berry Caffeine Free	1 can (11.5 oz)	40
Torocco Orange	1 can (11.5 oz)	45

FOOD	PORTION	CALS
Neuro		
Bliss	1 bottle (14.5 oz)	35
Gasm	1 bottle (14.5 oz)	35
Sleep	1 bottle (14.5 oz)	35
Sonic	1 bottle (14.5 oz)	35
Sport	1 bottle (14.5 oz)	35
Trim	1 bottle (14.5 oz)	35
NOS		
High Performance	1 bottle (11 oz)	150
Ocean Spray		
Cranergy Cranberry	8 oz	35
Cranergy Pomegranate Cranberry Lift	8 oz	35
Cranergy Raspberry Cranberry Lift	8 oz	20
Odwalla		
Berries GoMega	8 oz	160
Mo' Beta	8 oz	150
Super Protein Original	8 oz	190
Superfood	8 oz	130
Wellness	8 oz	150
OOBA		
All Flavors	8 oz	90
Palo		
Mamajuana	7 oz	50
Phase III Recovery		
Chocolate	1 bottle (14.5 oz)	330
Vanilla	1 bottle (14.5 oz)	320
Pimpjuice		
Energy Drink	1 can (8 oz)	140
PJ Tight	1 can (8 oz)	20
POMx		
Shot Antioxidant Supplement	1 bottle (3 oz)	100
Premier		
Nitro Shot	1 (1.8 oz)	75
Rocket Shot Berry Blast	1 (1.8 oz)	30
Purity Organic		
Acerola Cherry	1 bottle	60
Pomegranate Blueberry	1 bottle	60
Pomegranate Raspberry	1 bottle	60
Quench Aid		
Berry	1 pkg	10
Dragonfruit	1 pkg	10

FOOD	PORTION	CALS
Recharge		
Lemon as prep	8 oz	10
Tropical as prep	8 oz	10
Red Bull		
Original	1 can (8.3 oz)	110
Sugar Free	1 can (8.3 oz)	10
Rehab		
Recovery Supplement	1 can (12 oz)	150
Rockstar		
Energy Drink	8 oz	140
Simply Nutrilite		
Berry Antioxidant	1 can (8.4 oz)	120
SoCal		
Just Chill	1 can (8.4 oz)	50
Solixir		
Blackberry	1 can	50
Orange	1 can	55
Pomegranate	1 can	60
Source Burn		
2	8 oz	130
Energy Drink	8 oz	140
Sugar Free	8 oz	10
Steaz		
Organic Fuel	8 oz	90
Svelte		
Protein Drink All Flavors	1 bottle (15.9 oz)	260
T-Fusion		
Energy Tea	8 oz	0
Therafizz		
Energy	1 pkg	8
Vitamin C	1 pkg	5
UnderWay		
Appetite Suppressing All Flavors	8 oz	10
Unwind		
All Flavors	1 can (12 oz)	40
Venga		
Brainstorm	8 oz	130
Calorie Burn	8 oz	10
Energize	8 oz	100
Health&Zen	8 oz	80

FOOD	PORTION	CALS
VIB		
Chill-N	1 can (8 oz)	40
XOOD		
Endurance Drink All Flavors as prep	1 serv	135
Youth Juice		
Drink	2 oz	10
Zenergize		
Chill	1 tablet	2
Energy+	1 tablet	2
Hydrate	1 tablet	2
ENGLISH MUFFIN		
READY-TO-EAT		
crumpets	1 (1.5 oz)	80
plain	1 (2 oz)	129
whole wheat	1 (2.3 oz)	134
Aunt Gussie's		
Gluten Free Cinnamon Raisin	1 (3 oz)	200
Gluten Free Original	1 (3 oz)	200
Fiber One		
100% Whole Wheat	1 (2 oz)	100
Foods By George		
Gluten Free Multigrain	1 (3.6 oz)	220
Gluten Free No-Rye Rye	1 (3.6 oz)	210
Matthew's		
Golden White	1 (2.1 oz)	140
Milton's		
Healthy Multi-Grain	1 (2 oz)	150
Pepperidge Farm		
100% Whole Wheat	1	140
Original	1	130
Roman Meal		
English Muffin	1 (2.3 oz)	140
Rudi's Organic Bakery		
MultiGrain w/ Flax	1 (2 oz)	130
Whole Grain Wheat	1 (2 oz)	120
Sun-Maid		
Raisin	1 (2.5 oz)	170
Thomas'		
10 Grain	1 (2.1 oz)	130
100 Calories	1	100

FOOD	PORTION	CALS
100% Whole Wheat	1 (2 oz)	120
Griller Multi Grain	1 (3.2 oz)	210
Griller Onion	1 (3.2 oz)	200
Light Multi-Grain	1 (2 oz)	100
Multi-Grain	1 (2 oz)	150
Oatmeal & Honey	1	130
Original	1 (2 oz)	120
Raisin Cinnamon	1 (2.1 oz)	140
TAKE-OUT		
w/ butter	1 (2.2 oz)	189
w/ cheese & sausage	1 (4 oz)	365
w/ egg cheese & canadian bacon	1 (4.9 oz)	307
w/ egg cheese & sausage	1 (5.8 oz)	472

EPAZOTE

fresh	1 tbsp (1 g)	<1
fresh sprig	1 (2 g)	1

EPPAW

raw	½ cup	75

FALAFEL

Falafel Republic

Traditional	3 (3 oz)	210

Near East

Falafel Patties Vegetarian as prep	2.5	220

Veggie Patch

Falafel	4 (3 oz)	180

TAKE-OUT

falafel	1 (1.2 oz)	57

FAT (*see also* BUTTER, BUTTER SUBSTITUTES, MARGARINE, OIL)

bacon grease	1 tbsp	116
beef shortening	1 tbsp	115
beef suet	1 oz	242
chicken	1 tbsp (0.4 oz)	115
duck	1 tbsp (0.4 oz)	113
goose	1 oz	257
goose	1 tbsp	115
lamb new zealand	1 oz	182
lard	1 cup (7.2 oz)	1849
lard	1 tbsp (0.5 oz)	115

FOOD	PORTION	CALS
meat pan drippings	½ tbsp	124
pork raw	1 oz	230
salt pork	1 cube (1 oz)	215
shortening	1 cup	1812
shortening	1 tbsp	113
turkey	1 tbsp	116
ucuhuba butter	1 tbsp	120
whale blubber	1 oz	248
Crisco		
Butter Flavor	1 tbsp	110
Shortening	1 tbsp	110
Earth Balance		
Natural Shortening	1 tbsp	130
Nebraska Land		
Pork Fatback	½ oz	110
FAVA BEANS		
canned	½ cup	91
fava fresh cooked	½ cup	94
Progresso		
Fava Beans	½ cup (4.6 oz)	110
FEIJOA		
fresh	1 (1.75 oz)	25
puree	1 cup	119
FENNEL		
fresh bulb	1 (8.2 oz)	73
fresh sliced	1 cup	27
leaves	1 oz	7
seed	1 tsp	7
stir fried	1 cup	85
Ocean Mist		
Fennel Sweet Anise Sliced Fresh	1 cup	27
FENUGREEK		
seed	1 tsp	12
FIBER		
Benefiber		
Supplement	1 pkg (4 g)	20
Fiber Supreme		
Fiber	1 round tbsp (0.5 oz)	36

FOOD	PORTION	CALS
ND Labs		
Apple Fiber	1 round tbsp (7 g)	15
Liquid Fiber Flow	1 tbsp (0.5 oz)	42
UniFiber		
Natural Fiber	1 pkg (4 g)	4
Wellements		
Fiber-Psyll	1 scoop (0.5 oz)	55
FIDDLEHEAD FERNS		
fresh	3.5 oz	34
FIG JUICE		
Smart Juice		
Organic 100% Juice	8 oz	131
FIGS		
calimyrna	3 (5.4 oz)	120
canned in heavy syrup	½ cup	114
canned in light syrup	½ cup	87
canned water pack	½ cup	66
dried california	½ cup (3.5 oz)	200
dried cooked	½ cup	139
dried small	1 (1.4 oz)	30
dried whole	1 (8 g)	21
fresh large	1 (2.2 oz)	47
California Fresh		
Fresh	3 (5.4 oz)	120
Hermes		
Organic Adriatic Fig Spread	1 tbsp	60
Jenny		
Kalamata Crown Natural Sundried	4 (1.5 oz)	120
Nuta Figs		
Mission	¼ cup (1.4 oz)	110
Orchard Choice		
Mission	4–5 (1.4 oz)	110
Sun-Maid		
California Mission	4 (1.5 oz)	110
Calimyrna	3 (1.5 oz)	120
FIREWEED		
leaves chopped	¼ cup (0.2 oz)	6
plant	1 (0.8 oz)	23

FOOD	PORTION	CALS

FISH (see also INDIVIDUAL NAMES, SUSHI)
FROZEN

FOOD	PORTION	CALS
breaded fillet	1 (2 oz)	155
sticks	1 stick (1 oz)	76
Dr. Praeger's		
Fillets Lightly Breaded	1 (2.1 oz)	100
Fish Sticks Potato Crusted	3 (2.3 oz)	120
Fishies Lightly Breaded	3 (1.5 oz)	90
Gorton's		
Classic Crispy Battered Fillets	2	230
Classic Crunchy Golden Fillets	2	140
Fillets Beer Battered	2 (3.6 oz)	250
Fillets Breaded Lemon Herb	2 (3.6 oz)	240
Fillets Potato Crunch	2 (3.6 oz)	240
Fish Sticks Classic Breaded	6	290
Grilled Fillets Cajun Blackened	1 (3.8 oz)	100
Grilled Fillets Lemon Pepper	1 (3.7 oz)	100
Tenders Original Batter	3 pieces (3.6 oz)	230
SeaPak		
Popcorn	8 (3 oz)	190
Van de Kamp's		
Battered Tenders	4 (4 oz)	210
Crisp & Healthy Breaded Fish Sticks	6 (3.6 oz)	140
Crunchy Fillets	2 (3.5 oz)	230
Sticks	6 (4 oz)	260
TAKE-OUT		
amuk bok kum korean stir fried fish cake	1 cup (7.6 oz)	267
fish cake	1 (4.7 oz)	166
jamaican brown fish stew	1 serv	426
kedgeree	5.6 oz	242
mousse	1 serv (3.5 oz)	185
stew	1 cup (7.9 oz)	157
taramasalata	2 tbsp	124

FISH OIL

FOOD	PORTION	CALS
cod liver	1 tbsp	123
herring	1 tbsp	123
menhaden	1 tbsp	123
salmon	1 tbsp	123
sardine	1 tbsp	123

FOOD	PORTION	CALS
shark	1 oz	270
whale beluga	1 oz	256
whale bowhead	1 oz	252
Genesis Today		
Omega-3 Vitamin Super Chews	1	20
Nordic Naturals		
Nordic Omega-3 Gummies Tangerine Treats	2 pieces	20
Omega 3-6-9 Junior	2 pieces	9
Omega-3 Effervescent as prep	1 pkg (9.7 g)	39
FISH PASTE		
fish paste	2 tsp	15
FLAXSEED		
Arrowhead Mills		
Organic	3 tbsp (1 oz)	140
Bob's Red Mill		
Flaxseed Meal	2 tbsp	60
Carrington Farms		
Organic Flax Paks	1 pkg (0.4 oz)	50
Flax USA		
Flax Sprinkles	2 tbsp (0.5 oz)	70
Natural Ovens		
Flax Complete Supplement	1 tbsp (0.4 oz)	60
Tree Of Life		
Flax Seed	3 tbsp (1 oz)	140
FLOUNDER		
FRESH		
cooked	1 fillet (4.5 oz)	148
cooked	3 oz	99
FROZEN		
Mrs. Paul's		
Filets Lightly Breaded	1 (2.7 oz)	150
TAKE-OUT		
breaded & fried	3.2 oz	211
stuffed w/ crab	1 piece (7.6 oz)	332
FLOUR		
all-purpose enriched bleached	½ cup (2.2 oz)	228
all-purpose self-rising	½ cup (2.2 oz)	221
all-purpose unbleached	½ cup (2.2 oz)	228

FOOD	PORTION	CALS
arrowroot	½ cup (2.2 oz)	228
bread flour	½ cup (2.4 oz)	247
buckwheat whole groat	½ cup (2.1 oz)	201
cake	½ cup (2.4 oz)	248
carob	1 tbsp (0.2 oz)	13
carob	½ cup (1.8 oz)	114
chickpea besan	½ cup (1.6 oz)	178
peanut lowfat	½ cup (1.1 oz)	128
potato	½ cup (2.8 oz)	286
rice brown	½ cup (2.8 oz)	287
rice white	½ cup (2.8 oz)	289
rye dark	½ cup (2.2 oz)	207
rye light	½ cup (1.8 oz)	187
soy lowfat	½ cup (1.5 oz)	165
triticale whole grain	½ cup (2.3 oz)	220
whole wheat	½ cup (2.1 oz)	203
Arrowhead Mills		
Organic Barley	⅓ cup	95
Organic Brown Rice	⅓ cup	130
Organic Kamut	⅓ cup	130
Organic Oat	⅓ cup	120
Organic Rye	¼ cup	110
Organic Spelt	⅓ cup	130
Organic Unbleached White	¼ cup	120
Organic White Rice	⅓ cup	120
Azukar Organics		
Coconut	3.5 oz	413
Bob's Red Mill		
Brown Rice	¼ cup	140
Corn	¼ cup	160
Graham	¼ cup	120
Kamut Organic	¼ cup	94
Sorghum Sweet White Gluten Free	¼ cup	120
Spelt	¼ cup	120
Whole Wheat	¼ cup	110
Whole Wheat Hard White Organic	¼ cup	120
Ceresota		
100% Whole Wheat	¼ cup (1 oz)	100
All Purpose Unbleached	¼ cup (1 oz)	100

FOOD	PORTION	CALS
Domata Living Flour		
Gluten Free Casein Free	¼ cup	110
Gold Medal		
All Purpose	¼ cup (1 oz)	100
Self Rising	¼ cup (1 oz)	100
Wondra	¼ cup (1 oz)	100
Heckers		
100% Whole Wheat	¼ cup (1 oz)	100
All Purpose Unbleached	¼ cup (1 oz)	100
Lundberg		
Brown Rice	¼ cup	110
Manitoba Harvest		
Hemp Seed Flour	¼ cup	120
Pillsbury		
All Purpose	¼ cup (1.1 oz)	110
Bread Flour	¼ cup (1.1 oz)	110
Self Rising	¼ cup (1.1. oz)	100
Whole Wheat	¼ cup (1.1 oz)	110
FOOD COLORS		
blue	1 tsp	0
orange	1 tsp	0
red	1 tsp	<1
yellow	1 tsp	tr
FRENCH BEANS		
dried cooked	1 cup	228
FRENCH FRIES (see POTATO)		
FRENCH TOAST		
french toast frzn	1 slice (2 oz)	126
Aunt Jemima		
Cinnamon Sticks	4 (3.1 oz)	270
Homestyle	2 slices (4.1 oz)	220
Whole Grain	2 slices (4 oz)	210
Farm Rich		
Original Sticks	5 (4.2 oz)	330
Jimmy Dean		
French Toast Duos	1 serv (3.2 oz)	210
French Toast Griddlers Sandwich	1 (3.6 oz)	210

FOOD	PORTION	CALS
Weight Watchers		
Smart Ones French Toast w/ Turkey Sausage	1 pkg (4.4 oz)	280
TAKE-OUT		
plain	1 slice	151
sticks	5 (4.9 oz)	513
w/ butter	2 slices	356

FROG LEGS
frog legs	3 oz	175
TAKE-OUT		
as prep w/ seasoned flour & fried	1 (0.8)	70

FRUCTOSE
liquid	1 oz	84
powder	¼ cup (1.7 oz)	180
powder	1 tsp (4.2 g)	15
Bob's Red Mill		
Fructose	1 tsp	15
Tree Of Life		
Fructose	1 tsp (4 g)	15

FRUIT AND NUT BARS (see also CEREAL BARS, ENERGY BARS)
Cavewoman Bars		
Baklava	1 (2 oz)	190
PB&J	1 (2 oz)	210
Pineapple Upside Down Cake Raw	1 (2 oz)	190
Kind		
Apple Cinnamon Nut	1 (1.4 oz)	180
Blueberry Pecan + Fiber	1 (1.4 oz)	180
Blueberry Vanilla & Cashew	1 (1.4 oz)	180
Mango Macadamia	1 (1.4 oz)	190
Mini Bar Almond & Apricot	1 (0.8 oz)	110
Mini Bar Almond & Coconut + Omega-3	1 (0.8 oz)	107
Mini Bar Cranberry Almond + Antioxidants	1 (0.8 oz)	115
Mini Bar Fruit & Nut Delight	1 (0.8 oz)	108
Pomegranate Blueberry Pistachio + Antioxidants	1 (1.4 oz)	170
Orchard Bar		
Blueberry Pomegranate & Almond	1 (1.6 oz)	180
Pineapple Coconut & Macadamia	1 (1.6 oz)	190
Strawberry Raspberry & Walnut	1 (1.6 oz)	190

FOOD	PORTION	CALS
Pure		
Organic Apple Cinnamon	1 (1.7 oz)	190
Organic Chocolate Almond	1 (1.7 oz)	190
Organic Cranberry Orange	1 (1.7 oz)	190
Organic Peanut Raisin Crunch	1 (1.5 oz)	200
Organic Superfruit Nutty Crunch	1 (1.5 oz)	190
Organic Wild Blueberry	1 (1.7 oz)	190

FRUIT DRINKS (*see also* INDIVIDUAL NAMES, SMOOTHIES, YOGURT DRINKS)

FOOD	PORTION	CALS
FROZEN		
Chiquita		
Banana Colada as prep	8 oz	125
Mixed Berry as prep	8 oz	120
Peach Mango as prep	8 oz	120
Dole		
Orange Peach Mango not prep	¼ cup	120
MIX		
Aquafull		
Pomegranate Orange Dietary Supplement	1 pkg (9 g)	30
Bio Fruit		
Mix	1 scoop (8 g)	42
Crystal Light		
Fusion Fruit Punch as prep	8 oz	5
Immunity Cherry Pomegranate as prep	8 oz	5
South Beach		
Tide Me Over Strawberry Banana	1 pkg	30
Tide Me Over Tropical Breeze	1 pkg	30
READY-TO-DRINK		
fruit punch	6 oz	87
Apple & Eve		
100% Juice Cranberry Apple	8 oz	100
100% Juice Mango Passion	8 oz	120
Back To Nature		
100% Juice Berry	1 pkg (6 oz)	90
Bolthouse		
Bom Dia Acai Berry 100% Juice	8 oz	140
Brazsoy		
Fruit Juice w/ Soy	8 oz	94
Ceres		
100% Juice Apple Berry	8 oz	130
100% Juice Cherry Medley Of Fruits	8 oz	130

FOOD	PORTION	CALS
Crayons		
Kiwi Strawberry	1 bottle (12 oz)	130
Outrageous Orange Mango	1 bottle (12 oz)	140
Redder Than Ever Fruitpunch	1 bottle (12 oz)	130
Dole		
Orange Peach Mango	8 oz	120
Paradise Blend	8 oz	120
Pina Colada	8 oz	120
Strawberry Kiwi	8 oz	120
Drenchers		
Super Fruit Endurance Grape Apple	8 oz	120
Super Juice Fit N' Lean Heart Healthy Tropical Passion	8 oz	10
Super Juice Fit N' Lean Power Protein Orange Cream	8 oz	20
Super Juice Immunity Fruit & Veggie Berry	8 oz	110
EarthWise		
Orange Carrot Mango	8 oz	110
Essn		
Sparkling Blood Orange & Cranberry	1 can (8.4 oz)	160
Fizz Ed.		
Pomegranate Cherry	1 can (8.4 oz)	90
Fizzy Lizzy		
Raspberry Lemon	1 bottle (12 oz)	120
Frutzzo		
Organic 100% Juice Pomegranate Acai	1 bottle (12 oz)	140
Organic 100% Juice Pomegranate Passionfruit	1 bottle (12 oz)	140
Genesis Today		
Boost Pomegranate Berry 100% Juice	8 oz	130
GoodBelly		
Blueberry Acai Probiotic Drink	1 bottle (2.7 oz)	50
Cranberry Watermelon Probiotic Drink	8 oz	100
Peach Mango Probiotic Drink	1 bottle (2.7 oz)	50
Strawberry Rosehips Probiotic Drink	1 bottle (2.7 oz)	50
Honest Ade		
Superfruit Punch	8 oz	48
Honest Kids		
Organic Tropical Tango Punch	1 pkg (6.75 oz)	40
Juicy Juice		
Harvest Surprise Orange Mango	8 oz	130

FOOD	PORTION	CALS
Lakewood		
Lean Green	6 oz	90
Organic Acai Amazon Berry	6 oz	95
Land O'Lakes		
Juice Cranberry Apple	1 cup (8 oz)	120
Minute Maid		
Pomegranate Blueberry 100% Juice	8 oz	120
Moto Bar		
Strawberry Kiwi	8 oz	110
Mott's		
Apple Blueberry	8 oz	130
Fruit Medley	1 bottle (14 oz)	230
Nantucket Nectars		
100% Juice Peach Orange	8 oz	130
100% Juice Pomegranate Cherry	8 oz	120
Kiwi Berry	8 oz	120
Organic Banana Mango Carrot	8 oz	140
Pineapple Orange Guava	8 oz	120
Noble		
Organic 100% Juice Orange Tangerine	8 oz	120
Northland		
100% Juice Cranberry Pomegranate	8 oz	140
NutraShake		
Fruit Punch Plus Fiber	1 pkg (8 oz)	120
Ocean Spray		
100% Juice Cranberry & Concord Grape	8 oz	150
100% Juice Fruit & Veggie Tropical Citrus	8 oz	130
100% Juice Fruit & Veggie Tropical Citrus Light	8 oz	60
Cran-Apple	8 oz	130
Cran-Apple Light	8 oz	40
Cran-Cherry	8 oz	120
Cran-Grape	8 oz	120
Cran-Grape Light	8 oz	40
Cran-Pomegranate	8 oz	120
Cran-Pomegranate Light	8 oz	40
Cran-Raspberry	8 oz	110
Cran-Raspberry Light	8 oz	40
Ruby Tangerine	8 oz	110
White Cranberry Peach	8 oz	110

FOOD	PORTION	CALS
Odwalla		
Quenchers AntioxiDance	8 oz	90
Quenchers B Berrier	8 oz	120
Old Orchard		
100% Juice Acai Pomegranate	8 oz	130
100% Juice Berry Blend	8 oz	130
100% Juice Cherry Pomegranate	8 oz	130
Cranberry Grape Cocktail	8 oz	31
Healthy Balance Apple Kiwi Strawberry Cocktail	8 oz	31
Pomegranate Blueberry Acai Cocktail	8 oz	31
Very Cherry 100% Juice Tart Cherry Cranberry	8 oz	130
Pacific Chai		
Pomegranate Blueberry	8 oz	100
R.W. Knudsen		
Razzleberry 100% Juice	8 oz	120
Sensible Sippers Organic Fruit Punch	1 box (4.23 oz)	30
Sabor Latino		
Guava Mango Drink	1 box (7 oz)	110
Nectar Strawberry Banana + Calcium	8 oz	150
Pina Colada	8 oz	130
Santa Cruz		
Organic Cranberry Goji	8 oz	120
Smart Juice		
Organic 100% Juice Pomegranate Purple Carrot	8 oz	137
Snapple		
100% Juice Fruit Punch	8 oz	170
Juice Drink Acai Blackberry	8 oz	110
Juice Drink Cranberry Raspberry	8 oz	100
SSips		
Cherry Berry	1 box (7 oz)	110
Sun Shower		
100% Juice Nectarine Mango	8 oz	93
Sundia		
Tropical Medley	½ cup	70
Tree Ripe		
Organic Fruit Punch	8 oz	150
Tropical Grove		
Fruit Punch	8 oz	110

FOOD	PORTION	CALS
Tropicana		
Fruit Punch	1 cup	130
Fruit Punch Light	8 oz	10
Orange Tangerine Juice	8 oz	110
Orchard Berry	8 oz	110
Organic Orchard Medley	8 oz	120
Twister Berry Blast	8 oz	120
Twister Citrus Spark	8 oz	120
Twister Fruit Fury	8 oz	120
Twister Light Strawberry Spiral	8 oz	40
V8		
Light Peach Mango	8 oz	50
Splash Diet Berry Blend	8 oz	10
Splash Mango Peach	8 oz	80
V-Fusion Acai Mixed Berry	8 oz	110
V-Fusion Cranberry Blackberry	8 oz	110
V-Fusion Light Peach Mango	8 oz	50
Vruit		
Apple Carrot	1 box (8.45 oz)	120
Berry Veggie	1 box (8.45 oz)	110
Orange Veggie	1 box (8.45 oz)	110
Tropical Blend	1 box (8.45 oz)	110
Wadda Juice		
All Flavors	1 bottle (4 oz)	25
Walnut Acres		
Organic Orange Carrot	8 oz	110
Welch's		
100% Black Cherry Concord Grape	8 oz	160
Light Strawberry Mango	8 oz	50

FRUIT MIXED (*see also* INDIVIDUAL NAMES, FRUIT AND NUT BARS)
CANNED

FOOD	PORTION	CALS
fruit cocktail in heavy syrup	½ cup	93
fruit cocktail juice pack	½ cup	56
fruit cocktail water pack	½ cup	40
fruit salad in heavy syrup	½ cup	94
fruit salad in light syrup	½ cup	73
fruit salad juice pack	½ cup	62
fruit salad water pack	½ cup	37
mixed fruit in heavy syrup	½ cup	92
tropical fruit salad in heavy syrup	½ cup	110

FOOD	PORTION	CALS
Buddy Fruits		
100% Fruit Apple & Banana	1 pkg (3.2 oz)	50
Del Monte		
Carb Clever Fruit Cocktail	½ cup (4.2 oz)	40
Chunky Mixed Fruit In 100% Juice	½ cup (4.4 oz)	60
Chunky Mixed Fruit In Heavy Syrup	½ cup (4.5 oz)	100
Fruit Cocktail In 100% Juice	½ cup (4.4 oz)	60
Fruit Cocktail In Heavy Syrup	½ cup (4.5 oz)	100
Fruit Cocktail In Light Syrup	½ cup (4.5 oz)	60
Fruit Cocktail In Pear Juice	½ cup (4.4 oz)	60
Fruit Cocktail Lite	½ cup (4.4 oz)	60
Fruit Naturals Apples & Oranges	½ cup (4.4 oz)	70
Fruit Naturals Citrus Salad	½ cup (4.4 oz)	70
Fruit Naturals Tropical Medley	½ cup (4.4 oz)	70
Mixed Fruit In Cherry Gel	1 pkg (4.5 oz)	90
Mixed Fruit In Light Syrup	½ cup (4.4 oz)	80
Snack Cups Cherry Mixed Fruit	1 pkg (4 oz)	70
Superfruit Mixed Fruit Chunks Mango & Passion	1 pkg (6 oz)	120
Superfruit Peach Chunks Pomegranate & Orange	1 pkg (6 oz)	100
Superfruit Pear Chunks Acai & Blackberry	1 pkg (6 oz)	120
Tropical Fruit Salad	½ cup (4.3 oz)	60
Dole		
Cherry Mixed Fruit In Fruit Juice	1 pkg (4 oz)	70
Tropical Fruit In Fruit Juice	1 pkg (4 oz)	60
Homemade Harvey's		
Crushed Fruit Apple Pear & Spices	1 pkg (4.5 oz)	60
Crushed Fruit Mango Pineapple Banana & Passion Fruit	1 pkg (4.5 oz)	90
Crushed Fruit Strawberries Bananas & Kiwis	1 pkg (4.5 oz)	100
Mott's		
Healthy Harvest Pomegranate	1 pkg (3.9 oz)	50
Polar		
Mixed Fruit Light Syrup	½ cup (4.9 oz)	50
S&W		
Chunky Mixed In Sweetened Juice	½ cup (4.3 oz)	80
Fruit Cocktail	½ cup (4.4 oz)	80
DRIED		
mixed	11 oz pkg	712

FOOD	PORTION	CALS
Brothers-All-Natural		
Crisps Strawberry Banana	1 pkg (0.42 oz)	45
Crunchies		
Freeze Dried Mixed Fruit	¼ cup (7 g)	25
Elizabeth's Natural		
Fancy Mixed	5 pieces	80
Fruitaceuticals		
PomaCrans	¼ cup	100
Fun-Yums		
Fresh Crispy Mixed Fruit	1 serv (0.9 oz)	25
Mariani		
Berries 'N Cherries	¼ cup	140
Sun-Maid		
Fruit Bits	¼ cup (1.4 oz)	120
Mixed	¼ cup (1.4 oz)	100
Sunsweet		
Antioxidant Blend	¼ cup (1.4 oz)	130
Berry Blend	¼ cup (1.4 oz)	120
FRESH		
Chiquita		
Apple & Grape Bites	1 pkg (2.5 oz)	40
FROZEN		
mixed fruit sweetened	1 cup	245
FRUIT SNACKS		
fruit leather	1 bar (0.8 oz)	81
fruit leather pieces	1 pkg (0.9 oz)	92
fruit leather pieces	1 oz	97
fruit leather rolls	1 lg (0.7 oz)	73
fruit leather rolls	1 sm (0.5 oz)	49
Annie's Homegrown		
Orchard Fruit Bites Grape	1 pkg (0.6 oz)	60
Orchard Fruit Bites Strawberry	1 pkg (0.6 oz)	60
Organic Bunny Fruit Snacks Lemonade	1 pkg (0.6 oz)	70
Organic Bunny Fruit Tropical Treat	1 pkg (0.8 oz)	70
Bare Fruit		
Bananas & Cherries	1 pkg (0.6 oz)	55
Clif		
Twisted Fruit Grape	1 piece (0.7 oz)	70
Twisted Fruit Pineapple	1 piece (0.7 oz)	70
Twisted Fruit Tropical Twist	1 piece (0.7 oz)	70

FOOD	PORTION	CALS
Dole		
Real Fruit Bites Apple	1 pkg (0.7 oz)	80
Froose		
All Flavors	1 pkg (0.9 oz)	70
FruitziO		
Apples & Strawberries	1 pkg (0.9 oz)	100
Apricots	1 pkg (0.35 oz)	40
Peach	1 pkg (0.35 oz)	40
Strawberries	1 pkg (0.9 oz)	100
Funky Monkey		
Applemon	1 pkg (0.42 oz)	40
Bananamon	1 pkg (0.42 oz)	45
Carnaval Mix	1 pkg (0.42 oz)	45
Jivealime	1 pkg (0.42 oz)	45
MangoOJ	1 pkg (0.42 oz)	35
Pink Pineapple	1 pkg (0.42 oz)	45
Purple Funk	1 pkg (0.42 oz)	50
Jelly Belly		
Fruit Snacks	1 pkg (2.5 oz)	220
Kaia Foods		
Fruit Leather Lime Ginger	1 (1 oz)	50
Fruit Leather Vanilla Pear	1 (1 oz)	60
Kettle Valley		
100% Fruit Bar All Flavors	1 (0.7 oz)	70
Fruit Twists All Flavors	1 (0.6 oz)	60
Peeled Snacks		
Fruit & Nuts FigSated	⅓ cup	150
Fruit & Nuts Plu-what?	⅓ cup	150
Revolution Foods		
Organic Mashups Berry	1 pkg (3.2 oz)	40
Organic Mashups Strawberry Banana	1 pkg (3.2 oz)	60
Stretch Island		
Fruit Leather Bountiful Blueberry	1 pkg (0.5 oz)	45
Fruit Leather Harvest Grape	1 pkg (0.5 oz)	45
Fruit Leather Mango Sunrise	1 pkg (0.5 oz)	45
Fruit Leather Truly Tropical	1 pkg (0.5 oz)	45
Organic Smooshed Fruit Apple	1 piece (0.4 oz)	40
Organic Smooshed Fruit Strawberry	1 piece (0.4 oz)	40
Sun-Rype		
Fruit Bar Mango Strawberry	1 (1.3 oz)	120
Fruit Bar Strawberry	1 (1.3 oz)	130

FOOD	PORTION	CALS
Tahitian Noni		
Soft Chews Raspberry	1 pkg (2 oz)	240
Tasty		
All Flavors	1 pkg (0.8 oz)	130
That's It		
Bar 1 Apple + 1 Pear	1 (1.2 oz)	100
Bar 1 Apple + 10 Cherries	1 (1.2 oz)	100
Bar 1 Apple + 3 Apricots	1 (1.2 oz)	100
Tropicana		
Fruit Wise Bars All Flavors	1 bar (1.4 oz)	140
Fruit Wise Strips All Flavors	1 strip (0.7 oz)	70
Welch's		
Fruit'N Yogurt Strawberry	1 pkg (0.9 oz)	90
Mixed Fruit	1 pkg (0.9 oz)	80
GARLIC		
clove	1	4
fresh chopped	1 tbsp	18
powder	1 tsp	9
Jake & Amos		
Sweet Pickled Garlic	1 oz	36
McSweet		
Pickled	8 pieces (1 oz)	40
Spice World		
Ajo Garlic Clove	1 (3 g)	5
GEFILTE FISH		
sweet	1 piece (1.5 oz)	35
Mrs. Adler's		
Gefilte Fish	1 piece (1.8 oz)	50
Ungar's		
Gefilte Fish	2 slices (1.8 oz)	83
Lite	2 slices (2.4 oz)	80
No Sugar	2 slices (1.8 oz)	70
GELATIN		
READY-TO-EAT		
Dole		
Mixed Fruit In Cherry Gel Sugar Free	1 pkg (4.3 oz)	60
Mixed Fruit In Peach Gel	1 pkg (4.3 oz)	100
Pineapple In Lime Gel	1 pkg (4.3 oz)	90

FOOD	PORTION	CALS
Jell-O		
Sugar Free Lemon Lime	1 serv (3.2 oz)	10
Kozy Shack		
Gel Treats Sugar Free Strawberry	1 pkg (3.5 oz)	10
Smart Gels Cherry	1 pkg (3.5 oz)	80
Smart Gels Orange	1 pkg (3.5 oz)	80
Smart Gels Strawberry	1 pkg (3.5 oz)	80
Smart Gels Sugar Free Orange	1 pkg (3.5 oz)	5
Tropical	1 pkg (3.5 oz)	80
Tropical Sugar Free	1 pkg (3.5 oz)	5
Snack Pack		
Gels Cherry No Sugar Added	1 pkg (3.5 oz)	10
Gels Strawberry	1 pkg (3.5 oz)	100
GIBLETS		
capon simmered	1 cup (5 oz)	238
chicken fried	1 cup (5 oz)	402
chicken simmered	1 cup (5 oz)	289
turkey simmered	1 cup (5 oz)	243
GINGER		
ground	1 tsp	6
pickled	1 tbsp (0.3 oz)	9
preserved	1.5 oz	34
root fresh	5 slices	9
root fresh sliced	¼ cup	19
Dorot		
Crushed Cubes frzn	1 (3.5 g)	0
Tree Of Life		
Crystallized Pieces	7 (1.4 oz)	150
GINKGO NUTS		
canned	1 oz	32
dried	1 oz	99
raw	1 oz	52
GINSENG		
dried	1 oz	90
fresh	1 oz	28
GIZZARDS		
chicken simmered	1 cup (5 oz)	212
turkey simmered	1 (3 oz)	103

FOOD	PORTION	CALS
Foster Farms		
Chicken Gizzards & Hearts fresh	4 oz	150
Perdue		
Fresh Chicken	3 oz	130
GNOCCHI		
spinach	12 (4 oz)	220
Racconto		
Potato Whole Wheat as prep w/o salt	1 cup (5.8 oz)	248
Solterra		
Original Potato	¼ pkg (3 oz)	100
Spinach	¼ pkg (3 oz)	100
Vantia		
Gnocchi Whole Wheat	¾ cup	210
GOAT		
diced boiled	1 cup (4.7 oz)	190
fried boneless	3 oz	130
ribs cooked	3 (4.8 oz)	196
roasted boneless	3 oz	122
TAKE-OUT		
stew puerto rican style	1 cup (6.2 oz)	460
GOJI BERRIES		
dried	1 oz	106
Kopali		
Organic Dark Chocolate Covered	½ pkg (1 oz)	120
Navitas Naturals		
Dried	1 oz	90
Sunfood		
Organic	1 oz	90
Superfood Snacks		
Organic Chocolate Goji Treats	3 pieces (1.4 oz)	150
Tree Of Life		
Organic	1 oz	110
GOJI JUICE		
Arthur's		
Goji Plus	1 bottle (11 oz)	210
Gojilania		
Organic	8 oz	110

FOOD	PORTION	CALS
GOOSE		
boneless roasted	2.7 oz	231
meat only raw	6.5 oz	298
w/ skin & bone roasted	1 serv (6.6 oz)	573
wild boneless roasted diced	1 cup (4.9 oz)	426
GOOSEBERRIES		
canned in light syrup	1 cup	184
fresh	1 cup	66
Kopali		
Organic Goldenberry	1 pkg (1.8 oz)	150
Navitas Naturals		
Cape Gooseberry Dried	1 oz	80
GRAINS		
Kashi		
7 Whole Grain Pilaf Fiery Fiesta	1 cup (4.9 oz)	210
7 Whole Grain Pilaf Moroccan Curry	1 cup (4.9 oz)	220
7 Whole Grain Pilaf Original	1 cup (4.9 oz)	220
Village Harvest		
Wheatberry & Barley	½ cup	260
Whole Grain Creations w/ Cranberries & Almonds	¾ cup (4.3 oz)	220
Whole Grain Medley Farro & Red Rice	1 cup (5 oz)	290
GRAPE JUICE		
bottled unsweetened	1 cup	154
Apple & Eve		
Vintage Concord	8 oz	150
Cascadian Farm		
Organic frzn as prep	8 oz	150
Fizzy Lizzy		
Yakima Grape	1 bottle (12 oz)	120
Juicy Juice		
Harvest Surprise	8 oz	120
Kedem		
Organic	8 oz	140
Lakewood		
Organic Concord	6 oz	105
Mott's		
100% Juice Grape Medley	1 bottle (14 oz)	230

FOOD	PORTION	CALS
Nantucket Nectars		
Grapeade	8 oz	140
Organic Concord Grape	8 oz	130
Old Orchard		
100% Juice	8 oz	130
100% Juice White	8 oz	130
R.W. Knudsen		
100% Juice	8 oz	130
Santa Cruz		
Organic Concord Grape	8 oz	160
Snapple		
100% Juice Grape	8 oz	170
Grapeade	8 oz	100
Tree Ripe		
Organic 100% Juice	6 oz	120
Tropicana		
Grape	1 bottle (14 oz)	270
Walnut Acres		
Organic	8 oz	120
Welch's		
100% White	8 oz	160
GRAPE LEAVES		
canned	1 (4 g)	3
fresh raw	1 (3 g)	3
Galil		
Stuffed	5 (4.2 oz)	200
TAKE-OUT		
dolmas w/ beef & rice	1 (0.7 oz)	50
dolmas w/ lamb & rice	1 (0.7 oz)	56
dolmas w/ rice	1 (2 oz)	92
GRAPEFRUIT		
CANNED		
sections juice pack	½ cup (4.4 oz)	46
sections light syrup	½ cup (4.5 oz)	76
sections water pack	½ cup (4.3 oz)	44
Del Monte		
Fruit Bowls Grapefruit Duo	½ cup (4.4 oz)	60
Fruit Bowls Red	½ cup (4.4 oz)	60
SunFresh Red No Sugar Added	½ cup (4.2 oz)	40

FOOD	PORTION	CALS
FRESH		
pink or red	½ (4.6 oz)	52
sections pink or red	1 cup (8.1 oz)	97
sections white	1 cup (8.1 oz)	76
white	½ (4.1 oz)	39
Ocean Spray		
Sweet Ruby	½ med (5.4 oz)	60
GRAPEFRUIT JUICE		
canned sweetened	1 cup (8.8 oz)	115
canned unsweetened	1 cup (8.7 oz)	94
pink fresh	1 cup (8.7 oz)	96
white fresh	1 cup (8.7 oz)	96
Apple & Eve		
Ruby Red	8 oz	130
Fizzy Lizzy		
Grapefruit	1 bottle (12 oz)	100
Ocean Spray		
100% Juice Pink	8 oz	100
100% Juice White	8 oz	90
Ruby Drink Light	8 oz	40
Odwalla		
100% Juice	8 oz	90
Old Orchard		
Ruby Red Cocktail	8 oz	31
Sundia		
Ruby	½ cup	70
Tropicana		
Sweet	8 oz	130
GRAPES		
muscadine	10–12 (3.5 oz)	76
scuppernongs	10–12 (3.5 oz)	68
seedless red or green	1 cup	110
seedless red or green	20	69
thompson seedless in heavy syrup	½ cup	93
thompson seedless water pack	½ cup	49
with seeds red or green	20	80
with seeds red or green	1 cup	106
Chiquita		
Grapes	1 cup (3.2 oz)	62

FOOD	PORTION	CALS
Crunch Pak		
Sweet Seedless	⅕ pkg	40
Dole		
Fresh	26 (4.4 oz)	90
Earthbound Farms		
Organic Black	1½ cups	190
Revolution Foods		
Organic Mashups Grape	1 pkg (3.2 oz)	60
GRAVY		
CANNED		
beef	1 can (10 oz)	155
beef	1 cup	124
chicken	1 cup	189
mushroom	1 cup	120
turkey	1 cup	122
Campbell's		
Au Jus	¼ cup	5
Chicken	¼ cup	40
Fat Free Beef	¼ cup	15
Fat Free Turkey	¼ cup	20
Mushroom	¼ cup	20
Franco-American		
Fat Free Slow Roast Chicken	¼ cup	20
Slow Roast Chicken	¼ cup	20
Heinz		
Classic Chicken Fat Free	¼ cup	15
HomeStyle Classic Chicken	¼ cup	25
HomeStyle Roasted Turkey	¼ cup (2.1 oz)	25
Roasted Turkey Fat Free	¼ cup (2.1 oz)	20
MIX		
au jus as prep w/ water	1 cup	32
brown as prep w/ water	1 cup	75
chicken as prep	1 cup	83
mushroom as prep	1 cup	70
onion as prep w/ water	1 cup	77
pork as prep	1 cup	76
turkey as prep	1 cup	87
Bournvita		
Extract	2 heaping tsp	34

FOOD	PORTION	CALS
Bovril		
Extract	1 heaping tsp	9
Butterball		
Turkey	¼ cup (2 oz)	30
Knorr		
Au Jus Instant as prep	2 oz	10
Beef Instant as prep	2 oz	20
Brown Instant as prep	2 oz	25
Brown Low Sodium Instant as prep	2 oz	25
Chicken Instant as prep	2 oz	25
Chicken Low Sodium Instant as prep	2 oz	25
Leahey Gardens		
No Beef Brown Gluten Free	¼ cup	9
No Chicken Golden	¼ cup	18
Loney's		
Brown as prep	¼ cup (2.1 oz)	15
Turkey as prep	¼ cup (2.1 oz)	20
Marmite		
Extract	1 heaping tsp	9
Road's End Organics		
Savory Herb Cholesterol Free Gluten Free	¼ cup	25
TAKE-OUT		
au jus	1 cup	62
giblet gravy	¼ cup	45
GREAT NORTHERN BEANS		
canned	1 cup	299
dried cooked	1 cup	209
HamBeens		
Great Northerns as prep	½ cup	120
GREEN BEANS		
CANNED		
drained	1 cup	27
Allens		
No Salt	½ cup	15
Del Monte		
French Style	½ cup (4.2 oz)	20
Fresh Cut Italian	½ cup	30
Gertie's Finest		
Pickled	1 oz	15

FOOD	PORTION	CALS
Green Giant		
50% Less Sodium Cut	½ cup	20
Matiz		
Piparras	½ jar (1 oz)	5
McSweet		
Dilly Beans Whole	5 (1 oz)	30
S&W		
Cut	½ cup (4.2 oz)	20
Dilled	1 oz	20
FRESH		
cooked w/o salt	1 cup	44
raw	1 cup	34
raw whole beans	10	17
Ready Pac		
Fast 'N Fresh as prep	1 cup (3 oz)	30
FROZEN		
cooked	1 cup	38
Birds Eye		
Steamfresh Whole	1 cup (2.9 oz)	35
C&W		
French Cut	1 cup	30
Cascadian Farm		
Organic Petite Whole	1 cup	25
Green Giant		
Green Bean Casserole	⅔ cup	110
TAKE-OUT		
casserole w/ mushroom sauce	1 cup	108
pickled	½ cup	19
GREENS		
Allens		
Seasoned Mixed	½ cup	45
GROUNDCHERRIES		
fresh	½ cup	37
GROUPER		
cooked	3 oz	100
cooked	1 fillet (7.1 oz)	238
raw	3 oz	78

FOOD	PORTION	CALS
GUAR GUM		
Bob's Red Mill		
Guar Gum	1 tbsp	20
GUAVA		
fresh	1 (1.9 oz)	37
fresh cut up	1 cup (5.8 oz)	112
fresh strawberry	1 (6 g)	4
fresh strawberry cut up	1 cup (8.6 oz)	168
guava paste	1 piece (1.1 oz)	90
GUAVA JUICE		
nectar canned	8 oz	143
Apple & Eve		
Nectar	5 oz	130
Ceres		
100% Juice	8 oz	120
OKF		
Sparkling Fresh Guava	1 bottle (8.3 oz)	20
Sabor Latino		
Nectar + Calcium	8 oz	160
GUINEA HEN		
boneless w/o skin raw	½ hen (9.3 oz)	290
w/ skin raw	½ hen (12 oz)	545
Grimaud Farms		
Guinea Fowl	1 serv (3.7 oz)	130
HADDOCK		
fresh broiled	4 oz	127
roe raw	1 oz	37
smoked	1 oz	33
Van de Kamp's		
Battered Fillets	2 (3.6 oz)	210
TAKE-OUT		
breaded & fried	4 oz	229
HAGGIS		
scottish haggis	1 serv (6.4 oz)	473
Caledonian Kitchen		
Highland Beef	3 oz	173
Vegetarian	3 oz	190

FOOD	PORTION	CALS
House of Kenton		
Vegetarian	1 serv (3.5 oz)	249
MacSween		
Traditional	1 (8 oz)	260
Vegetarian	1 (8 oz)	238
HALIBUT		
atlantic & pacific cooked	½ fillet (5.6 oz)	223
atlantic & pacific cooked	3 oz	119
atlantic & pacific raw	3 oz	93
greenland baked	3 oz	203
greenland baked	5.6 oz	380
FROZEN		
Van de Kamp's		
Battered Fillets	3 (4 oz)	230
HAM		
boneless extra lean roasted	3 oz	123
boneless roasted	3 oz	151
canned extra lean roasted	3 oz	116
canned lean roasted	3 oz	142
center slice lean & fat roasted	3 oz	173
deviled	¼ cup	188
ham salad spread	2 tbsp	65
patty grilled	1 patty (2 oz)	205
prosciutto	4 slices (1.3 oz)	72
sliced	3 slices (2.9 oz)	137
sliced extra lean	3 slices (2.2 oz)	69
westphalian smoked	1 oz	105
whole roasted	3 oz	207
Applegate Farms		
Organic Uncured	2 oz	70
Carl Buddig		
Ham Sliced	2 oz	85
Honey Ham Sliced	2 oz	90
Dietz & Watson		
Boneless Old Fashioned	3 oz	110
Smoked	2 oz	80
Steak Our Traditional	5 oz	100
Healthy Ones		
Honey 97% Fat Free	7 slices (2 oz)	90

FOOD	PORTION	CALS
Hormel		
Chunk Ham canned	2 oz	90
Deli Cooked	4 slices (2 oz)	70
Deli Honey	4 slices (2 oz)	70
Deli Smoked	4 slices (2 oz)	60
Dinner	2 oz	70
Jones		
Steak Extra Lean	3 oz	100
Organic Prairie		
Hardwood Smoked Bone In Spiral Cut	3 oz	110
Oscar Mayer		
Ham Brown Sugar Thin Sliced	⅓ pkg (2 oz)	70
Virginia Shaved	2 oz	50
Sara Lee		
Virginia Baked	4 slices (1.8 oz)	60
Tyson		
Glazed Ham Maple & Brown Sugar	1 serv (5 oz)	180
Honey Ham	2 slices (1.6 oz)	50
TAKE-OUT		
croquette	1 (2.2 oz)	149
salad	½ cup	287
spam musubi	1 serv (6 oz)	253
thick slice fried	1 (2.2 oz)	140
HAMBURGER		
Applegate Farms		
Organic Beef Cooked	1 (3 oz)	195
Organic Turkey Burger	1 (4 oz)	190
Farm Rich		
Cheeseburgers Mini Bacon	2 (2.2 oz)	150
Foster Farms		
Cheeseburgers Mini Chicken w/ BBQ Sauce	1 (1.3 oz)	90
Hot Pockets		
Cheeseburger	1 (4.5 oz)	310
Lean Pockets		
Cheeseburger	1 (4.5 oz)	280
Oscar Mayer		
Lunchables All-Star Burgers	1 pkg	420
Quaker Maid		
Pure Beef Patties	1 (4 oz)	240

FOOD	PORTION	CALS
TAKE-OUT		
cheeseburger + condiments	1 reg (4.5 oz)	347
double hamburger + condiments	1 reg (5.8 oz)	384
single patty + condiments	1 reg (4 oz)	299
HAMBURGER SUBSTITUTES (*see also* MEAT SUBSTITUTES)		
Amy's		
All American Burger	1 (2.5 oz)	120
Cheddar Veggie Burger	1 (2.5 oz)	160
Texas Burger	1 (2.5 oz)	120
Asherah's Gourmet		
Organic Quinoa Vegan Burgers	1 (4 oz)	180
Dr. Praeger's		
Texmex	1 (4 oz)	170
Veggie Burger Bombay	1 (4 oz)	170
Veggie Burger California	1 (4 oz)	170
Veggie Burger California Slider	1 (1.6 oz)	80
Gardenburger		
Black Bean Chipotle	1 (2.5 oz)	80
Flame Grilled	1 (2.5 oz)	90
GardenVegan	1 (2.5 oz)	100
Original	1 (2.5 oz)	100
Portabella	1 (2.5 oz)	90
Harmony Valley		
Vegetarian Hamburger Mix as prep	1 (3 oz)	120
Morningstar Farms		
Classic Burger	1 (2.2 oz)	150
Okara Pattie	1 (2.2 oz)	120
Vegan Burger	1 (2.5 oz)	100
Sunshine		
Organic Garden Burger	1 (2.6 oz)	250
Sunshine Burgers		
Original	1 (2.6 oz)	190
Veggie Bites		
Garlic Portabella	1 (2.5 oz)	120
WildWood		
Organic Original Burgers Tofu-Veggie	1 (3.2 oz)	180
Yves		
Meatless Chicken Burger	1 (2.6 oz)	100

FOOD	PORTION	CALS
HAZELNUTS		
chocolate hazelnut spread	2 tbsp (1.3 oz)	200
chopped	¼ cup (1 oz)	181
ground	¼ cup (0.7 oz)	118
whole	¼ cup (1.2 oz)	212
whole nuts	21 (1 oz)	178
Chukar Cherries		
Chocolate Covered Spiced	3 tbsp (1.4 oz)	228
Fisher		
Chopped	¼ cup (1 oz)	180
Fundelina		
Choco-Hazelnut Spread All Flavors	2 tbsp (1.3 oz)	200
Love'n Bake		
Hazelnut Praline	2 tbsp	170
HEART		
beef simmered	3 oz	140
chicken cooked	1 (3 g)	5
chicken diced simmered	½ cup	134
lamb braised	3 oz	157
pork braised	1 (4.5 oz)	191
turkey simmered	½ cup	94
veal braised	3 oz	158
Rumba		
Beef	4 oz	130
HEARTS OF PALM		
canned	1 (1.2 oz)	9
canned	½ cup	20
Del Monte		
Hearts Of Palm	2–3 pieces (4.4 oz)	20
Native Forest		
Organic	1 oz	15
HEMP		
Living Harvest		
Organic Hemp Nuts	2 tbsp (1 oz)	170
Organic Protein Powder	2 scoops (1 oz)	110
Manitoba Harvest		
Hemp Seed Butter	2 tbsp	160
Organic Pro Fiber	4 tbsp (1 oz)	127

FOOD	PORTION	CALS
Organic Protein Dark Chocolate	4 tbsp (1 oz)	120
Shelled Seed	2 tbsp	160
Nutiva		
Organic Protein Powder	2 scoops (1 oz)	120
Shelled Hempseed	2 tbsp	110

HERBAL TEA (*see* TEA/HERBAL TEA)

HERBS/SPICES (*see also* INDIVIDUAL NAMES)

cajun seasoning	1 tbsp	19
chinese five spice	1 tsp	7
garam masala	1 tsp	8
poultry seasoning	1 tsp	5
pumpkin pie spice	1 tsp (1.7 g)	6
Bragg		
Herb & Spice Seasoning	¼ tsp	0
Dave's Gourmet		
Insanity Spice	¼ tsp (1 g)	5
Lawry's		
Spices & Seasonings Chimichurri Burrito Casserole	1 tbsp (7 g)	20
Spices & Seasonings Tuscan Chicken Marsala	1 tbsp (7 g)	20
McCormick		
Grill Mates Rub Applewood	2 tsp	15
Meat Tenderizer Seasoned	¼ tsp (1 g)	0
Perfect Pinch Salt Free Original	¼ tsp	0
Modern Day Masala		
Organic Garam Masala	1 tsp (3 g)	10
Mrs. Dash		
Grilling Blend Steak	¼ tsp (0.7 g)	0
Original Blend	¼ tsp (0.7 g)	0
Seasoning Blends Caribbean Citrus	¼ tsp (0.7 g)	0
Seasoning Blends Garlic & Herb	¼ tsp (0.7 g)	0
Seasoning Blends Italian Medley	¼ tsp (0.7 g)	0
Seasoning Blends Table Blend	¼ tsp (0.7 g)	0
Old Bay		
Seasoning	¼ tsp (0.6 g)	0
Seasoning 30% Less Sodium	¼ tsp (0.6 g)	0
Ribber City		
Rib-A-Dub-Rub Dry Rub Seasoning	¼ tsp (0.8 oz)	3

FOOD	PORTION	CALS
Spice Hunter		
All Purpose Blend	¼ tsp	0
Greek Seasoning Salt Free	¼ tsp	0
HERRING		
atlantic baked	4 oz	230
dried salted	1 fillet (1.4 oz)	161
pickled	1 oz	74
pickled in cream sauce	1 oz	72
roe	1 tbsp	39
smoked kippered	1 oz	62
TAKE-OUT		
breaded fried	1 serv (4 oz)	225
HIBISCUS		
flowers dried sweetened	⅓ cup	100
Santa Cruz		
Organic Hibiscus Cooler	8 oz	100
HICKORY NUTS		
dried	1 oz	187
HOMINY		
white canned	1 cup	119
yellow canned	½ cup	115
Allens		
White	½ cup	100
Bush's		
Golden	½ cup	60
HONEY		
honey	1 tbsp (0.7 oz)	64
honey	¼ cup (3 oz)	258
orange blossom	1 tbsp	60
wild honey	1 tbsp	60
Comfort Care		
Raw Clover	1 tbsp (0.7 oz)	60
Dutch Gold		
Clover	1 tbsp	60
Maple Grove Farms		
Honey Maple Spread	2 tbsp (1.5 oz)	160
Steel's		
Sugar Free	1 tbsp (0.5 oz)	24

FOOD	PORTION	CALS
SueBee		
Honey	1 tbsp (0.7 oz)	60
Tastes Like Honey		
Sugar Free	1 tbsp (0.7 oz)	21
Tree Of Life		
Alfalfa Honey Raw Unfiltered	1 tbsp	60
Avocado Honey Raw Unfiltered	1 tbsp (0.7 oz)	60
Buckwheat Honey Raw Unfiltered	1 tbsp	60
Tupelo Honey Raw Unfiltered	1 tbsp	60
Wholesome Sweeteners		
Organic Fair Trade Amber	1 tbsp	60
Organic Fair Trade Raw	1 tbsp (0.7 oz)	60
HONEYDEW		
balls frzn	1 cup (8 oz)	83
fresh cut up	1 cup	61
fresh wedge	⅛ melon (4.5 oz)	45
whole fresh	1 (35 oz)	360
Chiquita		
Fresh Cut Up	1 cup (6.2 oz)	64
Dole		
Fresh	⅒ med (4.7 oz)	50
HORSE		
roasted	3 oz	149
HORSERADISH		
japanese wasabi	¼ tsp	1
sauce	1 tbsp	7
wasabi root raw	1 (5.9 oz)	184
wasabi root raw sliced	½ cup (2.3 oz)	71
Dietz & Watson		
Cranberry Horseradish Sauce	1 tsp (5 g)	10
Gold's		
Horse Radish	1 tsp (5 g)	0
Robert Rothchild Farm		
Sauce	1 tsp	20
Zatarain's		
Prepared	1 tbsp (0.5 oz)	15
HOT CHOCOLATE		
mix not prep	1 pkg (1 oz)	111

FOOD	PORTION	CALS
mix w/ no calorie sweetener as prep w/ water	8 oz	72
mix w/ sugar as prep w/ nonfat milk	8 oz	209
mix w/ sugar as prep w/ water	8 oz	138
Hershey's		
Goodnight Hugs	1 pkg (1.2 oz)	140
Nestle		
Hot Cocoa Milk Chocolate	1 pkg (1 oz)	80
Hot Cocoa Rich Milk Chocolate as prep w/ water	1 pkg (0.7 oz)	80
Hot Cocoa Mix Fat Free as prep	1 pkg	20
Silhouette Solution		
Down East not prep	1 pkg (0.88 oz)	90
Starbucks		
Hot Cocoa Mix	1 pkg	130
Swiss Miss		
Cocoa Caramel as prep	1 pkg	120
Cocoa No Sugar Added as prep	1 pkg	60
Cocoa Rich Creamy as prep	1 pkg	110
Cocoa w/ Marshmallows as prep	1 pkg	120
Cocoa w/ Marshmallows Fat Free as prep	1 pkg	140
French Vanilla as prep	1 pkg	110
Milk Chocolate as prep	1 pkg	120
TAKE-OUT		
chocolate caliente w/ lowfat milk	1 serv (8.4 oz)	221
chocolate caliente w/ whole milk	1 serv (8.4 oz)	276
hot chocolate	1 cup (8.7 oz)	192
mexican hot chocolate	1 cup	173
HOT DOG (see also HOT DOG SUBSTITUTES)		
beef	1 (1.5 oz)	149
beef & pork	1 (1.5 oz)	137
beef lowfat	1 (2 oz)	133
chicken	1 (1.5 oz)	116
fat free	1 (2 oz)	62
low sodium	1 (2 oz)	180
lowfat	1 (2 oz)	88
pork and beef cheese smokie	1 (1.5 oz)	141
turkey	1 (1.5 oz)	102
Abeles&Heymann		
Beef Uncured Reduced Fat & Sodium	1 (1.7 oz)	120

FOOD	PORTION	CALS
Applegate Farms		
The Great Uncured Beef	1 (2 oz)	110
The Great Uncured Chicken	1 (1.7 oz)	70
The Great Uncured Turkey	1 (1.7 oz)	60
Uncured Big Apple	1 (2 oz)	110
Uncured Beef	1 (1.5 oz)	70
Dietz & Watson		
Beef Foot Long	1 (4 oz)	310
Black Forest Wieners	1 (2 oz)	180
Gourmet Lite	1 (2 oz)	60
Super Franks	1 (3.2 oz)	270
Foster Farms		
Chicken	1 (2 oz)	140
Corn Dog Chili Cheese	1 (2.6 oz)	190
Corn Dog Extreme Cheese	1 (2.6 oz)	200
Corn Dog Honey Crunchy	1 (2.6 oz)	180
Corn Dog Mini	4 (2.7 oz)	210
Turkey	1 (2 oz)	140
Healthy Ones		
Beef	1 (1.8 oz)	70
Franks	1 (1.8 oz)	70
Johnsonville		
Stadium Beef	1 (2.7 oz)	240
Organic Prairie		
Beef Uncured	1 (1.5 oz)	120
Oscar Mayer		
Beef	1 (1.6 oz)	140
Beef Light	1 (1.6 oz)	90
Cheese Dogs	1 (1.6 oz)	140
Corn Dogs	1	210
Smokies	1 (1.8 oz)	150
TAKE-OUT		
corndog	1	460
w/ bun chili	1	297
w/ bun plain	1	242

HOT DOG SUBSTITUTES
Health Is Wealth

FOOD	PORTION	CALS
Vegetarian Cocktail Franks	3 (2.4 oz)	220

FOOD	PORTION	CALS
Loma Linda		
Big Franks	1 (1.8 oz)	110
Big Franks Low Fat Vegan	1 (1.8 oz)	80
Morningstar Farms		
Veggie Dogs	1 (1.4 oz)	50
Yves		
Meatless Hot Dog	1	50
Tofu Dogs	1	45
HUMMUS		
Athenos		
Artichoke & Garlic	2 tbsp (0.9 oz)	50
Cucumber Dill	2 tbsp (0.9 oz)	50
Greek Style	2 tbsp (0.9 oz)	50
Original	2 tbsp (0.9 oz)	50
Roasted Red Pepper	2 tbsp (0.9 oz)	50
Cedar's		
Artichoke Spinach	2 tbsp (1 oz)	70
Emerald Valley		
Organic Greek Olive & Roasted Garlic	2 tbsp (1 oz)	60
Organic Original	2 tbsp (1 oz)	50
Organic Spinach Feta	2 tbsp (1 oz)	50
Fountain Of Health		
Traditional	1 oz	70
Guiltless Gourmet		
Original	2 tbsp (1.1 oz)	50
Margaritaville		
Cilantro Jalapeno	1 oz	70
Island Lemon	1 oz	70
Nasoya		
Super Classic Original	2 tbsp (1 oz)	50
Sabra		
Greek Olive	2 tbsp (1 oz)	70
Roasted Pine Nut	2 tbsp (1 oz)	80
Spinach & Artichoke	2 tbsp (1 oz)	70
Tribe		
40 Spices	2 tbsp	50
French Onion	2 tbsp	50
Organic Classic	2 tbsp	50
Organic Roasted Red Peppers	2 tbsp	40
Roasted Eggplant	2 tbsp	35

FOOD	PORTION	CALS
Scallion	2 tbsp	50
Zesty Lemon	2 tbsp	50
Wholesome Valley		
Organic Classic	2 tbsp (1 oz)	60
Wild Garden		
Hummus Dip	2 tbsp	35
WildWood		
Organic Low Fat	2 tbsp	50
Organic Mid-Eastern	2 tbsp	65
TAKE-OUT		
hummus	¼ cup (2.2 oz)	109

HYACINTH BEANS
dried cooked	1 cup	228

ICE CREAM AND FROZEN DESSERTS (see also ICES AND ICE POPS, SHERBET, YOGURT FROZEN)

FOOD	PORTION	CALS
chocolate	½ cup (4 fl oz)	143
dixie cup chocolate	1 (3.5 fl oz)	125
dixie cup strawberry	1 (3.5 fl oz)	112
dixie cup vanilla	1 (3.5 fl oz)	116
freeze dried ice cream chocolate strawberry & vanilla	1 pkg (0.75 oz)	158
strawberry	½ cup (4 fl oz)	127
vanilla	½ cup (4 fl oz)	132
vanilla soft serve	½ cup	111
Arctic Zero		
Chocolate	½ cup (2.6 oz)	37
Chocolate Coated Bars All Flavors	1 (2 oz)	85
Coffee	½ cup (2.6 oz)	37
Mint Chocolate Cookie	½ cup (2.6 oz)	37
Pumpkin Spice	½ cup (2.6 oz)	45
Vanilla Maple	½ cup (2.6 oz)	37
Breyers		
Butter Pecan	½ cup	150
Carb Smart Chocolate	½ cup	90
Carb Smart Fudge Bar	1 (3.5 oz)	100
Carb Smart Vanilla	½ cup	90
Carb Smart Vanilla Bar Chocolate Coated	1 (3 oz)	170
Cherry Vanilla	½ cup	130
Chocolate Crackle	½ cup	160

FOOD	PORTION	CALS
Chocolate Extra Creamy	½ cup	140
Coffee	½ cup	130
Cookies & Cream	½ cup	150
Double Churn½ Fat Chocolate Mocha Silk	½ cup	130
Double Churn½ Fat Creamy Vanilla	½ cup	100
Double Churn½ Fat Mint Chocolate Chip	½ cup	130
Double Churn½ Fat Rocky Road	½ cup	130
Double Churn Fat Free Chocolate Fudge Brownie	½ cup	110
Double Churn Fat Free Creamy Vanilla	½ cup	90
Double Churn Fat Free French Chocolate	½ cup	90
Double Churn No Sugar Added Vanilla	½ cup	80
Dulce De Leche	½ cup	150
French Vanilla	½ cup	140
Heath English Toffee	½ cup	160
Overload Very Chocolate Cherry	½ cup	120
Overload Waffle Cone	½ cup	130
Peach	½ cup	120
Sandwich Mrs. Fields Brownie	1 (6 oz)	450
Sandwich Mrs. Fields Cookie	1 (3 oz)	190
Sandwich Oreo	1 (3 oz)	170
Snicker	½ cup	170
Strawberry	½ cup	120
Strawberry Cheesecake Sara Lee	½ cup	150
Vanilla Fudge Brownie	½ cup	150
Vanilla Lactose Free	½ cup	130
Celestial Seasonings		
Tea Dreams Bars Chocolate Caramel Chai	1 (2.7 oz)	240
Tea Dreams Cinnamon Apple Spice	½ cup	140
Tea Dreams Vanilla Ginger Spice Chai	½ cup	140
Ciao Bella		
Gelato Chocolate	1 pkg (3.5 oz)	210
Gelato Hazelnut	1 pkg (3.5 oz)	210
Gelato Vanilla	1 pkg (3.5 oz)	184
Clemmy's		
Butter Pecan Sugar Free	½ cup	200
Chocolate Sugar Free	½ cup	200
Ice Cream Os Snack Size Sugar Free	1	100
Ice Cream Os Sugar Free	1	180
Toasted Almond Sugar Free	½ cup	220
Vanilla Bean Sugar Free	½ cup	200

FOOD	PORTION	CALS
Dippin' Dots		
Banana Split	½ cup	170
Chocolate	½ cup	165
Fudge Fat Free No Sugar Added	½ cup	92
Horchata	½ cup	170
Java Delight	½ cup	170
Root Beer Float	½ cup	111
Vanilla	½ cup	170
Fat Boy		
Casco Nut Sundae On A Stick	1 (3 oz)	310
Casco Nut Sundae On A Stick Cherry Cordial	1 (3 oz)	300
Sandwich Chocolate	1 (3 oz)	210
Sandwich Egg Nog	1 (3 oz)	220
Sandwich Jr. Vanilla	1 (1.6 oz)	120
Sandwich Vanilla	1 (3 oz)	220
Glace De Vino		
Chocolate Amarreto Cream Sherry	½ cup	180
Raspberry Merlot Cheesecake	½ cup	180
Good Humor		
Bar Chocolate Eclair	1 (3 oz)	160
Bar Cookies & Cream	1 (3 oz)	190
Bar King Heath	1 (4 oz)	310
Bar Vanilla Chocolate Coated	1 (4 oz)	260
Cone King Giant	1 (8 oz)	390
Cone King Vanilla	1 (4.6 oz)	250
Cone Sundae	1 (4.3 oz)	260
Sandwich Giant Vanilla	1 (6 oz)	220
Sandwich Oreo	1 (4.5 oz)	240
Sandwich Vanilla	1 (3 oz)	130
Swirlwind	1 (6 oz)	160
Haagen-Dazs		
Bailey's Irish Cream	½ cup (3.6 oz)	260
Bar Chocolate & Dark Chocolate	1 (3 oz)	290
Bar Vanilla & Almonds	1 (3 oz)	310
Bar Vanilla & Milk Chocolate	1 (3 oz)	290
Butter Pecan	½ cup (3.7 oz)	310
Caramel Cone	½ cup (4 oz)	320
Cherry Vanilla	½ cup (3.5 oz)	240
Chocolate Chip Cookie Dough	½ cup (3.6 oz)	310
Chocolate Peanut Butter	½ cup (3.8 oz)	360

FOOD	PORTION	CALS
Cookies & Cream	½ cup (3.6 oz)	270
Dulce De Leche	½ cup (3.7 oz)	290
Five Coffee	½ cup (3.6 oz)	220
Five Milk Chocolate	½ cup (3.6 oz)	220
Five Mint	½ cup (3.6 oz)	220
Five Passion Fruit	½ cup (3.6 oz)	220
Five Vanilla	½ cup (3.7 oz)	270
Green Tea	½ cup (3.6 oz)	250
Mango	½ cup (3.7 oz)	250
Reserve Amazon Valley Chocolate	½ cup (3.7 oz)	290
Reserve Caramelized Hazelnut Gianduja	½ cup (3.5 oz)	290
Reserve Fleur De Sel Caramel	½ cup (3.7 oz)	280
Reserve Hawaiian Lehua Honey & Sweet Cream	½ cup (3.8 oz)	270
Rocky Road	½ cup (3.6 oz)	300
Strawberry	½ cup (3.7 oz)	250
Vanilla Honey Bee	½ cup (3.6 oz)	270
Healthy Choice		
Bar Fudge	1 (2.2 oz)	80
Bar Low Fat Sorbet & Cream	1 (2.2 oz)	80
Sandwich Vanilla	1 (2.4 oz)	150
Hershey's		
Banana Split	½ cup (2.5 oz)	160
Chocolate	½ cup (2.5 oz)	140
Cookies And Cream	½ cup (2.5 oz)	160
Fudge Royale	½ cup (2.5 oz)	180
Mint Moose Tracks	½ cup (2.5 oz)	200
Raspberry	½ cup (2.5 oz)	170
Tally-Ho Low Fat Butter Pecan	½ cup (2.5 oz)	90
Vanilla	½ cup (2.5 oz)	150
Julie's		
Organic Gluten Free Sandwich Vanilla	1 (2.6 oz)	220
Klondike		
Bar Caramel Pretzel	1 (4 oz)	260
Bar Original Vanilla	1 (4.5 oz)	250
Bar Reese's	1 (4 oz)	260
Bar Whitehouse Cherry	1 (4.5 oz)	250
Cone Crunchy Vanilla	1 (4.3 oz)	280
Slim A Bear 100 Calorie Sandwich Vanilla	1 (3 oz)	100
Slim A Bear Bar Vanilla	1 (4 oz)	170

FOOD	PORTION	CALS
Lactaid		
Butter Pecan	½ cup (4 oz)	170
Chocolate	½ cup (2.5 oz)	160
Vanilla	½ cup (4 oz)	150
Land O'Lakes		
Vanilla	½ cup (2.4 oz)	150
Vanilla Light	½ cup (2.3 oz)	100
Lifeway		
Frozen Kefir Tart And Tangy Mango	½ cup (2.5 oz)	90
Frozen Kefir Tart And Tangy Original	½ cup (2.5 oz)	90
Frozen Kefir Tart And Tangy Pomegranate	½ cup (2.5 oz)	90
Frozen Kefir Tart And Tangy Strawberry	½ cup (2.5 oz)	90
Magnum		
Classic	1 bar (2.7 oz)	240
Dark	1 bar (2.7 oz)	240
Double Caramel	1 bar (3.2 oz)	320
White	1 bar (2.7 oz)	250
Molli Coolz		
Cup Banana Cream Pie	1	120
Cup Chocolate Fusion	1	140
Cup Chocolate Peanut Butter	1	160
Ionz Cotton Candy	1 cup	100
Ionz S'mores	1 cup	110
Rocks Cherry Blue Raz & Lemon	1 cup	80
Rocks Lemon Lime	1 cup	80
Shakers Chocolate	1 (10.2 oz)	250
Natural Choice		
Organic Double Chocolate	½ cup	230
Organic Strawberry	½ cup	210
Organic Vanilla	½ cup	220
Popsicle		
Creamsicle	1 (2.5 oz)	100
Purely Decadent		
Dairy Free Bar Chocolate Coated Vanilla	1 (2.7 oz)	200
Dairy Free Bar Chocolate Coated Vanilla Almond	1 (2.7 oz)	210
Organic Coconut Milk Chocolate	½ cup	150
Organic Coconut Milk Vanilla Bean	½ cup	150
Organic Dairy Free Belgian Chocolate	½ cup	180
Organic Dairy Free Chocolate Obsession	½ cup	210

FOOD	PORTION	CALS
Organic Dairy Free Gluten Free Cookie Dough	½ cup	230
Organic Dairy Free Mocha Almond Fudge	½ cup	200
Organic Dairy Free Snickerdoodle	½ cup	190
Organic Dairy Free Vanilla	½ cup	170
Rice Dream		
Bar Vanilla Chocolate Coating	1 (3 oz)	230
Bar Vanilla Nutty	1 (3.3 oz)	320
Carob Almond	½ cup	180
Frozen Pie Chocolate	1 (3.4 oz)	330
Mint Carob Chip	½ cup	170
Strawberry	½ cup	160
Sheer Bliss		
Bar Pomegranate	1 (3.1 oz)	260
Blissbites	2 (1.1 oz)	100
Blisswich	1 (3.3 oz)	270
Freedom	½ cup (4 oz)	290
Mediterranean Coffee	½ cup (4 oz)	260
Pomegranate	½ cup (4 oz)	290
Vanilla	½ cup (4 oz)	300
Skinny Cow		
Bar Dippers Vanilla & Caramel	1	80
Bar Truffle Caramel	1	100
Bar Truffle French Vanilla	1	100
Cone Chocolate w/ Fudge	1	150
Cone Vanilla w/ Caramel	1	150
Fudge Bar	1	100
Sandwich Chocolate Peanut Butter	1	150
Sandwich Cookies 'N Cream	1	150
Sandwich Vanilla	1	140
Sandwich Vanilla No Sugar Added	1	140
SoDelicious		
Dairy Free Sandwich Minis Pomegranate	1 (1.4 oz)	90
Dairy Free Sandwich Mint	1 (2.2 oz)	150
Dairy Free Sandwich Vanilla	1 (2 oz)	150
Dairy Free Sugar Free Chocolate Coated Vanilla Bar	1 (2.2 oz)	150
Dairy Free Sugar Free Fudge Bar	1 (2 oz)	80
Organic Dairy Free Sandwich Neapolitan	1 (2.2 oz)	150
Soy Dream		
Butter Pecan	½ cup	140

FOOD	PORTION	CALS
Sandwich Lil' Dreamers Chocolate	1 (1.4 oz)	100
Vanilla	½ cup	140
Starbucks		
Caramel Macchiato	½ cup (3.6 oz)	240
Coffee	½ cup (3.5 oz)	210
Java Chip Frappuccino	½ cup (3.5 oz)	250
Mocha Frappuccino	½ cup (3.5 oz)	220
Mocha Bar	1	280
Stonyfield Farm		
Gotta Have Java	1 serv (4 oz)	250
Strawberry Licious	1 serv (4 oz)	220
Vanilla Chai	1 serv (4 oz)	240
Straus		
I'm Organic Coffee	4 oz	240
I'm Organic Raspberry	½ cup (4 oz)	230
I'm Organic Vanilla Bean	4 oz	240
Organic Brown Sugar Banana	½ cup (3.2 oz)	250
The Greek Gods		
Pagoto Ice Krema Baklava	½ cup (4 oz)	240
Pagoto Ice Krema Chocolate Fig	½ cup (4 oz)	240
Pagoto Ice Krema Honey Pomegranate	½ cup (4 oz)	230
Tofutti		
Cuties Chocolate	1 (1.3 oz)	130
Cuties Vanilla	1 (1.3 oz)	130
Flowers Chocolate Covered	1 (1.4 oz)	180
Marry Me Dessert Bars	1 bar (2.5 oz)	168
Yours Truly Cones	1 (2.6 oz)	220
Turkey Hill		
Banana Split	½ cup	150
Choco Mint Chip	½ cup	160
Chocolate All Natural	½ cup	150
Chocolate Marshmallow	½ cup	160
Coconut Cream Pie	½ cup	170
Cookies 'N Cream	½ cup	150
Duetto Cherry	½ cup	120
Duetto Lemon	½ cup	120
Duetto Root Beer	½ cup	120
French Vanilla	½ cup	140
Light Banana Split	½ cup	110
Light Dulce De Chocolate	½ cup	120

FOOD	PORTION	CALS
Light Moose Tracks	½ cup	140
Light Vanilla Bean	½ cup	100
No Sugar Added Cherry Fudge Ripple	½ cup	80
No Sugar Added Vanilla Bean	½ cup	70
Original Vanilla	½ cup	140
Peanut Butter Ripple	½ cup	170
Rocky Road	½ cup	170
Sandwich Chocolate Chunk	1 (3.2 oz)	320
Sandwich Vanilla Bean	1 (2.5 oz)	190
Sandwich Light Vanilla Bean	1 (2.5 oz)	160
Sundae Cone Vanilla Fudge	1 (3.3 oz)	320
Tin Roof Sundae	½ cup	150
Weight Watchers		
Smart Ones Sundae Chocolate Fudge Brownie	1 (2.3 oz)	140
Smart Ones Sundae Turtle	1 (2.2 oz)	130
TAKE-OUT		
cone vanilla light soft serve	1 (4.6 oz)	164
gelato chocolate hazelnut	½ cup (5.3 oz)	370
gelato vanilla	½ cup (3 oz)	211
ice cream pie no crust	1 slice (3.4 oz)	218
mud pie	⅛ pie (8 oz)	698
sundae caramel	1 (5.4 oz)	303
sundae hot fudge	1 (5.4 oz)	284
sundae strawberry	1 (5.4 oz)	269

ICE CREAM CONES AND CUPS

FOOD	PORTION	CALS
brown sugar cone	1 (10 g)	40
wafer cone	1	17
waffle cone	1 lg	121
Keebler		
Cone Sugar	1	50
Ice Creme Cone	1	15
Waffle Bowl	1	50
Waffle Cone	1	50

ICE CREAM TOPPINGS

FOOD	PORTION	CALS
butterscotch	2 tbsp (1.4 oz)	103
caramel	2 tbsp (1.4 oz)	103
marshmallow cream	1 oz	88
marshmallow cream	1 jar (7 oz)	615
nuts in syrup	2 tbsp	184

FOOD	PORTION	CALS
pineapple	1 cup (11.5 oz)	861
pineapple	2 tbsp (1.5 oz)	106
strawberry	2 tbsp (1.5 oz)	107
strawberry	1 cup (11.5 oz)	863
Hershey's		
Sundae Syrup Caramel	2 tbsp (1.4 oz)	100
Smucker's		
Plate Scrapers Chocolate Fudge	2 tbsp (1.4 oz)	120
Steel's		
Sugar Free Fudge Sauce	2 tbsp (0.9 oz)	110

ICED TEA
MIX
Aquafull

Zesty Lemon Dietary Supplement	1 pkg (9 g)	20
Crystal Light		
Antioxidant Sugar Free Green Tea Raspberry as prep	8 oz	5
On The Go White Peach Tea as prep	8 oz	5
Pure Sugar Free Mixed Berry as prep	8 oz	15
Lipton		
Tea To Go Green Sugar Free Mandarin Mango	½ pkg (0.7 oz)	0
Nestea		
Lemon Liquid Concentrate as prep	8 oz	80
Peach Liquid Concentrate as prep	8 oz	90
Sugar Free w/ Lemon	2 tsp	5
Sweetened w/ Lemon	1⅓ tbsp	60
Unsweetened w/ Lemon	2 tsp	5

READY-TO-DRINK
Arizona

Black & White	8 oz	50
Diet Black Tea Peach	8 oz	0
Green Tea Lemonade	8 oz	50
Organic Green Tea	8 oz	50
Bina		
Lemon	8 oz	70
Peach	8 oz	114
Bolthouse Farms		
Perfectly Protein Vanilla Chai Tea w/ Soy	8 oz	160
Bombilla & Gourd		
Organic Eco Teas All Flavors	8 oz	40

FOOD	PORTION	CALS
Cafe Sepia		
Matcha Latte	1 can (8.6 oz)	130
Delta Blues		
Tea Punch Black Tea Sumptuous Spearmint	8 oz	90
Tea Punch Green Tea Peach & Delectable Lemongrass	8 oz	90
Tea Punch Green Tea Peach Apricot Pineapple Quince	8 oz	100
Fuze		
Antioxidant Tea	8 oz	60
Green Tea	8 oz	60
White Tea	8 oz	60
Gold Peak Tea		
Green Tea Sweetened	1 bottle (16.9 oz)	170
Hawaiian		
Iced Tea	1 can (11.5 oz)	120
Honest Tea		
Assam Black	8 oz	17
Green Dragon	8 oz	30
Green Tea Zero Calorie Passion Fruit	8 oz	0
Half & Half	8 oz	48
Heavenly Lemon Tulsi	8 oz	30
Jasmine Green Energy	8 oz	17
Just Green	8 oz	0
Pearfect White	8 oz	35
White Mango Acai	8 oz	35
Ito En		
Dark Green Tea Oi Ocha	8 oz	0
Golden Oolong	8 oz	0
Green Tea Jasmine	8 oz	0
Green Tea Oi Ocha	8 oz	0
Sencho Shot Japanese Green Tea	1 can (6.4 oz)	0
Kombucha		
Wonder Drink Asian Pear Ginger	1 bottle (8.5 oz)	65
Wonder Drink Rooibus Red Peach	1 bottle (8.5 oz)	60
Lipton		
Diet Green Tea w/ Citrus	8 oz	0
Diet Green Tea w/ Watermelon	8 oz	0
Green Tea 100% Natural Citrus	8 oz	70
Green Tea 100% Natural Passionfruit Mango	8 oz	50

FOOD	PORTION	CALS
Nantucket Nectars		
Half & Half	8 oz	90
Original Lemon	8 oz	80
Nestea		
Green Tea Diet Peach	8 oz	0
Green Tea Peach	1 bottle (20 oz)	220
Lemon	1 bottle (20 oz)	210
Lemon Diet	8 oz	0
Sweetened	8 oz	60
Sweetened Diet Green Tea	8 oz	0
Sweetened Green Tea	8 oz	80
Old Orchard		
Green Tea w/ Lemon & Honey	8 oz	45
Red Tea w/ Currant	8 oz	45
Osteo		
Fruit Tea All Flavors	1 can (12 oz)	120
Pixie		
Black Tea Mate Lemon Ginger	8 oz	35
Yerba Mate Authentic	8 oz	30
POMx		
Green Tea Pomegranate Lychee	8 oz	70
Light Green Tea Pomegranate Hibiscus	8 oz	35
Rooibee Red Tea		
Lemon Honey	1 bottle (12.5 oz)	80
Peach	1 bottle (12.5 oz)	80
Unsweet	1 bottle (12.5 oz)	0
Santa Cruz		
Organic Lemon	8 oz	60
Organic Peppermint	8 oz	60
Organic TeaZer Passionfruit	1 bottle (12 oz)	90
Organic TeaZer Pear	1 bottle (12 oz)	90
Snapple		
Black Tea Lemon	8 oz	80
Diet Lemon Tea	8 oz	10
Diet Lemonade Iced Tea	8 oz	10
Diet Peach	8 oz	0
Diet Plum-A-Granate	8 oz	5
Green Tea Mango Metabolism	8 oz	60
Peach	8 oz	90
Red Tea Pomegranate Raspberry	8 oz	80
White Tea Apple Plum	8 oz	80

FOOD	PORTION	CALS
Sokenbicha		
All Flavors	1 bottle	0
SSips		
Diet Green Tea w/ Honey & Ginseng	1 box (7 oz)	0
Green Tea w/ Honey & Ginseng	1 box (7 oz)	60
Lemon	8 oz	100
Sweet Leaf		
Diet Mint & Honey Green Tea	8 oz	0
Lemon & Lime Unsweet	8 oz	0
Original Sweet	8 oz	70
Pomegranate Green Tea	8 oz	60
Swiss Tea		
Diet	8 oz	0
Diet Decafe	8 oz	0
Green Tea w/ Ginseng & Honey	8 oz	80
Sweet Tea Southern Style w/ Lemon	8 oz	90
White Tea Sweetened w/ Raspberry	8 oz	90
Teas' Tea		
Green Hoji	8 oz	0
Lemongrass Green	8 oz	0
Pure Black	8 oz	0
Pure Green	8 oz	0
True Brew		
Cranberry Orange	8 oz	72
Green Tea	8 oz	64
Sweet Tea	8 oz	76
Turkey Hill		
Decaffeinated	8 oz	80
Diet Decaffeinated	8 oz	0
Nature's Accents Blueberry Oolong	8 oz	100
Nature's Accents Chai Spiced Zero Calorie	8 oz	0
Nature's Accents Green Tea	8 oz	70
Southern Brew Extra Sweet	8 oz	90
VidaTea		
All Flavors	1 can	90
VitaZest		
Green Tea Vitamin Enriched	8 oz	0
Weil For Tea		
Gyokuro	1 can (8.6 oz)	0
Turmeric	1 can (8.6 oz)	0

FOOD	PORTION	CALS
ICES AND ICE POPS		
Breeze Freeze		
100% Fruit Juice	1 (8 oz)	54
Fruit Granita	1 (8 oz)	120
Breyers		
Pure Fruit Pop Lemon Lime	1 (1.75 oz)	40
Pure Fruit Pop Pomegranate Blends	1 (1.75 oz)	40
Dippin' Dots		
Cherry Berry	½ cup	90
Watermelon	½ cup	90
Dole		
Fruit Bars Strawberry	1 (2.75 oz)	90
Super Fruit Bars Acai Blueberry	1 (2.75 oz)	90
Haagen-Dazs		
Fat Free Sorbet Mango	½ cup (4 oz)	120
Fat Free Sorbet Raspberry	½ cup (3.7 oz)	120
Fat Free Sorbet Zesty Lemon	½ cup (4 oz)	110
Lowfat Sorbet Chocolate	½ cup (3.7 oz)	130
Luigi's		
Italian Ice Cherry	1 (6 oz)	130
Italian Ice Lemon Strawberry	1 (6 oz)	120
Italian Ice No Sugar Added Lemon	1 (6 oz)	60
Italian Ice Pina Colada	1 (6 oz)	130
Swirl Blue Ribbon Lemonade	1 (6 oz)	150
Mr. J		
All Flavors	1 bar (2.25 oz)	50
Natural Choice		
Organic Vegan Fruit Bars Coconut	1 (2.75 oz)	90
Organic Vegan Fruit Bars Pink Lemonade	1 (2.75 oz)	50
Organic Vegan Grape	1 (2.75 oz)	50
Organic Vegan Sorbet Blueberry	½ cup	110
Organic Vegan Sorbet Lemon	½ cup	110
Organic Vegan Sorbet Mango	½ cup	110
PickleSickle		
Pop	1 (2 oz)	3
Popsicle		
Creamsicle Pop No Sugar Added	2 (1.65 oz)	45
Creamsicle Pop Sugar Free	2 (1.65 oz)	40
Diet Soda Pops	1 (1.6 oz)	15
Firecracker	1 (1.6 oz)	35

FOOD	PORTION	CALS
Fudgsicle Bar	1 (2.5 oz)	100
Fudgsicle Pops No Sugar Added	1 (1.65 oz)	40
Lifesavers Pop	1 (3.5 oz)	90
Pop Ups Orange Burst	1 (2.75 oz)	90
Rainbow Pops	1 (1.65 oz)	40
Snow Cone	1 (7 oz)	30
Power Of Fruit		
Fruit Bar Banana Berry	1 (1.75 oz)	27
Fruit Bar Original	1 (1.75 oz)	28
Fruit Bar Tropical	1 (1.75 oz)	30
SoDelicious		
Dairy Free Creamy Orange Bar	1 (2.2 oz)	80
Sweet Nothings		
Bar Mango Raspberry	1 (2.6 oz)	100
Turkey Hill		
Venice Mango	½ cup	100
Venice Pomegranate Blueberry w/ Acai	½ cup	100

INDIAN FOOD (see ASIAN FOOD)

JACKFRUIT

canned in syrup	½ cup (3.1 oz)	82
fresh sliced	1 cup (5.8 oz)	157

JALAPENO (see PEPPERS)

JAM/JELLY/PRESERVES

apple butter	1 tbsp (0.6 oz)	31
jam all flavors	1 tbsp (0.7 oz)	56
jam all flavors	1 pkg (0.5 oz)	39
jam apricot	1 tbsp (0.7 oz)	48
jam diet all flavors	1 tbsp (0.5 oz)	18
jelly all flavors	1 tbsp (0.7 oz)	51
jelly diet all flavors	1 tbsp (0.7 oz)	25
jelly reduced sugar all flavors	1 tbsp (0.7 oz)	34
orange marmalade	1 tbsp (0.7 oz)	49
preserves all flavors	1 tbsp (0.7 oz)	56
Beth's Farm Kitchen		
Apple Butter	2 tbsp (1 oz)	15
Jam Gooseberry	2 tbsp (1 oz)	45
Jam Sour Cherry	2 tbsp (1 oz)	15
Jam Strawberry Rhubarb	2 tbsp (1 oz)	40
Marmalade Bitter Orange	2 tbsp (1 oz)	40

FOOD	PORTION	CALS
Cascadian Farm		
Organic Fruit Spread Blackberry	1 tbsp	45
Organic Fruit Spread Raspberry	1 tbsp	45
Organic Sweet Orange Marmalade	1 tbsp	45
Chukar Cherries		
Preserves No Sugar Added Cherry Amaretto	1 tbsp	24
Preserves Red Sour Cherry	1 tbsp	40
Preserves Vanilla Peach	1 tbsp	28
Columbia Empire Farms		
Marionberry Seedless Preserves	1 tbsp	60
Comfort Care		
Country Apple Butter	1 tbsp (1 oz)	40
Delicia		
Fruit Spread Black Cherry	1 tbsp (0.7 oz)	40
Gedney		
State Fair Preserves Strawberry Rhubarb	1 tbsp	50
Hero		
Swiss Preserves Black Cherry	1 tbsp (0.7 oz)	50
Jake & Amos		
Jam Fig	1 tbsp (0.5 oz)	35
Jam Hot Pepper	1 tbsp	43
Jam Rhubarb	1 tbsp (0.7 oz)	40
Jenkins Jellies		
Hell Fire Pepper Jelly	1 tbsp (0.7 oz)	40
Polaner		
All Fruit w/ Fiber Grape	1 tbsp (0.6 oz)	30
Revolution Foods		
Organic Jelly Grape	1 tbsp (0.7 oz)	60
Organic Preserves Strawberry	1 tbsp (0.7 oz)	60
Robert Rothchild Farm		
Preserves Cherry Acai	1 tbsp	35
Sarabeth's		
Spreadable Fruit Blood Orange Marmalade	1 tbsp (0.7 oz)	35
Spreadable Fruit Chunky Apple	1 tbsp (0.7 oz)	30
Spreadable Fruit Orange Apricot Marmalade	1 tbsp (0.7 oz)	30
Spreadable Fruit Pineapple Mango	1 tbsp (0.7 oz)	35
Spreadable Fruit Strawberry Peach	1 tbsp (0.7 oz)	30
Spreadable Fruit Strawberry Rhubarb	1 tbsp (0.7 oz)	40
Smucker's		
Jam Blackberry	1 tbsp (0.7 oz)	50

FOOD	PORTION	CALS
Jam Concord Grape	1 tbsp (0.7 oz)	50
Jam Red Plum	1 tbsp (0.7 oz)	50
Jam Seedless Red Raspberry	1 tbsp (0.7 oz)	50
Jelly Apple	2 tbsp (0.7 oz)	50
Jelly Concord Grape	1 tbsp (0.7 oz)	50
Jelly Strawberry	1 tbsp (0.7 oz)	50
Orange Marmalade Low Sugar	2 tbsp (0.7 oz)	25
Preserves Apricot Low Sugar	1 tbsp (0.6 oz)	25
Simply Fruit Black Cherry	1 tbsp (0.7 oz)	40
Simply Fruit Peach	1 tbsp (0.7 oz)	40
Simply Fruit Strawberry	1 tbsp (0.7 oz)	40
Trappist		
Jelly Pomegranate	1 tbsp (0.7 oz)	50
Tree Of Life		
Organic Fruit Spread Grape	1 tbsp (0.6 oz)	30
Organic Fruit Spread Peach	1 tbsp (0.6 oz)	30
Welch's		
Grape Jelly	1 tbsp (1 oz)	50

JAPANESE FOOD (see ASIAN FOOD, SUSHI)

JELLY (see JAM/JELLY/PRESERVES)

JELLYFISH

pickled	½ cup	10

JERKY

beef	1 oz	122
pork	1 oz	122
venison	1 oz	119
Applegate Farms		
Natural Joy Stick	1 (1 oz)	100
Dakota Gourmet		
Fruit Jerky Strawberry Kiwi	1	70
Frank's RedHot		
Chile'N Lime Steak Strips	1 oz	80
Original Beef	1 oz	80
Gary West		
Beef Strips Hickory Smoked	1 oz	70
Buffalo Strips	½ pkg (1 oz)	60
Elk Strips	½ pkg (1 oz)	70

FOOD	PORTION	CALS
Jerky For Life		
Beef Steak Black Pepper & Garlic	¼ pkg (1 oz)	50
Beef Steak Jalapeno	¼ pkg (1 oz)	50
King Kalibur		
Black Angus Beef Sticks	1 (1.2 oz)	93
Matador		
Beef Original	1 pkg (1.4 oz)	110
Snack Stick Original	1 (1 oz)	150
Ostrim		
Stick Beef & Ostrich	1 (1.5 oz)	80
Outpost		
Beef	1 oz	70
Beef Steak	1 pkg (0.9 oz)	60
Beef Stick	1 (0.4 oz)	60
Primal		
Meatless Vegan Hickory Smoke	1 pkg (1 oz)	99
Meatless Vegan Mesquite Lime	1 pkg (1 oz)	74
Meatless Vegan Texas BBQ	1 pkg (1 oz)	81
Meatless Vegan Thai Peanut	1 pkg (1 oz)	74
Slim Jim		
Beef	7 pieces	130
Beef Jerky Hickory Smoked	1 oz	80
Classic Handipack	1 box	210
Giant Caddy Pepperoni	1 pkg	150
Twin Pack Cheese & Pepperoni	1 pkg	150
Sunrich Naturals		
Fruit Bar Sour Apple	1 (0.7 oz)	70
Fruit Bar Strawberry Kiwi	1 (0.7 oz)	70
Tanka		
Natural Buffalo Cranberry Bar	1 (1 oz)	70
Natural Buffalo Cranberry Bite	1 (0.5 oz)	35
Tony's Smokehouse		
Salmon	1 pkg (0.5 oz)	40
Umpqua Indian Foods		
Brew Pub Steak Jerky Beef Flavored	¼ pkg (1 oz)	90
Steak Jerky Original	¼ pkg (1 oz)	60
JICAMA		
fresh	1 sm (12.8 oz)	139
raw sliced	1 cup	46

FOOD	PORTION	CALS
JUJUBE		
dried	1 oz	82
JUTE		
cooked	1 cup	32
KALE		
chopped cooked w/o salt	1 cup	36
fresh cooked w/ fat	1 cup	69
scotch chopped cooked w/o salt	1 cup	36
Allens		
Seasoned	½ cup	35
Glory		
Fresh Greens	1 serv (2.8 oz)	40
Seasoned canned	½ cup	35
KANGAROO		
kangaroo	3 oz	120
KEFIR		
kefir	8 oz	98
Evolve		
Plain	8 oz	120
Strawberry	8 oz	180
Green Valley		
Organic Lactose Free Blueberry Pom Acai	1 pkg (6 oz)	150
Organic Lactose Free Plain	8 oz	90
Helios		
Organic Blueberry	8 oz	160
Organic Nonfat Plain w/ Omega 3s	8 oz	80
Organic Plain	8 oz	120
Organic Raspberry	8 oz	160
Lifeway		
BioKefir Shot Digestion Vanilla	1 bottle (3.5 oz)	60
BioKefir Shot Heart Health Black Cherry	1 bottle (3.5 oz)	60
BioKefir Shot Heart Health Blackberry	1 bottle (3.5 oz)	60
Greek Style	8 oz	210
Lowfat Blueberry	8 oz	140
Lowfat Cappuccino	8 oz	140
Lowfat Pomegranate	8 oz	140
Nonfat Peach	8 oz	180
Nonfat Plain	8 oz	90

FOOD	PORTION	CALS
Nonfat Raspberry	8 oz	150
Organic Lowfat Plain	8 oz	110
Organic Lowfat Wildberry	8 oz	160
Original	8 oz	150
Plain Lowfat	8 oz	110
Plain Whole Milk	8 oz	160
Probugs Goo-Berry Pie	1 bottle (5 oz)	130
Slim6 Mixed Berry	8 oz	110
Slim6 Plain	8 oz	110
Nancy's		
Organic Lowfat Blackberry	1 cup	180
Organic Lowfat Plain	1 cup	110
Organic Lowfat Raspberry	1 cup	180
Yakult		
Drink	1 bottle (2.7 oz)	50
KETCHUP		
banana	1 tsp	10
ketchup	1 tbsp	15
ketchup	1 pkg (0.2 oz)	6
low sodium	1 tbsp	15
Annie's Homegrown		
Organic	1 tbsp (0.6 oz)	15
Fischer & Wieser		
Chipotle Chili	1 tbsp (0.7 oz)	15
Heinz		
Ketchup	1 tbsp	15
No Salt Added	1 tbsp (0.6 oz)	20
Reduced Sugar	1 tbsp (0.6 oz)	5
Hunt's		
Ketchup No Salt Added	1 tbsp (0.6 oz)	25
Squeeze	1 tbsp (0.6 oz)	20
Muir Glen		
Organic	1 tbsp	20
Nature's Hollow		
Sugar Free	1 tbsp (0.7 oz)	0
OrganicVille		
No Added Sugar	1 tbsp (0.6 oz)	20
Texas Sassy		
Tequila Ketchup	1 tbsp (0.5 oz)	20

FOOD	PORTION	CALS
Tree Of Life		
Organic	1 tbsp (0.6 oz)	20
Walden Farms		
Calorie Free	1 tbsp (0.5 oz)	0
Wholemato		
Organic Agave	1 tbsp	15
KIDNEY		
beef simmered	3 oz	134
lamb braised	3 oz	116
pork braised	3 oz	128
veal braised	3 oz	139
Rumba		
Beef	4 oz	120
KIDNEY BEANS		
canned	½ cup	108
dried cooked w/o salt	½ cup	112
B&M		
Red Kidney Baked Beans	½ cup (4.6 oz)	200
Progresso		
Cannellini	½ cup (4.6 oz)	110
Van Camp's		
New Orleans	½ cup	90
KIWI		
fresh	1 med (2.6 oz)	46
fresh	1 lg (3.2 oz)	56
Chiquita		
Fresh	1 (2.7 oz)	46
FruitziO		
Kiwi	1 pkg (0.88 oz)	40
KIWI JUICE		
Auna		
Kiwifruit Juice	1 bottle (12 oz)	120
KNISH		
Gabila's		
Potato	1 (4.5 oz)	180
TAKE-OUT		
cheese	1 (2.1 oz)	205
meat	1 (1.8 oz)	174

FOOD	PORTION	CALS
potato	1 sm (2.1 oz)	212
potato	1 lg (6 oz)	639

KOHLRABI

raw sliced	1 cup	36
sliced cooked w/o salt	1 cup	48

TAKE-OUT

creamed	1 cup	150

KRILL

fresh	1 oz	22

KUMQUATS

canned in syrup	1	13
fresh	1	13

LAMB

cubed lean & fat braised	4 oz	253
cubed lean broiled	4 oz	211
ground broiled	4 oz	321
leg roasted	4 oz	213
loin chop lean & fat broiled	1 chop (4 oz)	222
rib chop lean & fat broiled	1 chop	165
rib roast baked	4 oz	386
shank lean & fat braised	4 oz	360
shoulder chop lean & fat cooked	1 chop (5.5 oz)	274
shoulder w/ bone braised	4 oz	231

LAMB DISHES
TAKE-OUT

keema w/ coconut milk	1 serv (8 oz)	380
moroccan pilaf w/ bulgur	1 serv	327
moussaka	4 in sq (16 oz)	659
shepherd's pie	1 (21.3 oz)	742
stew w/ potatoes & vegetables	1 cup	260

LAMBSQUARTERS

chopped cooked w/ salt	1 cup	58

LECITHIN

lecithin	1 tbsp	104
Bob's Red Mill		
Lecithin Granules	1 tbsp	60

FOOD	PORTION	CALS
Tree Of Life		
Granules	1 tbsp (0.3 oz)	55
LEEKS		
chopped cooked w/o salt	¼ cup	8
cooked	1 (4.4 oz)	38
freeze dried	1 tbsp	1
LEMON		
fresh	1 med (4 oz)	22
peel	1 tbsp	3
peel	1 tsp	1
wedge	1 (7 g)	2
True Lemon		
Crystallized Lemon	1 pkg (1 g)	0
LEMON CURD		
lemon curd made w/ egg	2 tsp	29
Robert Rothchild Farm		
Lemon Curd & Tart Filling	1 tbsp	50
LEMON JUICE		
bottled	1 oz	6
bottled	1 tbsp	3
fresh	1 oz	8
from 1 lemon	1.6 oz	12
from wedge	6 g	1
Canarino		
Italian Hot Lemon Beverage as prep	1 cup	0
Essn		
Sparkling Meyer Lemon Juice	1 can (8.4 oz)	170
Italian Volcano		
Organic	2 tbsp (1 oz)	9
Izze		
Esque Sparkling Limon	1 bottle (12 oz)	50
Natalie's Orchid Island Juice		
100% Juice	1 tsp	1
Santa Cruz		
Organic 100% Juice	1 tsp	0
Volcano		
Organic Lemon Burst	2 tbsp (1 oz)	0

FOOD	PORTION	CALS
LEMONADE		
MIX		
Crystal Light		
Sugar Free as prep	8 oz	5
Hansen's		
Fruit Stix Strawberry Lemonade	½ pkg (2 g)	5
READY-TO-DRINK		
Apple & Eve		
Organic	8 oz	130
EarthWise		
Harvest Lemonade	8 oz	100
Honest Ade		
Classic Zero Calorie	8 oz	0
Mike's		
Hard Lemonade	1 bottle (12 oz)	220
Minute Maid		
Lemonade	1 can (12 oz)	150
Nantucket Nectars		
Lemonade	8 oz	110
Natalie's Orchid Island Juice		
Lemonade	8 oz	130
Odwalla		
PomaGrand	8 oz	110
Pure Squeezed	8 oz	120
Raaw		
Carrot Lemonade	8 oz	110
Santa Cruz		
Organic Sparkling	8 oz	110
Simply		
Lemonade	8 oz	120
SSips		
Lemonade	8 oz	110
Sweet Leaf		
Half & Half Lemonade Tea	8 oz	85
Original	8 oz	90
Tropicana		
Light	1 cup	10
Orchard Style	8 oz	120
Trop50 Raspberry	8 oz	50
Twister Light	8 oz	50

FOOD	PORTION	CALS
Turkey Hill		
Lemonade	8 oz	120
Uncle Matt's		
Organic	8 oz	120

LEMONGRASS
fresh	1 tbsp	5

LENTILS
dried cooked	1 cup	230
Near East		
Lentil Pilaf	1 cup	200
TastyBite		
Jodhpur Lentils	½ pkg (5 oz)	106
Madras Lentils	½ pkg (5 oz)	120
TruRoots		
Organic Sprouted Green not prep	¼ cup (1.4 oz)	140
TAKE-OUT		
lentil loaf	1 slice (1.6 oz)	83
middle eastern lentil salad	1 serv (4.5 oz)	158
yemiser selatta ethiopian lentil salad	1 serv (3 oz)	115

LETTUCE (see also SALAD)
arugula	6 leaves (0.4 oz)	3
arugula shredded	1 cup	5
boston	1 head (5.7 oz)	21
boston chopped	6 leaves	7
cornsalad field salad	1 cup (1.9 oz)	7
iceberg	6 med leaves	7
iceberg	1 lg head (26.5 oz)	106
iceberg shredded	1 cup	10
looseleaf outer leaves	6 (5 oz)	22
looseleaf shredded	1 cup	5
red leaf	6 leaves (3.6 oz)	16
red leaf shredded	1 cup	4
romaine	3 leaves (3 oz)	14
romaine heart	6 leaves (1.3 oz)	6
romaine shredded	1 cup	8
Dole		
Just Lettuce	1½ cups (3 oz)	15
Romaine Chopped	1½ cups (3 oz)	15

FOOD	PORTION	CALS
Earthbound Farms		
Organic Baby Romaine Salad	2 cups	15
Fresh Express		
5 Lettuce Mix	3 cups	15
Lettuce Trio	2½ cups	15
Organic Baby Arugula	3 cups	20
Organic Hearts Of Romaine	1½ cups	15
Premium Romaine	2 cups	15
Shreds Iceberg	1½ cups	15
Sweet Butter	2½ cups	10
Mann's		
Green Leaf Singles	6 leaves (3 oz)	15
Ocean Mist		
Butter Leaf Shredded	1 cup (2 oz)	7
Green Or Green Leaf Shredded	1 cup (1.3 oz)	5
Iceberg	⅙ head (3 oz)	15
Ready Pac		
Baby Arugula	4 cups (3 oz)	20
Shredded Iceberg	1 cup (3 oz)	10
Simply Lettuce	2½ cups (3 oz)	15

LILY ROOT
dried	1 oz	89
fresh	1 oz	32

LIMA BEANS
CANNED
lima beans	½ cup	95
Allens		
Baby Butter Beans	½ cup	120
Medium Green	½ cup	140
East Texas Fair		
Green	½ cup	120
Hanover		
Butter Beans In Sauce	½ cup	100
DRIED		
cooked	½ cup	150
FROZEN		
C&W		
Baby	½ cup	110

FOOD	PORTION	CALS
Green Giant		
Baby & Butter Sauce as prep	⅔ cup	100
LIME		
fresh	1 (2.4 oz)	20
wedge	1 (8 g)	2
True Lime		
Crystallized Lime	1 pkg	0
LIME JUICE		
bottled	1 oz	6
fresh	1 oz	8
from 1 lime	1.1 oz	11
Angostura		
Lime Mixer	1 tsp	5
Honest Ade		
Limeade	8 oz	48
Natalie's Orchid Island Juice		
100% Juice	1 tsp	0
Sabor Latino		
Limeade	8 oz	160
Santa Cruz		
Organic 100% Juice	1 tsp	0
Simply		
Limeade	8 oz	120
Sweet Leaf		
Limeade Cherry	8 oz	90
Turkey Hill		
Limonade	8 oz	120
Volcano		
Organic Lime Burst	2 tbsp (1 oz)	0
LING		
blue raw	3.5 oz	83
fresh baked	3 oz	95
fresh fillet baked	5.3 oz	168
LINGCOD		
baked	3 oz	93
fillet baked	5.3 oz	164

FOOD	PORTION	CALS

LIQUOR (see ALCOHOL DRINKS, BEER AND ALE, CHAMPAGNE, MALT, WINE)

LITCHI JUICE
Ceres

100% Juice	8 oz	120

LIVER (see also PATE)

beef braised	1 slice (2.4 oz)	130
beef pan-fried	1 slice (2.8 oz)	142
chicken fried	3 oz	146
chicken simmered	3 oz	142
duck raw	1 (1.5 oz)	60
goose raw	1 (3.3 oz)	125
lamb braised	3 oz	187
lamb fried	3 oz	202
moose braised	3 oz	132
pork braised	3 oz	140
turkey simmered	1 liver (2.9 oz)	227
veal braised	1 slice (2.8 oz)	154
veal pan fried	1 slice (2.4 oz)	129

Organic Prairie

Beef	2 oz	80

Perdue

Chicken Fresh	4 oz	130

Rumba

Beef	4 oz	160

TAKE-OUT

calves liver w/ onions	1 serv (5 oz)	177

LLAMA

llama	3 oz	120

LOBSTER

northern cooked	3 oz	83
northern cooked	1 cup	142
northern raw	3 oz	77
northern raw	1 lobster (5.3 oz)	136
spiny steamed	3 oz	122
spiny steamed	1 (5.7 oz)	233

TAKE-OUT

newburg	1 cup	485

FOOD	PORTION	CALS
LOGANBERRIES		
fresh	½ cup (2.5 oz)	40
frzn thawed	½ cup (2.6 oz)	40
LONGANS		
fresh	1	2
LOQUATS		
fresh	1 sm (0.5 oz)	6
fresh	1 lg (0.7 oz)	9
fresh cubed	½ cup (2.6 oz)	35
LOTUS		
root raw sliced	10 slices	45
root sliced cooked	10 slices	59
seeds dried	1 oz	94
LOX (see SALMON)		
LUPINES		
dried cooked	1 cup	197
LYCHEES		
canned in syrup	½ cup (4.4 oz)	114
canned in syrup	1 (0.7 oz)	19
dried	1 (2.5 g)	7
fresh	1 (0.3 oz)	6
fresh cut up	½ cup (3.3 oz)	63
Polar		
Lychee	1	110
MACA ROOT		
Navitas Naturals		
Powder Gelatanized	1 tsp (5 g)	20
Raw Powder	1 tsp (5 g)	20
MACADAMIA NUTS		
dry roasted w/ salt	11 nuts (1 oz)	200
oil roasted	1 oz	204
Chukar Cherries		
Extra Dark Chocolate Covered	3 tbsp (1.4 oz)	216
Emily's		
Milk Chocolate Covered	4 (1.5 oz)	260

FOOD	PORTION	CALS
Fisher		
Macadamia Nuts	¼ cup (1 oz)	200
Hawaiian Host		
White Choco	3 pieces (1.4 oz)	230
Mauna Loa		
Dry Roasted Salted	¼ cup (1 oz)	230
Dry Roasted Unsalted	¼ cup (1 oz)	230
Honey Roasted	¼ cup (1 oz)	200
Kona Coffee	¼ cup (1 oz)	180
Maui Onion & Garlic	1 pkg (1.2 oz)	230
MACE		
ground	1 tsp	8
MACKEREL		
CANNED		
jack	1 can (12.7 oz)	563
jack	1 cup	296
Chicken Of The Sea		
Jack In Water	⅓ cup	90
Polar		
Jack	⅓ cup	90
FRESH		
atlantic cooked	3 oz	223
atlantic raw	3 oz	174
jack baked	3 oz	171
jack fillet baked	6.2 oz	354
king baked	3 oz	114
king fillet baked	5.4 oz	207
pacific baked	3 oz	171
pacific fillet baked	6.2 oz	354
spanish cooked	3 oz	134
spanish fillet cooked	1 (5.1 oz)	230
spanish raw	3 oz	118
SMOKED		
atlantic	3.5 oz	296
MAHI MAHI		
fresh baked	4 oz	192
MALANGA		
dasheen mashed	1 cup	226

FOOD	PORTION	CALS
dasheen pieces boiled	1 cup	212
pieces fried	1 cup	304
root raw	1 (10.7 oz)	299
MALT		
malt liquor	1 bottle (12 oz)	148
nonalcoholic	1 bottle (12 oz)	133
MALTED MILK		
chocolate as prep w/ milk	1 cup	179
chocolate flavor powder	3 heaping tsp (0.7 oz)	79
natural flavor as prep w/ milk	1 cup	186
natural flavor powder	3 heaping tsp (0.7 oz)	87
MAMMY APPLE		
fresh	1	431
MANGO		
dried	1 slice (5 g)	16
dried	½ cup (1.8 oz)	74
fresh	1 (7.3 oz)	135
fresh sliced	½ cup (3 oz)	54
pickled	1 slice (1 oz)	38
C&W		
Chunks	¾ cup	90
Crispy Green		
Crispy Mangoes	1 pkg (0.35 oz)	40
Crunchies		
Freeze Dried	¼ cup (6 g)	20
Crunchy N'Yummy		
Organic Freeze Dried	1 pkg (1 oz)	100
Del Monte		
SunFresh In Extra Light Syrup	½ cup (4.4 oz)	70
Dole		
Chunks frzn	¾ cup (4.9 oz)	90
Fresh	½ (3.6 oz)	70
Kopali		
Organic Dried	1 pkg (1.8 oz)	140
Peeled Snacks		
Fruit Picks Go-Mango-Man-Go	1 pkg (1.4 oz)	120
Phillippine Brand		
Dried	6 pieces	160
Dried Green	1 pkg (0.7 oz)	75

FOOD	PORTION	CALS
Polar		
Sliced	3 pieces (5 oz)	100
Sunsweet		
Philippine dried	6 pieces (1.4 oz)	130
MANGO JUICE		
nectar canned	1 cup (8.8 oz)	128
Ceres		
100% Juice	8 oz	120
GoodBelly		
Mango Probiotic Drink	8 oz	100
Old Orchard		
Nectar Cocktail	8 oz	75
Snapple		
Juice Drinks Mango Madness	8 oz	100
Ultra Lo-Gly		
Mango Mojito	1 bottle (10 oz)	35
MANGOSTEEN		
canned in syrup	½ cup (3.4 oz)	72
Xango		
Single Supplement	1 pkg (1 oz)	13
MARGARINE		
margarine butter blend	1 tbsp (0.5 oz)	101
squeeze	1 pkg (0.2 oz)	36
squeeze liquid	1 tbsp (0.5 oz)	102
stick	1 tbsp (0.5 oz)	100
stick	1 stick (4 oz)	810
tub diet	1 tbsp (0.5 oz)	26
tub fat free	1 tbsp (0.5 oz)	27
tub light	1 tbsp (0.5 oz)	59
tub salted	1 tbsp (0.5 oz)	101
whipped salted	1 tbsp (0.3 oz)	67
Benecol		
Spread Light	1 tbsp	50
Spread Regular	1 tbsp	70
Brummel & Brown		
Creamy Fruit Spread Strawberry	1 tbsp	50
Spread w/ Natural Yogurt	1 tbsp (0.5 oz)	45
Country Crock		
Light	1 tbsp (0.5 oz)	50

FOOD	PORTION	CALS
Regular	1 tbsp (0.5 oz)	90
Spread w/ Calcium + Vitamin D	1 tbsp (0.5 oz)	50
Earth Balance		
Butter Blend Salted	1 tbsp	100
Buttery Spread Original	1 tbsp	100
Buttery Spread Soy Garden	1 tbsp	100
Buttery Sticks Vegan	1 tbsp	100
I Can't Believe It's Not Butter		
Original	1 tbsp (0.5 oz)	70
Original Soft	1 tbsp (0.5 oz)	70
Original Squeeze	1 tbsp (0.4 oz)	60
Spray	2 sprays (1 g)	0
Land O'Lakes		
Soft	1 tbsp (0.5 oz)	100
Stick	1 tbsp (0.5 oz)	100
Move Over Butter		
Spread	1 tbsp	50
Parkay		
Original Spread	1 tbsp (0.4 oz)	70
Spray	5 sprays (1 g)	0
Squeeze	1 tbsp (0.5 oz)	70
Stick	1 tbsp (0.5 oz)	80
Promise		
Buttery Spread	1 tbsp (0.5 oz)	80
Buttery Spread Activ	1 tbsp	70
Fat Free	1 tbsp	5
Light	1 tbsp	45
Light Activ	1 tbsp	45
Smart Balance		
Butter Blend Stick	1 tbsp (0.5 g)	100
Buttery Spread 37% Light	1 tbsp (0.5 oz)	45
Buttery Spread 67%	1 tbsp (0.5 oz)	80
Buttery Spread Low Sodium	1 tbsp (0.4 oz)	65
Buttery Spread Omega Plus	1 tbsp (0.5 oz)	80
Buttery Spread Omega-3 w/ Extra Virgin Olive Oil	1 tbsp (0.4 oz)	60
Buttery Spread w/ Flax Oil	1 tbsp (0.5 oz)	80
Spray Buttery Burst w/ Organic Soy	5 sprays (1 g)	0

MARINADE (*see* SAUCE)

FOOD	PORTION	CALS
MARJORAM		
dried	1 tsp	2
MARLIN		
raw	3 oz	110
MARSHMALLOW		
chocolate coated	1 (0.4 oz)	41
coconut coated	1 (0.4 oz)	33
marshmallow regular	1 (0.3 oz)	23
miniatures	1 cup (1.8 oz)	159
miniatures	10 (0.3 oz)	22
MATZO		
brie	1 piece (0.5 oz)	54
egg	1 (1 oz)	109
matzo ball	1 med (1.2 oz)	48
plain	1 (1 oz)	111
whole wheat	1 (1 oz)	98
Holiday Candies		
Dark Chocolate Coated	1 oz	130
Manischewitz		
Egg & Onion	1 (1 oz)	100
Matzo Ball Mix	2 tbsp	50
Yehuda		
Organic	1 (1 oz)	110
MAYONNAISE		
diet	1 tbsp	36
imitation	1 tbsp	35
mayonnaise	1 tbsp	99
Baconnaise		
Lite	1 tbsp (0.5 oz)	30
Regular	1 tbsp (0.5 oz)	80
Cains		
All Natural	1 tbsp	100
Light	1 tbsp	50
Dietz & Watson		
Mixed Pepper Mayo	1 tbsp (0.5 oz)	100
Hellman's		
Light	1 tbsp (0.5 oz)	35
Real	1 tbsp	90

FOOD	PORTION	CALS
Real Canola No Cholesterol	1 tbsp	90
Reduced Fat	1 tbsp	20
W/ Extra Virgin Olive Oil	1 tbsp	50
Hollywood		
Canola	1 tbsp	100
Safflower	1 tbsp	100
Kraft		
Mayo	1 tbsp	90
Mayo w/ Olive Oil	1 tbsp	45
Miracle Whip		
Free	1 tbsp	15
Light	1 tbsp	25
Original	1 pkg (0.4 oz)	35
Nasoya		
Nayonaise Original	1 tbsp (0.5 oz)	35
NatureNaise		
Organic Spread	1 tbsp (0.5 oz)	40
Smart Balance		
Omega Plus Light	1 tbsp (0.5 oz)	50
Vegenaise		
Grapeseed Oil	1 tbsp (0.5 oz)	90
Organic	1 tbsp (0.5 oz)	90
Original	1 tbsp (0.5 oz)	90

MEAT SUBSTITUTES (*see also* BACON SUBSTITUTES, CANADIAN BACON SUBSTITUTES, CHICKEN SUBSTITUTES, HAMBURGER SUBSTITUTES, MEATBALL SUBSTITUTES, SAUSAGE SUBSTITUTES, TURKEY SUBSTITUTES)

FOOD	PORTION	CALS
Amy's		
Veggie Loaf w/ Mashed Potatoes & Vegetables	1 pkg (10 oz)	290
Gardein		
BBQ Pulled Shreds	1 serv (4.5 oz)	160
Beefless Tips	1 serv (3.5 oz)	120
Seasoned Bites	1 serv (4.4 oz)	130
Gardenburger		
BBQ Riblets w/ Sauce	1 serv (5 oz)	240
Helen's Kitchen		
GardenSteak Tofu Steak	1 (3 oz)	150
Loma Linda		
Dinner Cuts	2 slices (3.2 oz)	90
Swiss Stake	1 piece (3.2 oz)	130

FOOD	PORTION	CALS
Morningstar Farms		
Meal Starters Steak Strips	12 pieces (3 oz)	140
Veat		
Gourmet Bites	1 serv (2.5 oz)	90
Vegetarian Fillet	1 (1.8 oz)	170
Vjana		
Cowgirl Veggie Steaks	1 (3.7 oz)	260
Veggie Doner Kebab	½ cup (3 oz)	210
Veggie Gyros	24 pieces (3 oz)	220
Worthington		
Bolono	3 slices (2 oz)	80
Choplets	2 slices (3.2 oz)	90
Corned Beef Vegetarian	3 slices (2 oz)	140
Dinner Roast	1 slice (3 oz)	180
Multigrain Cutlets	2 slices (3.2 oz)	100
Prime Stakes	1 piece (3.2 oz)	120
Vegetable Skallops	½ cup (3 oz)	90
Wham	2 slices (2 oz)	110
Yves		
Meatless Beef Skewers	1 (2.8 oz)	100
Meatless Bologna	4 slices	60
Meatless Pepperoni	6 slices	90
Meatless Ground Round Original	⅓ cup	60

MEATBALL SUBSTITUTES

FOOD	PORTION	CALS
meatless	2 (1.3 oz)	71
Franklin Farms		
Portabella Veggiballs Gluten Free	3 (3 oz)	140
Gardenburger		
Mama Mia Meatballs	6 (3 oz)	110
Loma Linda		
Tender Rounds	6 (2.8 oz)	120
Morningstar Farms		
Meal Starters Veggie Meatballs	5 (2.8 oz)	130
Veggie Patch		
Meatless	4 (3 oz)	120
Vjana		
Veggie Cevapcici	4 (2.8 oz)	240

MEATBALLS

FOOD	PORTION	CALS
beef cocktail	1 (0.2 oz)	18

FOOD	PORTION	CALS
beef lg	1 (1.5 oz)	111
beef med	1 (1 oz)	74
chicken cocktail	1 (0.2 oz)	12
chicken lg	1 (1.5 oz)	71
chicken med	1 (1 oz)	47
turkey med	1 (1 oz)	47
venison	1 (1.5 oz)	69
Butterball		
Seasoned Italian frzn	6 (3 oz)	170
Coleman		
Chicken Buffalo Style	4	160
Chicken Chipotle Cheddar	4 (2.6 oz)	180
Chicken Italian w/ Parmesan	7 (2.6 oz)	150
Chicken Pesto Parmesan	4 (2.6 oz)	170
Chicken Spinach Fontina Cheese & Roasted Garlic	4 (2.6 oz)	130
Chicken Sun-Dried Tomato Basil & Provolone	4 (2.6 oz)	150
DelGrosso		
Italian Style	3 (3 oz)	180
Farm Rich		
Original	6 (3 oz)	240
Turkey	5 (3.1 oz)	150
Foster Farms		
Turkey	3 (2.9 oz)	150
Hans All Natural		
Chicken Buffalo Style	4	160
Chicken Sweet Basil Parmesan	4	170
Honeysuckle White		
Turkey Italian Style frzn	3 (3 oz)	190
Mama Lucia		
Homestyle	4	207
Italian Style	4	280
Sausage Beef	8	220
Mom Made		
Bite-Size Turkey	9 (3 oz)	140
Organic Classics		
Italian Beef	3 (3 oz)	180
Perdue		
Turkey Italian Style	4 (3 oz)	180

FOOD	PORTION	CALS
Shady Brook		
Turkey Meatballs Appetizer Size + Sweet & Sour Sauce	6 + 2 tbsp sauce	235
Tyson		
Italian Style Chicken	6 (3 oz)	180
TAKE-OUT		
albondigas w/ sauce	3 + sauce (5.3 oz)	372
porcupine + tomato sauce	3 + sauce	160
swedish w/ cream sauce	3 + sauce (4.7 oz)	215
sweet & sour	3 + sauce (4.5 oz)	188

MELON

FOOD	PORTION	CALS
sprite	1 (10.6 oz)	110

MEXICAN FOOD (see SALSA, SPANISH FOOD, TORTILLA)

MILK

FOOD	PORTION	CALS
CANNED		
condensed sweetened	1 tbsp (0.7 oz)	61
condensed sweetened	1 cup (10.7 oz)	982
evaporated nonfat	1 tbsp (0.5 oz)	12
evaporated nonfat	1 cup (9 oz)	200
Borden		
Sweetened Condensed	2 tbsp (1.4 oz)	130
Sweetened Condensed Low Fat	2 tbsp	120
Carnation		
Evaporated	2 tbsp (1 oz)	40
Evaporated Fat Free	2 tbsp (1 oz)	25
Evaporated Lowfat 2%	2 tbsp (1 oz)	25
Meyenberg		
Goat Evaporated	4 oz	145
DRIED		
buttermilk	¼ cup (1 oz)	111
buttermilk	1 tbsp (0.2 oz)	25
nonfat instant	1 tbsp (0.6 oz)	61
nonfat instant	1 pkg (3.2 oz)	326
whole milk	¼ cup (1.1 oz)	159
Alba		
Instant Non-Fat as prep	1 cup	80
Bob's Red Mill		
Buttermilk Sweet Cream as prep	8 oz	60
Non Fat as prep	8 oz	80

FOOD	PORTION	CALS
Carnation		
Instant Nonfat as prep	1 cup	80
Meyenberg		
Powdered Goat	1 scoop (1 oz)	90
Organic Valley		
Buttermilk	3 tbsp	110
Nonfat	3 tbsp	90
Sanalac		
Powder	¼ cup (0.8 oz)	80
REFRIGERATED		
1%	1 cup (8.6 oz)	102
2%	1 cup (8.6 oz)	122
buffalo	7 oz	224
buttermilk lowfat	1 cup (8.6 oz)	98
camel	7 oz	160
donkey	7 oz	86
fat free	1 cup (8.6 oz)	83
goat	1 cup (8.6 oz)	168
human	1 cup (8.6 oz)	172
indian buffalo	1 cup (8.6 oz)	237
mare	7 oz	98
sheep	1 cup (8.6 oz)	265
whole	1 cup (8.6 oz)	146
Active Lifestyle		
Fat Free w/ Plant Sterols	8 oz	90
Dairy Ease		
Fat Free Lactose Free	1 cup (8 oz)	90
Reduced Fat 2% Lactose Free	1 cup (8 oz)	130
Whole Lactose Free	1 cup (8 oz)	160
Farmland		
Buttermilk	8 oz	160
Fat Free	8 oz	80
Special Request 1% Plus Omega-3	8 oz	130
Special Request Skim Plus	8 oz	110
Special Request Skim Plus 100% Lactose Free	8 oz	110
Whole	8 oz	160
Friendship		
Buttermilk Lowfat	1 cup	120
Horizon		
Fat Free	8 oz	90

FOOD	PORTION	CALS
Lowfat 1%	8 oz	100
Reduced Fat 2%	8 oz	120
Whole	8 oz	150
Lactaid		
Fit & Creamy Lowfat	8 oz	120
Whole	8 oz	160
Land O'Lakes		
1%	1 cup (8 oz)	100
2%	1 cup (8 oz)	120
Skim	1 cup (8 oz)	90
Whole	1 cup (8 oz)	150
Meyenberg		
Goat Low Fat	8 oz	89
Goat Whole	8 oz	142
Organic Valley		
Buttermilk Lowfat 1%	1 cup	100
Fat Free	1 cup	90
Lactose Free Fat Free	1 cup	90
Whole Nonhomogenized	1 cup	150
Over The Moon		
Fat Free	8 oz	100
Low Fat	8 oz	120
Smart Balance		
1% Lowfat w/ HeartRight	1 cup (8 oz)	120
1% Lowfat w/ Omega-3s & Vitamin E	1 cup (8 oz)	140
Fat Free w/ Omega-3s & Vitamin E	1 cup (8 oz)	120
Straus		
Organic Cream Top Whole	8 oz	150
Organic Fat Free	8 oz	90
Organic Whole Milk	8 oz	170
SunMilk		
Heart Healthy 1% Sunflower Oil	8 oz	120
Heart Healthy 2% Sunflower Oil	8 oz	120
Turkey Hill		
Cool Moos Whole Milk	8 oz	160
Valio		
100% Lactose Free 0% Fat	8 oz	80
100% Lactose Free 2% Fat	8 oz	120
Welsh Farms		
Fat Free	8 oz	80

FOOD	PORTION	CALS
SHELF-STABLE		
Parmalat		
2% Reduced Fat	8 oz	130
Fat Free	8 oz	80
Lactose Free 2% Reduced Fat	8 oz	130
MILK DRINKS		
chocolate milk	1 cup (8.8 oz)	208
chocolate milk lowfat	1 cup (8.8 oz)	158
Bravo!		
Blenders Creamy Double Chocolate	1 bottle (11 oz)	180
Blenders Creamy French Vanilla	1 bottle (11 oz)	160
Cocio		
Chocolate Milk	8 oz	140
Dove		
Bravo! Dark Chocolate	1 bottle	310
Bravo! Milk Chocolate	1 bottle	310
DrSears		
Cool Fuel Chocolate	1 pkg (8 oz)	190
Cool Fuel Chocolate Banana	1 pkg (8 oz)	190
Cool Fuel Vanilla	1 pkg (8 oz)	190
Farmland		
Really Really Good! Chocolate Milk	8 oz	160
Horizon Organic		
Lowfat Chocolate Milk	8 oz	170
Strawberry	8 oz	200
Lactaid		
Chocolate Milk 1% Fat	8 oz	150
Land O'Lakes		
2% Swiss Chocolate	1 cup (8.4 oz)	190
Chocolate Skim	1 cup (8 oz)	160
Strawberry	1 cup (8 oz)	190
MojoMilk		
Chocolate Mix not prep	1 pkg (4.5 g)	20
Probiotic Chocolate Milk not prep	1 pkg (4.5 g)	20
Nesquik		
Chocolate Powder No Sugar Added as prep w/ lowfat milk	1 cup (8 oz)	160
Chocolate Powder as prep w/ lowfat milk	1 cup (8 oz)	180
Ready-To-Drink Banana	1 cup (8 oz)	200
Ready-To-Drink Chocolate	1 cup (8 oz)	200

FOOD	PORTION	CALS
Ready-To-Drink Strawberry	1 cup (8 oz)	200
Ready-To-Drink Vanilla	1 cup (8 oz)	200
Strawberry Powder as prep w/ lowfat milk	1 cup (8 oz)	190
Strawberry Powder not prep	2 tbsp (0.6 oz)	60
Over The Moon		
Chocolate Milk Fat Free	8 oz	150
Parmalat		
Chocolate Milk 2% Reduced Fat	1 cup	190
Sipahh		
Straw Banana	1 straw	15
Straw Cookies and Cream	1 straw	15
TruMoo		
Chocolate Milk Fat Free	8 oz	130
Chocolate Milk Lowfat	8 oz	150
Strawberry Milk Fat Free	8 oz	130
Turkey Hill		
Cool Moos 2% Reduced Fat	8 oz	120
Cool Moos Chocolate	8 oz	180
MILK SHAKE		
chocolate	1 serv (10.6 oz)	357
malted milk shake	1 serv (10 oz)	402
vanilla	1 (11 oz)	351
Buffy's Cool Cow		
Chocolate	1 pkg (8 oz)	150
Vanilla	1 pkg (8 oz)	150
Lean Body		
Hi-Protein Chocolate Ice Cream	1 (17 oz)	260
Molli Coolz		
Shakers Vanilla as prep w/ skim milk	1 (10.2 oz)	240
Nesquik		
Ready-To-Drink Chocolate	1 cup (8 oz)	170
Silhouette Solution		
Colossal Chocolate not prep	1 pkg (1.05 oz)	110
Vanilla Creme not prep	1 pkg (1.02 oz)	100
MILK SUBSTITUTES		
soy milk	1 cup	79
Brazsoy		
Condensed Soy Milk	1 serv (0.7 oz)	54
Soy Cream	1 tbsp (0.5 oz)	27

FOOD	PORTION	CALS
Living Harvest		
Hempmilk Original	1 cup	130
Hempmilk Vanilla	1 cup	130
Lundberg		
Organic Drink Rice Original	8 oz	120
Manitoba Harvest		
Hemp Bliss Chocolate	8 oz	160
Hemp Bliss Original	1 cup	110
Hemp Bliss Vanilla	8 oz	150
Odwalla		
Soy Smart Chai	8 oz	150
Soy Smart Vanilla	8 oz	120
Soymilk Plain	8 oz	110
Soymilk Vanilla Being	8 oz	100
Organic Valley		
Soy Original	1 cup	100
Soy Unsweetened	1 cup	80
Pacific Foods		
7 Grain Original Organic	1 cup (8 oz)	140
Almond Original Unsweetened Organic	8 oz	35
Hazelnut Original	8 oz	110
Hemp Original	8 oz	140
Oat Original Organic	1 cup (8 oz)	130
Rice All Natural Plain	1 cup (8 oz)	130
Soy Original Unsweetened Organic	1 cup (8 oz)	90
Soy Ultra Plain	1 cup (8 oz)	120
Pearl		
Organic Soymilk Coffee	8 oz	150
Organic Soymilk Green Tea	8 oz	110
Organic Soymilk Original	8 oz	110
Rice Dream		
Carob	8 oz	150
Heartwise Vanilla	8 oz	140
Horchata	8 oz	130
Original	8 oz	120
Original Enriched	8 oz	120
Vanilla Enriched	8 oz	130
Silk		
Chocolate	1 cup (8 oz)	140
Plain	8 oz	100

FOOD	PORTION	CALS
Soy Heart Health	1 cup	80
Soy Plain Light	1 cup	70
Soy Plus DHA Omega-3	1 cup	110
Soy Pumpkin Spice	1 cup	170
Soy Unsweetened	1 cup	80
Vanilla	1 cup (8 oz)	100
Sol		
Sunflower Original	8 oz	70
Sunflower Unsweetened	8 oz	45
Sunflower Vanilla	8 oz	90
Soy Dream		
Classic Vanilla	8 oz	140
Original Enriched	8 oz	100
Sunrich Naturals		
Soymilk Original Plain	8 oz	110
Soymilk Vanilla	8 oz	130
Vitasoy		
Organic Lite Plus Original	8 oz	60
Organic Lite Plus Vanilla	8 oz	80
Organic Mint Chocolate	8 oz	160
Organic Original	8 oz	90
Organic Vanilla	8 oz	110
WildWood		
Organic Probiotic Soymilk Blueberry	8 oz	190
Organic Probiotic Soymilk Pomegranate	8 oz	180
Organic Soymilk Plain	8 oz	100
Organic Soymilk Unsweetened	8 oz	72
ZenSoy		
Soy Milk Cappuccino	8 oz	150
Soy Milk Chocolate	8 oz	170
Soy Milk Plain	8 oz	90
Soy Milk Vanilla	8 oz	110
Soy On The Go Vanilla w/ Omega 3	1 pkg (8.25 oz)	110
MILKFISH (AWA)		
baked	4 oz	215
MILLET		
cooked	1 cup (6.1 oz)	207
Arrowhead Mills		
Organic Hulled not prep	¼ cup	150

FOOD	PORTION	CALS

MINERAL WATER (see WATER)

MISO
dried	1 oz	86
miso	½ cup	284

MOLASSES
blackstrap	1 tbsp (0.7 oz)	47
molasses	¼ cup (3 oz)	244
molasses	1 tbsp (0.7 oz)	58

Tree Of Life
Blackstrap Unsulphured	1 tbsp	45

MONKFISH
baked	3 oz	82

MOOSE
roasted	4 oz	142

MOTH BEANS
dried cooked	1 cup	207

MOUSSE
TAKE-OUT
chocolate	½ cup	454
fish timbale	1 cup	329

MUFFIN
MIX
Betty Crocker
Banana Nut as prep	1	120
Blueberry as prep	1	120
Cornbread Muffin as prep	1	160
Fiber One Banana Nut as prep	1	170
Fiber One Blueberry as prep	1	160
Lemon Poppyseed as prep	1	200

Duncan Hines
Blueberry Streusel as prep	1	210
Cinnamon Swirl 100% Whole Grain as prep	1	220
Triple Chocolate Chunk 100% Whole Grain as prep	1	240

Glory
Golden Sweet Corn as prep	1	170

FOOD	PORTION	CALS
Martha White		
Whole Grain Apple Cinnamon not prep	¼ cup (1.2 oz)	140
Whole Grain Blueberry not prep	¼ cup (1.2 oz)	140
Yellow Corn not prep	¼ cup (1.2 oz)	140
Miracle Muffins		
Banana w/ Splenda as prep	1	86
VitaMuffin		
Deep Chocolate as prep	1 (2 oz)	100
Golden Corn as prep	1 (2 oz)	100
READY-TO-EAT		
Do Goodie		
Gluten Free Banana Nut	1	180
Foods By George		
Gluten Free Blueberry	1 (2.8 oz)	220
Hostess		
100 Calorie Pack Mini Banana Streusel	1 pkg (1.2 oz)	100
100 Calorie Pack Mini Blueberry Streusel	1 pkg (1.2 oz)	100
Udi's		
Gluten Free Double Chocolate	1 (4 oz)	350
Uncle Wally's		
Apple Cinnamon Rich & Moist	1 (4 oz)	380
Blueberry Rich & Moist	1 (4 oz)	370
Cheesecake Rich & Moist	1 (4 oz)	390
Chocolate Passion Fat Free	½ (2 oz)	120
Corn Rich & Moist	1 (4 oz)	400
Cranberry Apple Smart Portion	1 (1.1 oz)	80
Cranberry Orange Supreme Fat Free	½ (2 oz)	140
Fiber One Banana Chocolate Chip	1 (2.3 oz)	180
Fiber One Wild Blueberry & Oats	1 (2.3 oz)	170
Honey Raisin Bran Fat Free	½ (2 oz)	140
My Sweet Multi Bran Sugar Free	1 (2 oz)	120
Pineapple Coconut Rich & Moist	1 (4 oz)	390
Sweet Chocolate Dreams Sugar Free	1 (2 oz)	130
Wild Blueberry Bliss Fat Free	½ (2 oz)	110
VitaMuffin		
Banana Nut	1 (2 oz)	100
Banana Nut Sugar Free	1 (2 oz)	90
VitaTop		
Apple Crumb	1 (2 oz)	100
BlueBran	1 (2 oz)	100

FOOD	PORTION	CALS
CranBran	1 (2 oz)	100
Deep Chocolate	1 (2 oz)	100
Golden Corn	1 (2 oz)	100
Raisin Bran	1 (2 oz)	100
TAKE-OUT		
blueberry	1 (5 oz)	546
corn	1 lg (5 oz)	424
oat bran	1 lg (5 oz)	375
pumpkin w/ raisins & nuts	1 med (4 oz)	351
MULBERRIES		
fresh	½ cup (2.5 oz)	30
fresh	20 (1 oz)	13
Kopali		
Organic Dark Chocolate Covered	½ pkg (1 oz)	140
Organic Dried	1 pkg (1.7 oz)	240
Navitas Naturals		
Dried	1 oz	91
MULLET		
striped cooked	3 oz	127
striped raw	3 oz	99
MUNG BEANS		
dried cooked	1 cup	213
TruRoots		
Organic Sprouted not prep	¼ cup (1.4 oz)	140
MUNGO BEANS		
dried cooked	1 cup	190
MUSHROOMS		
CANNED		
caps	8 (1.6 oz)	12
caps pickled	6 (0.8 oz)	5
chanterelle	3.5 oz	12
pickled	1 cup	33
pieces	½ cup	20
straw	1 cup	58
Green Giant		
Pieces & Stems	½ cup	25
Jake & Amos		
Pickled Dill Mushrooms	1 serv (1 oz)	5

FOOD	PORTION	CALS
Polar		
Straw	½ cup	20
Whole Button	½ cup	30
Whole Shiitake	½ cup	30
DRIED		
chanterelle	1 oz	25
shiitake	1 (3.6 g)	11
tree ear	½ cup (0.4 oz)	36
wood ear mok yee	½ cup (0.4 oz)	25
Ocean Spring		
Fresh Crispy Mixed Mushrooms	1 serv (0.9 oz)	113
FRESH		
brown italian or crimini sliced	1 cup	19
brown italian or crimini whole	1 (0.7 oz)	5
chanterelle	3.5 oz	11
enoki raw	1 lg (5 g)	2
enoki sliced	1 cup	29
enoki whole	1 cup	28
maitake diced	1 cup	26
maitake whole	1 (6.6 g)	2
morel	3.5 oz	9
oyster	1 sm (0.5 oz)	5
oyster sliced	1 cup	30
portabella raw	1 cap (3 oz)	22
portabella sliced grilled	1 cup (4.2 oz)	42
shiitake cooked	4 (2.5 oz)	40
shiitake pieces cooked	1 cup	81
white	1 (0.6 oz)	4
white sliced cooked	1 cup	28
white sliced raw	½ cup	8
Dole		
Raw	½ cup (1.2 oz)	9
Giorgio		
Mushrooms	3 oz	20
Golden Gourmet		
Beech Brown	4 oz	20
Beech White	4 oz	13
King Trumpet	4 oz	20
Maitake	4 oz	20

FOOD	PORTION	CALS
Hokto		
Organic Bunashimeji Beech Mushrooms	1 pkg (3.5 oz)	30
Organic Maitake Hen Of The Wood	1 pkg (3.5 oz)	30
FROZEN		
Farm Rich		
Breaded	5 (3 oz)	120
TAKE-OUT		
battered fried	1 lg (0.6 oz)	39
creamed	1 cup	171
stuffed	1 (0.8 oz)	67
MUSKRAT		
roasted	3 oz	199
MUSSELS		
blue raw	1 cup	129
blue raw	3 oz	73
fresh blue cooked	3 oz	147
Polar		
Mussels	2 oz	60
MUSTARD		
dry mustard	1 tsp	15
hot chinese	1 tsp	3
organic yellow	1 tsp	5
seed	1 tsp	15
yellow prepared	1 tbsp	3
Annie's Homegrown		
Organic Dijon	1 tsp (5 g)	5
Bone Suckin'		
Fat Free Gluten Free	1 tbsp	25
Dave's Gourmet		
Insanity	1 tsp (5 g)	5
Dietz & Watson		
Champagne Dill	1 tsp (5 g)	5
Yellow	1 tsp (5 g)	0
D'Oni		
Bold As Love Honey Habanero	1 tsp	5
French's		
Classic Yellow	1 tsp	0
Honey	1 tsp	10
Honey Dijon	1 tsp	10

FOOD	PORTION	CALS
Horseradish	1 tsp	5
Spicy Brown	1 tsp	5
Gulden's		
Spicy Brown	1 tsp	5
Hellman's		
Deli	1 tsp	5
Dijonnaise	1 tsp	5
Honey Mustard	1 tsp	10
Jack & Amos		
Sweet Dipping	1 tbsp (0.5 oz)	30
Robert Rothchild Farm		
Champagne Garlic	1 tsp	6
School House Kitchen		
Sweet Smooth Hot	1 tsp	15
Texas Sassy		
Mustard Sauce	2 tbsp (1 oz)	15
Vivi's		
Classic	1 tbsp (0.5 oz)	15
Sizzlin' Chipotle	1 tbsp (0.5 oz)	15
Zatarain's		
Creole	1 tsp (7 g)	10

MUSTARD GREENS

canned	1 cup	23
fresh as prep w/ fat	1 cup	50
fresh chopped boiled w/o salt	1 cup	21
fresh raw chopped	1 cup	15
frozen chopped boiled w/o salt	1 cup	28
Allen's		
Seasoned	½ cup	45
Glory		
Seasoned	½ cup	35
Sylvia's		
Specially Seasoned	½ cup	30

NATTO
House

Natto	2 oz	120

NAVY BEANS

canned	1 cup	296
dried cooked	1 cup	259

FOOD	PORTION	CALS
NECTARINE		
fresh	1 sm (4.5 oz)	57
fresh	1 lg (5.5 oz)	69
fresh sliced	1 cup (5 oz)	63
Chiquita		
Fresh	1 (5 oz)	63
Dole		
Fresh	1 med (5 oz)	60
NECTARINE JUICE		
Sun Shower		
100% Juice	8 oz	93
NEUFCHATEL		
neufchatel	1 pkg (3 oz)	215
neufchatel	1 oz	72
Organic Valley		
Soft	2 tbsp	70
NONI JUICE		
Lakewood		
Noni Pure Juice	2 oz	8
Snapple		
Juice Drink Low Calorie Metabolism Noni Berry	8 oz	15
Tree Of Life		
100% Juice Concentrate	2 tbsp	15
NOODLES		
cellophane	1 cup	492
chow mein	1 cup (1.6 oz)	237
egg	1 cup (38 g)	145
egg cooked	1 cup (5.6 oz)	213
japanese soba cooked	1 cup (4 oz)	113
japanese somen cooked	1 cup (6.2 oz)	231
korean acorn noodles not prep	2 oz	195
rice cooked	1 cup (6.2 oz)	192
spinach/egg cooked	1 cup (5.6 oz)	211
Gluten Free Cafe		
Asian Noodles	1 pkg (9.2 oz)	340
House		
Shirataki Tofu Noodles	2 oz	20
Shirataki Yam Noodles	2 oz	5

FOOD	PORTION	CALS
Krasdale		
Egg Wide not prep	1 cup (2 oz)	210
La Choy		
Chow Mein Noodles	½ cup (1 oz)	130
Rice	½ cup	130
Light 'N Fluffy		
Egg Extra Wide not prep	⅙ pkg (2 oz)	210
No Yolks		
Dumplings	2 oz	210
NoOodle		
All Natural	1 serv (1.6 oz)	0
Pennsylvania Dutch		
Fine Egg not prep	1 cup (2 oz)	220
Ronzoni		
Healthy Harvest Whole Grain Extra Wide not prep	2 oz	180
Streit's		
Egg Wide not prep	1¾ cups (2 oz)	210
NUTMEG		
ground	1 tsp	12
nutmeg butter	1 tbsp	120

NUTRITION SUPPLEMENTS (*see also* CEREAL BARS, ENERGY BARS, ENERGY DRINKS)

Be Happy		
Health Guard	1 bottle (2 oz)	40
Cirku		
Beverage Mix Summer Citrus	1 pkg (0.23 oz)	15
Clif		
Shot Bloks Black Cherry	3 (1 oz)	100
Shot Bloks Cola	3 (1 oz)	100
Shot Bloks Margarita	3 (1 oz)	90
Shot Bloks Orange	3 (1 oz)	100
Ensure		
Shake Creamy Milk Chocolate	1 bottle (8 oz)	250
Shake Strawberries & Cream	1 bottle (8 oz)	250
Glowelle		
Beauty Drink All Flavors	1 bottle	100
Glucerna		
Shake Creamy Chocolate Delight	1 bottle (8 oz)	200
Shake Homemade Vanilla	1 bottle (8 oz)	200

FOOD	PORTION	CALS
Jelly Belly		
Sport Beans Lemon Lime	1 pkg (1 oz)	100
Joint Juice		
Cranberry Pomegranate	1 bottle (8 oz)	20
Easy Shot Glucosamine Chondrotin	2.5 tbsp (1.25 oz)	15
Easy Shot Hyal-Joint	2.5 tbsp (1.25 oz)	15
On The Go Blueberry Acai	1 pkg (6 g)	20
Luna		
Electrolyte Splash	1 pkg	80
Moons Energy Chews Watermelon	6 (1 oz)	100
Recovery Smoothie	1 pkg	120
Orgain		
Organic Meal Replacement All Flavors	1 pkg (11 oz)	255
Oxylent		
Oxygenating Multivitamin Drink	1 pkg	10
Premier		
Protein Shake Chocolate	1 (11 oz)	160
Protein Shake Strawberry	1 (11 oz)	160
Protein Shake Vanilla	1 (11 oz)	160
S/7		
Prenatal Vitamin Drink Berry	1 pkg (0.5 oz)	45
Slim-Fast		
Optima Ready-To-Drink Creamy Milk Chocolate	1 can (11 oz)	190
To Go		
Extreme Berries	½ pkg (3.15 g)	12
NUTS MIXED (see also individual names)		
dry roasted w/ peanuts salted	¼ cup	203
dry roasted w/ peanuts w/o salt	¼ cup	203
mixed nuts chocolate covered	¼ cup (1.5 oz)	240
oil roasted w/o peanuts salted	¼ cup	221
oil roasted w/o peanuts w/o salt	¼ cup	221
Back To Nature		
Tuscan Herb Roast	1 oz	170
Dave's Gourmet		
Burning Nuts	1 oz	200
Emily's		
Roasted Mixed Nuts	¼ cup (1.3 oz)	230
Frito Lay		
Deluxe Mixed	¼ cup	170

FOOD	PORTION	CALS
Mauna Loa		
Mixed Nuts	¼ cup (1 oz)	180
NuttZo		
Multi-Nut Butter Organic	2 tbsp (1.1 oz)	180
Planters		
Bar Big Triple Nut	1 (1.6 oz)	220
Lightly Salted	1 oz	170
Mixed	1 oz	170
Unsalted	1 oz	170
True North		
Clusters Pecan Almond Peanut	8 (1 oz)	170
OCTOPUS		
dried boiled	3 oz	144
fresh steamed	3 oz	139
smoked	1 oz	40
Matiz		
Pulpo In Olive Oil	½ pkg (2 oz)	107
TAKE-OUT		
ensalada de pulpo	1 cup	299
OHELOBERRIES		
fresh	1 cup	39
OIL		
almond	1 cup	1927
almond	1 tbsp	120
apricot kernel	1 tbsp	120
apricot kernel	1 cup	1927
avocado	1 cup	1927
avocado	1 tbsp	124
babassu palm	1 tbsp	120
butter oil	1 tbsp	112
butter oil	1 cup	1795
canola	1 tbsp	124
canola	1 cup	1927
coconut	1 tbsp	117
corn	1 cup	1927
corn	1 tbsp	120
cottonseed	1 cup	1927
cottonseed	1 tbsp	120
cupu assu	1 tbsp	120

FOOD	PORTION	CALS
garlic oil	1 tbsp	150
grapeseed	1 tbsp	120
hazelnut	1 cup	1927
hazelnut	1 tbsp	120
mustard	1 cup	1927
mustard	1 tbsp	124
oat	1 tbsp	120
olive	1 cup	1909
olive	1 tbsp	119
palm	1 tbsp	120
palm	1 cup	1927
palm kernel	1 tbsp	117
palm kernel	1 cup	1879
peanut	1 tbsp	119
peanut	1 cup	1909
peppermint	1 tsp	42
poppyseed	1 tbsp	120
pumpkin seed	1 oz	217
rice bran	1 tbsp	120
safflower	1 cup	1927
safflower	1 tbsp	120
sesame	1 tbsp	120
sheanut	1 tbsp	120
soybean	1 tbsp	120
soybean	1 cup	1927
sunflower	1 cup	1927
sunflower	1 tbsp	120
teaseed	1 tbsp	120
tomatoseed	1 tbsp	120
vegetable	1 tbsp	120
vegetable	1 cup	1927
walnut	1 cup	1927
walnut	1 tbsp	120
wheat germ	1 tbsp	120
Annie's Homegrown		
Basil Oil	1 tbsp (0.5 oz)	120
Dipping Oil	1 tbsp (0.5 oz)	100
Azukar Organics		
Virgin Coconut	1 tbsp (0.5 oz)	125

FOOD	PORTION	CALS
Bell Plantation		
Extra Virgin Roasted Peanut	1 tbsp	120
Bella Sun Luci		
Olive Extra Virgin Cold Pressed	1 tbsp (0.5 oz)	120
Bragg		
Olive Extra Virgin	1 tbsp	120
Carapelli		
Grapeseed	1 tbsp	120
Olive Extra Virgin	1 tbsp	120
Carotino		
Palm Fruit Oil	1 tbsp (0.5 oz)	121
Red Palm & Canola	1 tbsp	120
Colavita		
Olive Extra Virgin	1 tbsp (0.5 oz)	120
Crisco		
Cooking Spray Original	⅓ sec spray	0
Frying Oil Blend	1 tbsp	130
Light Olive	1 tbsp	120
Peanut	1 tbsp	120
Pure Vegetable	1 tbsp	120
Gaea		
Olive Carbon Neutral	1 tbsp (0.5 oz)	130
Gourme Mist		
Extra Virgin Olive Cold Pressed	1 sec spray	4
Hollywood		
Canola Enriched	1 tbsp	120
Peanut Enriched Gold	1 tbsp	120
Safflower Expeller Pressed	1 tbsp	120
House Of Tsang		
Mongolian Fire	1 tsp	45
Wok Oil	1 tbsp	130
Kinloch Plantation		
100% Virgin Pecan	1 tbsp	130
Living Harvest		
Organic Hemp Oil	2 tbsp	250
LouAna		
Canola	1 tbsp (0.5 oz)	120
Lucini		
Extra Virgin Premium Select	1 tbsp (0.5 oz)	120

FOOD	PORTION	CALS
Manitoba Harvest		
Hemp Seed Oil	1 tbsp	126
Martinis		
Kalamata Olive Extra Virgin Cold Pressed	1 tbsp (0.5 oz)	120
Mazola		
Corn	1 tbsp	120
Monini		
Grapeseed	1 tbsp (0.5 oz)	120
Navitas Naturals		
Organic Virgin Coconut	1 tbsp (0.5 oz)	120
Nutiva		
Organic Coconut Extra Virgin	1 tbsp	120
Organic Hemp Cold Pressed	1 tbsp	120
Olivo		
Spray Olive Oil 100% Extra Virgin	⅓ sec spray	0
Pam		
All Varieties	¼ sec spray	0
Penny's PopSurprise		
Organic Extra Virgin Olive Spicy	1 tbsp (0.5 oz)	130
Pillsbury		
Baking Spray w/ Flour	⅙ sec spray	0
Planters		
100% Pure Peanut	1 tbsp (0.5 oz)	120
Pompeian		
Olive	1 tbsp	130
Robert Rothchild Farm		
Basil Infused	1 tbsp	120
Smart Balance		
Omega Oil	1 tbsp (0.5 oz)	120
Tree Of Life		
Almond Expeller Pressed	1 tbsp (0.5 oz)	120
Avocado Expeller Pressed	1 tbsp (0.5 oz)	120
Macadamia Nut Expeller Pressed	1 tbsp (0.5 oz)	120
Organic Coconut Expeller Pressed	1 tbsp	120
Walnut Expeller Pressed	1 tbsp (0.5 oz)	120
Wesson		
Canola	1 tbsp	120
OKRA		
CANNED		
pickled	6 pods (2.3 oz)	18

FOOD	PORTION	CALS
Allens		
Cut	½ cup	30
McIlhenny		
Spicy Pickled	1 oz	10
Trappey's		
Creole Gumbo	½ cup	35
FRESH		
cooked w/ salt	8 pods	19
luffa chinese okra cooked	1 cup	39
sliced cooked w/ salt	½ cup	18
TAKE-OUT		
batter dipped fried	10 pieces (2.6 oz)	142
OLIVES		
black	2 med (0.3 oz)	8
greek	1 (0.5 oz)	16
green	2 extra lg (0.5 oz)	19
green	2 med (0.2 oz)	10
green	2 lg (0.3 oz)	11
green	1 sm (0.2 oz)	8
green chopped	¼ cup (1.2 oz)	48
green olive tapenade	1 tbsp	25
green stuffed	2 sm (0.2 oz)	9
green stuffed	¼ cup (1.3 oz)	47
green stuffed	2 lg (0.3 oz)	12
green stuffed	2 med (0.3 oz)	10
ripe	2 lg (0.3 oz)	10
ripe	2 sm (0.2 oz)	7
ripe	2 extra lg (0.4 oz)	12
ripe sliced	¼ cup (1.2 oz)	35
spanish stuffed	5 (0.5 oz)	15
Dave's Gourmet		
Olives In Pain	⅛ jar (0.5 oz)	15
Martinis		
Kalamata Pitted	4 (0.5 oz)	40
Matiz		
Olivada Spread Sweet	2 tbsp	87
Olivada Spread Traditional & Hot	2 tbsp	114
Peloponnese		
Amfissa	3	45
Ionian Green	3	25

FOOD	PORTION	CALS
Kalamata Pitted	5	45
Kalamata Spread	1 tsp	15
Priorat Natur		
Natural Olives	10	30
Progresso		
Tapenade	1 tbsp (0.5 oz)	20
Stonewall Kitchen		
Mixed Olive Spread	1 tbsp	35
Zatarain's		
Cocktail	7 (0.5 oz)	25
Stuffed	6 (0.5 oz)	25
ONION		
CANNED		
cocktail	½ cup	41
Dietz & Watson		
Sweet Vidalia In Sauce	1 tbsp (0.5 oz)	12
French's		
Original French Fried	2 tbsp	45
McSweet		
Pickled Onions	4 (1 oz)	10
The Gracious Gourmet		
Balsamic Four Onion Spread	1 tbsp (0.5 oz)	20
DRIED		
flakes	1 tbsp	17
powder	1 tsp	7
shallots	1 tbsp	3
Bob's Red Mill		
Minced	1 tbsp	40
Seneca		
Crisp Onions	1 tbsp (7 g)	40
FRESH		
cooked w/o salt	1 sm (2 oz)	26
cooked w/o salt	1 med (3.3 oz)	41
cooked w/o salt	1 lg (4.5 oz)	56
cooked w/o salt chopped	1 tbsp	7
raw chopped	1 tbsp	4
raw chopped	½ cup	32
raw slice	1 (0.5 oz)	6
raw sliced	½ cup	23
scallions raw	1 med (0.5 oz)	5

FOOD	PORTION	CALS
scallions raw chopped	¼ cup	8
shallots raw chopped	¼ cup	29
sweet whole raw	1 (11.6 oz)	106
whole raw	1 sm (2.5 oz)	28
whole raw	1 med (4 oz)	44
whole raw	1 lg (5.3 oz)	60
Bland Farms		
Vidalia Sweet	1 (5 oz)	60
Blue Ribbon		
Yellow	1 med (5.2 oz)	60
Earthbound Farms		
Organic Green Onions	¼ cup	10
Organic Red	1 med (5.2 oz)	60
Ocean Mist		
Green Onions Chopped	¼ cup	10
OsoSweet		
Onion	1 med (5 oz)	60
RealSweet		
Vidalia	1 (5.2 oz)	45
FROZEN		
C&W		
Petite Whole	⅔ cup (3 oz)	30
Farm Rich		
Petals Breaded + Sauce	10 (3 oz)	200
TAKE-OUT		
creamed	1 cup	187
fried	½ cup	57
rings breaded & fried	8 to 9 (3 oz)	276

OPOSSUM

roasted	3 oz	188

ORANGE
CANNED
Del Monte

Mandarin In Lite Orange Gel	1 pkg (4.5 oz)	60
SunFresh Mandarin In Light Syrup	½ cup (4.5 oz)	70
Dole		
Mandarin In Fruit Juice	1 pkg (4 oz)	80
FRESH		
california valencia	1 (4.2 oz)	59

FOOD	PORTION	CALS
california valencia sections	½ cup (3.2 oz)	44
florida	1 (5.3 oz)	69
florida sections	½ cup (3.2 oz)	43
fresh	1 sm (3.4 oz)	45
fresh	1 med (4.6 oz)	62
fresh	1 lg (6.5 oz)	86
navel	1 (4.9 oz)	69
navel sections	1 cup (5.8 oz)	81
peel	1 tbsp (0.2 oz)	3
Darling		
Mandarine	1 med (3.8 oz)	50
Dole		
Orange	1 med (4.2 oz)	60
Sunkist		
Cara Cara	1 med (5.4 oz)	80
ORANGE JUICE		
chilled bottled	1 cup (8.7 oz)	112
fresh	1 cup (8.7 oz)	112
mandarin orange	7 oz	94
Dole		
100% Juice w/ Calcium	8 oz	120
Florida's Natural		
Calcium & Vitamin D	8 oz	110
Gensis Today		
Omega Orange 100% Juice	8 oz	90
Italian Volcano		
Organic Blood Orange	8 oz	101
Izze		
Esque Sparkling Mandarin	1 bottle (12 oz)	50
Land O'Lakes		
Juice	1 cup (8 oz)	110
Juice w/ Calcium	1 cup (8 oz)	120
Mott's		
100% Juice Sunkist Orange Sensation	1 bottle (14 oz)	210
Mr. J		
100% Juice Calcium Fortified	1 pkg (4 oz)	60
NutraBalance		
Fortified	1 pkg (4 oz)	60
Ocean Spray		
Juice	8 oz	100

FOOD	PORTION	CALS
Odwalla		
100% Juice	8 oz	110
Old Orchard		
100% Juice	8 oz	130
Organic Valley		
W/ Calcium	1 cup	110
Simply		
Orange Calcium Fortified	8 oz	110
Orange Original	8 oz	110
Snapple		
Orangeade	8 oz	100
SSips		
Orangeade	8 oz	120
Tree Ripe		
100% Juice + Calcium & Vitamins	8 oz	120
Tropicana		
Antioxidant Advantage	8 oz	110
Calcium + Vitamin D	8 oz	110
Fiber	8 oz	120
Healthy Heart	8 oz	120
Healthy Kids	8 oz	110
Light'n Healthy w/ Calcium	8 oz	50
No Pulp	8 oz	110
Orangeade	8 oz	111
Organic	8 oz	120
Trop50 Orange Juice Beverage	8 oz	50
Uncle Matt's		
Organic 100% Juice Pulp Free	8 oz	110
Organic 100% Juice w/ Pulp	8 oz	110
Welsh Farms		
Juice	8 oz	110
TAKE-OUT		
orange julius	1 cup (9.2 oz)	212
OREGANO		
crumbled	1 tsp	3
ground	1 tsp	6

ORGAN MEATS (*see* BRAINS, GIBLETS, GIZZARDS, HEART, KIDNEY, LIVER, SWEETBREAD)

FOOD	PORTION	CALS
OSTRICH		
cooked	4 oz	195
cooked diced	1 cup (4.7 oz)	215
Natural Frontier Foods		
Filets	1 (4 oz)	130
Ground Lean	4 oz	130
OYSTERS		
canned eastern	1 cup	112
eastern baked	6 med	47
eastern raw	6 med	50
eastern sauteed	6 med	76
smoked	6	33
Chicken Of The Sea		
Smoked In Oil	1 can (3.75 oz)	170
Whole	¼ can (2 oz)	80
Polar		
Whole	¼ cup	70
Whole Smoked	⅓ cup	95
TAKE-OUT		
breaded & fried	6	368
fritter	1 (1.4 oz)	121
oysters rockefeller	1 cup	302
stew	1 cup	208
PANCAKE/WAFFLE SYRUP		
light	¼ cup	98
pancake syrup	¼ cup	209
pancake syrup	1 pkg (2 oz)	156
Aunt Jemima		
Butter Lite	¼ cup (2.1 oz)	100
Log Cabin		
Lite	¼ cup (2 oz)	100
Naturally Fresh		
Maple Mountain Sugar Free	2 tbsp	0
Smucker's		
Breakfast Syrup Sugar Free	¼ cup (2.1 oz)	20
Wholesome Sweeteners		
Organic	¼ cup	240

FOOD	PORTION	CALS

PANCAKES
FROZEN
Aunt Jemima

FOOD	PORTION	CALS
Blueberry	3 (3.7 oz)	260
Buttermilk	3 (3.7 oz)	250
Buttermilk Lowfat	3 (3.6 oz)	200
Oatmeal	3 (3.7 oz)	230
Whole Grain	3 (3.6 oz)	240
Dr. Praeger's		
Broccoli	1 (2 oz)	80
Potato	1 (2.2 oz)	100
Sweet Potato Bites	1 (2 oz)	80
Golden		
Potato Latkes	1 (1.3 oz)	70
Zucchini	1 (1.3 oz)	70
Jimmy Dean		
Breakfast Bowls Pancake & Sausage Links	1 pkg	710
Griddle Cake Sandwich Sausage Egg & Cheese	1 (4 oz)	370
Griddle Sticks	1 (2.5 oz)	160
Pillsbury		
Blueberry	3 (4 oz)	230
Buttermilk	3 (4 oz)	240
Original	3 (4 oz)	250
Ratner's		
Potato Latkes	1 (1.5 oz)	80
MIX		
Arrowhead Mills		
Gluten Free Pancake & Waffle as prep	2 (5 in)	240
Batter Blaster		
Organic Original Pancake & Waffle Batter not prep	¼ cup (2 oz)	112
Bisquick		
Shake 'N Pour Buttermilk as prep	3	220
Maple Grove Farms		
Buttermilk & Honey as prep	1	220
Mix Gluten Free as prep	1	200
TAKE-OUT		
bu chu jun korean w/ vegetables	1 (4 oz)	83
buckwheat	1 (7 in)	142
norwegian lefse	1 (9 in) (2.7 oz)	163

FOOD	PORTION	CALS
pindaettok korean mung bean	1 (3.9 oz)	204
plain	1 (7 in)	183
potato	1 (1.3 oz)	70
w/ butter & syrup	2 (8.1 oz)	520
whole wheat	1 (7 in)	183

PANCREAS (see SWEETBREAD)

PANINI (see SANDWICHES)

PAPAYA

canned in syrup	½ cup (2.3 oz)	50
dried	1 strip (0.8 oz)	59
fresh	1 sm (5.3 oz)	59
fresh	1 lg (13.3 oz)	148
fresh cubed	1 cup (4.9 oz)	55
green cooked	½ cup (2.3 oz)	18
Crunchy N'Yummy		
Organic Papaya	1 pkg (1 oz)	55
Dole		
Fresh	½ (4.9 oz)	60

PAPAYA JUICE

nectar	1 cup (8.8 oz)	142
Ceres		
100% Juice	8 oz	120
Lakewood		
Red	8 oz	80
Yellow	8 oz	105
Old Orchard		
Nectar Cocktail	8 oz	75

PAPRIKA

dried	1 tsp	1
Bob's Red Mill		
Hungarian	½ tsp	11

PARSLEY

dried	1 tbsp	4
freeze dried	1 tbsp	1
fresh chopped	¼ cup	5
fresh chopped	1 tbsp	1
fresh sprigs	5 (1.8 oz)	18

FOOD	PORTION	CALS
PARSNIPS		
fresh sliced cooked w/o salt	½ cup (2.7 oz)	55
whole cooked	1 (5.6 oz)	114
TAKE-OUT		
creamed	1 cup (8 oz)	237
PASSION FRUIT		
fresh	1 (0.6 oz)	17
fresh cut up	½ cup (4.1 oz)	114
PASSION FRUIT JUICE		
nectar	1 cup (8.8 oz)	168
yellow lilikoi	1 cup (8.7 oz)	138
Ceres		
100% Juice	8 oz	130
EarthWise		
Passionfruit Aloe	8 oz	110
Santa Cruz		
Organic 100% Juice Nectar	8 oz	150
PASTA (*see also* NOODLES, PASTA DINNERS, PASTA SALAD)		
DRY		
corn cooked	1 cup (4.9 oz)	176
elbows not prep	1 cup	389
elbows cooked	1 cup (4.9 oz)	197
shells small cooked	1 cup (4 oz)	162
spaghetti cooked	1 cup (4.9 oz)	197
spinach spaghetti cooked	1 cup (4.9 oz)	182
spirals cooked	1 cup (4.7 oz)	189
vegetable cooked	1 cup (4.7 oz)	172
whole wheat all shapes cooked	1 cup	174
Amish Natural		
Fettuccine Fiber Rich not prep	2 oz	200
Fettuccine not prep	2 oz	201
Fettuccine Whole Wheat not prep	2 oz	210
Barilla		
Lasagne not prep	2 pieces (1.8 oz)	180
Piccolini Mini Penne not prep	2 oz	210
Plus Spaghetti not prep	2 oz	210
Rotini Whole Grain not prep	2 oz	200
Spaghetti Whole Grain not prep	⅐ box (2 oz)	200
Tortellini Three Cheese	⅔ cup (2 oz)	230

FOOD	PORTION	CALS
DeBoles		
Angel Hair Rice Pasta not prep	¼ pkg (2 oz)	210
Elbow Corn Pasta Wheat Free not prep	⅙ pkg (2 oz)	200
Fettuccine not prep	¼ pkg (2 oz)	210
Organic Angel Hair Whole Wheat not prep	¼ pkg (2 oz)	210
Organic Eggless Ribbon not prep	1 cup (2 oz)	210
Organic Fettucini Spinach not prep	¼ pkg (2 oz)	210
Organic Lasagna not prep	¼ pkg (2.5 oz)	260
Organic Rigatoni Whole Wheat not prep	1 cup (2 oz)	210
Rigatoni not prep	¼ pkg (2 oz)	210
Dreamfields		
Lasagna not prep	2 pieces (2 oz)	190
Rotini not prep	⅔ cup (2 oz)	190
Gillian's		
Penne Brown Rice Pasta Wheat Gluten Egg Free not prep	2 oz	200
Heartland		
Gluten Free not prep	2 oz	200
Naturals Penne not prep	¾ cup (2 oz)	210
Perfect Balance Elbow Macaroni not prep	½ cup (2 oz)	200
Whole Wheat Rotini not prep	¾ cup (2 oz)	210
Jovial		
Organic Einkorn All Shapes	2 oz	200
Organic Einkorn White All Shapes	2 oz	200
Organic Gluten Free Brown Rice All Shapes	2 oz	210
Lundberg		
Organic Spaghetti Brown Rice not prep	2 oz	210
Maddy's		
Gluten Free not prep	4 oz	310
MagNoodles		
Organic Smart not prep	2 oz	204
Mara's Pasta		
100% Whole Wheat not prep	2 oz	190
Mueller's		
Elbow Macaroni not prep	½ cup	210
Racconto		
Essentials Heart Health not prep	2 oz	190
Essentials Heart Health Rigatoni not prep	⅙ pkg (2 oz)	190
Ronzoni		
Alphabets not prep	⅓ cup (2 oz)	210

FOOD	PORTION	CALS
Bow Ties not prep	1 cup (2 oz)	210
Elbows not prep	½ cup (2 oz)	210
Garden Delight Radiatore not prep	2 oz	190
Garden Delight Spaghetti not prep	2 oz	190
Quick Cook Penne Rigate not prep	¾ cup (2 oz)	210
Smart Taste Angel Hair not prep	½ pkg (2 oz)	170
Smart Taste Rotini not prep	2 oz	180
Thai Kitchen		
Stir-Fry Rice Linguini not prep	2 oz	210
Wacky Mac		
Veggie Bows not prep	⅙ pkg (2 oz)	200
FRESH		
cooked	2 oz	75
spinach cooked	2 oz	74
Buitoni		
Angel Hair	⅓ pkg (2.8 oz)	230
Ravioli Four Cheese	1 serv (3.7 oz)	340
Reserva Quattro Formaggi Agnolotti	1 serv (4.4 oz)	360
Tortellini Spinach Cheese	1 serv (3.7 oz)	320
Tortelloni Whole Wheat Cheese	1 serv (3.7 oz)	330
Monterey Gourmet		
Whole Wheat Ravioli Vegetable & Cheese	1 cup (3.5 oz)	240
Whole Wheat Tortellini Italian Cheese	1 cup (3.5 oz)	290
Nasoya		
Pasta Zero Plus Silken	⅔ cup (4 oz)	20
Pasta Prima		
Ravioli Butternut Squash	½ pkg (4 oz)	250
Ravioli Gluten Free Butternut Squash	1 cup (3.5 oz)	180
Ravioli Gluten Free Five Cheese	1 cup (3.5 oz)	230
Ravioli Italian Sausage	½ pkg (4 oz)	290
Ravioli Lobster	½ pkg (4 oz)	250
Ravioli Spinach & Cheese	1 cup (3.5 oz)	210
FROZEN		
Pasta Prima		
Ravioli Spinach & Mozzarella	1 cup (4 oz)	200
Solterra		
Fettuccine Gluten Free	⅓ pkg (4 oz)	330
Tofutti		
Ravioli Dairy Free	4 (3.2 oz)	210

FOOD	PORTION	CALS

PASTA DINNERS (see also PASTA SALAD)
CANNED
Annie's Homegrown

Organic Cheesy Ravioli	1 cup (8.5 oz)	180
Organic P'sghetti Loops	1 cup (8.4 oz)	190

Campbell's

Spaghettio's Slice Franks	1 cup (8.8 oz)	220

Chef Boyardee

Beef Ravioli	1 cup (8.6 oz)	230
Beefaroni	1 cup (8.7 oz)	240
Mini Ravioli	1 cup (8.8 oz)	250
Mini-Bites Spaghetti & Meatballs	1 cup (8.8 oz)	240
Spaghetti & Meat Balls	1 cup (9 oz)	260

Hormel

Kid's Kitchen Microwave Meals Cheezy Mac 'N Beef	1 pkg (7.5 oz)	250
Kid's Kitchen Microwave Meals Cheezy Mac 'N Cheese	1 pkg (7.5 oz)	270
Kid's Kitchen Microwave Meals Mini Beef Ravioli	1 pkg (7.5 oz)	240
Kid's Kitchen Microwave Meals Spaghetti Rings & Franks	1 pkg (7.5 oz)	240
Lasagna w/ Meat Sauce	1 pkg (7.5 oz)	210
Spaghetti w/ Meat Sauce	1 pkg (7.5 oz)	210

SpaghettiOs

A to Z's w/ Meatballs	1 cup	260
A to Z's w/ Sliced Franks	1 cup	230
Mini Beef Ravioli In Meat Sauce	1 cup	260
Pasta	1 cup	180
Plus Calcium	1 cup	170

FROZEN
4Real

Mac+Cheese	1 pkg (8 oz)	230
Meat Sauce w/ Beef Ravioli	1 pkg (8 oz)	190
Spaghetti Rings	1 pkg (8 oz)	180

Amy's

Bowls Baked Ziti	1 pkg	390
Bowls Stuffed Pasta Shells	1 pkg	310
Lasagna Cheese	1 pkg (10.2 oz)	380
Lasagna Tofu Vegetable	1 pkg (9.4 oz)	310

FOOD	PORTION	CALS
Macaroni & Cheese	1 pkg (8.9 oz)	410
Macaroni & Cheese Light In Sodium	1 pkg (8.9 oz)	400
Macaroni & Soy Cheese	1 pkg (8.9 oz)	370
Rice Mac & Cheese	1 pkg (9 oz)	400
Banquet		
Lasagna Family Entree	1 cup	510
Macaroni & Cheese	1 cup	200
Noodles & Beef	1 cup	160
Birds Eye		
Steamfresh Meals For Two Shrimp Alfredo	½ pkg (11.9 oz)	420
Steamfresh Meals For Two Shrimp Pasta Primavera	½ pkg (11.9 oz)	450
Blue Horizon Organic		
Penne Alfredo w/ Shrimp	½ pkg (9.9 oz)	430
Penne Alla Vodka w/ Shrimp	½ pkg (9.9 oz)	270
Pesto Farfalle w/ Shrimp	½ pkg (9.9 oz)	280
Scampi Rotini w/ Shrimp	½ pkg (9.9 oz)	410
Buitoni		
Braised Beef & Sausage Ravioli w/ Creamy Marinara Sauce	½ pkg (11.9 oz)	590
Chicken & Mushroom Ravioli w/ Marsala Wine Sauce	½ pkg (10.9 oz)	530
Four Cheese & Spinach Ravioli w/ Tomato Basil Sauce	½ pkg (12.9 oz)	550
Grilled Chicken w/ Spinach Cannelloni w/ Alfredo Sauce	½ pkg (10.9 oz)	560
Caesar's		
Gluten Free Lasagna Cheese In Marinara Sauce	1 pkg (11.5 oz)	520
Gluten Free Lasagna Vegetable In Marinara Sauce	1 pkg (11.5 oz)	510
Gluten Free Manicotti w/ Cheese In Marinara Sauce	1 pkg (11 oz)	380
Gluten Free Stuffed Shells w/ Cheese In Marinara Sauce	1 pkg (11 oz)	370
Candle Cafe		
Macaroni & Vegan Cheese	1 pkg (9 oz)	300
Tofu Spinach Ravioli	1 pkg (9 oz)	320
Cedarlane		
Zone Chicken & Vegetables Pasta & Ginger	1 pkg (10 oz)	340
Zone Lasagna Vegetable	1 pkg (10.9 oz)	310

FOOD	PORTION	CALS
Celentano		
Cheese Ravioli	4 (4.3 oz)	220
Contessa		
Ravioli Portabello	6 (6.7 oz)	360
Glory		
Macaroni & Cheese	1 pkg	480
Gluten Free Cafe		
Fettuccini Alfredo	1 pkg (9.2 oz)	400
Pasta Primavera	1 pkg (9.2 oz)	270
Glutino		
Gluten Free Duo Mushroom Penne	1 pkg (10.5 oz)	380
Gluten Free Macaroni & Cheese	1 pkg (8.8 oz)	430
Gluten Free Penne Alfredo	1 pkg (9.1 oz)	340
Green Giant		
Skillet Meal Chicken & Cheesy Pasta as prep	1¼ cups	270
Healthy Choice		
Chicken Fettuccini Alfredo	1 pkg (11.4 oz)	300
Hearty Beef Stroganoff	1 pkg (10.9 oz)	280
Lobster Cheese Ravioli	1 pkg (8.9 oz)	270
Roasted Red Pepper Marinara	1 pkg (8.5 oz)	270
Tortellini Primavera Parmesan	1 pkg (8.9 oz)	240
Helen's Kitchen		
Farfalle & Basil Pasta w/ Tofu Steaks	1 pkg (9 oz)	320
Joy Of Cooking		
Al Dente Cavatappi Bolognese	1 cup (7.7 oz)	280
Best Loved Macaroni & Cheese	1 cup (5.4 oz)	280
Cheese Ravioli Pomodoro	1 cup (7.7 oz)	250
Creamy Fettuccine Carbonara	1 cup (7.5 oz)	330
Kashi		
Chicken Pasta Pomodoro	1 pkg (10 oz)	280
Lean Cuisine		
Cafe Cuisine Three Cheese Stuffed Rigatoni	1 pkg (9 oz)	230
Dinnertime Selects Chicken Fettuccini	1 pkg (12 oz)	330
Market Creations Tortelloni Mushroom	1 pkg (10 oz)	280
Simple Favorites Alfredo Pasta w/ Chicken & Broccoli	1 pkg (10 oz)	300
Simple Favorites Angel Hair Pomodoro	1 pkg (10 oz)	250
Simple Favorites Cheese Ravioli	1 pkg (8.5 oz)	220
Simple Favorites Chicken Fettuccini	1 pkg (9.25 oz)	270
Simple Favorites Fettuccini Alfredo	1 pkg (9.25 oz)	330

FOOD	PORTION	CALS
Simple Favorites Lasagna Chicken Florentine	1 pkg (10 oz)	280
Simple Favorites Lasagna Classic Five Cheese	1 pkg (11.5 oz)	350
Simple Favorites Lasagna w/ Meat Sauce	1 pkg (10.5 oz)	320
Simple Favorites Macaroni & Cheese	1 pkg (10 oz)	290
Simple Favorites Spaghetti w/ Meat Sauce	1 pkg (11.5 oz)	300
Simple Favorites Spaghetti w/ Meatballs	1 pkg (9.5 oz)	270
Spa Cuisine Ravioli Butternut Squash	1 pkg (9.9 oz)	260
Marie Callender's		
Fettucine Chicken & Broccoli	1 meal	630
Meat Lasagna	1 cup	240
Meals To Live		
Turkey Meatballs w/ Marinara Sauce & Whole Wheat Spaghetti	1 pkg (11 oz)	300
Milton's		
Lasagna Vegetable w/ Multi-Grain Pasta	1 cup (8 oz)	340
Mom Made		
Cheesy Mac	1 pkg (7 oz)	200
Spaghetti w/ Turkey Meatballs & Sauce	1 pkg (7 oz)	180
Mon Cuisine		
Vegetarian Spaghetti & Meatballs	1 pkg (10 oz)	360
Moosewood		
Organic Vegetarian Broccoli & Pasta Parmesan	1 pkg (10 oz)	380
Organic Vegetarian Farfalle & Spinach Pesto Sauce	1 pkg (10 oz)	370
Organic Vegetarian Spicy Penne Puttanesca	1 pkg (10 oz)	300
New York Ravioli		
Jolie Kid Shapes Ravioli Cheese	1 cup	330
Jolie Kid Shapes Ravioli Cheese & Broccoli	1 cup	340
Ravioli Four Cheese	1 cup	360
Ravioli Tomato Basil & Mozzarella	1 cup	340
Organic Bistro		
Pasta Puttanesca	1 pkg (12.15 oz)	330
Organic Classics		
Cajun Chicken Tetrazzine w/ Penne Pasta	1 pkg (10 oz)	370
Chicken Cacciatore w/ Penne Pasta	1 pkg (10 oz)	270
Macaroni & Meat Sauce	1 pkg (10 oz)	340
Plum Organics		
Bowtie Pasta	1 pkg (6.9 oz)	230
Cheese Filled Spinach Tortellini	1 pkg (6.9 oz)	190

FOOD	PORTION	CALS
Putney Pasta		
Ravioli Butternut Squash & Vermont Maple Syrup	1 cup	200
Ravioli Portabello & Grilled Onion	7 (5.2 oz)	240
Ravioli Whole Wheat Spinach & Cheese	9 (5 oz)	300
Skillet Meal Chicken Piccata	1 serv (9 oz)	300
Skillet Meal Shrimp Pesto	1 serv (9 oz)	540
Tortellini Spinach Mozzarella & Walnuts	1 cup	360
Tortellini Tri-Color Three Cheese	1 cup	340
Stouffer's		
Cheesy Spaghetti Bake	1 pkg (12 oz)	460
Chicken Parmigiana	1 pkg (13.13 oz)	460
Homestyle Chicken & Noodles	1 pkg (12 oz)	340
Italian Sausage Stuffed Rigatoni	1 pkg (9.13 oz)	380
Lasagna Bake w/ Meat Sauce	1 pkg (11.5 oz)	380
Lasagna Vegetable	1 pkg (10.5 oz)	390
Macaroni & Beef	1 pkg (11.5 oz)	330
Macaroni & Cheese	1 cup (6 oz)	350
Manicotti Cheese	1 pkg (9 oz)	360
Shrimp Scampi	1 pkg (14 oz)	410
Tuna Noodle Casserole	1 pkg (10 oz)	350
Turkey Tettrazini	1 pkg (10 oz)	380
Tabatchnick		
Macaroni & Cheese	1 serv (7.5 oz)	250
Taste Above		
Meatless Thai Peanut Coconut Sauce w/ Veggie Chicken & Vermicelli	1 pkg (10 oz)	320
Meatless Tuscan Marinara Sauce w/ Veggie Chicken & Penne Pasta	1 pkg (10 oz)	320
Weight Watchers		
Smart Ones Lasagna w/ Meat Sauce	1 pkg (10.5 oz)	300
Smart Ones Ziti w/ Meatballs & Cheese	1 pkg (11.7 oz)	390
Yves		
Meatless Lasagna	1 pkg (10.5 oz)	300
MIX		
Annie's Homegrown		
Gluten Free Rice Pasta & Cheddar as prep	1 cup	280
Mac & Cheese Lower Sodium as prep	1 cup	280
Organic 5-Grain Elbows & White Cheddar as prep	1 cup	270

FOOD	PORTION	CALS
Organic Classic Mac & Cheese as prep	1 cup	280
Organic Peace Pasta & Parmesan as prep	1 cup	270
Organic Shells & Real Aged Wisconsin Cheddar as prep	1 cup	270
Organic Skillet Meals Beef Stroganoff as prep	1 cup	360
Organic Skillet Meals Cheesy Lasagna as prep	1 cup	440
Organic Skillet Meals Tuna Spirals as prep	1 cup	320
Shells & White Cheddar as prep	1 cup	270
Back To Nature		
Crazy Bugs Macaroni & Cheese as prep	1 cup	370
Harvest Wheat Elbows & Cheddar as prep	½ pkg	380
Organic Shells & Cheese as prep	½ pkg	380
Carapelli		
Penne Alfredo as prep	1 cup	240
Spirals Creamy Tomato as prep	1 cup	240
DeBoles		
Organic Macaroni & Cheese Whole Wheat as prep	1 cup	410
Pasta & Cheese as prep	1 cup	420
Rice Shells & Cheddar as prep	½ cup	260
Hamburger Helper		
Cheesy Jambalaya as prep	1 cup	330
Knorr		
Pasta & Sauce Jalapeno Jack as prep	1 cup	230
Pasta Sides w/ Whole Grains Alfredo as prep	⅔ cup	300
Kraft		
Macaroni & Cheese White Cheddar as prep	⅓ pkg	380
La Bella Vita		
Chicken & Lemon Borsellini as prep	1 cup	270
Near East		
Basil & Herb as prep	1 cup	240
Spicy Tomato as prep	1 cup	230
Pasta Roni		
Angel Hair w/ Herbs as prep	1 cup	310
Chicken as prep	1 cup	300
Chicken Quesadilla as prep	1 cup	310
Fettuccine Alfredo as prep	1 cup	450
Nature's Way Mushrooms In Cream Sauce as prep	1 cup	280
Sour Cream & Chives as prep	1 cup	310
Stroganoff as prep	1 cup	350

FOOD	PORTION	CALS
Road's End Organics		
Mac & Cheese Dairy Free Gluten Free as prep	1 cup	310
Shells & Cheese as prep	1 cup	330
Simply Shari's		
Mac & Cheese Gluten Free as prep	¼ pkg (4 oz)	280
Thai Kitchen		
Stir-Fry Rice Noodles Thai Peanut as prep	½ pkg	310
REFRIGERATED		
Country Crock		
Elbow Macaroni & Cheese	1 cup (8 oz)	370
Four Cheese Pasta	1 cup (8 oz)	380
NoOodle		
Mamma Mia! Marinara	1 pkg (10 oz)	70
Say Cheese Pleeeze!	1 pkg (10 oz)	100
Terri-Yaki Chicken	1 pkg (10 oz)	80
Ultra-Lite Primavera	1 pkg (10 oz)	30
Rozzano		
Organic Ravioli Grilled Vegetable	1 cup (3.5 oz)	200
Simply Sensible		
Lasagna w/ Meat Sauce	½ pkg (8 oz)	200
Mediterranean Style Chicken	1½ cups (7.2 oz)	250
SHELF-STABLE		
Allergaroo		
Gluten Free Spaghetti	1 pkg (8 oz)	220
Gluten Free Spyglass Noodles	1 pkg (8 oz)	230
Betty Crocker		
Bowl Appetit! Cheddar Broccoli Pasta	1 bowl (2.8 oz)	330
Bowl Appetit! Garlic Parmesan Pasta	1 bowl (2.8 oz)	320
Healthy Choice		
Balsamic Vegetable Medley	1 pkg (6.9 oz)	290
Fresh Mixers Rotini & Zesty Marinara Sauce	1 pkg (9.9 oz)	300
Fresh Mixers Ziti & Meat Sauce	1 pkg (6.9 oz)	340
Pasta Margherita	1 pkg (6.9 oz)	270
Hormel		
Compleats Microwave Meals Chicken & Noodles	1 pkg (9.9 oz)	240
TastyBite		
Peanut Sauce w/ Noodles	1 pkg (10 oz)	530
TAKE-OUT		
lasagna meatless	1 piece (9 oz)	356

FOOD	PORTION	CALS
lasagna w/ meat	1 piece (8 oz)	362
lasagna w/ vegetables	1 serv (9 oz)	315
macaroni & cheese w/ ham	1 cup	542
manicotti cheese w/ marinara sauce	1 (5 oz)	229
manicotti cheese w/ meat sauce	1 (5 oz)	239
pasta w/ pesto sauce	1 cup	370
ravioli cheese & spinach w/ cream sauce	1 cup	362
ravioli cheese w/ tomato sauce	1 cup	335
ravioli meat w/ marinara sauce	1 cup	372
rigatoni w/ sausage sauce	¾ cup	260
spaghetti w/ red clam sauce	1 cup	285
spaghetti w/ sauce & meatballs	2 cups	670
spaghetti w/ white clam sauce	1 cup	456
tortellini cheese w/ tomato sauce	1 cup	332
tortellini meat w/ marinara sauce	1 cup	281
tortellini spinach w/ marinara sauce	1 cup	238

PASTA SALAD
MIX
Suddenly Salad

Caesar as prep	1 cup (1.8 oz)	310
Classic as prep	¾ cup	250
Creamy Italian as prep	¾ cup	350
Creamy Parmesan as prep	¾ cup	370

TAKE-OUT

pasta salad w/ crab vegetables & mayonnaise	1 cup	317
pasta salad w/ shrimp vegetables & mayonnaise	1 cup (6.2 oz)	335
tortellini salad cheese filled w/ vinaigrette dressing	1 cup	333

PATE

chicken liver canned	1 tbsp	26
duck pate	1 oz	96
fish pate	1 oz	76
liver w/ truffle	1 serv (2 oz)	183
mushroom pate	1 can (2.25 oz)	130
pate de foie gras smoked canned	1 tbsp	60
pork pate	1 oz	107
pork pate en croute	1 oz	91
rabbit pate	1 oz	66
shrimp pate	1 (2.25 oz)	140

FOOD	PORTION	CALS
Patchwork		
All Flavors	2 oz	270
PEACH		
CANNED		
halves in heavy syrup	½ cup (2.6 oz)	85
halves in light syrup	1 half (3.4 oz)	53
halves juice pack	1 half (3.4 oz)	43
peach sauce	½ cup	120
pickled	½ cup (4.2 oz)	143
pickled whole	1 (3.1 oz)	104
slices juice pack	½ cup (4.4 oz)	55
slices light syrup	½ cup (4.4 oz)	68
slices water pack	½ cup (4.3 oz)	29
spiced in heavy syrup	½ cup (4.2 oz)	91
Del Monte		
Carb Clever Sliced	½ cup (4.2 oz)	30
Chunks Raspberry Flavor	½ cup (4.4 oz)	80
Clingstone Sliced In Light Syrup	½ cup (4.4 oz)	70
Fruit Bowls	½ cup (4.4 oz)	70
Fruit Cup Diced In Water No Sugar Added	1 pkg (3.75 oz)	25
Fruit Naturals Chunks No Sugar Added	½ cup (4.2 oz)	40
Orchard Select Cinnamon Spiced	½ cup (4.4 oz)	80
Orchard Select Sliced Cling No Sugar Added	½ cup (4.2 oz)	40
Peaches In Peach Gel	1 pkg (4.5 oz)	90
Polar		
White	½ cup	70
S&W		
Slices Natural Style	½ cup (4.4 oz)	80
DRIED		
halves	1 (0.5 oz)	31
halves	½ cup (2.8 oz)	191
halves cooked w/o sugar	½ cup (4.5 oz)	99
Mrs. May's		
Fruit Chips	1 pkg	35
Stoneridge Orchards		
Whole	⅓ cup (1.4 oz)	140
FRESH		
peach	1 lg (6.1 oz)	68
peach	1 med (5.3 oz)	58
sliced	½ cup (2.7 oz)	30

FOOD	PORTION	CALS
Dole		
Peach	1 lg (5.2 oz)	60
FROZEN		
C&W		
Ultimate Sliced	¾ cup	50
Dole		
Sliced	¾ cup (4.9 oz)	50
REFRIGERATED		
Dole		
Fruit Crisp Peach	1 pkg (4 oz)	150
Parfait Peaches & Creme	1 pkg (4.3 oz)	120
PEACH JUICE		
nectar	1 cup (8.7 oz)	134
Ceres		
100% Juice	8 oz	120
Froose		
Playful Peach	1 box (4.2 oz)	80
OKF		
Sparkling Fresh Peach	1 bottle (8.3 oz)	50
Santa Cruz		
Organic Nectar	8 oz	120
PEANUT BUTTER		
chunky	2 tbsp (1.1 oz)	188
no sugar added	2 tbsp (1.1 oz)	208
reduced sodium	2 tbsp (1.1 oz)	202
smooth	2 tbsp (1.1 oz)	188
Arrowhead Mills		
Organic Creamy	2 tbsp	190
Organic Honey Sweetened Creamy	2 tbsp	190
Organic Natural Crunchy	2 tbsp	190
Better'n Peanut Butter		
Creamy	2 tbsp (1.1 oz)	100
Low Sodium	2 tbsp (1.1 oz)	100
Chet's		
Chocolate	2 tbsp	180
Roasted Nut	2 tbsp	180
Earth Balance		
Creamy or Chunky	1 tbsp	190

FOOD	PORTION	CALS
Jake & Amos		
Schmier	1 tbsp (0.6 oz)	60
Jif		
Simply	2 tbsp (1.1 oz)	190
Justin's		
Organic Cinnamon	2 tbsp (1.1 oz)	180
Organic Classic	2 tbsp (1.1 oz)	150
Maple Grove Farms		
Crunchy No Salt Added	2 tbsp (1.1 oz)	190
Naturally More		
Natural	2 tbsp	169
Organic	2 tbsp	170
PB2		
Powdered Chocolate	2 tbsp	52
Powdered Chocolate Chip	2 tbsp	53
Peanut Butter & Co.		
Cinnamon Raisin Swirl	2 tbsp (1.1 oz)	160
Dark Chocolate Dreams	2 tbsp (1.1 oz)	170
Old Fashioned Crunchy	2 tbsp (1.1 oz)	190
The Bee's Knees	2 tbsp (1.1 oz)	180
Reese's		
Creamy	2 tbsp (1.1 oz)	190
Peanut Butter Chips	1 tbsp (0.5 oz)	80
Revolution Foods		
Organic Creamy & Crunchy	1 tbsp (1.1 oz)	200
Santa Cruz		
Organic Creamy	2 tbsp (1.1 oz)	210
Skippy		
Creamy	2 tbsp (1.3 oz)	190
Extra Chunky Super Chunk	2 tbsp (1.1. oz)	190
Reduced Fat Creamy	2 tbsp (1.3 oz)	180
Roasted Honey Nut Creamy	2 tbsp (1.1 oz)	190
Smart Balance		
Omega Creamy & Chunky	2 tbsp (1.1 oz)	200
Smucker's		
Chunky	2 tbsp (1.1 oz)	200
Creamy Honey	2 tbsp (1.2 oz)	200
Creamy No Salt Addded	2 tbsp (1.1 oz)	210
Creamy Reduced Fat	2 tbsp (1.2 oz)	190
Goober Grape	3 tbsp (1.9 oz)	240
Goober Peanut Butter & Chocolate Spread	3 tbsp (2 oz)	230

FOOD	PORTION	CALS
Wonder		
Peanut Spread	2 tbsp	100
Peanut Spread Low Sodium	2 tbsp	100
PEANUT BUTTER SUBSTITUTES		
NoNuts		
Golden Peabutter	1 tbsp	93
PEANUTS		
chocolate coated	1	21
chocolate coated	¼ cup	193
cooked w/ salt	½ cup	286
dry roasted w/ salt	28 (1 oz)	164
dry roasted w/o salt	¼ cup	214
dry roasted w/o salt	28 (1 oz)	164
honey roasted	¼ cup	191
sugar coated	¼ cup	203
yogurt coated	¼ cup	230
Fisher		
Butter Toffee	¼ cup (1 oz)	140
Honey Roasted	¼ cup (1 oz)	170
Frito Lay		
Salted In Shells	1 oz	160
Lance		
Salted	1 pkg (1.1 oz)	200
Nuts Are Good		
Buffalo	1 oz	120
Pina Colada	1 oz	130
Raspberry	1 oz	130
Vanilla Rum	1 oz	130
Planters		
Bar Big Double	1 (1.6 oz)	220
Dry Roasted	1 oz	160
Dry Roasted Lightly Salted	1 oz	160
Dry Roasted Unsalted	1 oz	170
Five Alarm Chili Dry Roasted	39 (1 oz)	160
Honey & Dry Roasted	1 oz	160
Roasted In Milk Chocolate	¼ cup (1.4 oz)	210
Sunfood		
Organic Wild Jungle	1 oz	174

FOOD	PORTION	CALS
SunRidge Farms		
Chocolate Toffee	6 (1.4 oz)	200
Yogurt Clusters	4 (1.4 oz)	220
True North		
Clusters	6 (1 oz)	170
PEAR		
CANNED		
halves in heavy syrup	1 (1.7 oz)	36
halves in heavy syrup	½ cup (3.5 oz)	74
halves in juice pack	1 (2.7 oz)	38
halves in juice pack	½ cup (4.4 oz)	62
halves in light syrup	1 (2.7 oz)	43
halves in light syrup	½ cup (4.4 oz)	72
halves in water pack	1 (2.7 oz)	22
Del Monte		
Halves In 100% Juice	½ cup (4.4 oz)	60
Halves In Heavy Syrup	½ cup (4.6 oz)	100
Halves In Light Syrup	½ cup (4.4 oz)	80
Orchard Select Sliced Bartlett	½ cup (4.4 oz)	70
Dole		
Diced In Fruit Juice	1 pkg (4 oz)	90
Liberty Gold		
Bartlett In Heavy Syrup	½ cup (4.5 oz)	90
S&W		
Halves Light Syrup	½ cup (4.4 oz)	80
DRIED		
halves	5 (3 oz)	229
halves	1 (0.6 oz)	47
halves	½ cup (3.2 oz)	236
halves cooked w/o sugar	½ cup (4.5 oz)	162
Bare Fruit		
Organic	1 pkg (0.6 oz)	46
Brothers-All-Natural		
Crisps Asian Pear	1 pkg (0.35 oz)	40
Crispy Green		
Crispy Asian Pears	1 pkg (0.35 oz)	40
Crunchies		
Freeze Dried	¼ cup (6 g)	20
FRESH		
asian	1 med (4.3 oz)	51

FOOD	PORTION	CALS
asian	1 lg (9.6 oz)	116
pear	1 sm (5.2 oz)	86
pear	1 med (6.2 oz)	103
pear	1 lg (8.1 oz)	133
sliced w/ skin	1 cup (4.9 oz)	81
Chiquita		
Pear	1 (6.2 oz)	103
Dole		
Pear	1 med (5.8 oz)	100
PEAR JUICE		
nectar canned	1 cup (8.8 oz)	150
Ceres		
100% Juice	8 oz	120
Froose		
Perfect Pear	1 box (4.2 oz)	80
Santa Cruz		
Organic Nectar	8 oz	120
Smart Juice		
Organic 100% Juice	8 oz	110
PEAS		
CANNED		
green	½ cup (4.4 oz)	66
green low sodium	½ cup (4.4 oz)	66
Del Monte		
Sweet No Salt Added	½ cup	60
Green Giant		
50% Less Sodium Young Tender Sweet	½ cup	60
Young Tender Sweet	½ cup	60
Le Sueur		
Very Young Small	½ cup (4.2 oz)	60
S&W		
Petit Pois	½ cup (4.4 oz)	60
DRIED		
split cooked w/o salt	1 cup (6.9 oz)	231
Arrowhead Mills		
Organic Green Split not prep	¼ cup	160
Crunchies		
Freeze Dried Organic	¼ cup (0.5 oz)	50

FOOD	PORTION	CALS
Goya		
Green Split Peas not prep	¼ cup (1.6 oz)	110
HamPeas		
Green Split Peas as prep	½ cup	120
Jack Rabbit		
Green Split	¼ cup (1.6 oz)	110
Snapea Crisps		
Baked Original	22 (1 oz)	70
SunRidge Farms		
Wasabi Roasted	¼ cup (1 oz)	120
Tree Of Life		
Wasabi Peas	¼ cup (1.1 oz)	120
FRESH		
green cooked w/o salt	½ cup (2.8 oz)	67
green raw	½ cup (2.5 oz)	59
snap peas cooked w/o salt	1 cup (5.6 oz)	67
snap peas raw	1 cup (2.2 oz)	26
snap peas raw	10 (1.2 oz)	14
Dole		
Sugar Snap Peas	1 cup (3 oz)	35
Mann's		
Snow Peas	1 serv (3 oz)	35
FROZEN		
creamed	1 cup (4.3 oz)	132
green cooked w/o salt	½ cup (2.8 oz)	62
Birds Eye		
Steamfresh Garlic Baby Peas & Mushrooms	¾ cup	80
Steamfresh Singles Sweet Peas	1 pkg (3.2 oz)	70
C&W		
Alfredo	½ cup	110
Early Harvest Petite No Salt Added	⅔ cup	70
Sugar Snap	⅔ cup	40
Green Giant		
Early June No Sauce	⅔ cup	50
SHELF-STABLE		
TastyBite		
Agra Peas & Greens	½ pkg (5 oz)	138
PECANS		
candied	1 oz	190
dry roasted	1 oz	187

FOOD	PORTION	CALS
dry roasted salted	1 oz	187
halves dry roasted w/ salt	20 (1 oz)	200
halves dried	1 cup	721
oil roasted	1 oz	195
oil roasted salted	1 oz	195
Emily's		
Roasted & Salted	¼ cup (1 oz)	210
Fisher		
Roasted & Salted	¼ cup (1 oz)	200
Planters		
Halves	1 oz	200
PECTIN		
powder	1 pkg (1.75 oz)	162
Sure Jell		
Fruit Pectin	1 pkg (1.75 oz)	0
PEPEAO		
dried	¼ cup	18
raw sliced	1 cup	25
PEPPER		
black	1 tsp	5
cayenne	1 tsp	6
white	1 tsp	7
McCormick		
Lemon Pepper w/ Garlic & Onion California Style	¼ tsp (0.6 g)	0
PEPPERMINT		
fresh chopped	2 tbsp	2
PEPPERS		
CANNED		
chili green	1 cup (5.5 oz)	29
chili green hot chopped	½ cup	17
chili pepper paste	1 tbsp	6
chili red hot	1 (2.6 oz)	18
chili red hot chopped	½ cup	17
green halves	½ cup	13
jalapeno chopped	½ cup	17
red halves	½ cup	13

FOOD	PORTION	CALS
Costa Peruana		
Organic Aji Paste All Flavors	1 tbsp (0.5 oz)	10
Dietz & Watson		
Sweet Roasted	1 oz	5
Gedney		
Hot & Sweet Jalapeno Peppers	¼ cup	30
Hot Banana Pepper Rings	¼ cup	10
Gertie's Finest		
Piquillo	1 oz	10
Jake & Amos		
Mild Sweet Stuffed	2 tbsp	15
Matiz		
Organic Piquillo Peppers	2	20
Pace		
Green Chiles Diced	2 tbsp	10
DRIED		
ancho	1 (0.6 oz)	48
ancho	1 tsp	3
casabel	1 tsp	3
chipotle smoked	1 tsp	3
green	1 tbsp	1
guajillo	1 tsp	3
mulato	1 tsp	3
pasilla	1 (7 g)	24
pasilla	1 tsp	3
red	1 tbsp	1
FRESH		
banana	1 (4 in) (1.2 oz)	9
banana	1 cup (4.4 oz)	33
chili green hot	1	18
chili green hot chopped	½ cup	30
chili red chopped	½ cup	30
chili red hot	1 (1.6 oz)	18
green	1 (2.6 oz)	20
green chopped	½ cup	13
green chopped cooked	½ cup	19
green cooked	1 (2.6 oz)	20
habanero	1 tsp	9
hungarian	1 (0.9 oz)	8
jalapeno	1 (0.5 oz)	4
jalapeno sliced	1 cup (3.2 oz)	27

FOOD	PORTION	CALS
red	1 (2.6 oz)	20
red chopped	½ cup	13
red chopped cooked	½ cup	19
red cooked	1 (2.6 oz)	20
serrano	1 (6 g)	2
serrano chopped	1 cup (3.7 oz)	34
yellow	1 (6.5 oz)	50
yellow	10 strips	14
FROZEN		
green chopped	1 oz	6
red chopped	1 oz	6
C&W		
Strips	¾ cup	25
Farm Rich		
Stuffed Jalapeno	2 (1.7 oz)	120
PERCH		
FRESH		
cooked	3 oz	99
cooked	1 fillet (1.6 oz)	54
ocean perch atlantic cooked	1 fillet (1.8 oz)	60
ocean perch atlantic cooked	3 oz	103
ocean perch atlantic raw	3 oz	80
raw	3 oz	77
red raw	3.5 oz	114
FROZEN		
Bell		
Cajun Nuggets	12 (4.5 oz)	170
Fillets Breaded	1 piece (4.5 oz)	170
Fillets Unbreaded	1 piece (3.5 oz)	80
PERSIMMONS		
dried japanese	1 (1.2 oz)	93
fresh	1 (6 oz)	118
PHEASANT		
breast boneless cooked	½ (4.4 oz)	312
cooked diced	1 cup	332
drumstick & thigh cooked	1 (2.6 oz)	184
PHYLLO		
sheet	1 (0.7 oz)	57

FOOD	PORTION	CALS
Athens		
Mini Fillo Shells	2 (7 g)	25
Ekizian		
Sheets	2 (4 oz)	433
The Fillo Factory		
Kataifi Shredded Fillo	1 (2 oz)	180
Organic	2 sheets (1.5 oz)	130
Organic Whole Wheat	2 sheets (1.8 oz)	140
Shells Large	1 (0.7 oz)	80

PICANTE (*see* SALSA)

PICKLES

FOOD	PORTION	CALS
bread & butter	6 slices	39
dill	1 lg (4.7 oz)	24
dill low sodium	1 med (2.3 oz)	12
dill sliced	6 slices	7
sweet gherkin	1 (1.2 oz)	41
tsukemono japanese pickles sliced	¼ cup	10
Claussen		
Bread 'N Butter Chips	1 oz	20
Kosher Dills Halves	1 (1 oz)	5
Sandwich Slices Hearty Garlic	2 (1.2 oz)	5
Sweet Gerkins	1 (0.9 oz)	30
Dietz & Watson		
New Half Sours	2 pieces (1 oz)	0
Gedney		
Baby Dills	3 (1 oz)	5
Organic Baby Dills	2 (1 oz)	5
Jake & Amos		
Bread & Butter Chips	2 tbsp	20
Mt. Olive		
Bread & Butter Spears	⅔ spear (1 oz)	20
Texas Sassy		
Pickle Chips	1 tbsp (0.5 oz)	30
Tree Of Life		
Organic Sweet Bread & Butter Chips	4 (1 oz)	30
Vlasic		
Kosher Dill Spears Reduced Sodium	⅔ spear (1 oz)	0
Stackers Kosher Dill	1 (1 oz)	0
Stackers Kosher Dill Reduced Sodium	1 (1 oz)	0

FOOD	PORTION	CALS

PIE (*see also* PIE CRUST, PIE FILLING)
FROZEN
Edwards

FOOD	PORTION	CALS
Pie Slices Key Lime	1 slice (3.25 oz)	330

Mom Made

Munchie Apple	1 (2.5 oz)	220

Mrs. Smith's

Bake & Serve No Sugar Added Apple	1 slice (4.6 oz)	310
Blueberry Crumb	1 slice (4.2 oz)	320
Cherry	1 slice (4.6 oz)	330
Cinnabon Apple Crumb	1 slice (4.6 oz)	350
Classic Cream Key Lime	1 slice (4.2 oz)	410
Coconut Custard	1 slice (4.4 oz)	300
Deep Dish Berry Burst	1 slice (4.2 oz)	340
Dutch Apple Crumb	1 slice (4.6 oz)	370
Pumpkin Custard	1 slice (4.6 oz)	300
Soda Shoppe Boston Cream	1 slice (2.7 oz)	220
Soda Shoppe Chocolate Cream	1 slice (4.6 oz)	350
Soda Shoppe Lemon Meringue	1 slice (4.2 oz)	300

READY-TO-EAT
Foods By George

Gluten Free Pecan Tarts	1 (4 oz)	470

Lance

Pecan	1 (3 oz)	350

Lifestream

| Pie Oh-My Apple | 1 (3.5 oz) | 280 |
| Pie Oh-My Pineapple | 1 (3.5 oz) | 280 |

TAKE-OUT

apple one crust	1 slice (5.3 oz)	363
apple tart	1 (4.2 oz)	370
apple two crust	1 slice (5.3 oz)	356
apricot tart	1 (4.2 oz)	356
apricot two crust	1 slice (5.3 oz)	417
banana cream	1 slice (5.1 oz)	387
blackberry one crust	1 slice (4.4 oz)	341
blackberry two crust	1 slice (5.3 oz)	394
blueberry one crust	1 slice (4.8 oz)	292
blueberry tart	1 (4.2 oz)	346
blueberry two crust	1 slice (5.3 oz)	348
cherry one crust	1 slice (4.8 oz)	312

FOOD	PORTION	CALS
cherry two crust	1 slice (5.3 oz)	390
chess	1 slice (3 oz)	365
chocolate cream	1 slice (5 oz)	380
coconut creme	1 slice (5 oz)	429
custard	1 slice (4.8 oz)	286
grasshopper	1 slice (3.5 oz)	341
key lime	1 slice (5 oz)	420
lemon meringue	1 slice (4.8 oz)	367
lemon meringue tart	1 (4.1 oz)	298
mince two crust	1 slice (5.3 oz)	434
peach two crust	1 slice (5.3 oz)	334
pear two crust	1 slice (5.3 oz)	400
pecan	1 slice (4 oz)	456
pineapple two crust	1 slice (5.3 oz)	394
plum two crust	1 slice (5.3 oz)	441
prune one crust	1 slice (5.3 oz)	450
pumpkin	1 slice (5.4 oz)	323
raisin tart	1 (4.2 oz)	348
raisin two crust	1 slice (5.3 oz)	376
raspberry one crust	1 slice (4.8 oz)	330
raspberry two crust	1 slice (5.3 oz)	422
rhubarb two crust	1 slice (5.3 oz)	444
shoo-fly	1 slice (4 oz)	404
strawberry rhubarb two crust	1 slice (5.3 oz)	422
strawberry two crust	1 slice (6 oz)	386
sweet potato	1 piece (5.4 oz)	276

PIE CRUST

baked	⅙ crust (1 oz)	147
chocolate wafer	⅛ crust (1.2 oz)	177
chocolate wafer tart shell	1 (0.8 oz)	111
deep dish frzn	⅛ crust (1.8 oz)	266
graham cracker	⅙ crust (1.2 oz)	172
graham cracker tart shell	1 (0.8 oz)	109
puff pastry shell	1 (1.4 oz)	223
tart shell	1 (1 oz)	149

Honey Maid

Graham Cracker Crumbs as prep	⅛ pie	160

Keebler

Graham Reduced Fat	⅛ pie (0.7 oz)	100
Ready Crust Chocolate	⅛ pie (0.7 oz)	100

FOOD	PORTION	CALS
Ready Crust Graham	1/10 pie (0.9 oz)	130
Ready Crust Shortbread	1/8 pie (0.7 oz)	110
Mrs. Smith's		
Deep Dish Shell frzn	1 slice (1 oz)	130
Nilla Wafers		
Pie Crust	1/6 (1 oz)	140
Pepperidge Farm		
Puff Pastry Sheets frzn	1/6 sheet	170
Puff Pastry Shell frzn	1	190
Pillsbury		
Crusts Just Unroll	1/8 (1 oz)	110
Deep Dish frzn	1/8 (0.7 oz)	90
Pet Ritz Deep Dish frzn	1/8 (0.6 oz)	90
PIE FILLING		
apple	1 cup	155
blueberry	1 cup	474
cherry	1 cup	317
lemon	1 cup	923
pumpkin pie mix canned	1 cup (9.5 oz)	281
Chukar Cherries		
Triple Cherry	1/2 cup	190
Comstock		
Country Cherry Original	1/3 cup (3.1 oz)	90
Farmer's Market		
Organic Pumpkin Pie Mix	1/2 cup	100
PIEROGI		
potato	1 (1.3 oz)	70
Mrs. T's		
Mini Potato & Cheddar	7 (3 oz)	130
Potato & Cheddar	4 (4 oz)	170
Potato & Onion	3 (4 oz)	160
Potato Broccoli & Cheddar	3 (4 oz)	190
Sauerkraut	3 (4 oz)	140
Sour Cream & Chive	3 (4 oz)	190
PIGEON PEAS		
dried cooked	1 cup	204
dried cooked w/ salt	1/2 cup (2.9 oz)	102

PIGNOLIA (see PINE NUTS)

FOOD	PORTION	CALS
PIG'S FEET		
cooked	1	201
pickled	1	177
Hormel		
Pigs Feet	2 oz	80
PIKE		
northern cooked	½ fillet (5.4 oz)	176
northern cooked	3 oz	96
northern raw	3 oz	75
roe raw	1 oz	37
walleye baked	3 oz	101
walleye fillet baked	4.4 oz	147
PILLNUTS		
canarytree dried	1 oz	204
PIMIENTOS		
canned	1 slice	0
canned	1 tbsp	3
PINE NUTS		
pine nuts dried	¼ cup (1.2 oz)	277
pinyon dried	20 (2 g)	13
pinyon dried	1 oz	178
Fisher		
Pine Nuts	¼ cup (1 oz)	190
PINEAPPLE		
CANNED		
in heavy syrup crushed sliced or chunks	1 cup (8.9 oz)	198
in heavy syrup slice	1 (1.7 oz)	38
in juice crushed sliced or chunks	1 cup (8.7 oz)	149
in light syrup crushed sliced or chunks	1 cup (8.8 oz)	131
in light syrup slice	1 (1.7 oz)	25
in water crushed sliced or chunks	1 cup (8.6 oz)	79
juice pack slice	1 (1.6 oz)	28
water pack slice	1 (1.6 oz)	15
Del Monte		
Chunks In Heavy Syrup	½ cup (4.3 oz)	90
Chunks In Its Own Juice	½ cup (4.3 oz)	70
Crushed In Heavy Syrup	½ cup (4.3 oz)	90
Crushed In Its Own Juice	½ cup (4.3 oz)	70

FOOD	PORTION	CALS
Fruit Naturals Chunks	½ cup (4.4 oz)	70
Slices In Heavy Syrup	2 (4 oz)	60
Dole		
Crushed In Heavy Syrup	½ cup (4.3 oz)	90
Crushed Juice Pack	½ cup (4.3 oz)	70
Slices In Heavy Syrup	2 (4.1 oz)	90
Slices Juice Pack	2 (4 oz)	60
Gefen		
Chunks In Juice	½ cup (4.9 oz)	80
Liberty Gold		
Chunks Natural Juice	½ cup (4.7 oz)	80
Slices Natural Juice	½ cup	80
DRIED		
dried	1 piece (1 oz)	71
Brothers-All-Natural		
Crisps	1 pkg (0.53 oz)	60
Crispy Green		
Crispy Pineapple	1 pkg (0.35)	35
Crunchies		
Freeze Dried	1 pkg (9 g)	35
Crunchy N'Yummy		
Organic Freeze Dried	1 pkg (1 oz)	100
Kopali		
Organic	1 pkg (1.7 oz)	170
Mrs. May's		
Fruit Chips	1 pkg	35
Sunsweet		
Philippine	⅓ cup (1.4 oz)	130
FRESH		
chunks	1 cup (5.8 oz)	82
slice	1 slice (3 oz)	42
whole	1 (2 lbs)	452
Chiquita		
Bites	1 piece (2.8 oz)	40
Cut Up	1 cup (5.8 oz)	82
Dole		
Pineapple	2 slices (3.9 oz)	60
FROZEN		
chunks sweetened	1 cup (8.6 oz)	211

FOOD	PORTION	CALS
Dole		
Chunks	¾ cup (4.9 oz)	70
Tropical Gold	1 pkg (3 oz)	45
PINEAPPLE JUICE		
canned unsweetened w/ vitamin C	1 cup (8.8 oz)	132
frzn unsweetened as prep w/ water	1 cup (8.8 oz)	130
Ceres		
100% Juice	8 oz	120
Dole		
100% Juice	1 can (6 oz)	90
Fizzy Lizzy		
Pineapple	1 bottle (12 oz)	100
Sundia		
Purely	½ cup	60
Walnut Acres		
Organic	8 oz	130
PINK BEANS		
dried cooked	1 cup	252
PINTO BEANS		
dried cooked	1 cup	245
Arrowhead Mills		
Organic Dried not prep	¼ cup	150
HamBeens		
Dried as prep	½ cup	120
Tree Of Life		
Organic	½ cup (4.6 oz)	120
TAKE-OUT		
stewed w/ viandas	1 cup	222
PISTACHIOS		
dry roasted w/ salt	49 nuts (1 oz)	161
dry roasted w/o salt	49 nuts (1 oz)	162
in shells	½ cup	165
Fisher		
Shelled	¼ cup (1 oz)	160
Love'n Bake		
Pistachio Paste	2 tbsp	160
Planters		
Dry Roasted	1 oz	170

FOOD	PORTION	CALS
True North		
Sea Salted In Shells	½ cup	170
Wonderful		
Roasted & Salted In Shells	½ cup	160
PITANGA		
fresh	1 cup	57
fresh	1	2
PIZZA (see also PIZZA CRUST)		
4Real		
Cheese	1 (4.2 oz)	220
Cheesy Pizza Quesadilla	1 (2.5 oz)	160
Turkey Pepperoni	1 (4.2 oz)	220
A.C.LaRocco		
Thin Crust Whole Grain Cheese & Garlic	⅓ pie (4.8 oz)	250
Thin Crust Whole Grain Greek Sesame	⅓ pie (4.4 oz)	250
Thin Crust Whole Grain Tomato & Feta	⅓ pie (4.8 oz)	250
Ultra Thin Sprouted Grain Bruschetta	½ pie (3.5 oz)	170
Ultra Thin Sprouted Grain Old World Veggie	½ pie (3.6 oz)	170
Amy's		
Cheese & Pesto Whole Wheat Crust	⅓ pie (4.6 oz)	360
Margherita	1 pie (6.2 oz)	360
Non Dairy Cheese Rice Crust	1 pie (6 oz)	460
Pocket Sandwich Spinach Feta	1 (4.5 oz)	260
Roasted Vegetable No Cheese	⅓ pie (4 oz)	270
Single Serve Spinach Light In Sodium	1 (7.2 oz)	440
Soy Cheese	⅓ pie (4.3 oz)	290
Toaster Pops Cheese Pizza	5–6 pieces	160
Bellatoria		
Fire Grilled Flatbread Buffalo Chicken	⅓ pie (5.8 oz)	340
Fire Grilled Flatbread Chicken Ranch w/ Uncured Bacon	¼ pie (4.5 oz)	270
Ultra Thin Crust Margherita	⅓ pie (4.9 oz)	280
Ultra Thin Crust Ultimate Pepperoni	¼ pie (4.3 oz)	300
Bold Organics		
Deluxe	½ pie (6.7 oz)	460
Meat Lovers	½ pie (6 oz)	450
Vegan Cheese	½ pie (5.5 oz)	380
Veggie Lovers	½ pie (6.2 oz)	390
Cedarlane		
Zone Cheese	1 (6.5 oz)	380

FOOD	PORTION	CALS
Dayeinu		
Passover Pizza	1 slice (4 oz)	325
DiGiorno		
Crispy Flatbread Tuscan Chicken	⅓ pie (4.6 oz)	280
For One Thin Crust Grilled Chicken & Vegetable	1 (8.4 oz)	520
For One Traditional Crust Supreme	1 (9.9 oz)	790
Four Cheese	⅙ pie (4.7 oz)	310
Garlic Bread Pepperoni	⅙ pie (5 oz)	380
Rising Crust Four Cheese	⅓ pie (4 oz)	270
Rising Crust Italian Sausage	⅙ pie (5 oz)	350
Rising Crust Spinach Mushroom Garlic	⅙ pie (5 oz)	290
Rising Crust Three Meat	⅙ pie (5 oz)	350
Stuffed Crust Pepperoni	⅕ pie (5.3 oz)	380
Thin Crispy Crust Pepperoni	⅕ pie (4.4 oz)	320
Thin Crispy Crust Spinach Mushroom Garlic	⅕ pie (4.6 oz)	250
Ultimate Topping Four Meat	⅕ pie (5 oz)	380
Ultimate Topping Supreme	⅕ pie (5.3 oz)	360
Farm Rich		
Pizza Slices Pepperoni	2 (3.5 oz)	280
Foods By George		
Gluten Free Cheese	1 pie (6.5 oz)	400
Glutino		
Gluten Free Duo Cheese	1 (6.1 oz)	420
Gluten Free Spinach & Feta	1 (6.1 oz)	430
Health Is Wealth		
Vegetarian Mini Pizza Bagels	4 (3.1 oz)	150
Hot Pockets		
Croissant Five Cheese	1 (4.5 oz)	350
Croissant Pepperoni	1 (4.5 oz)	380
Sausage	1 (4.5 oz)	330
Jeno's		
Crisp 'N Tasty Cheese	1 pie (6.8 oz)	440
Crisp 'N Tasty Pepperoni	1 (6.7 oz)	490
Crisp 'N Tasty Supreme	1 (7.2 oz)	490
Kraft		
Rising Crust Three Meat	⅓ pie (4.4 oz)	320
Lean Cuisine		
Casual Cuisine Deep Dish Roasted Vegetable	1 pkg (6 oz)	320
Casual Cuisine Deep Dish Spinach & Mushroom	1 pkg (6 oz)	340
Casual Cuisine Deep Dish Three Meat	1 pkg (6.4 oz)	390

FOOD	PORTION	CALS
Casual Cuisine Flatbread Melts Chicken Philly	1 pkg (6.5 oz)	350
Casual Cuisine Traditional Deluxe	1 pkg (6 oz)	340
Casual Cuisine Traditional Four Cheese	1 pkg (6 oz)	350
Casual Cuisine Traditional Mushroom	1 pkg (6 oz)	300
Casual Cuisine Traditional Pepperoni	1 pkg (6 oz)	380
Casual Cuisine Wood Fire Bacon Alfredo	1 pkg (6 oz)	320
Casual Cuisine Wood Fire Margherita	1 pkg (6 oz)	310
Simple Favorites French Bread Cheese	1 pkg (6 oz)	340
Lean Pockets		
Pepperoni	1 (4.5 oz)	260
Sausage & Pepperoni	1 (4.5 oz)	280
Lunchables		
Extra Cheesy	1 pkg	280
Pizza w/ Pepperoni	1 pkg	310
Mom Made		
Munchie Cheese Pizza	1 (2.5 oz)	160
Pacific Foods		
BBQ Chicken	⅓ pie (4.5 oz)	270
Herb Garlic Chicken	⅓ pie (4.5 oz)	270
Supreme	⅓ pie (4.8 oz)	270
Red Baron		
Classic Crust 4 Cheese	1 pie (8.6 oz)	740
Simply Shari's		
Gluten Free Cheese	½ pie (5 oz)	290
Gluten Free Pepperoni	½ pie (5 oz)	320
Gluten Free Pesto Margherita	½ pie (5 oz)	340
Gluten Free Spinach Feta	¼ pkg (5 oz)	280
Gluten Free Vegetable Margherita	¼ pie (5 oz)	220
Solterra		
Cheese Margherita	½ pie (4.1 oz)	200
Vegan	½ pie (4.1 oz)	210
Stouffer's		
Corner Bistro Flatbread Margherita	1 pkg (9.13 oz)	540
Corner Bistro Flatbread Shrimp & Roasted Garlic	1 pkg (9.33 oz)	600
French Bread Grilled Vegetable	1 pkg (11.63 oz)	340
French Bread Sausage	1 pkg (4.2 oz)	420
French Bread Sausage & Pepperoni	1 pkg (4.2 oz)	460
French Bread White Pizza	1 pkg (10.13 oz)	470
Tandoor Chef		
Naan Pizza Margherita	½ pie (4 oz)	220

FOOD	PORTION	CALS
Naan Pizza Roasted Eggplant	½ pie (4.6 oz)	320
Naan Pizza Spinach & Paneer Cheese	½ pie (4.2 oz)	290
Tofutti		
Pan Crust Pizzaz Dairy Free	1 slice (2.7 oz)	180
Totino's		
Crisp Crust Canadian Bacon	½ pie (5.1 oz)	320
Crisp Crust Combination	½ pie (5.3 oz)	380
Crisp Crust Pepperoni Trio	½ pie (5 oz)	370
Crisp Crust Three Meat	½ pie (5.2 oz)	350
Pizza Rolls Combination	6 (3 oz)	220
Pizza Rolls Mega Ultimate Combination	3 (3.3 oz)	200
Pizza Rolls Supreme	6 (3 oz)	210
TAKE-OUT		
cheese	⅛ of 16 in pie	423
cheese deep dish individual	1 (5.5 oz)	460
cheese & vegetables	⅛ of 16 in pie	428
ground beef	16 in pie	3753
ham & pineapple	⅛ of 16 in pie	439
no cheese	⅛ of 16 in pie	262
pepperoni	⅛ of 16 in pie	469
white pizza	⅛ of 16 in pie	484

PIZZA CRUST

FOOD	PORTION	CALS
crust	1 slice (1.7 oz)	130
whole wheat	⅛ crust (2 oz)	120
Boboli		
100% Whole Wheat	⅕ crust (2 oz)	150
Original	⅛ crust (1.8 oz)	140
Original Mini	½ crust (2.5 oz)	190
Thin Crust	⅕ crust (2 oz)	170
French Meadow Bakery		
Gluten Free	¼ pie (1.9 oz)	160
Martha White		
Mix not prep	¼ pkg	160
Pillsbury		
Classic	⅙ crust (2.3 oz)	160
Udi's		
Gluten Free	½ crust (4.2 oz)	300

PLANTAINS

FOOD	PORTION	CALS
cooked mashed	1 cup	232
sliced cooked	1 cup	179

FOOD	PORTION	CALS
Dole		
Fresh cooked	½ med (3.2 oz)	100
Grab Em Snacks		
Chips Black Pepper	1 oz	150
Isleno		
Chips	1 oz	150
TAKE-OUT		
mofongo	1 serv	320
ripe fried	1 serv (2.8 oz)	214
sweet baked w/ ice cream	1 serv	285
PLUM JUICE		
Nantucket Nectars		
Red Plum	8 oz	120
Sunsweet		
PlumSmart Light	8 oz	60
PlumSmart w/ Extra Fiber	8 oz	160
PLUMS		
canned purple in heavy syrup	1 cup	163
canned purple juice pack	1 cup	146
canned purple water pack	1 cup	102
dried japanese	1	9
fresh	1	30
pickled	1	34
Chiquita		
Fresh	1 (2.3 oz)	30
Dole		
Fresh	2 (5.3 oz)	70
Oregon		
Whole In Heavy Syrup	½ cup (4.6 oz)	100
Sunsweet		
Plumsweets Dried	14 pieces (1 oz)	120
POI		
poi	1 cup	240
POKEBERRY SHOOTS		
cooked	½ cup	16
fresh	½ cup	18

FOOD	PORTION	CALS

POLENTA
Bob's Red Mill
Corn Grits Polenta not prep | ¼ cup | 130

POLLACK
atlantic baked | 3 oz | 100
atlantic fillet baked | 5.3 oz | 178

POMEGRANATE
fresh | 1 (5.4 oz) | 105
Navitas Naturals
Pomegranate Powder | 1 tbsp (0.5 oz) | 50

POMEGRANATE JUICE
Apple & Eve
Organic | 8 oz | 130
Arthur's
Pom Plus | 1 bottle (11 oz) | 220
Frutzzo
Organic 100% Juice | 1 bottle (12 oz) | 130
Langers
100% Juice | 8 oz | 150
Odwalla
PomaGrand 100% Juice | 8 oz | 160
POM
100% Juice | 8 oz | 160
Pomegranate Blueberry | 8 oz | 160
Pomegranate Mango | 8 oz | 140
Smart Juice
Organic 100% Juice | 8 oz | 149
Tart Is Smart
Concentrate | 0.5 oz | 37
Ultra Lo-Gly
Pomegranate | 1 bottle (10 oz) | 45
Pomegranate Mojita | 1 bottle (10 oz) | 40

POMPANO
smoked | 2 oz | 109
steamed or poached | 4 oz | 156
TAKE-OUT
battered & fried | 4 oz | 304
breaded & fried | 4 oz | 242

FOOD	PORTION	CALS
POPCORN		
air popped	1 cup (0.3 oz)	31
caramel coated	1 cup (1.2 oz)	152
caramel coated w/ peanuts	⅔ cup (1 oz)	114
cheese	1 cup (0.4 oz)	58
oil popped	1 cup (0.4 oz)	55
Bachman		
Regular	2¾ cups (1 oz)	160
Chip'ins		
Chips Hot Buffalo Wing	18 (1 oz)	130
Chips Jalapeno Ranch	18 (1 oz)	130
Chips Sea Salt	18 (1 oz)	120
Chips White Cheddar	18 (1 oz)	130
Cracker Jack		
The Original	½ cup (1 oz)	120
Deep River Snacks		
Sharp White Cheddar	1 oz	150
Divvies		
Caramel Corn Vegan	½ cup	80
I.M. Healthy		
Roasted Sweet Corn Original Lightly Salted	1 oz	120
Jay's		
Caramel	¾ cup	110
Ok-Ke-Doke Cheese	1 oz	160
Lance		
White Cheddar	1 pkg (0.7 oz)	100
Mrs. Fields		
Clusters Butter Toffee Crunch	⅔ cup	170
Orville Redenbacher's		
Microwave Smart Pop 94% Fat Free as prep	1 cup	15
Popcorn Indiana		
Kettle Corn Original	2 cups (1 oz)	130
Kettle Corn Smoked Cheddar	2 cups (1 oz)	120
Movie Theater	2 cups (1 oz)	150
Sea Salt	3 cups (1 oz)	130
PopCorners		
Butter	1 oz	120
Jalapeno	1 oz	130
Kettle	1 oz	120
SeaSalt	1 oz	130
White Cheddar	1 oz	130

FOOD	PORTION	CALS
Poppycock		
Cashew Lovers	½ cup (1.1 oz)	148
Original	½ cup (1.1 oz)	160
Pecan Delight	½ cup (1.1 oz)	150
Smart Balance		
Movie Style as prep	1 cup	35
Smart 'N Healthy as prep	1 cup	20
Smartfood		
Kettle Corn	1¼ cups (1 oz)	140
Reduced Fat White Cheddar	3 cups (1 oz)	130
White Cheddar	1¾ cups (1 oz)	160
Snyder's Of Hanover		
Butter	0.6 oz	100
The Whole Earth		
Organic Kettle Corn Salty & Sweet	2 cups (1 oz)	120
Tree Of Life		
Organic Lightly Salted	4 cups	100
Utz		
Butter	2 cups	170
Cheese	2 cups	160
Puff'n Corn Original Hulless	2 cups	150
POPOVER		
home recipe as prep w/ 2% milk	1 (1.4 oz)	87
home recipe as prep w/ whole milk	1 (1.4 oz)	90
mix as prep	1 (1.2 oz)	67
POPPY SEEDS		
poppy seeds	1 tbsp	47
Bob's Red Mill		
Poppy Seeds	3 tbsp	170
Love'n Bake		
Poppy Seed Filling	2 tbsp	120
PORGY		
fresh	3 oz	77
PORK (see also HAM, JERKY, PORK DISHES)		
FRESH		
boneless loin lean & fat roasted	3.5 oz	195
center loin chop bone in broiled	1 (3 oz)	178
center rib chop lean & fat bone in broiled	1 (3 oz)	189
country style ribs bone in lean & fat braised	3.5 oz	288

FOOD	PORTION	CALS
dehydrated oriental style	1 cup (0.8 oz)	135
fresh ham rump half lean & fat roasted	4 oz	278
fresh ham shank half lean & fat roasted	4 oz	319
fresh ham whole lean & fat roasted	4 oz	302
ground cooked	4 oz	328
ham hock cooked	1	167
shoulder chop bone in braised	1 (3 oz)	229
sirloin roast lean & fat bone in roasted	4 oz	231
spareribs bone in roasted	3 oz	304
tail simmered	3 oz	336
tenderloin roast boneless lean & fat roasted	4 oz	145
top loin chop boneless lean & fat broiled	1 (3.5 oz)	195
Boar's Head		
Smoked Shoulder Butt Roast	3 oz	170
Dietz & Watson		
Chops Boneless Smoked	3 oz	110
Shoulder Butt	3 oz	150
Spare Ribs Canadian Center Cut	1 serv (5 oz)	300
Hatfield		
Chop Center Cut Boneless	1 (4 oz)	130
Hormel		
Always Tender Loin Filet Honey Mustard	1 serv (4 oz)	140
Always Tender Tenderloin Apple Bourbon	1 serv (4 oz)	140
Pork Roast Au Jus	1 serv (2 oz)	90
Organic Prairie		
Chop Bone In	1 (3.3 oz)	220
Smithfield		
Boneless Smoked Pork Chop	3 oz	110
Smoked Pork Chop	3 oz	100
Tyson		
Baby Back Ribs Buffalo	4 oz	300
Ground Reduced Fat	4 oz	260
Half Loin Boneless	4 oz	190
Loin Chops Bone-In Center Cut	4 oz	190
Spareribs	4 oz	290
Stew Meat	4 oz	130
FROZEN		
Organic Prairie		
Ribs Boneless Country Style	1 (4 oz)	160
Tenderloin	4 oz	150

FOOD	PORTION	CALS
TAKE-OUT		
char siu chinese style	1 piece (0.4 oz)	28
chicharrones pork cracklings fried	1 cup	492
chop breaded & fried	1 lg (5 oz)	441
chop breaded & fried	1 med (3.4 oz)	304
chop stewed	1 lg (4.6 oz)	315

PORK DISHES
A La Carte Gourmet
Pork Loin w/ Cream Spinach Feta Stuffing	1 serv (5 oz)	200

Tyson
Roast Pork w/ Vegetables	1 serv (4 oz)	190

Ventera
Pork Carnitas	1 serv (5 oz)	190

TAKE-OUT

kalua pork	1 cup (7 oz)	497
pork satay w/ peanut sauce	5 sticks (3.5 oz)	214
pulled pork w/ barbecue sauce	1 serv (5 oz)	240
spareribs barbecue w/ sauce	2 med (2.8 oz)	248
tourtiere	1 piece (4.9 oz)	451

PORK RINDS (*see* SNACKS)

POT PIE
Amy's
Broccoli	1 (7.5 oz)	430
Shepherd's	1 (8 oz)	160
Shepherd's Pie Light In Sodium	1 (8 oz)	160
Vegetable	1 (7.5 oz)	360

Banquet
Beef	1	450
Chicken	1	370
Chicken w/ Broccoli	1	350
Turkey	1	390

Bell & Evans
Chicken	1 cup (7.9 oz)	520

Hot Pockets
Pot Pie Express Chicken	1 (4.5 oz)	330

Marie Callender's
Beef	½ pie	540
Cheesy Chicken	½ pie	600
Chicken	1	670

FOOD	PORTION	CALS
Creamy Mushroom & Chicken	½ pie	560
Turkey	1	670
Mon Cuisine		
Vegan	1 pkg (9 oz)	650
Pacific Foods		
Organic Beef	1 cup (8 oz)	410
Organic Turkey	1 cup (8 oz)	400
Pepperidge Farm		
Chili Beans & Cornbread	1 cup	360
Reduced Fat Roasted White Meat Chicken	1 cup	470
Roasted White Meat Chicken	1 cup	510
Stouffer's		
Chicken White Meat	1 pkg (10 oz)	660
TAKE-OUT		
beef	1 (14.6 oz)	938
chicken	1 (14.6 oz)	897
ham	1 serv (11 oz)	752
oyster	1 serv (11.5 oz)	817
puerto rican pastelon de carne	1 piece (5 oz)	666
st. stephen's day pie	1 serv (16.7 oz)	549
tuna	1 (27 oz)	1715
vegetarian w/ meat substitute	1 (8 oz)	511

POTATO (*see also* CHIPS, KNISH, PANCAKES)

FOOD	PORTION	CALS
CANNED		
potatoes	½ cup	54
Butterfield		
Whole White	3.5 pieces (5.8 oz)	90
Del Monte		
Savory Sides Au Gratin	½ cup	80
S&W		
New Whole	2 (5.5 oz)	60
Sunshine		
Whole White	3 pieces (5.9 oz)	90
FRESH		
baked skin only	1 skin (2 oz)	115
baked w/ skin	1 (6.5 oz)	220
baked w/o skin	½ cup	57
baked w/o skin	1 (5 oz)	145
boiled	½ cup	68
microwaved	1 (7 oz)	212

FOOD	PORTION	CALS
microwaved w/o skin	½ cup	78
raw w/o skin	1 (3.9 oz)	88
Dole		
Idaho	1 (5.3 oz)	110
Green Giant		
Klondike Gourmet	5 sm (5.3 oz)	110
Masser's		
Roasted Russet Triple Washed	1 (5.3 oz)	110
Melissa's		
Dutch Yellow Baby diced	¾ cup (3.9 oz)	80
FROZEN		
french fries	10 strips	111
french fries thick cut	10 strips	109
hash browns	½ cup	170
potato puffs	1	16
potato puffs	½ cup	138
Alexia		
Sweet Potato Puffs	⅔ cup (3 oz)	130
Birds Eye		
Steamfresh Roasted Red Potatoes w/ Garlic Butter Sauce	1¼ cups (5.1 oz)	190
Cascadian Farm		
Organic Country Style	¾ cup	50
Organic Hash Browns	1 cup	60
Funster		
BBQ Lite	14 pieces (3 oz)	140
Cheddar	14 pieces (3 oz)	135
Original	14 pieces (3 oz)	135
Green Giant		
Roasted Potatoes w/ Garlic & Herb Sauce as prep	½ cup	90
Health Is Wealth		
Twice Baked Cheddar Cheese	1 (5 oz)	200
Vegetarian Potato Skins	2 (2.7 oz)	110
Joy Of Cooking		
Elegant Scalloped	1 cup (8 oz)	300
Red Skin Mashed	1 cup (4.2 oz)	160
Lean Cuisine		
Simple Favorites Cheddar Potato w/ Broccoli	1 pkg (10.25 oz)	210
McCain		
5 Minute Fries	1 serv (3 oz)	120

FOOD	PORTION	CALS
Farmer's Kitchen Oven Baked Crinkles	12 pieces (2 oz)	50
Purely Potatoes Whole Baby Skin On	1 serv (3 oz)	100
MIX		
au gratin as prep	½ cup	160
instant mashed flakes as prep w/ whole milk & butter	½ cup	118
instant mashed flakes not prep	½ cup	78
instant mashed granules as prep w/ whole milk & butter	½ cup	114
instant mashed granules not prep	½ cup	372
scalloped	½ cup	105
Betty Crocker		
Au Gratin as prep	⅔ cup	150
Cheddar & Bacon as prep	⅔ cup	120
Cheesy Scalloped as prep	½ cup	120
Julienne as prep	⅔ cup	140
Mashed Creamy Butter as prep	⅔ cup	80
Mashed Four Cheese as prep	½ cup	170
Mashed Sour Cream & Chives as prep	½ cup	170
Scalloped as prep	½ cup	130
Seasoned Skillets Hash Browns as prep	½ cup	120
Idahoan		
Mashed Buttery Homestyle as prep	½ cup	110
Mashed Buttery Yukon as prep	½ cup	110
Mashed Original as prep	½ cup	170
Mashed Roasted Garlic & Parmesan as prep	½ cup	110
REFRIGERATED		
Bob Evans		
Mashed Potatoes Original	½ cup (4.4 oz)	150
Country Crock		
Garlic Mashed	⅔ cup (5 oz)	160
Homestyle Mashed	⅔ cup (5 oz)	160
Loaded Mashed	⅔ cup (5 oz)	200
Diner's Choice		
Mashed	⅔ cup	110
Reser's		
Potato Express Red Skinned Mashed	½ cup	140
Simply Potatoes		
Traditional Mashed	½ cup (4.4 oz)	120

FOOD	PORTION	CALS
SHELF-STABLE		
TastyBite		
Bombay Potatoes	½ pkg (5 oz)	105
TAKE-OUT		
au gratin w/ cheese	½ cup	178
baked topped w/ cheese sauce	1	475
baked topped w/ cheese sauce & bacon	1	451
baked topped w/ cheese sauce & broccoli	1 (12 oz)	403
baked topped w/ cheese sauce & chili	1	481
baked topped w/ sour cream & chives	1	394
cheese fries w/ ranch dressing	1 serv	3010
french fries	1 reg	235
hash browns	½ cup (2.5 oz)	151
indian yogurt potatoes	1 serv	315
mashed	½ cup	111
o'brien	1 cup	157
potato pancakes	1 (1.3 oz)	101
potato salad	½ cup	179
red new boiled	5 sm (5 oz)	120
scalloped	½ cup	127
twice baked w/ cheese	1 half (10 oz)	392
POTATO STARCH		
potato starch	1 oz	96
Bob's Red Mill		
Potato Starch	1 tbsp	40
POUT		
ocean baked	3 oz	87
ocean fillet baked	1 (4.8 oz)	140
PRETZELS		
chocolate covered	1 (0.4 oz)	47
soft	1 lg (5 oz)	483
twists salted	10 (2.1 oz)	229
twists w/o salt	10 (2.1 oz)	229
whole wheat	2 sm (1 oz)	103
yogurt covered	1 cup (3 oz)	391
yogurt covered	1 (4 g)	19
Annie's Homegrown		
Organic Bunnies	32 (1 oz)	100

FOOD	PORTION	CALS
Bachman		
Honey Wheat Splits	9 (1 oz)	110
Mini Low Sodium	17 (1 oz)	110
Original Twist	5 (1 oz)	100
Rolled Rods	2 (1 oz)	110
Thin N Rights	12 (1 oz)	120
Better Balance		
Cinnamon Toast Gluten Free	1 oz	120
Golden Butter Twists Gluten Free	1 oz	110
Jalapeno Mustard Gluten Free	1 oz	120
Braids		
Honey Wheat	7 (1 oz)	110
Mini Knots	17 (1 oz)	110
Farm Rich		
Stuffed Bites frzn	3 (1.7 oz)	110
Glenny's		
Organic Original Salted	8 (1 oz)	110
Organic Sourdough	6 (1 oz)	110
Glutino		
Gluten Free All Shapes	44 (1.4 oz)	190
New York Style		
Pretzel Flatz Original Salt	12	110
Rold Gold		
Braided Twists Honey Wheat	8 (1 oz)	110
Rods	3 (1 oz)	110
Sourdough	1 (0.8 oz)	90
Sticks	53 (1 oz)	100
Tiny Twists Fat Free	18 (1 oz)	110
Salba Smart		
Omega-3 Enriched	1 oz	110
Snyder's Of Hanover		
100 Calorie Pack Snaps	1 pkg (0.9 oz)	100
Dips Milk Chocolate	1 oz	140
Dips Special Dark Chocolate	1 oz	140
Gluten Free Sticks	30 (1 oz)	110
Mini Unsalted	1 oz	110
MultiGrain Sticks Lightly Salted	1 oz	120
MultiGrain Twists	1 oz	120
Nibblers Sourdough	1 oz	120
Old Tyme	1 oz	120
Organic Honey Wheat	1 oz	130

FOOD	PORTION	CALS
Organic Oat Bran	1 oz	120
Pieces Garlic Bread	1 oz	140
Pieces Honey Mustard & Onions	1 oz	140
Pieces Hot Buffalo Wing	1 oz	140
Pretzel Sandwich Peanut Butter	1 oz	140
Rods	1 oz	120
Snaps	1 oz	120
Sourdough Unsalted	1 oz	100
Sticks 12 Multi Grain	1 oz	130
Superpretzel		
Mozzarella	2 (1.8 oz)	130
Pretzelfils Pizza	2 (1.8 oz)	130
Soft	1 (2.25 oz)	160
Soft Bites	5 (1.9 oz)	150
Softstix	2 (1.8 oz)	130
Tom Sturgis		
Little Cheesers	17 (1 oz)	120
Little Ones	17 (1 oz)	110
Utz		
Braided Twists Baked Honey Wheat	1 oz	110
Chocolate Covered	6 (1.1 oz)	140
Hard	1	90
Special	1 oz	110
Special Multigrain	1 oz	110
Sticks Organic Whole Grain	1 oz	120
PRUNE JUICE		
jarred	1 cup	182
Lakewood		
Organic	8 oz	165
Sunsweet		
100% Juice	8 oz	180
Tree Of Life		
Organic 100% Juice	8 oz	180
PRUNES		
cooked w/o sugar	½ cup	133
dried	1	20
Del Monte		
Dried Pitted	5 (1.5 oz)	100
Earthbound Farms		
Organic Dried Plums	5	110

FOOD	PORTION	CALS
Love'n Bake		
Prune Lekvar	2 tbsp	90
Sunsweet		
Ones	4 (1.4 oz)	100
Pitted	5 (1.4 oz)	100
Pitted 60 Calorie Pack	1 pkg (0.9 oz)	60

PUDDING
READY-TO-EAT
Jell-O

FOOD	PORTION	CALS
100 Calorie Pack Fat Free Chocolate Vanilla Swirl	1 pkg (4 oz)	100
100 Calorie Pack Fat Free Tapioca	1 pkg (4 oz)	100
Boston Cream Pie Sugar Free	1 pkg (4 oz)	60
Dulce De Leche Sugar Free	1 pkg (3.7 oz)	60
Vanilla	1 serv (4 oz)	110
Kozy Shack		
Banana	1 pkg (4 oz)	130
Bread Pudding Apple Cinnamon	1 pkg (3.5 oz)	150
Chocolate No Sugar Added	1 pkg (4 oz)	60
Old Fashioned Tapioca	1 pkg (4 oz)	130
Original Rice	1 pkg (4 oz)	130
Real Chocolate	1 pkg (4 oz)	140
Rice No Sugar Added	1 pkg (4 oz)	70
Soy Chocolate	1 pkg (4.4 oz)	120
Soy Vanilla	1 pkg (4.4 oz)	110
Tapioca No Sugar Added	1 pkg (4 oz)	70
Vanilla	1 pkg (4 oz)	130
Vanilla No Sugar Added	1 pkg (4 oz)	90
Snack Pack		
Banana Cream Pie	1 pkg (3.5 oz)	110
Butterscotch	1 pkg (3.5 oz)	110
Caramel Cream	1 pkg (3.5 oz)	120
Chocolate	1 pkg (3.5 oz)	130
Chocolate Daredevil Triples	1 pkg (3.5 oz)	130
Chocolate Fat Free	1 pkg (3.5 oz)	80
Chocolate No Sugar Added	1 pkg (3.5 oz)	70
Lemon	1 pkg (3.5 oz)	130
Tapioca	1 pkg (3.5 oz)	120
Tapioca Fat Free	1 serv (3.5 oz)	80
Vanilla	1 pkg (3.5 oz)	120

FOOD	PORTION	CALS
SoYummi		
GoLite Bavarian Cream	1 pkg (3.5 oz)	86
Mousse All Flavors	1 pkg (4.4 oz)	137
Swiss Miss		
Chocolate	1 pkg	150
Chocolate Low Fat	1 pkg	130
Pie Lover's Banana Cream	1 pkg	130
Pie Lover's Lemon Meringue	1 pkg	140
Swirl Chocolate Vanilla	1 pkg	140
ZenSoy		
Banana	1 pkg (4 oz)	100
Chocolate	1 pkg (4 oz)	130
Vanilla	1 pkg (4 oz)	110
TAKE-OUT		
blancmange	1 serv (4.7 oz)	154
bread w/ raisins	1 cup	306
coconut	1 cup	291
corn	1 cup	328
guinataan coconut milk pudding	1 cup (9 oz)	331
indian pudding	½ cup	156
noodle pudding kugel	1 cup	297
plum pudding	1 slice (1.5 oz)	125
pumpkin	½ cup (4.6 oz)	139
queen of puddings	1 serv (4.4 oz)	266
rice pudding	1 cup	302
sweet potato	½ cup	107
tapioca	1 cup	236
yorkshire	1 serv (3 oz)	177
PUFFERFISH		
raw	3 oz	72
PUMMELO		
fresh white	1 (21.4 oz)	231
sections white	1 cup (6.7 oz)	72
PUMPKIN		
butter	1 tbsp	32
canned w/o salt	1 cup (8.6 oz)	83
cooked mashed w/o salt	1 cup (8.6 oz)	49
flowers cooked w/o salt	1 cup (4.7 oz)	20
leaves cooked w/o salt	1 cup (2.5 oz)	15

FOOD	PORTION	CALS
Farmer's Market		
Organic Puree	½ cup (4.3 oz)	50
Jake & Amos		
Pumpkin Butter	1 tbsp (0.5 oz)	5
Libby's		
Pumpkin	½ cup (4.3 oz)	40
Tree Of Life		
Organic Puree	½ cup (4.3 oz)	50
TAKE-OUT		
indian sago	1 serv (2.3 oz)	75
pumpkin fritters	1 (1.2 oz)	84
PUMPKIN SEEDS		
kernels dried	¼ cup (1.1 oz)	180
kernels roasted w/o salt	¼ cup (1 oz)	169
whole roasted w/o salt	¼ cup (0.5 oz)	71
David		
Kernels	1 pkg (2.5 oz)	280
Mrs. May's		
Pumpkin Crunch	1 oz	164
Spitz		
Seasoned Hulled	¼ cup (1 oz)	180
Sunrich Naturals		
Pepitas Lightly Salted	1 pkg (1 oz)	160
Tree Of Life		
Seeds Roasted & Salted	¼ cup (2 oz)	300
PURSLANE		
cooked	1 cup	21
fresh	1 cup	7
QUAIL		
cooked bone removed	1 (2.7 oz)	177
QUICHE		
Mrs. Smith's		
Pour-A-Quiche Bacon & Onion	1 serv (4.3 oz)	230
TAKE-OUT		
cheese pie	⅛ (9 in)	566
lorraine pie	⅛ (9 in)	568
mushroom	1 slice (3 oz)	256
spinach pie	⅛ (9 in)	342

FOOD	PORTION	CALS
QUINCE		
fresh	1	53
Matiz		
Quince Pasta	2 tbsp	83
QUINCE JUICE		
Smart Juice		
Organic 100% Juice	8 oz	110
QUINOA		
cooked	1 cup (6.5 oz)	222
quinoa not prep	¼ cup (1.5 oz)	156
Alti Plano Gold		
Natural	1 pkg	170
Ancient Harvest Quinoa		
Flakes not prep	¼ cup	159
Organic Inca Red not prep	¼ cup	163
Organic Traditional not prep	¼ cup	172
Simply Shari's		
Quinoa + Marinara Gluten Free as prep	¼ pkg (4 oz)	175
TruRoots		
Organic not prep	¼ cup (1.6 oz)	172
Village Harvest		
Whole Grain Medley Golden Quinoa	¾ cup (5 oz)	220
Whole Grain Medley Red Quinoa & Brown Rice	1 cup (5 oz)	300
RABBIT		
domestic w/o bone roasted	3 oz	167
wild w/o bone stewed	3 oz	147
RACCOON		
roasted	3 oz	217
RADICCHIO		
raw shredded	½ cup	5
RADISHES		
chinese dried	½ cup	157
chinese raw	1 (12 oz)	62
chinese raw sliced	½ cup	8
chinese sliced cooked	½ cup	13
daikon dried	½ cup	157
daikon raw	1 (12 oz)	62

FOOD	PORTION	CALS
daikon raw sliced	½ cup	8
daikon sliced cooked	½ cup	13
red raw	10	7
red sliced	½ cup	10
white icicle raw	1 (0.5 oz)	2
white icicle raw sliced	½ cup	7
Cadis		
Fresh	6 (2.6 oz)	12
TAKE-OUT		
korean kimchee	½ cup	31
moo namul saengche korean salad	1 serv (3.7 oz)	34

RAISINS

FOOD	PORTION	CALS
cinnamon coated	¼ cup	108
cooked	¼ cup	162
golden seedless	¼ cup	109
jumbo golden	¼ cup	130
milk chocolate coated	28 (1 oz)	109
milk chocolate coated	¼ cup	176
seedless	55 (1 oz)	86
sultanas	1 oz	88
Amazin' Raisin		
All Flavors	1 pkg (1 oz)	84
Bob's Red Mill		
Unsulfured	⅓ cup	130
Dole		
Golden Seedless	¼ cup (1.4 oz)	120
Earthbound Farms		
Organic Jumbo Flame Seedless	¼ cup	120
Emily's		
Milk Chocolate Covered	29 (1.4 oz)	180
Fool		
Cinnamon Raisin Spread	1 tbsp	20
Godiva		
Milk Chocolate Covered	1 pkg (1.2 oz)	150
Revolution Foods		
Organic	1 pkg (1.2 oz)	100
Sun-Maid		
Chocolate Covered	30 (1.4 oz)	170
Golden	¼ cup (1.4 oz)	130
Jumbo	¼ cup (1.4 oz)	130

FOOD	PORTION	CALS
Seedless	¼ cup (1.4 oz)	130
Snack Box	1 (1 oz)	90

RAMBUTAN
canned in syrup	1 (0.3 oz)	7
canned in syrup	1 cup (4.3 oz)	123
puerto rican fresh	5 (1.6 oz)	34
Polar		
In Syrup	½ cup	68

RASPBERRIES
black fresh	1 cup	70
canned in heavy syrup	½ cup	116
canned water pack	1 cup	43
fresh	1 pt	162
fresh	1 cup	64
frzn sweetened	1 cup	129
frzn unsweetened	1 cup	65
C&W		
Ultimate Red	¾ cup	70
Cascadian Farm		
Organic frzn	1¼ cup	60
Dole		
Fresh	1 cup (4.3 oz)	60
Raspberries frzn	1 cup (4.9 oz)	70
Oregon		
In Heavy Syrup	½ cup	120
Stoneridge Orchards		
Dried Whole	⅓ cup (1.4 oz)	130

RASPBERRY JUICE
Izze		
Esque Sparkling Black Raspberry	1 bottle (12 oz)	50
Old Orchard		
100% Juice	8 oz	130

RED BEANS
Allens		
Red Beans	½ cup	100

RELISH
hamburger	1 tbsp	19
hamburger	½ cup	158

FOOD	PORTION	CALS
hot dog	1 tbsp	14
hot dog	½ cup	111
piccalilli	1.4 oz	13
sweet	½ cup	159
sweet	1 tbsp	19
tomato	¼ cup (2.8 oz)	119
Cascadian Farm		
Organic Sweet Relish	1 tbsp (0.5 oz)	15
Claussen		
Sweet Pickle	1 tbsp (0.5 oz)	15
Gedney		
Hot Dog	1 tbsp	18
Organic Sweet	1 tbsp	15
Jake & Amos		
Chow Chow Sweet & Sour	1 serv (4 oz)	140
Corn	2 tbsp	40
Green Tomato	1 serv (1 oz)	25
Patak's		
Brinjal Eggplant Sweet Spicy	1 tbsp	70
Garlic	1 tbsp	45
Lime Mild	1 tbsp	30
Mango Mild	1 tbsp	40
Peloponnese		
Sun Dried Tomato	1 tbsp	25
Texas Sassy		
Pickle Relish	1 tbsp (0.5 oz)	30
Tree Of Life		
Organic Sweet Pickle	1 tbsp (0.5 oz)	15
RENNIN		
tablet	1 (0.9 g)	1
RHUBARB		
fresh	½ cup	13
frzn	½ cup	60
frzn as prep w/ sugar	½ cup	139
RICE (see also RICE CAKES, WILD RICE)		
arborio	½ cup	100
brown long grain cooked	1 cup (6.8 oz)	216
brown medium grain cooked	1 cup (6.8 oz)	218
glutinous cooked	1 cup (6.1 oz)	169

FOOD	PORTION	CALS
starch	1 oz	98
white long grain cooked	1 cup (5.5 oz)	205
white long grain instant cooked	1 cup (5.8 oz)	162
white medium grain cooked	1 cup (6.5 oz)	242
white short grain cooked	1 cup (6.5 oz)	242
Amy's		
Bowls Brown Rice Black-Eyed Peas & Veggies	1 pkg (8.9 oz)	290
Bowls Brown Rice & Vegetables	1 pkg (9.9 oz)	260
Arrowhead Mills		
Organic Brown Basmati not prep	¼ cup	140
Organic Long Grain Brown not prep	¼ cup	160
Betty Crocker		
Bowl Appetit! Teriyaki Rice	1 bowl (2.5 oz)	260
Birds Eye		
Steamfresh Whole Grain Brown Rice as prep	1 cup (4.8 oz)	150
Carolina		
White Medium Grain as prep	1 cup	160
Country Crock		
Cheddar Broccoli Rice	1 cup (7 oz)	270
Gourmet House		
Indian Basmati as prep	¾ cup	160
Italian Arborio as prep	¾ cup	160
Organic Brown as prep	¾ pkg	150
Organic White as prep	¾ cup	150
Goya		
Yellow Rice not prep	¼ cup (1.6 oz)	160
Green Giant		
Rice Pilaf	1 pkg (9.9 oz)	200
White & Wild & Green Beans	1 pkg (9.9 oz)	260
Knorr		
Asian Side Dish Chicken Fried Rice as prep	1 cup	240
Rice Sides Rice Medley as prep	1 cup	250
Rice Sides Sesame Chicken w/ Whole Grains as prep	⅔ cup	300
Lundberg		
Eco-Farmed Black Japonica not prep	¼ cup	170
Eco-Farmed California Brown Basmati not prep	¼ cup	160
Eco-Farmed White California Arborio not prep	¼ cup	160
Organic Brown Golden Rose not prep	¼ cup	160

FOOD	PORTION	CALS
Organic Rice Sensations Ginger Miso not prep	½ cup	116
Organic Risotto Porcini Mushroom not prep	½ cup	143
Organic White Sushi Rice not prep	¼ cup	150
Organic Wild Blend not prep	¼ cup	150
RiceXpress Chicken Herb	½ pkg (4.4 oz)	250
RiceXpress Santa Fe Grill	½ pkg (4.4 oz)	260
Risotto Butternut Squash not prep	½ cup	143
Mahatma		
Jasmine as prep	¾ cup	160
White as prep	¾ cup	150
Whole Grain Brown as prep	¾ cup	150
Marrakesh Express		
Pilaf Tomato & Basil as prep	1 cup	190
Risotto Parmesan as prep	1 cup	200
Minute		
Brown as prep	⅔ cup	150
Ready To Serve Brown & Wild Rice	1 pkg (4.4 oz)	230
Ready To Serve Pilaf	1 pkg (4.4 oz)	220
Ready To Serve Spanish Rice	1 pkg (4.4 oz)	230
Ready To Serve Whole Grain Brown	1 pkg (4.4 oz)	230
Steamers Broccoli & Cheese	1 cup (6.4 oz)	200
Steamers Fried Rice	1 cup (6.5 oz)	280
White as prep	1 cup	200
Near East		
Long Grain & Wild Original as prep	1 cup	220
Pilaf Curry as prep	1 cup	220
Pilaf Original as prep	1 cup	220
Pilaf Sesame Ginger as prep	1 cup	270
Pilaf Spanish Rice as prep	1 cup	310
Whole Grains Brown Rice as prep	1 cup	210
Patak's		
Basmati	1 pkg	430
Coconut	1 pkg	500
Yellow	1 pkg	440
Rice A Roni		
Beef as prep	1 cup	310
Chicken as prep	1 cup	310
Express Asian Fried	1 cup	280
Fried Rice as prep	1 cup	320
Garden Vegetable as prep	1 cup	270

FOOD	PORTION	CALS
Long Grain & Wild as prep	1 cup	250
Lower Sodium Chicken as prep	1 cup	270
Parmesan Chicken as prep	1 cup	370
Red Beans & Rice as prep	1 cup	290
Savory Whole Grain Blends Spanish as prep	1 cup	250
Spanish as prep	1 cup	260
River Rice		
Brown as prep	¾ cup	150
Stahlbush Island Farms		
Organic Brown Rice & Black Beans frzn	1 cup (6.2 oz)	200
Success		
Boil-In-Bag Jasmine as prep	¾ cup	150
Boil-In-Bag White as prep	1 cup	190
Ready To Serve Brown	1 cup	170
TastyBite		
Pilaf Multigrain	½ pkg (5 oz)	200
Pilaf Tandoori	½ pkg (5 oz)	183
Thai Kitchen		
Jasmine not prep	2 tbsp (1.5 oz)	160
Uncle Ben's		
Boil-In-Bag Whole Grain Brown Rice	1 cup	170
Long Grain & Wild Herb Roasted Chicken as prep	1 cup	190
Long Grain & Wild Sun-Dried Tomato Florentine as prep	1 cup	180
Ready Rice Spanish	1 cup (5 oz)	200
Ready Rice Whole Grain Medley	1 cup (5 oz)	210
Ready Rice Whole Grain Medley Roasted Garlic	1 cup (4.9 oz)	200
Whole Grain White Broccoli Cheddar as prep	1 cup	200
Whole Grain White Creamy Chicken as prep	1 cup	200
Whole Grain White Garden Vegetable as prep	1 cup	180
Whole Grain White Long Grain as prep	1 cup	170
Whole Grain White Sweet Tomato as prep	1 cup	210
Whole Grain White Taco as prep	1 cup	160
Village Harvest		
Whole Grain Creations w/ Corn & Black Beans	¾ cup (4.3 oz)	140
Whole Grain Medley Brown Red & Wild Rice frzn	1 cup (5 oz)	250
Water Maid		
Medium Grain as prep	¾ cup	160

FOOD	PORTION	CALS
Zatarain's		
Black Eyed Peas & Rice as prep	1 cup	220
Caribbean Rice Mix as prep	1 cup	160
Cheddar Broccoli as prep	1 cup	220
Yellow as prep	1 cup	190
TAKE-OUT		
coconut rice	1 serv	500
congee	½ cup (4.1 oz)	44
dirty rice w/ chicken giblets	1 cup (6.9 oz)	291
nasi goreng indonesian rice & vegetables	1 cup (4.9 oz)	130
pea palau rice & peas fried in ghee	1 serv	144
pilaf	½ cup	84
rice & black beans	1 cup (5.1 oz)	220
risotto	1 serv (6.6 oz)	426
spanish	¾ cup	363

RICE CAKES
Hain		
Mini Munchies Apple Cinnamon	9 (0.5 oz)	60
Lundberg		
Eco-Farmed Apple Cinnamon	1 (0.7 oz)	80
Eco-Farmed Brown Rice Salt Free	1 (0.7 oz)	70
Eco-Farmed Toasted Sesame	1 (0.7 oz)	70
Organic Caramel Corn	1 (0.7 oz)	80
Organic Green Tea w/ Lemon	1 (0.7 oz)	80
Organic Mochi Sweet	1 (0.7 oz)	70
Mother's		
Caramel	1 (0.5 oz)	45
Plain Salted	1 (0.3 oz)	35
Plain Unsalted	1 (0.3 oz)	35
Salted Butter	1 (0.3 oz)	35
Quaker		
Mini Delights Chocolatey Drizzle	1 pkg (0.7 oz)	90
Riceworks		
Sweet Chili	10 (1 oz)	140
Wasabi	10 (1 oz)	140

ROCKFISH
pacific cooked	1 fillet (5.2 oz)	180
pacific cooked	3 oz	103
pacific raw	3 oz	80

FOOD	PORTION	CALS
ROE (*see also* INDIVIDUAL FISH NAMES)		
fresh baked	1 oz	58
ROLL		
FROZEN		
Joy Of Cooking		
Ciabatta Olive Oil Rosemary	1 (1.7 oz)	120
French Baguettes Mini	1 (1.6 oz)	100
Pillsbury		
Dinner Rolls Crusty French	1 (1.2 oz)	90
Dinner Rolls Crusty Sourdough	1 (1.2 oz)	90
Dinner Rolls Whole Wheat	1 (1.2 oz)	90
READY-TO-EAT		
bialy	1 (2.2 oz)	138
brioche sweet roll	1 (3.5 oz)	410
cheese	1 (2.3 oz)	238
cinnamon raisin	1 (2.1 oz)	223
dinner	1 (1 oz)	78
egg	1 (1.2 oz)	107
french	1 (1.3 oz)	105
garlic	1 (1.5 oz)	133
hamburger or hot dog	1 (1.5 oz)	120
hamburger or hot dog multi grain	1 (1.5 oz)	113
hamburger or hot dog reduced calorie	1 (1.5 oz)	84
hamburger or hot dog whole wheat	1 (1.5 oz)	114
hard	1 (2 oz)	167
hoagie or submarine roll whole wheat	1 (4.7 oz)	359
hot cross bun	1	202
mexican bolillo	1 (4.1 oz)	305
oat bran	1 (1.2 oz)	78
oatmeal	1 (1.3 oz)	103
pumpernickel	1 (1.3 oz)	100
rye	1 med (1.3 oz)	103
sourdough	1 (1.6 oz)	130
wheat	1 (1 oz)	76
whole wheat	1 med (1.3 oz)	96
Arnold		
Whole Grains Sandwich 100% Whole Wheat	1 (2.2 oz)	160
Calise		
Kaiser 100% Whole Wheat	1 (2.5 oz)	190

FOOD	PORTION	CALS
Ecce Panis		
Focaccia	1 (3.2 oz)	260
French Meadow Bakery		
Gluten Free Italian	1 (4.4 oz)	340
J.J. Cassone		
Sandwich	1 (2.5 oz)	190
Mrs Baird's		
Home Bake	1 (1 oz)	80
Natural Ovens		
Better Wheat Buns	1 (2.2 oz)	170
Nature's Own		
100% Whole Grain Sugar Free	1 (1.9 oz)	110
Butter Buns	1 (1.7 oz)	120
Pepperidge Farm		
Deli Flats Soft 100% Whole Wheat	1 (1.5 oz)	100
Hamburger 100% Whole Wheat	1 (1.5 oz)	120
Hoagie Soft w/ Sesame Seeds	1	210
Hot & Crusty Sourdough	1	100
Hot Dog	1	140
Hot Dog Whole Grain White	1	110
Parker House Dinner	1	80
Premium Wheat	1	220
Sandwich Buns Sesame Seeds	1 (1.6 oz)	130
Rudi's Organic Bakery		
100% Whole Wheat	1 (2.3 oz)	160
Hot Dog Spelt	1 (2 oz)	140
Hot Dog Wheat	1 (2 oz)	150
Hot Dog White	1 (2 oz)	150
S. Rosen's		
Brat & Sausage Rolls	1 (2.1 oz)	160
Klassic Kaiser	1 (2.6 oz)	230
Stroehmann		
Hot Dog Wheat	1 (1.8 oz)	140
Udi's		
Gluten Free Cinnamon	1 (3 oz)	260
Weight Watchers		
Sandwich Wheat	1 (2 oz)	140
REFRIGERATED		
crescent	1 (1 oz)	78

FOOD	PORTION	CALS
Pillsbury		
Crescent Big & Buttery	1 (1.7 oz)	170
Crescent Butter Flake	1 (1 oz)	110
Crescent Original	1 (1 oz)	110
Crescent Reduced Fat	1 (1 oz)	90
ROSE APPLE		
fresh	3.5 oz	32
ROSE HIP		
fresh	1 oz	26
ROSELLE		
fresh	1 cup	28
ROSEMARY		
dried	1 tsp	4
fresh	1 tbsp	1
ROUGHY		
orange baked	3 oz	75
RUBS (see HERBS/SPICES)		
RUTABAGA		
cooked mashed	1 cup	94
cubed cooked	1 cup	66
Glory		
Cut Fresh	1 cup	50
Sunshine		
Diced	½ cup	30
SABLEFISH		
baked	3 oz	213
fillet baked	5.3 oz	378
smoked	3 oz	218
smoked	1 oz	72
SAFFLOWER		
seeds dried	1 oz	147
SAFFRON		
dried	1 tsp	2

FOOD	PORTION	CALS
SAGE		
ground	1 tsp	2
SALAD (see also SALAD TOPPINGS)		
Dole		
American Blend	1½ cups (3 oz)	15
Butter Bliss	1½ cups (3 oz)	15
European Blend	1½ cups (3 oz)	15
Field Greens	1½ cups (3 oz)	20
Italian Blend	1½ cups (3 oz)	15
Kit Asian Island Crunch as prep	1½ cups (3.5 oz)	130
Seven Lettuces	1½ cups (3 oz)	20
Spring Mix	1½ cups (3 oz)	20
Very Veggie Blend	1½ cups (3 oz)	20
Earthbound Farms		
Organic Baby Arugula Salad	2 cups	20
Organic Baby Lettuce Salad	2 cups	15
Organic Baby Spinach Salad	2 cups	10
Organic Fresh Herb Salad	2 cups	15
Organic Mixed Baby Greens	2 cups	15
Fresh Express		
50/50 Mix	3 cups	10
Asian Supreme w/ Dressing as prep	2½ cups	170
Caesar Lite w/ Dressing as prep	2½ cups	100
Caesar w/ Dressing as prep	2½ cups	150
Fancy Field Greens Caribbean	3 cups	20
Gourmet Cafe Chicken as prep	1 pkg (3.5 oz)	120
Gourmet Cafe Chicken Caesar w/ Crostini as prep	1 pkg (3.5 oz)	150
Gourmet Cafe Chopped Turkey Chef as prep	1 pkg (3.5 oz)	120
Gourmet Cafe Orchard Harvest as prep	1 pkg (3.5 oz)	230
Gourmet Cafe Tuscan Pesto Chicken as prep	1 pkg (3.5 oz)	130
Gourmet Cafe Waldorf Chicken as prep	1 pkg (3.5 oz)	190
More Carrots American	1½ cups	15
Organic Italian	2½ cups	15
Original Iceberg Garden With Zip	1½ cups	15
Pacifica! Veggie Supreme w/ Dressing as prep	3 cups	220
Spring Mix	3 cups	15
Sweet Baby Greens	3 cups	10
Veggie Lover's	2 cups	20

FOOD	PORTION	CALS
Lifestyle Foods		
Asian w/ Chicken	1 pkg (8.9 oz)	340
Casear	1 pkg (5 oz)	210
Garden	1 pkg (6.6 oz)	180
Greek	1 pkg (6 oz)	130
Mann's		
Rainbow	1 serv (3 oz)	25
Ready Pac		
All American	2 cups (3 oz)	15
American Blue Cheese Mix as prep	1¾ cups (3.5 oz)	110
Baby Romaine Blend	4½ cups (3 oz)	20
Baby Spinach Mix as prep	2 cups (3.5 oz)	140
Chef	1 pkg (7.7 oz)	270
Cobb	1 pkg (7.2 oz)	300
Garden	2 cups (3 oz)	15
Grand Asian Mix as prep	1¼ cups (3.5 oz)	130
Spinach Bacon	1 pkg (4.7 oz)	240
Spring Mix	4½ cups	20
Spring Mix Spinach	5 cups (3 oz)	20
Veggie Medley	2 cups (3 oz)	15
TAKE-OUT		
7-layer salad	2 cups	557
caesar	4 cups	734
chef salad w/o dressing	3 cups	535
cobb w/ dressing	4 cups	645
greek w/ dressing	4 cups	424
mixed salad greens shredded	1 cup	9
somen w/ lettuce egg fish pork	2 cups	550
spinach w/o dressing	4 cups	429
tossed w/ avocado w/o dressing	2 cups	90
tossed w/ chicken w/o dressing	3 cups	194
tossed w/ egg w/o dressing	2 cups	93
tossed w/ shrimp w/o dressing	1½ cups (8.3 oz)	106
tossed w/ shrimp & egg w/o dressing	3 cups	185
tossed w/o dressing	2 cups	22
waldorf	1 cup	242
wilted lettuce w/ bacon dressing	1 cup	99

FOOD	PORTION	CALS

SALAD DRESSING (*see also* SALAD TOPPINGS)
MIX
Good Seasons

FOOD	PORTION	CALS
Italian as prep	2 tbsp	130
Italian not prep	⅛ pkg (3 g)	5
J&D's		
Bacon Ranch as prep	2 tbsp	120
READY-TO-EAT		
blue cheese	1 tbsp	77
french	1 tbsp	67
french reduced calorie	1 tbsp	22
italian	1 tbsp	69
italian reduced calorie	1 tbsp	16
japanese ginger salad dressing	2 tbsp	90
russian	1 tbsp	76
russian reduced calorie	1 tbsp	23
sesame seed	1 tbsp	68
thousand island	1 tbsp	59
thousand island reduced calorie	1 tbsp	24
Annie's Homegrown		
Cowgirl Ranch	2 tbsp (1 oz)	90
Tuscany Italian	2 tbsp (1 oz)	100
Vinaigrette Lite Gingerly	2 tbsp (1.1 oz)	40
Vinaigrette Lite Honey Mustard	1 tbsp (1.1 oz)	40
Vinaigrette Mango Fat Free	2 tbsp (1.1 oz)	20
Vinaigrette Roasted Red Pepper	2 tbsp (1.1 oz)	60
Bernstein's		
Chunky Blue Cheese	2 tbsp	120
Creamy Caesar	2 tbsp	120
Italian Restaurant Recipe	2 tbsp	120
Light Fantastic Roasted Garlic Balsamic	2 tbsp	45
Red Wine & Garlic Italian	2 tbsp	110
Bragg		
Ginger & Sesame	2 tbsp	150
Organic Vinaigrette	2 tbsp	150
Cains		
Caesar Creamy	2 tbsp	170
Caesar Fat Free	2 tbsp	30
Caesar Light	2 tbsp	70
Chianti Vinaigrette	2 tbsp	130

FOOD	PORTION	CALS
Creamy Dill Cucumber Fat Free	2 tbsp	35
French	2 tbsp	120
French Light	2 tbsp	80
Greek	2 tbsp	160
Italian Fat Free	2 tbsp	15
Ranch	2 tbsp	180
Ranch Light	2 tbsp	80
David's Unforgettables		
Balsamic Vinaigrette Low Fat	1 tbsp (0.5 oz)	40
Balsamic Vinaigrette Original	1 tbsp (0.5 oz)	70
Follow Your Heart		
Lemon Herb	2 tbsp (1 oz)	100
Sesame Miso	2 tbsp (1 oz)	64
Thousand Island	2 tbsp (1 oz)	80
Gotta Luv It		
Chipotle Lime	2 tbsp	110
Raspberry Balsamic Vinaigrette	2 tbsp	150
Sweet & Tangy Italian	2 tbsp	140
Jake & Amos		
Bacon	2 tbsp (1 oz)	90
Ken's		
Light Vinaigrette Balsamic	2 tbsp (1 oz)	60
Kraft		
Honey Dijon	2 tbsp	100
Italian Creamy	2 tbsp	100
Light Done Right Caesar	2 tbsp	60
Light Done Right Red Wine Vinaigrette	2 tbsp	45
Ranch Garlic	2 tbsp	120
Special Collection Classic Italian Vinaigrette	2 tbsp	60
Special Collection Parmesan Romano	2 tbsp	140
Special Collection Tangy Tomato Bacon	2 tbsp	100
Thousand Island w/ Bacon	2 tbsp	100
LiteHouse		
Bleu Cheese Bacon	2 tbsp	150
Organic Vinaigrette Raspberry Lime	2 tbsp	40
Ranch Homestyle	2 tbsp	120
Ranch Lite	2 tbsp	70
Sesame Ginger	2 tbsp	35
Spinach Salad	2 tbsp	50
Vinaigrette Huckleberry	2 tbsp	20
Vinaigrette Lite Honey Dijon	2 tbsp	130

FOOD	PORTION	CALS
Lucini		
Delicate Cucumber & Shallots	2 tbsp (1 oz)	120
Fig & Walnut Savory Balsamic	2 tbsp (1 oz)	110
Roasted Hazelnut & Extra Virgin Olive Oil	2 tbsp (1 oz)	120
Maple Grove Farms		
Asiago & Garlic	2 tbsp (1 oz)	40
Caesar Lite	2 tbsp (1 oz)	50
Cranberry Balsamic Fat Free	2 tbsp (1 oz)	30
Creamy Ranch Sugar Free	2 tbsp (1 oz)	100
Honey Dijon Fat Free	2 tbsp (1 oz)	35
Poppyseed Fat Free	2 tbsp (1 oz)	35
Sesame Ginger	2 tbsp (1 oz)	45
Strawberry Balsamic	1 tbsp (1 oz)	30
Sweet'n Sour	2 tbsp (1 oz)	90
Vidalia Onion Fat Free	2 tbsp (1 oz)	20
Vinaigrette Balsamic Sugar Free	2 tbsp (1 oz)	5
Vinaigrette Champagne	2 tbsp (1 oz)	100
Marie's		
Blue Cheese Lite Chunky	2 tbsp	80
Blue Cheese Vinaigrette	2 tbsp	120
Caesar	2 tbsp	170
Coleslaw	2 tbsp	120
Creamy Ranch	2 tbsp	170
Red Wine Vinaigrette	2 tbsp	60
Sesame Ginger	2 tbsp	70
Naturally Fresh		
Balsamic Vinaigrette	2 tbsp	10
Bleu Cheese	2 tbsp	170
Bleu Cheese Bacon	2 tbsp	170
Bleu Cheese Lite	2 tbsp	100
Buffalo Ranch	2 tbsp	110
Classic Oriental	2 tbsp	100
Ginger	2 tbsp	70
Greek Feta	2 tbsp	100
Honey French	2 tbsp	100
Honey Mustard	2 tbsp	140
Orange Miso	2 tbsp	100
Ranch Classic	2 tbsp	150
Ranch Lite	2 tbsp	80
Slaw	2 tbsp	90

FOOD	PORTION	CALS
Newman's Own		
Lighten Up Light Balsamic Vinaigrette	2 tbsp (1 oz)	45
OrganicVille		
Herbs De Provence	2 tbsp (1 oz)	100
Miso Ginger	2 tbsp (1 oz)	100
Orange Cranberry	2 tbsp (1 oz)	100
Pomegranate	2 tbsp (1 oz)	100
Ranch Non Dairy	2 tbsp (1 oz)	90
Sesame Goddess	2 tbsp (1 oz)	130
Petrini's		
Italian Original	2 tbsp (1 oz)	106
Italian Ranch	2 tbsp (1 oz)	140
School House Kitchen		
Balsamic Vinaigrette Basico	2 tbsp	160
Soy Vay		
Cha-Cha Chinese Chicken	3 tbsp	190
Texas Sassy		
Vinaigrette	2 tbsp (1 oz)	80
Three Acre Kitchen		
Balsamic Vinaigrette	2 tbsp (1.1 oz)	130
Vino De Milo		
Gorgonzola Pear Riesling	2 tbsp	80
Pomegranate Port	2 tbsp	90
Walden Farms		
Sesame Ginger Calorie Free	2 tbsp (1 oz)	0
Wild Thymes Farm		
Salad Refreshers Black Currant	1 tbsp	36
Salad Refreshers Meyer Lemon	1 tbsp	35
Salad Refreshers Morello Cherry	1 tbsp	34
Salad Refreshers Pomegranate	1 tbsp	33
Vinaigrette Mandarin Orange Basil	1 tbsp	43
Vinaigrette Raspberry Pear	1 tbsp	43
Vinaigrette Roasted Apple Shallot	1 tbsp	42
Vinaigrette Toasted Sesame Wasabi	1 tbsp	42
Wishbone		
Bountifuls Berry Delight	2 tbsp	35
Bountifuls Tuscan Romano Basil	2 tbsp	25
Western	2 tbsp (1 oz)	160
Western Fat Free	2 tbsp (1 oz)	50
Western Light Just 2 Good	2 tbsp (1 oz)	70

FOOD	PORTION	CALS
TAKE-OUT		
vinegar & oil	1 tbsp	72
SALAD TOPPINGS		
Fresh Gourmet		
Crispy Onions Garlic Pepper	1½ tbsp	35
Tortilla Strips Lightly Salted	2 tbsp	35
Wonton Strips Wasabi Ranch	2 tbsp	35
McCormick		
Salad Toppins	1.3 tbsp (7 g)	35
Salad Toppins Garden Vegetable	1.3 tbsp (7 g)	35
Naturally Fresh		
Fruit & Nut Mix	½ tbsp	45
Glazed Almond & Pecan Pieces	½ tbsp	40
SALBA		
Salba Smart		
Ground	2 tbsp	65
Whole Grain	1 tbsp	65
SALMON		
CANNED		
w/ bone	½ cup	106
Chicken Of The Sea		
Pink	¼ cup (2.2 oz)	90
Pink Skinless & Boneless	⅓ pkg (2 oz)	60
Pink Smoked Pacific	1 pkg (3 oz)	120
Red	¼ cup	110
Polar		
Pink	¼ cup	90
Sockeye Red	¼ cup	110
Tonnino		
Wild Sockeye In Olive Oil	2 oz	220
Wild Planet		
Salmon Wild Alaskan Pink	2 oz	65
Salmon Wild Alaskan Sockeye	2 oz	85
FRESH		
atlantic farmed baked	4 oz	233
coho wild poached	4 oz	209
pink baked	4 oz	169
roe raw	1 oz	59
sockeye baked	4 oz	245

FOOD	PORTION	CALS
FROZEN		
Gorton's		
Fillets Classic Grilled	1 (3 oz)	100
SeaPak		
Burgers	1 (3.2 oz)	110
Herb Butter Fillet	1 (5 oz)	350
SMOKED		
lox	1 oz	33
Kasilof Fish Co.		
Wild Alaska Fillet	1 pkg (2 oz)	90
TAKE-OUT		
guisado salmon stew	1 serv (7.4 oz)	320
roulette w/ spinach stuffing	1 serv (4 oz)	160
salmon cake	1 (4.2 oz)	264
salmon loaf	1 slice (3.7 oz)	206
SALSA		
black bean & corn	2 tbsp	15
citrus	2 tbsp (1 oz)	10
peach	2 tbsp	15
tomatoless corn & chile	2 tbsp	45
Amy's		
Organic Black Bean & Corn	2 tbsp (1 oz)	15
Organic Medium	2 tbsp (1 oz)	10
Bone Suckin'		
Fat Free Gluten Free	2 tbsp	40
Chi-Chi's		
Fiesta Mild	2 tbsp	10
Chukar Cherries		
Peach Cherry	1 tbsp	13
Clint's		
Texas Medium	2 tbsp (1 oz)	5
Dave's Gourmet		
Insanity	2 tbsp (1 oz)	15
Dei Fratelli		
Casera Mild	2 tbsp (1.1 oz)	5
DelGrosso		
Chunky Hot	2 tbsp (1.1 oz)	10
Chunky Mild	2 tbsp (1.1 oz)	10
Emerald Valley		
Organic Fiesta	1 tbsp (1 oz)	20

FOOD	PORTION	CALS
Organic Green	2 tbsp (1 oz)	10
Frontera		
Chipotle Hot	2 tbsp (1 oz)	10
Corn & Poblano Medium	2 tbsp (1 oz)	10
Guajillo Medium	2 tbsp (1 oz)	10
Spanish Olive Mild	2 tbsp (1 oz)	10
Jake & Amos		
Black Bean	2 tbsp (1 oz)	15
Peach	2 tbsp (1 oz)	20
Jala-Fresca		
Green Stuff Medium	2 tbsp	10
Margaritaville		
Medium	2 tbsp	10
Peppadew Chipotle Garlic	1 oz	10
Peppadew Mild	1 oz	10
Muir Glen		
Organic Medium	2 tbsp	10
Number 9		
Black Bean & Corn	2 tbsp (1.1 oz)	20
Hot	2 tbsp (1.1 oz)	15
Mild	2 tbsp (1.1 oz)	15
OrganicVille		
Mild	2 tbsp (1 oz)	15
Pineapple	2 tbsp (1 oz)	15
Pace		
Black Bean & Corn	2 tbsp	25
Organic Picante	2 tbsp	10
Thick & Chunky	2 tbsp	10
Ready Pac		
Pico De Gallo	2 tbsp (1 oz)	5
Robert Rothchild Farm		
Tomatillo & Pepper	2 tbsp	20
Salba Smart		
Organic Omega-3 Enriched	2 tbsp	12
Snyder's Of Hanover		
Sweet	2 tbsp	20
Tostitos		
All Natural Chunky Mild	2 tbsp (1.2 oz)	10
Con Queso	2 tbsp	40
Utz		
Sweet	2 tbsp	10

FOOD	PORTION	CALS
Walnut Acres		
Organic Fiesta Cilantro	2 tbsp	10
Organic Sweet Southwestern Peach	2 tbsp	20
SALSIFY		
fresh sliced cooked	½ cup	46
SALT SUBSTITUTES		
gomasio sesame salt	2 tsp	34
AlsoSalt		
Butter Flavored	¼ tsp	1
Garlic Flavored	¼ tsp	1
Original	¼ tsp	1
French's		
No Salt	¼ cup	0
Nu-Salt		
Salt Substitute	1 pkg (1 g)	0
SALT/SEASONED SALT		
kosher	¼ tsp	0
salt	1 dash (0.4 g)	0
salt	1 tsp (6 g)	0
salt	1 tbsp (0.6 oz)	0
sea salt coarse	1 tsp	0
sea salt fine	¼ tsp	0
BaconSalt		
Original	¼ tsp (1 g)	0
Peppered	¼ tsp (1 g)	0
Bob's Red Mill		
Garlic Salt Blend	¼ tsp	0
Sea Salt	¼ tsp	0
David's		
Kosher Salt	¼ tsp (1.5 g)	0
Falksalt		
Flake Salt All Flavors	¼ tsp (1.5 g)	0
Lawry's		
Original Seasoned Salt	¼ tsp	0
Maine Coast		
Sea Salt w/ Sea Veg	¼ tsp	0
McCormick		
Grinder Garlic Sea Salt	¼ tsp	0
Grinder Sea Salt	¼ tsp	0

FOOD	PORTION	CALS
Morton		
Iodized	¼ tsp	0
NutraSalt		
African Medley	1 serv (1g)	0
Sea Salt	1 serv (1g)	0
Seasoned Salt	1 serv (1g)	0
Ocean's Flavor		
Natural Sea Salt	¼ tsp	0
Spice Hunter		
Celery Salt	¼ tsp	0
Garlic Salt	¼ tsp	0

SANDWICHES
Alexia
FOOD	PORTION	CALS
Panini Tuscan Four Cheese w/ Roasted Tomato & Basil	1 pkg (6 oz)	380
Panini Tuscan Grilled Chicken w/ Mozzarella	1 pkg (6 oz)	400
Panini Tuscan Grilled Steak w/ Mushrooms & Onions	1 pkg (6 oz)	370
Panini Tuscan Smoked Chicken w/ Fire Roasted Vegetables & Parmesan	1 pkg (6 oz)	410
Amy's		
Pocket Sandwich Tofu Scramble	1 (4 oz)	180
Pocket Sandwich Vegetable Pie	1 (5 oz)	300
Wrap Indian Somosa	1 (5 oz)	250
Aunt Jemima		
Biscuit Sausage Egg & Cheese	1 (4 oz)	340
Griddlecake Sausage Egg & Cheese	1 (4.4 oz)	350
Sausage Egg & Cheese On French Toast	1 (4.7 oz)	310
Aunt Trudy's		
Fillo Pocket Cheese & Tomato	1 (5 oz)	320
Fillo Pocket Classic Samosa	1 (5 oz)	280
Fillo Pocket Mediterranean Olive & Veggies	1 (5 oz)	270
Organic Fillo Pocket Roasted Sweet Potato	1 (5 oz)	310
Cedarlane		
Wrap Low Fat Couscous & Vegetable Veggie	1 (6 oz)	220
DiGiorno		
Flatbread Melts Chicken Parmesan	1 (6 oz)	380
Farm Rich		
Philly Cheese Steak	2 (3 oz)	220
Sandwich Melts	2 (4.2 oz)	290

FOOD	PORTION	CALS
Gardenburger		
Wrap Black Bean Chipotle	1 (4.7 oz)	240
Wrap Pizza 100% Meatless Margherita	1 (4.7 oz)	240
Guiltless Gourmet		
Wrap Black Bean Chipotle	1 (5.7 oz)	270
Wrap California Veggie	1 (5.7 oz)	300
Wrap Mediterranean Spinach	1 (5.7 oz)	270
Hot Pockets		
Bacon Egg & Cheese	1 (2.2 oz)	160
Barbecue Beef	1 (4.5 oz)	310
Biscuit Sausage Egg & Cheese	1 (4.5 oz)	270
Calzone Four Meat & Four Cheese	½ (4.2 oz)	300
Calzone Pepperoni & Three Cheese	½ (4.2 oz)	330
Chicken Melt	1 (4.5 oz)	300
Croissant Chicken Parmesan	1 (4.5 oz)	340
Croissant Turkey Bacon Club	1 (4.5 oz)	320
Ham & Cheese	1 (4.5 oz)	290
Meatballs & Mozzarella	1 (4.5 oz)	300
Philly Steak & Cheese	1 (4.5 oz)	270
Steak Fajita	1 (4.5 oz)	280
Turkey & Ham w/ Cheese	1 (4 .5 oz)	280
Jimmy Dean		
Bagel Sausage Egg & Cheese	1 (4.8 oz)	380
Biscuit Sausage Egg & Cheese	1 (4.5 oz)	440
Croissant Sausage Egg & Cheese	1 (4.5 oz)	430
D-Lights Croissants Turkey Sausage Egg White & Cheese	1 (4.8 oz)	300
D-Lights Honey Wheat Muffin Canadian Bacon Egg White & Cheese	1 (4.5 oz)	230
Muffin Sausage Egg & Cheese	1 (4.6 oz)	350
Lean Cuisine		
Casual Cuisine Panini Chicken Club	1 pkg (6 oz)	360
Casual Cuisine Panini Spinach Artichoke Chicken	1 pkg (6 oz)	320
Casual Cuisine Panini Steak Cheddar & Mushroom	1 pkg (6 oz)	340
Lean Pockets		
Bacon Egg & Cheese	1 (2.2 oz)	150
Barbecue Beef	1 (4.5 oz)	290
Chicken Cheddar & Broccoli	1 (4.5 oz)	260

FOOD	PORTION	CALS
Chicken Fajita	1 (4.5 oz)	240
Chicken Parmesan	1 (4.5 oz)	290
Ham & Cheese	1 (4.5 oz)	270
Meatballs & Mozzarella	1 (4.5 oz)	260
Philly Steak & Cheese	1 (4.5 oz)	270
Sausage Egg & Cheese	1 (2.2 oz)	140
Steak Fajita	1 (4.5 oz)	250
Three Cheese & Chicken Quesadilla	1 (4.5 oz)	260
Turkey & Ham w/ Cheddar	1 (4.5 oz)	280
Turkey Broccoli & Cheese	1 (4.5 oz)	270
Lunchables		
Cracker Stackers Bologna & American	1 pkg	390
Cracker Stackers Ham & Cheddar	1 pkg	410
Sub Sandwich Ham & American	1 pkg	240
Sub Sandwich Turkey & Cheddar	1 pkg	230
Mom Made		
Munchie Turkey Sausage	1 (2.5 oz)	220
Munchies Chicken	1 (2.5 oz)	220
Oscar Mayer		
Deli Creations Honey Ham & Swiss	1 pkg (6.8 oz)	440
Deli Creations Steakhouse Cheddar	1 pkg (7.1 oz)	450
Deli Creations Turkey & Cheddar Dijon	1 pkg (6.7 oz)	430
PBJammerz		
Peanut Butter & Jelly All Flavors	1 (2 oz)	220
Pillsbury		
Toaster Scrambles Cheese Egg & Bacon	1 (1.6 oz)	180
Toaster Scrambles Cheese Egg & Sausage	1 (1.6 oz)	180
Smucker's		
Uncrustables Peanut Butter & Grape Jelly On Whole Wheat	1 (2 oz)	210
Uncrustables Peanut Butter & Strawberry Jam	1 (2 oz)	210
Uncrustables Peanut Butter On Wheat Bread	1 (2 oz)	210
Stouffer's		
Corner Bistro Panini Philly Style Steak & Cheese	1 pkg (6 oz)	340
Corner Bistro Panini Southwestern Chicken	1 pkg (6 oz)	360
The Fillo Factory		
Organic Fillo Pocket Asian Vegetable	1 (5 oz)	240

FOOD	PORTION	CALS
Van's		
Breakfast In A Pocket Sandwich Ham Egg & Cheese	1 (4.5 oz)	370
Breakfast In A Pocket Sandwich Veggie Egg & Cheese	1 (4.5 oz)	340
Breakfast Panini Huevos Rancheros	1 (4.5 oz)	270
Breakfast Panini Sausage Egg & Cheese	1 (4.5 oz)	290
TAKE-OUT		
bacon & egg	1 (6.2 oz)	388
bacon lettuce & tomato w/ mayo	1 (5.8 oz)	344
beef barbecue w/ bun	1 (6.7 oz)	417
calzone beef & cheese	1 (14 oz)	1476
calzone cheese	1 (15 oz)	1632
chicken fillet	1 (6.4 oz)	515
chicken fillet w/ cheese	1 (8 oz)	632
chicken salad	1 (5 oz)	333
crab cake w/ bun	1	308
crispy chicken fillet w/ lettuce tomato & mayo	1 (7.7 oz)	537
croque monsieur	1 (12.4 oz)	765
egg salad	1 (5.6 oz)	485
french dip w/ roll	1 (6.8 oz)	357
fried egg	1 (3.4 oz)	226
grilled cheese	1 (2.9 oz)	290
gyro	1 (13.7 oz)	593
ham & egg	1 (4.4 oz)	272
ham w/ cheese lettuce & mayo	1 (5.4 oz)	369
hot turkey w/ gravy	1	389
peanut butter	1 (3.3 oz)	342
peanut butter & banana	1	617
peanut butter & jelly	1 (3.3 oz)	327
reuben w/ sauerkraut & cheese	1 (6.4 oz)	463
roast beef w/ gravy	1 (7.8 oz)	386
sloppy joe pork on bun	1 (6.5 oz)	318
tuna melt	1 (5.3 oz)	350
tuna salad w/ lettuce	1 (5.9 oz)	289
turkey w/ mayo	1 (5 oz)	329

SAPODILLA

fresh	1	140
fresh cut up	1 cup	199

FOOD	PORTION	CALS
SAPOTES		
fresh	1	301
SARDINES		
CANNED		
atlantic in oil w/ bone	1 can (3.2 oz)	192
atlantic in oil w/ bone	2	50
pacific in tomato sauce w/ bone	1 can (13 oz)	658
pacific in tomato sauce w/ bone	1 (1.3 oz)	68
Chicken Of The Sea		
In Hot Sauce	1 can (3.75 oz)	120
In Oil Lightly Smoked	1 can (3.75 oz)	150
In Tomato Sauce	1 can (3.75 oz)	90
In Water	1 can (3.75 oz)	90
King Oscar		
In Extra Virgin Olive Oil	1 can (3.75 oz)	150
Skinless Boneless In Soya Oil	3 pieces (1.9 oz)	120
Matiz		
In Olive Oil	½ pkg (2 oz)	120
Polar		
In Mustard	1 can (4.5 oz)	170
In Tomato Sauce	1 can (4.5 oz)	120
In Water	1 can (3 oz)	100
Wild Planet		
Sardines Wild In Extra Virgin Olive Oil	2 oz	110
Sardines Wild In Marinara Sauce	2 oz	60
Sardines Wild In Oil w/ Lemon	2 oz	110
Sardines Wild In Spring Water	2 oz	73
FRESH		
raw	3.5 oz	135
SAUCE (see also BARBECUE SAUCE, CURRY, GRAVY, SPAGHETTI SAUCE)		
adobo fresco	2 tbsp	81
bearnaise	1 oz	177
cheese mix as prep w/ milk	1 cup	307
enchilada sauce green	¼ cup	46
enchilada sauce red	¼ cup	79
fish sauce chinese	1 tbsp	9
fish sauce vietnamese nuoc mam	1 tbsp	6
hoisin	1 tbsp	35
moroccan tagine	½ cup (4 oz)	70

FOOD	PORTION	CALS
mushroom mix as prep w/ milk	1 cup	228
oyster	1 tbsp	8
plum sauce	0.5 oz	42
satay peanut sauce	1 oz	77
sour cream mix as prep w/ milk	1 cup	509
stroganoff mix as prep	1 cup	271
sweet & sour mix as prep	1 cup	294
teriyaki	1 tbsp	15
teriyaki mix as prep	1 cup	131
white sauce mix as prep w/ milk	1 cup	241
Ahh!Gourmet		
Perky Savory Coffee Sauce	4 tbsp	71
Ritzy Kumquat Plum Sauce	4 tbsp	98
Spicy Garlicky Sweet Sauce Paste	4 tbsp	101
Spicy Ginger Soy Sauce Paste	4 tbsp	137
Annie's Homegrown		
Organic Worchestershire	1 tsp (5 g)	5
Asian Creations		
Marvelous Mango	¼ cup	20
Pad Thai Pizzazz	2 oz	110
Peanut Passion	¼ cup	130
Bear-Man		
Sap-Happy Golden Bear	2 tbsp	60
Bone Suckin'		
Hiccuppin' Hot	1 tsp	10
Yaki Stir Fry	1 tbsp	30
Burbon Chicken		
Marinade Original	1 tbsp (0.6 oz)	5
Cains		
Tartar	2 tbsp	160
Chef Hymie Grande		
New Mexico Sweet Basting Sauce	2 tbsp (1.2 oz)	35
China Pride		
Duck Sauce Sweet & Pungent	2 tbsp	80
Dave's Gourmet		
Hot Sauce Roasted Garlic	1 tsp (5 g)	0
Insanity Sauce	1 tsp (5 g)	10
Jammin' Jerk	1 tsp (5 g)	5
Steak Sauce	1 tbsp (0.6 oz)	20

FOOD	PORTION	CALS
Dei Fratelli		
Sloppy Joe Sauce	¼ cup (2.2 oz)	35
DelGrosso		
Sloppy Joe Sauce	¼ cup (2.2 oz)	60
D'Oni		
Happy Together Orange Chili Garlic	2 tbsp	50
Moondance Marinade	1 tbsp	10
Ethnic Gourmet		
Punjab Saag Spinach	4 oz	60
Simmer Sauce Calcutta Masala	4 oz	90
Simmer Sauce Delhi Korma	4 oz	100
Fischer & Wieser		
Bourbon Charred Pineapple	1 tbsp (0.7 oz)	35
Chipotle Original Roasted Raspberry	1 tbsp (0.7 oz)	40
Grilling Chipotle Plum	1 tbsp (0.7 oz)	40
Grilling Spicy Garlic Steak	1 tbsp (0.7 oz)	20
Habanero Mango Ginger	1 tbsp (0.7 oz)	40
Marinade All Purpose Vegetable & Meat	1 tbsp (0.7 oz)	35
Onion Glaze Sweet & Savory	1 tbsp (0.7 oz)	45
Roasted Blackberry Chipotle	1 tbsp (0.7 oz)	35
Soppin' Big Bold Red	1 tbsp (0.7 oz)	35
Fortun's		
Asian Style Pepper	¼ cup (2 oz)	40
Lemon Dill Caper w/ White Wine	¼ cup (2 oz)	20
Marsala & Mushroom	¼ cup (2 oz)	40
Spicy Mustard w/ Brandy	¼ cup (2 oz)	35
Stroganoff	¼ cup (2 oz)	45
Frank's		
RedHot Chile & Lime Sauce	1 tsp	0
RedHot Original Cayenne Pepper Sauce	1 tsp	0
RedHot X-tra Hot	1 tsp	0
French's		
Worcestershire	1 tsp	0
Frontera		
Hot Sauce Habanero	1 tsp	5
Good Clean Food		
Simmer Sauce Balsamic Mushroom	⅜ cup (3 oz)	100
Simmer Sauce Cacciatore	⅜ cup (3 oz)	70
Simmer Sauce Creole	⅜ cup (3 oz)	45
Simmer Sauce Dill	⅜ cup (3 oz)	60

FOOD	PORTION	CALS
Simmer Sauce French Tarragon	⅜ cup (3 oz)	90
Simmer Sauce Mediterranean	⅜ cup (3 oz)	50
Hot Squeeze		
Original	2 tbsp (1 oz)	110
House Of Tsang		
General Tsao	1 tsp	45
Hoisin	1 tsp	15
Kobe Steak Grill	1 tbsp	50
Korean Teriyaki Stir Fry	1 tbsp	35
Peanut Sauce Bangkok Padang	1 tbsp	45
Spicy Brown Bean	1 tbsp	15
Sweet & Sour	1 tbsp	35
Sweet Ginger Sesame	1 tbsp	40
Thai Peanut	1 tbsp	50
Kikkoman		
Black Bean w/ Garlic	1 tbsp (1.2 oz)	50
Hoisan	2 tbsp (1.2 oz)	80
Katsu	1 tbsp (0.6 oz)	20
Marinade Quick & Easy Honey & Mustard	1 tbsp (0.6 oz)	30
Oyster	1 tbsp (0.6 oz)	25
Peanut Sauce Thai Style	2 tbsp (1.2 oz)	80
Plum	2 tbsp (1.2 oz)	80
Stir-Fry	1 tbsp (0.6 oz)	20
Sweet & Sour	2 tbsp (1.2 oz)	35
Teriyaki Less Sodium	1 tbsp (0.5 oz)	15
Teriyaki Sauce & Marinade	1 tbsp (0.5 oz)	15
Teriyaki Takumi Original	1 tbsp (0.6 oz)	30
Knorr		
Alfredo Mix as prep	2 oz	60
Bearnaise Mix as prep	2 oz	35
Demi-Glace Mix as prep	2 oz	30
Green Peppercorn Mix as prep	2 oz	35
Hollandaise Mix as prep	2 oz	35
Mango Habanero	1 oz	20
Sweet Red Chili	1 oz	80
White Mix as prep	2 oz	20
La Choy		
Sweet & Sour	2 tbsp (1.2 oz)	60
Teriyaki	1 tbsp (0.6 oz)	40

FOOD	PORTION	CALS
Latino Chef		
Chimichurri Sun Dried Tomato	2 tbsp	120
Sofrito	2 tbsp	20
Lawry's		
Marinade Szechuan Sweet & Sour BBQ	1 tbsp (0.5 oz)	35
Marinade Tuscan Sun-Dried Tomato	1 tbsp (0.5 oz)	15
Lea & Perrins		
Worcestershire	1 tsp (0.2 oz)	5
Loney's		
Bar-B-Q Chicken as prep	¼ cup (2.1 oz)	15
Manwich		
Sloppy Joe Original	¼ cup (2.2 oz)	40
Margaritaville		
ConQueso In Paradise	1 oz	45
Matiz		
Paella Sofrito	¼ cup	137
McCormick		
Cocktail For Seafood Original	¼ cup (2.1 oz)	90
Seafood Sauce Asian	2 tbsp (1.2 oz)	50
Seafood Sauce Cajun Style	1 tbsp (1.1 oz)	15
Seafood Sauce Scampi	1 tbsp (1 oz)	160
Tartar Fat Free	2 tbsp (1.1 oz)	30
Tartar Original	2 tbsp (1 oz)	140
Mrs. Dash		
10 Minute Marinade Lemon Herb Peppercorn	1 tbsp (0.5 oz)	25
10 Minute Marinade Mesquite Grille	1 tbsp (0.5 oz)	25
10 Minute Marinade Spicy Teriyaki	1 tbsp (0.5 oz)	25
10 Minute Marinade Zesty Garlic Herb	1 tbsp (0.5 oz)	25
Naturally Fresh		
Seafood Cocktail	2 tbsp	25
Tartar Sauce	2 tbsp	130
Old Bay		
Tartar Sauce	2 tbsp (1.1 oz)	130
Old El Paso		
Enchilada Mild	¼ cup	25
OrganicVille		
Island Teriyaki	1 tbsp (0.5 oz)	25
Pace		
Taco Sauce Green	1 tbsp	5
Taco Sauce Red	2 tbsp	10

FOOD	PORTION	CALS
Patak's		
Jalfrezi Sweet Peppers & Coconut	½ cup	140
Korma Rich Creamy Coconut	½ cup	240
Rogan Josh Spicy Tomato & Cardamon	½ cup	90
Tikka Masala Tangy Lemon & Cilantro	½ cup	120
Progresso		
Bruschetta	2 tbsp (1 oz)	10
Road's End Organics		
Alfredo Style Dairy Free Gluten Free	⅓ pkg	35
Cheddar Style Dairy Free	⅓ pkg	35
Robert Rothchild Farm		
Anne Mae's Smoky Sweet Chipotle	2 tbsp	35
Saucy Susan		
Peach Apricot	2 tbsp (1.3 oz)	80
Simply Boulder		
Coconut Peanut	2 tbsp (1 oz)	90
Lemon Pesto	2 tbsp (1 oz)	50
Zesty Pineapple	2 tbsp (1 oz)	45
Soy Vay		
Hoisin Garlic Asian Glaze & Marinade	1 tbsp	40
Veri Veri Teriyaki	1 tbsp	35
Steel's		
Cocktail w/ Dill & Lemon Sugar Free Gluten Free	¼ cup (2.4 oz)	35
Hoisin No Sugar Added Gluten Free	2 tbsp (1 oz)	30
Tabasco		
Pepper Sauce	1 tsp	0
Texas Sassy		
Marinade Salsa	1 tbsp (0.5 oz)	15
Pickle Sauce	1 tbsp (0.5 oz)	30
Thai Kitchen		
Pineapple & Chili	2 tbsp (1 oz)	25
Premium Fish Sauce	1 tbsp (0.5 oz)	10
Sweet Red Chili	2 tbsp (1 oz)	70
Thai Chili & Ginger	2 tbsp (1 oz)	40
The Gracious Gourmet		
Pesto Lemon Artichoke	2 tbsp (1 oz)	50
The Wizard's		
Organic Worcestershire Vegetarian Wheat Free	1 tsp	0

FOOD	PORTION	CALS
Three Acre Kitchen		
Marinade Balsamic w/ Juniper & Rosemary	1 tbsp (0.5 oz)	50
Walden Farms		
Calorie Free Scampi Sauce	2 tbsp (1 oz)	0
Wild Thymes Farm		
Marinade Hawaiian Teryaki	1 tbsp	19
Marinade Korean Ginger Scallion	1 tbsp	20
Marinade New Orleans Creole	1 tbsp	11
WildWood		
Aioli	1 tbsp	80
Pesto Basil & Pine Nuts	¼ cup	230
Wingers		
Hotter Than Hot	1 tsp	0
World Harbors		
Buccaneer Blends Pirate's Original	1 tbsp (0.6 oz)	20
Chimichurri	2 tbsp (1.2 oz)	40
Fajita	2 tbsp (1.1 oz)	45
Jerk	2 tbsp (1 oz)	70
Lemon Pepper & Garlic	2 tbsp (1 oz)	35
Thai	2 tbsp (1 oz)	40
TAKE-OUT		
cucumber yogurt sauce	1½ tbsp	20
SAUERKRAUT		
canned	½ cup	22
Ba-Tampte		
Kosher	2 tbsp (1 oz)	5
Dei Fratelli		
Sauerkraut	2 tbsp (1 oz)	5
Gedney		
Sauerkraut	½ cup	15
Tree Of Life		
Organic	½ cup (3.6 oz)	15
SAUSAGE		
beef & pork	1 link (2.3 oz)	196
beef & pork w/ cheddar cheese	1 link (2.7 oz)	228
bierschinken	3.5 oz	174
bierwurst	3.5 oz	258
blutwurst uncooked	3.5 oz	424
bockwurst	3.5 oz	276

FOOD	PORTION	CALS
bratwurst chicken cooked	1 (3 oz)	148
bratwurst pork cooked	1 link (2.5 oz)	226
brotwurst pork & beef	1 link (2.5 oz)	226
chipolata	3.5 oz	342
chorizo	1 link (2.1 oz)	273
fleischwurst	3.5 oz	305
free range chicken breakfast	2 links (2.7 oz)	110
gelbwurst uncooked	3.5 oz	363
italian pork cooked	1 (2.4 oz)	230
italian turkey smoked	1 (2 oz)	88
jagdwurst	3.5 oz	211
knockwurst pork & beef	1 (2.5 oz)	221
mettwurst uncooked	3.5 oz	483
plockwurst uncooked	3.5 oz	312
polish kielbasa	2 oz	127
pork cooked	2 links (1.7 oz)	163
regensburger uncooked	3.5 oz	354
smoked beef cooked	1 (1.4 oz)	134
venison patty	1 (1 oz)	84
vienna canned	1 can (4 oz)	260
vienna canned	1 link (0.5 oz)	37
weisswurst uncooked	3.5 oz	305
zungenwurst (tongue)	3.5 oz	285
Applegate Farms		
Organic Andouille	1 (3 oz)	120
Armour		
Sizzle & Serve Turkey	3 (1.8 oz)	130
Banquet		
Brown'N Serve Lite Maple	3 (2 oz)	130
Brown'N Serve Lite Original	3 (2.1 oz)	120
Brown'N Serve Turkey	3 (2.1 oz)	110
Butterball		
Bratwurst Turkey	1 (3.2 oz)	140
Breakfast Turkey	3 (3 oz)	130
Polska Kielbasa Turkey	2 oz	100
Sweet Italian Turkey	1 (3.2 oz)	140
Coleman		
Bratwurst	1 (3 oz)	240
Chicken Spicy Chorizo	1 (3 oz)	150

FOOD	PORTION	CALS
Dietz & Watson		
Italian	1 (2 oz)	160
Italian Chicken	1 (3.4 oz)	130
Jerk Chicken	1 (3.4 oz)	130
Polska Kielbasa	1 (2 oz)	150
Scrapple Philadelphia	2 oz	120
Foster Farms		
Turkey Breakfast Links	2 (2 oz)	120
Hans All Natural		
Breakfast Links Skinless Chicken	2 (1.7 oz)	60
Chicken Spinach & Feta	1 (2.7 oz)	130
Healthy Ones		
Smoked	2 oz	80
High Plains Bison		
Bratwurst Beer & Cheddar	1 (3.2 oz)	280
Cocktail	1 (2 oz)	180
Wild Rice & Asiago	1 (3.2 oz)	260
Honeysuckle White		
Turkey Roll Mild Italian	2.5 oz	100
Jimmy Dean		
Fully Cooked Original Links	3 (2.4 oz)	240
Fully Cooked Original Patties	2 (2.4 oz)	240
Fully Cooked Turkey Links	3 (2.4 oz)	120
Fully Cooked Turkey Patties	2 (2.4 oz)	120
Original Links	3 (2 oz)	170
Original Patties cooked	2 (2.4 oz)	240
Pork All Natural cooked	2 oz	190
Pork Light cooked	2 oz	140
Johnsonville		
Bratwurst Original	1 (3 oz)	270
Breakfast Patty Original	2 (2 oz)	180
Grilling Chorizo	1 (3 oz)	280
Italian Mild	1 (3 oz)	270
Original Summer	1 (2 oz)	170
Polish	1 (2.7 oz)	240
Pork	2 oz	180
Smoked Turkey	1 (3 oz)	110
Jones		
All Natural Light	3 (2.1 oz)	130

FOOD	PORTION	CALS
Libby's		
Vienna Sausage BBQ	3	140
Murray's		
Chicken Spinach & Garlic	3 oz	130
Perdue		
Turkey Breakfast	2 oz	80
Turkey Sweet Italian cooked	1 link (2.8 oz)	150
Wampler		
Bratwurst as prep	1 (2.5 oz)	230
Breakfast Links as prep	2 (1.2 oz)	130
Breakfast Patties as prep	1 (1.1 oz)	120
Italian as prep	1 (2.5 oz)	230

SAUSAGE DISHES
TAKE-OUT

italian sausage w/ peppers & onions	1 cup	210
sausage roll	1 (2.3 oz)	311

SAUSAGE SUBSTITUTES

meatless	1 link (0.9 oz)	64
meatless	1 patty (1.3 oz)	98
Gardenburger		
Veggie Breakfast	1 patty (1.5 oz)	45
Harmony Valley		
Vegetarian Breakfast Sausage Mix as prep	1 (2 oz)	90
Morningstar Farms		
Breakfast Patties	1 (1.3 oz)	80
Worthington		
Saucettes Breakfast Links	1 (1.3 oz)	90
Yves		
Veggie Brats Classic	1 (3.3 oz)	160

SAVORY

ground	1 tsp	4

SCALLOP

raw	3 oz	75
Mrs. Paul's		
Fried	13 (3.7 oz)	260
TAKE-OUT		
breaded & fried	2 lg	67

FOOD	PORTION	CALS
SCONE		
TAKE-OUT		
apricot	1	232
blueberry	1 (3 oz)	270
cheese	1 (3.5 oz)	364
orange poppy	1 (3 oz)	260
plain	1 (3.5 oz)	362
raisin	1 (3 oz)	270
SCUP		
fresh baked	3 oz	115
SEA BASS (see BASS)		
SEA CUCUMBER		
dried	1 oz	74
fresh	1 oz	20
SEA URCHIN		
canned	1 oz	39
fresh	1 oz	36
roe paste	1 tbsp	19
SEATROUT (see TROUT)		
SEAWEED		
agar dried	1 oz	87
agar fresh	1 oz	<1
furikake	1 tbsp (5 g)	15
hijiki dried	1 tbsp	9
hijiki rehydrated	1 tbsp (3 g)	1
irishmoss fresh	1 oz	14
kelp fresh	1 oz	12
konbu dried	1 piece (5 g)	11
konbu fresh	1 oz	12
laver fresh	1 oz	10
nori fresh	1 oz	10
nori sheet dried	1 (8 x 8 in)	5
ogo fresh	1 cup (2.8 oz)	24
seahair dried	1 tbsp	13
spirulina dried	1 oz	83
spirulina fresh	1 oz	7
tangle fresh	1 oz	12
wakame rehydrated	1 tbsp (3 g)	1

FOOD	PORTION	CALS
Annie Chun's		
Roasted Snacks Sesame	1 pkg (1.5 g)	5
Roasted Snacks Wasabi	1 pkg (1.5 g)	10
Maine Coast		
Organic Alaria Whole Leaf	⅓ cup	18
Organic Dulse Granules	1 tsp	6
Organic Dulse Whole Leaf	½ cup	19
Organic Kelp Granules	½ tsp	5
Organic Kelp Whole Leaf	⅓ cup	17
Organic Laver Whole Leaf	⅓ cup	22

SEEDS
SaviSeed
Cocoa Kissed	⅕ pkg (1 oz)	170
Karmalized	⅕ pkg (1 oz)	160
Oh Natural	⅕ pkg (1 oz)	190

SEMOLINA
dry	1 cup (5.9 oz)	601

SEITAN (see WHEAT)

SESAME
seeds	1 tsp	16
sesame butter	1 tbsp	95
sesame crunch candy	1 oz	146
sesame crunch candy	20 pieces (1.2 oz)	181
tahini from roasted & toasted kernels	1 tbsp	89
tahini from stone ground kernels	1 tbsp	86
tahini from unroasted kernels	1 tbsp	85
Arrowhead Mills		
Organic Seeds	¼ cup	210
Organic Tahini	2 tbsp	190
Mrs. May's		
Black Sesame Crunch	1 oz	165
Peloponnese		
Tahini	1 tbsp	100
Tree Of Life		
Organic Sesame Tahini	2 tbsp	108
Seeds	¼ cup (1.3 oz)	210

SESBANIA
flower	1	1

FOOD	PORTION	CALS
flowers	1 cup	5
flowers cooked	1 cup	23

SHAD

american baked	3 oz	214
cooked	1 oz	55
roe baked w/ butter & lemon	1 oz	36

SHALLOTS (see ONION)

SHARK

fin dried	1 oz	32
raw	3 oz	111
TAKE-OUT		
batter-dipped & fried	3 oz	194

SHEEPSHEAD FISH

cooked	1 fillet (6.5 oz)	234
cooked	3 oz	107
raw	3 oz	92

SHELLFISH (see INDIVIDUAL NAMES, SHELLFISH SUBSTITUTES)

SHELLFISH SUBSTITUTES

crab imitation	1 cup (4.4 oz)	144
scallop imitation	3 oz	84
shrimp imitation	3 oz	86
surimi	3 oz	84
Louis Kemp		
Crab Delights Flake Style	½ cup (3 oz)	90
Crab Delights Leg Style	½ cup (3 oz)	90
Crab Delights Snack Delights	1 stick (1.5 oz)	35
Lobster Delights Chunk Style	½ cup (3 oz)	90
TAKE-OUT		
crab salad	1 cup	395

SHELLIE BEANS

canned	½ cup	37

SHERBET

orange	½ gal	2158
orange	½ cup (4 fl oz)	132
orange	1 bar (2.75 fl oz)	91

FOOD	PORTION	CALS
Ciao Bella		
Lemon	1 pkg (3.5 oz)	120
Mango	1 pkg (3.5 oz)	100
Raspberry	1 pkg (3.5 oz)	110
Dippin' Dots		
Lemon Lime	½ cup	97
Hershey's		
Lemon	½ cup (3.4 oz)	100
Orange	½ cup (3.4 oz)	100
Strawberry	½ cup (3.4 oz)	110
Hola Fruta		
Bar Pomegranate & Blueberry	1 (2.5 oz)	100
Mango	½ cup	130
Margarita	½ cup	140
Peach	½ cup	130
Pomegranate	½ cup	140
Land O'Lakes		
Orange	½ cup (3.2 oz)	130
Turkey Hill		
Fruit Rainbow	½ cup	120
Orange Grove	½ cup	120
SHRIMP (*see also* ASIAN FOOD, EGG ROLLS)		
CANNED		
canned drained	10 (1.1 oz)	32
canned drained	1 cup (4.5 oz)	128
chinese shrimp paste	1 tbsp	46
Chicken Of The Sea		
Medium	½ can (2 oz)	45
Small	½ can (2 oz)	45
Tiny	½ can (2 oz)	45
Polar		
Tiny Peeled	¼ cup (2 oz)	44
Wild Planet		
Shrimp Wild Pink	2 oz	50
DRIED		
dried	1 oz	72
dried	10 (5 g)	13
FRESH		
broiled jumbo	3 (1 oz)	44
broiled small	3 (0.4 oz)	18

FOOD	PORTION	CALS
broiled tiny popcorn	3 (3 g)	4
prawn broiled	3 (0.6 oz)	27
steamed jumbo	3 (1 oz)	41
steamed large	3 (0.6 oz)	25
steamed medium	3 (0.5 oz)	21
Chicken Of The Sea		
Ring w/ Cocktail Sauce	⅓ pkg (3 oz)	100
FROZEN		
Blue Horizon Organic		
Garlic Shrimp	1 serv (3.5 oz)	160
Panko Shrimp	1 serv (3.5 oz)	160
Popcorn Shrimp	1 serv (3.5 oz)	160
Tempura Shrimp	1 serv (3.5 oz)	160
Chicken Of The Sea		
Tempura w/ Soy Dipping Sauce	3	200
Contessa		
Orange Shrimp	11 to 13 (6 oz)	250
Ragin' Cajun	8 to 10 (4 oz)	170
Shrimp Scampi	8 to 10 (4 oz)	290
Gorton's		
Popcorn Crunchy Golden	20 (3.2 oz)	240
Temptations Breaded Butterfly	5 (3.5 oz)	250
Temptations Scampi Sauced	1 serv (4 oz)	120
Margaritaville		
Island Lime	6 (4 oz)	240
Jammin' Jerk	7 (4 oz)	210
Plum Crazy + Sauce	7 + 2 oz sauce	270
Mrs. Paul's		
Butterfly	7 (4 oz)	250
SeaPak		
Butterfly	7 (3 oz)	210
Coconut + Sauce	4 (3.7 oz)	310
Popcorn	15 (3 oz)	210
Scampi	8 (4 oz)	350
Tempura + Sauce	4 (4.1 oz)	240
Shrimp Burgers		
Cajun	1 (4 oz)	160
Original	1 (4 oz)	160
Teriyaki	1 (4 oz)	150

FOOD	PORTION	CALS
Van de Kamp's		
Battered	6 (4 oz)	200
Breaded Popcorn	20 (4 oz)	260
TAKE-OUT		
battered jumbo	3 (3 oz)	268
battered large	3 (1.8 oz)	152
battered medium	3 (1.2 oz)	98
battered small	3 (0.6 oz)	54
battered tiny popcorn	3 (6 g)	18
breaded & fried	1 lg (0.6 oz)	44
cocktail w/ cocktail sauce	4 shrimp (3.2 oz)	78
creole w/o rice	1 cup (8.6 oz)	335
gingered	4	80
jambalaya w/ rice	1 cup (8.5 oz)	294
scampi	1 cup	310
shish kabob w/ vegetables	1 (7.1 oz)	184
shrimp cake	1 (4.2 oz)	238
shrimp egg patty torta de cameron seco	2 (1.3 oz)	152
shrimp in garlic sauce	1 cup (7.4 oz)	649
shrimp newburg	1 cup (8.6 oz)	605
shrimp salad	1 cup (6.4 oz)	258
shrimp w/ crab stuffing	3 (1.7 oz)	94
tempura	1 (0.9 oz)	65
toast fried	3 pieces (2.5 oz)	219

SMELT

FOOD	PORTION	CALS
rainbow cooked	3 oz	106
rainbow raw	3 oz	83

SMOOTHIES (see also FRUIT DRINKS, YOGURT DRINKS)

FOOD	PORTION	CALS
Arizona		
Smoothie Mix Orchard Peach as prep	8 oz	150
Arthur's		
Carrot Energizer	1 bottle (11 oz)	200
Green Energy	1 bottle (11 oz)	230
Bolthouse Farms		
Green Goodness	8 oz	140
Mango Lemonade	8 oz	120
Passion Fruit Apple Carrot Juice	8 oz	120
C&W		
Berry Blend	½ cup	90
Peach	½ cup	80

FOOD	PORTION	CALS
Del Monte		
Ready-To-Blend Mango Pineapple	1 (6 oz)	115
Ready-To-Blend Strawberry Peach	1 (6 oz)	120
Ready-To-Blend Strawberry Peach Lite	1 (6 oz)	80
Dole		
Shakers Mixed Berry not prep	1 pkg (4 oz)	100
Horizon Organic		
Tropical Punch	1 bottle (6.2 oz)	120
Jamba Juice		
Mango-A-Go-Go not prep	½ pkg (4 oz)	70
Razzmatazz not prep	½ pkg (4 oz)	60
Strawberries Wild not prep	½ pkg (4 oz)	60
Kidz Dream		
Orange Cream	1 box	120
Main St Cafe		
Protein Smoothie Mixed Berry	1 bottle (11 oz)	270
Protein Smoothie Peach	1 bottle (11 oz)	260
Protein Smoothie Strawberry	1 bottle (11 oz)	280
Nutiva		
Organic HempShake Amazon Acai not prep	4 tbsp	100
Organic HempShake Chocolate not prep	4 tbsp	80
Odwalla		
Bluberry B Monster	8 oz	140
Citrus C Monster	8 oz	150
Mango Tango	8 oz	150
Sambazon		
Acai Amazon Cherry	8 oz	156
Acai Mango Banana	8 oz	190
Acai Mango Uprising	8 oz	190
Acai Protein Warrior Vanilla	8 oz	215
Acai Shaman's Immunity	8 oz	90
Acai Soy Energy	8 oz	210
Acai Strawberry Sensation	8 oz	210
Acai Supergreens Revolution	8 oz	200
Organic Acai	1 bottle	155
Soy Fusion		
Berry	1 box (8.45 oz)	120
Matcha Green Tea	1 box (8.45 oz)	110
Tropicana		
Fruit Smoothie Mixed Berry	1 bottle (11 oz)	220
Fruit Smoothie Tropical Fruit	1 bottle (11 oz)	220

FOOD	PORTION	CALS
V8		
Splash Tropical Colada	8 oz	100
SNACKS		
cheese puffs	1 oz	122
oriental mix	1 oz	155
pork skins	1 oz	154
pork skins barbecue	1 oz	152
Annie's Homegrown		
Organic Cheddar Snack Mix	40 pieces (1 oz)	140
Organic Pizza Snack Mix	½ cup (1 oz)	140
Bachman		
Baked Cheese Curls	23 (1 oz)	140
Onion Rings	½ pkg (1 oz)	130
Baken-ets		
Pork Skins Hot 'N Spicy	9 (0.5 oz)	80
Pork Skins Traditional	9 (0.5 oz)	80
Barbara's Bakery		
Cheese Puffs Bakes Original	¾ cup	160
Cheese Puffs Original	¾ cup (1 oz)	150
Better Balance		
Kruncheeze White Cheddar Gluten Free	1 oz	130
Carole's		
Soycrunch Cinnamon & Raisins	½ cup	110
Soycrunch Original	½ cup	120
Soycrunch Toffee	½ cup	110
Cheetos		
Baked Crunchy	34 (1 oz)	130
Corn BBQ	29 (1 oz)	150
Natural White Cheddar	1 oz	150
Puffs	13 (1 oz)	160
Cheez It		
Right Bites Party Mix	1 pkg (0.74 oz)	100
Chester's		
Puffcorn Butter	1 oz	160
Snack Mix Crazy Cheddar	1¼ cups (1 oz)	140
DrSears		
Popumz BBQ	1 pkg (0.74 oz)	70
Popumz Caramel Drizzle	1 pkg (0.75 oz)	90
Popumz Cheddar	1 pkg (0.74 oz)	80

FOOD	PORTION	CALS
Popumz Cool Ranch	1 pkg (0.74 oz)	80
Popumz Vanilla Drizzle	1 pkg (0.74 oz)	90
Fullbites		
Bold Cheddar	1 pkg (1.3 oz)	150
Savory BBQ	1 pkg (1.3 oz)	150
Funyuns		
Onion Rings	13 (1 oz)	140
Kay's Naturals		
Snack Mix Sweet BBQ Gluten Free	1 oz	120
Lance		
Cheese Puffs	9 (1 oz)	170
Gold-N-Chees	1 oz	150
Lifestyle Foods		
Awake	1 pkg (5 oz)	170
Essential	1 pkg (5.6 oz)	200
Miami	1 pkg (7.5 oz)	180
Power Up	1 pkg (6.7 oz)	170
Medora Snacks		
Corners Sea Salt	1 oz	130
Pucci Garlic	1 oz	120
Pucci Tomato Basil	1 oz	120
Sotos Cheese Olive Oil & Lemon	1 oz	120
Michael Season's		
Cheese Puffs & Curls	1½ cups	180
Munchies		
Snack Mix Totally Ranch	¾ cup (1 oz)	140
Robert's American Gourmet		
Booty Barbeque	1 oz	130
Booty Pirate's	1 oz	130
Booty Veggie	1 oz	130
Smart Puffs	1 oz	130
Tings	1 oz	160
Sabritones		
Puffed Wheat Chili & Lime	23 pieces (1 oz)	150
Silhouette Solution		
Puffs BBQ	1 pkg (1.06 oz)	120
Snikiddy		
Puffs Grilled Cheese	1 pkg (0.6 oz)	80
Puffs Rockin' Ranch	1 pkg (0.6 oz)	83

FOOD	PORTION	CALS
Snyder's Of Hanover		
CheddAirs	1 oz	130
MultiGrain Cheese Puffs	1 oz	130
SunRidge Farms		
Mocha Marble Crunch	¼ pkg (1.4 oz)	220
Sweet Emotions		
Chocolate Passion	1 pkg (0.5 oz)	60
Cinnamon Joy	1 pkg (0.5 oz)	60
T.G.I. Friday's		
Mozzarella Sticks	20 (1 oz)	150
Utz		
Cheese Balls	50 (1 oz)	150
Cheese Curls	18 (1 oz)	150
Onion Rings	41 (1 oz)	130
Party Mix	1 oz	150
Pork Cracklins	0.5 oz	90
Pork Rinds Original	0.5 oz	80
SNAIL		
cooked	3 oz	233
raw	3 oz	117
TAKE-OUT		
escargot cooked	5	25
SNAKE		
fresh	3 oz	78
SNAPPER		
cooked	1 fillet (6 oz)	217
cooked	3 oz	109
raw	3 oz	85
SODA		
club	12 oz	0
cola	12 oz	151
cream	12 oz	191
diet cola	12 oz	2
ginger ale	12 oz	124
grape	12 oz	161
lemon lime	12 oz	149
orange	12 oz	177
pepper type	12 oz	151

FOOD	PORTION	CALS
quinine	12 oz	125
root beer	12 oz	152
shirley temple	1 serv	159
tonic water	12 oz	125
Ale 8 One		
Soft Drink	1 bottle (12 oz)	120
Barq's		
Diet French Vanilla Creme	8 oz	1
Diet Red Creme	8 oz	4
Diet Root Beer	8 oz	1
Floatz	8 oz	127
French Vanilla Creme	8 oz	112
Red Creme	8 oz	115
Root Beer	8 oz	111
Cape Cod Dry		
Cranberry	8 oz	120
Diet Cranberry	8 oz	10
Carver's		
Ginger Ale	8 oz	94
Celsius		
Cola	1 bottle (12 oz)	5
Coca-Cola		
C2	8 oz	45
Classic	8 oz	97
W/ Lime	8 oz	98
Coke		
Cherry	8 oz	104
Diet	8 oz	1
Diet Cherry	8 oz	1
Diet Plus	8 oz	0
Diet Vanilla	8 oz	1
Diet w/ Lime	8 oz	2
Vanilla	8 oz	100
DRY		
Juniper Berry	1 bottle (12 oz)	55
Vanilla Bean	1 bottle (12 oz)	60
Fanta		
Apple	8 oz	121
Citrus	8 oz	91
Orange	8 oz	111

FOOD	PORTION	CALS
Fresca		
Soda	8 oz	2
Fresh Ginger		
Ginger Ale Jasmine Green Tea	1 bottle (12 oz)	160
Ginger Ale Original	1 bottle (12 oz)	160
Ginger Ale Pomegranate w/ Hibiscus	1 bottle (12 oz)	160
Goya		
Ginger Beer	1 bottle (12 oz)	190
GuS		
Dry Cola	1 bottle (12 oz)	95
Dry Crimson Grape	1 bottle (12 oz)	90
Dry Pomegranate	1 bottle (12 oz)	98
Star Ruby Grapefruit	1 bottle (12 oz)	90
Hansen's		
Blackberry	1 bottle	150
Health Cola		
Soda	1 bottle (12 oz)	140
HotLips		
Apple	1 bottle	136
Boysenberry	1 bottle	152
Pear	1 bottle	142
Inca Kola		
Diet	8 oz	1
Soda	8 oz	96
Jones Soda		
Blue Bubble Gum	1 bottle (12 oz)	190
Cream	1 bottle (12 oz)	190
Crushed Melon	1 bottle (12 oz)	190
FuFu Berry	1 bottle (12 oz)	190
Green Apple	1 bottle (12 oz)	180
Orange Cream	1 bottle (12 oz)	180
Lucozade		
Soda	7 oz	136
Manzana Mia		
Soda	8 oz	99
Mello Yellow		
Diet	8 oz	3
Soda	8 oz	118
Mr. Pibb		
Diet	8 oz	1

FOOD	PORTION	CALS
Northern Neck		
Diet Ginger Ale	8 oz	4
Ginger Ale	8 oz	94
Nutrisoda		
Calm Sparkling Wild Berry & Citron	1 can (8.7 oz)	0
Flex Sparkling Black Cherry & Apple	1 can (8.7 oz)	5
Immune Sparkling Tangerine & Lime	1 can (8.7 oz)	15
Slender Sparkling Guava & Grapefruit	1 can (8.7 oz)	10
Oogave Natural		
All Flavors	8 oz	68
Orangina		
Sparkling Citrus	8 oz	100
Pepsi		
Cola	8 oz	100
Diet	8 oz	0
Diet Vanilla	8 oz	0
One	8 oz	1
Wild Cherry	8 oz	100
Pibb		
Zero	8 oz	2
Polar		
Birch Beer	8 oz	110
Bitter Lemon Mixer	8 oz	120
Collins Mixer	8 oz	90
Cream	8 oz	120
Diet Pomegranate Dry	8 oz	10
Orange	8 oz	130
Pomegranate Dry	8 oz	120
Seltzer All Flavors	8 oz	0
Strawberry	8 oz	120
Tonic Water	8 oz	90
Vichy Water	8 oz	0
Red Flash		
Soda	8 oz	105
Reed's		
Ginger Brew Original	1 bottle (12 oz)	145
Santa Cruz		
Organic Cherry	1 can (12 oz)	140
Organic Ginger Ale	1 can (12 oz)	150
Organic Root Beer	1 can (12 oz)	150
Organic Vanilla Creme	1 can (12 oz)	160

FOOD	PORTION	CALS
Sprite		
Diet Zero	8 oz	0
ReMix Aruba Jam	8 oz	97
Soda	8 oz	96
Steaz		
Organic Green Tea Soda Cola	8 oz	90
Organic Green Tea Soda Diet Black Cherry	8 oz	20
Organic Green Tea Soda Ginger Ale	8 oz	90
Organic Green Tea Soda Lemon	8 oz	90
Stewart's		
Birch Beer	1 bottle (12 oz)	170
Stirrings		
Ginger Ale	8 oz	120
Tab		
Soda	8 oz	1
Tava		
Sparkling Brazilian Samba	8 oz	0
Sparkling Mediterranean Fiesta	8 oz	0
Thomas Kemper		
Black Cherry	1 bottle (12 oz)	170
Ginger Ale	1 bottle (12 oz)	150
Orange Cream	1 bottle (12 oz)	170
Root Beer	1 bottle (12 oz)	160
Root Beer Low Calorie	1 bottle (12 oz)	20
Vanilla Cream	1 bottle (12 oz)	150
Tropicana		
Twister Orange	1 can (12 oz)	180
Vignette		
Wine Country Soda Chardonnay	1 bottle (12 oz)	130
Wine Country Soda Pinot Noir	1 bottle (12 oz)	130
Virgil's		
Micro Brewed Root Beer	1 bottle (12 oz)	160
Zevia		
Dr. Zevia	1 can (12 oz)	0
SOLE		
cooked	3 oz	99
cooked	1 fillet (4.5 oz)	148
lemon raw	3.5 oz	85
TAKE-OUT		
breaded & fried	3.2 oz	211

FOOD	PORTION	CALS
SORGHUM		
sorghum	1 cup (6.7 oz)	651
SOUFFLE		
Garden Lites		
Roasted Vegetable	1 pkg (7 oz)	140
Heavenly Souffle		
Chocolate	1 (2.6 oz)	262
TAKE-OUT		
cheese	1 cup	194
chicken	1 cup (5.6 oz)	278
corn	1 cup	257
lime chilled	1 cup	388
seafood	1 cup	245
spinach	1 cup	124
SOUP		
CANNED		
Allens		
Chicken Broth	1 cup	10
Amy's		
Organic Butternut Squash Light In Sodium	1 cup (8.6 oz)	100
Organic Chunky Tomato Bisque	1 cup (8.4 oz)	120
Organic Chunky Tomato Bisque Light In Sodium	1 cup (8.6 oz)	120
Organic Cream Of Mushroom	¾ cup (6.5 oz)	150
Organic Lentil Light In Sodium	1 cup (8.6 oz)	180
Organic No Chicken Noodle Soup	1 cup (8.6 oz)	100
Organic Pasta & 3 Bean	1 cup (8.6 oz)	150
Organic Southwestern Vegetable	1 cup (8.7 oz)	140
Organic Split Pea	1 cup (8.6 oz)	100
Split Pea Light In Sodium	1 cup (8.6 oz)	100
Tom Kha Phak Thai Coconut	1 cup (7 oz)	140
Butterball		
Chicken Broth 99% Fat Free	1 cup	10
Campbell's		
25% Less Sodium Chicken Noodle as prep	1 cup	60
25% Less Sodium Cream Of Mushroom as prep	1 cup	110
98% Fat Free Cream Of Celery as prep	1 cup	60
98% Fat Free Cream Of Chicken as prep	1 cup	70

FOOD	PORTION	CALS
Cheddar Cheese as prep	1 cup	110
Chicken & Stars as prep	1 cup	70
Chicken Alphabet as prep	1 cup	70
Chicken Noodle O's as prep	1 cup	90
Chunky Creamy Chicken & Dumplings	1 cup (8.4 oz)	170
Chunky Healthy Request Chicken Noodle	1 cup (8.4 oz)	120
Chunky Italian Wedding	1 cup (8.4 oz)	130
Chunky Roadhouse Beef & Bean Chili	1 cup	230
Chunky Split Pea & Ham	1 cup (8.4 oz)	170
Curly Noodle as prep	1 cup	80
Double Noodle Chicken as prep	1 cup	110
Goldfish Pasta Meatball as prep	1 cup	90
Healthy Request Cream Of Chicken as prep	1 cup (8.4 oz)	80
Healthy Request Tomato as prep	1 cup	90
Italian Wedding Light as prep	1 cup (8.4 oz)	80
Just For Kids Goldfish Pasta as prep	1 cup	80
Light Chicken Gumbo as prep	1 cup (8.4 oz)	70
Low Sodium Chicken Broth	1 can	25
Mega Noodle as prep	1 cup	90
Microwavable Bowl Chicken Noodle	1 cup	70
Minestrone as prep	1 cup (8.4 oz)	90
Select Italian Sausage w/ Pasta & Pepperoni	1 cup	150
Select Mexican Chicken Tortilla	1 cup	130
Select Vegetable Beef	1 cup	110
Select Harvest Caramelized French Onion	1 cup (8.4 oz)	80
Select Harvest Chicken Tuscany	1 cup	90
Select Harvest Chicken w/ Egg Noodles	1 cup	100
Select Harvest Chicken w/ Whole Grain Pasta	1 cup (8.4 oz)	100
Select Harvest Creole Chicken w/ Red Beans & Rice	1 cup (8.4 oz)	130
Select Harvest Harvest Tomato w/ Basil	1 cup (8.4 oz)	100
Select Harvest Light Minestrone w/ Whole Grain Pasta	1 cup	80
Select Harvest Light Savory Chicken w/ Vegetables	1 cup	80
Select Harvest Light Southwestern Style Vegetable	1 cup	50
Select Harvest Light Vegetable & Pasta	1 cup (8.4 oz)	60
Select Harvest Light Vegetable Beef & Barley	1 cup (8.4 oz)	80
Select Harvest Southwest White Chicken Chili	1 cup (8.4 oz)	140

FOOD	PORTION	CALS
Slow Kettle Burgundy Beef Stew w/ Baby Bella Mushrooms & Roasted Garlic	1 cup (8.4 oz)	160
Slow Kettle Portobello Mushroom & Madeira Bisque w/ Shallots	1 cup (8.4 oz)	230
Slow Kettle Southwest Chicken Chile w/ Black Beans & Sweet Corn	1 cup (8.4 oz)	190
Slow Kettle Tuscan Chicken & White Bean w/ Asiago Cheese Thyme & Rosemary	1 cup (8.4 oz)	140
Soup At Hand 25% Less Sodium Chicken w/ Mini Noodles	1 pkg (10.75 oz)	80
Soup At Hand Vegetable Medley	1 pkg (10.75 oz)	100
Soup At Hand Velvety Potato	1 pkg (10.75 oz)	160
Tomato as prep	1 cup (8.4 oz)	90
V8 Garden Broccoli	1 cup (8.4 oz)	90
V8 Golden Butternut Squash	1 cup	140
V8 Sweet Red Pepper	1 cup	120
V8 Tomato Herb	1 cup	90
College Inn		
Beef Broth 99% Fat Free	1 cup (8.4 oz)	25
Beef Broth Fat Free Lower Sodium	1 cup (8.4 oz)	15
Bold Stock Rotisserie Chicken	1 cup (8.4 oz)	30
Bold Stock Tender Beef	1 cup (8.4 oz)	45
Chicken Broth 99% Fat Free	1 cup (8.5 oz)	15
Chicken Broth Light & Fat Free 50% Less Sodium	1 cup (8.4 oz)	5
Chicken Broth w/ Roasted Garlic	1 cup (8.5 oz)	20
Chicken Broth w/ Roasted Vegetables & Herbs	1 cup (8.5 oz)	20
Culinary Broth Thai Coconut Curry	1 cup (8.4 oz)	20
Culinary Broth Wine & Herbs	1 cup (8.4 oz)	5
Garden Vegetable Broth	1 cup (8.4 oz)	25
Turkey Broth	1 cup (8.4 oz)	20
Comfort Care		
Hearty Beef Barley	1 cup (8 oz)	190
Savory Chicken	1 cup (8 oz)	200
Tomato Cheddar Jack	1 cup (8 oz)	90
Dr. McDougall's		
Chunky Tomato Gluten Free	1 cup (8.6 oz)	90
Lentil	1 cup (8.6 oz)	115
Organic Black Bean Lower Sodium	1 cup (8.6 oz)	150
Organic Tortilla	1 cup (8.6 oz)	100

FOOD	PORTION	CALS
Split Pea	1 cup (8.6 oz)	110
Vegetable Gluten Free Vegan	1 cup (3.3 oz)	230
Frontera		
Gourmet Mexican Classic Tortilla	1 cup (8.6 oz)	80
Gourmet Mexican Roasted Vegetable	1 cup (8.6 oz)	80
Go Appetit		
Carrot Bisque	8 oz	110
Gazpacho	8 oz	100
Mango Melange	8 oz	150
Health Valley		
Beef Broth Fat Free	1 cup	10
Chicken Broth Fat Free	1 cup	20
Chicken Broth Fat Free No Salt Added	1 cup	35
Chicken Broth Low Fat	1 cup	35
Clam Chowder Manhattan	1 cup	90
Clam Chowder New England	1 cup	110
Corn & Vegetable Fat Free	1 cup	70
Garden Vegetable Fat Free	1 cup	80
Lentil & Carrot Fat Free	1 cup	100
Organic Black Bean	1 cup	130
Organic Cream Of Mushroom	1 cup	90
Organic Minestrone	1 cup	100
Organic Minestrone No Salt Added	1 cup	70
Organic Mushroom Barley	1 cup	70
Organic Mushroom Barley No Salt Added	1 cup	70
Organic Split Pea No Salt Added	1 cup	110
Organic Tomato	1 cup	80
Organic Tomato No Salt Added	1 cup	80
Tomato Vegetable Fat Free	1 cup	80
Vegetable Broth Fat Free	1 cup	20
Healthy Choice		
Bean & Ham	1 cup (8.7 oz)	180
Chicken & Dumplings	1 cup (8.8 oz)	150
Chicken w/ Rice	1 cup (8.4 oz)	110
Garden Vegetable	1 cup (8.6 oz)	130
Italian Wedding	1 cup (8.6 oz)	120
New England Clam Chowder	1 cup (8.4 oz)	110
Split Pea & Ham	1 cup (8.8 oz)	160
Tomato Basil	1 cup (8.8 oz)	100

FOOD	PORTION	CALS
Hormel		
Bean & Ham	1 pkg (7.5 oz)	190
Beef Vegetable	1 pkg (7.5 oz)	100
Chicken Noodle	1 pkg (7.5 oz)	100
Chicken w/ Rice	1 pkg (7.5 oz)	110
New England Clam Chowder	1 pkg (7.5 oz)	140
Imagine		
Lobster Bisque	1 cup	130
Organic Creamy Butternut Squash	1 cup	90
Organic Creamy Chicken	1 cup	70
Organic Creamy Sweet Corn	1 cup	120
Organic Sweet Potato	1 cup	110
Organic Bistro Cuban Black Bean Bisque	1 cup	170
Organic Broth Beef	1 cup	20
Organic Broth Free Range Chicken Vegetable	1 cup	10
Organic Broth	8 oz	20
Lucini		
Roman Tomato Cream	1 cup (8.6 oz)	170
Umbrian Lentil	1 cup (8.6 oz)	160
Manischewitz		
Beef Broth	1 cup (8.4 oz)	150
Chicken Broth	1 cup (8.4 oz)	15
Chicken Broth Low Sodium	1 cup (8.4 oz)	15
Muir Glen		
Organic Garden Vegetable	1 cup	80
Organic Southwest Black Bean	1 cup	140
New England Country Soup		
Caribbean Black Bean	1 cup (8.8 oz)	210
Chicken Pomodoro	1 cup (8.6 oz)	140
Nana's Chicken	1 cup (8.6 oz)	120
Sweet Chicken Curry	1 cup (8.8 oz)	160
Yankee White Bean	1 cup (9.3 oz)	380
Original SoupMan		
Italian Wedding	1 cup	120
New England Clam Chowder	1 cup	290
Organic Butternut Squash	1 cup	250
Tomato Basil	1 cup	140
Turkey Chili	1 cup	210
Pacific Foods		
Beef Broth Organic	1 cup (8 oz)	20

FOOD	PORTION	CALS
Butternut Squash Organic	1 cup (8 oz)	90
Cashew Carrot Ginger Bisque	1 cup (8.4 oz)	130
Chicken Broth Free Range	1 cup (8 oz)	10
Chicken Broth Free Range Low Sodium Organic	1 cup (8 oz)	15
Cream Of Celery	1 cup (8.6 oz)	70
Curried Red Lentil	1 cup (8 oz)	140
French Onion Organic	1 cup (8 oz)	30
Minestone w/ Chicken Meatballs	1 cup (8.8 oz)	130
Mushroom Broth Organic	1 cup (8 oz)	5
Organic Pho Vegetarian Soup Base	1 cup (8 oz)	25
Organic Broth Pho Beef	1 cup (8 oz)	35
Polano Pepper & Corn Chowder	1 cup (8.7 oz)	190
Red Pepper & Tomato Light Sodium Organic	1 cup (8 oz)	110
Rosemary Potato Chowder	1 cup (8.7 oz)	230
Thai Sweet Potato	1 cup (8.6 oz)	160
Tomato Light Sodium Organic	1 cup (8 oz)	100
Vegetable Broth Organic	1 cup (8 oz)	15
Progresso		
40% Less Sodium Italian Style Wedding	1 cup (8.7 oz)	90
50% Less Sodium Garden Vegetable	1 cup (8.8 oz)	100
High Fiber Chicken Tuscany	1 cup (8.7 oz)	130
High Fiber Creamy Tomato Basil	1 cup (8.8 oz)	130
Light Beef Pot Roast	1 cup (8.4 oz)	80
Light Chicken Vegetable Rotini	1 cup (8.3 oz)	70
Light Chicken Noodle	1 cup (8.3 oz)	70
Light Italian Style Vegetable	1 cup (8.6 oz)	60
Light Savory Vegetable Barley	1 cup (8.5 oz)	60
Light Vegetable	1 cup (8.4 oz)	60
Light Vegetable & Noodle	1 cup (8.7 oz)	60
Reduced Sodium Chicken Gumbo	1 cup (8.7 oz)	110
Reduced Sodium Chicken Noodle	1 cup (8.4 oz)	90
Rich & Hearty Beef Pot Roast	1 cup (8.7 oz)	120
Rich & Hearty Chicken & Homestyle Noodles	1 cup (8.6 oz)	100
Rich & Hearty Chicken Pot Pie	1 cup (8.6 oz)	170
Rich & Hearty Savory Beef Barley Vegetable	1 cup (8.6 oz)	130
Rich & Hearty Sirloin Steak & Vegetables	1 cup (8.5 oz)	130
Rich & Hearty Slow Cooked Vegetable Beef	1 cup (8.6 oz)	120
Rich & Hearty Steak & Roasted Russet Potatoes	1 cup (8.6 oz)	140
Traditional Beef & Vegetable	1 cup (8.7 oz)	120
Traditional Beef Barley	1 cup (8.5 oz)	120

FOOD	PORTION	CALS
Traditional Chickarina	1 cup (8.3 oz)	120
Traditional Chicken & Wild Rice	1 cup (8.4 oz)	100
Traditional Chicken Noodle	1 cup (8.3 oz)	100
Traditional Italian Style Wedding	1 cup (8.4 oz)	100
Traditional Manhattan Clam Chowder	1 cup (8.4 oz)	100
Traditional New England Clam Chowder	1 cup (8.4 oz)	180
Traditional Potato Broccoli & Cheese	1 cup (8.8 oz)	180
Traditional Split Pea w/ Ham	1 cup (8.5 oz)	140
Traditional Turkey Noodle	1 cup (8.4 oz)	80
Vegetable Classics Creamy Mushroom	1 cup (8.1 oz)	130
Vegetable Classics French Onion	1 cup (8 oz)	50
Vegetable Classics Hearty Black Bean	1 cup (8.5 oz)	160
Vegetable Classics Hearty Tomato	1 cup (8.6 oz)	110
Vegetable Classics Lentil	1 cup (8.5 oz)	160
Vegetable Classics Vegetable	1 cup (8.4 oz)	80
World Recipes Caldo De Pollo	1 cup (8.6 oz)	90
Snow's		
Clam Chowder	1 cup (8.4 oz)	200
Spoonful Of Comfort		
Chicken Soup	1 serv (8 oz)	80
Swanson		
50% Low Sodium Beef Broth	1 cup	15
Beef Broth	1 cup	15
Beef Stock	1 cup	30
Chicken Broth	1 cup	10
Chicken Stock	1 cup	20
Vegetable Broth	1 cup	15
Tabatchnick		
Garden Fresh Vegetable Broth	⅔ cup (5.5 oz)	10
Wisconsin Cheddar Cheese	⅔ cup (5.5 oz)	150
FROZEN		
Kettle Cuisine		
Angus Beef Steak Chili w/ Beans Gluten Free Dairy Free	1 pkg (10 oz)	250
Chicken w/ Rice Noodles Gluten Free	1 pkg (10 oz)	140
Roasted Vegetable Gluten Free Dairy Free	1 pkg (10 oz)	140
Thai Curry Chicken Gluten Free Dairy Free	1 pkg (10 oz)	330
Three Bean Chili Gluten Free	1 pkg (10 oz)	220
Tabatchnick		
Cabbage	1 serv (7.5 oz)	90

FOOD	PORTION	CALS
Chicken Broth w/ Noodles & Dumplings	1 serv (7.25 oz)	150
Corn Chowder	1 serv (7.5 oz)	130
Organic Vegetarian Chili	1 serv (7.5 oz)	180
Soup Singles Split Pea	1 bowl (10.9 oz)	210
Split Pea	1 serv (7.5 oz)	140
Vegetable	1 serv (7.5 oz)	90
Vegetable Low Sodium	1 serv (7.5 oz)	90
Wilderness Wild Rice	1 serv (7.5 oz)	80
Yankee Bean	1 serv (7.5 oz)	180
MIX		
beef broth cube	1 cube	6
chicken broth cube	1 cube (4.8 g)	9
Annie Chun's		
Ramen Soy Ginger as prep	1 pkg (4.9 oz)	230
Ramen Spring Vegetable as prep	1 pkg (4.9 oz)	230
Dr. McDougall's		
Black Bean & Lime not prep	1 pkg (3.3 oz)	340
Chicken Noodle Light Sodium not prep	1 pkg (1.4 oz)	140
Chinese Chicken Noodle Light Sodium not prep	1 pkg (1.4 oz)	140
Minestone & Pasta not prep	1 pkg (2.3 oz)	200
Tamale w/ Baked Chips not prep	1 pkg (2.4 oz)	200
Tortilla w/ Baked Chips not prep	1 pkg (2 oz)	200
White Bean & Pasta Light Sodium not prep	1 pkg (1.8 oz)	170
Edward & Sons		
Bouillon Cubes Not-Beef	½ cube	20
Bouillon Cubes Not-Chicken	½ cube	15
Veggie Low Sodium	½ cup	20
HamBeens		
15 Bean as prep	½ cup	120
15 Bean Beef as prep	½ cup	120
15 Bean Cajun as prep	½ cup	120
15 Bean Chicken as prep	½ cup	120
Spanish American Black Bean as prep	½ cup	120
Herb Ox		
Instant Chicken Bouillon	1 pkg (4 g)	5
Kikkoman		
Instant Tofu Miso	1 pkg (6 g)	15
Instant Wakame Seaweed	1 pkg (10 g)	35
Leahey Gardens		
No Beef Noodle as prep	1½ cups	89
No Chicken Noodle as prep	1½ cups	94

FOOD	PORTION	CALS
Manischewitz		
Lentil as prep	1 cup	150
Matzo Ball Soup as prep	1 cup	40
Southwestern Black Bean as prep	1 cup	90
Split Pea w/ Barley as prep	1 cup	110
Vegetable & Pasta as prep	1 cup	90
Miso-Cup		
Golden Vegetable as prep	1 cup	30
Japanese Restaurant Style as prep	1 cup	60
Organic Traditional w/ Tofu as prep	1 cup	35
Reduced Sodium as prep	1 cup	25
Savory Seaweed as prep	1 cup	30
Nissin		
Chicken Vegetable as prep	1 pkg	290
White Cheddar as prep	1 pkg	290
Silhouette Solution		
Mediterranean Tomato	1 pkg (1.16 oz)	110
Newbury Chicken Cream	1 pkg (1.3 oz)	110
Streit's		
Matzo Ball as prep	1 cup	50
Thai Kitchen		
Rice Noodle Bowl Lemongrass & Chili as prep	½ pkg	110
Rice Noodle Bowl Thai Ginger as prep	½ pkg	120
REFRIGERATED		
Moosewood		
Organic Creamy Potato & Corn Chowder	1 cup (8.4 oz)	170
Organic Hungarian Vegetable Noodle	1 cup (8.4 oz)	80
Organic Savannah Sweet Potato Bisque	1 cup (8.4 oz)	200
Organic Texas Two Bean Chili	1 cup (8.4 oz)	200
Organic Tuscan White Bean & Vegetable	1 cup (8.4 oz)	130
Organic Classics		
French Onion w/ Croutons	1 cup	140
Seafood Chowder	1 cup	160
TAKE-OUT		
ban mien fish head	1 serv (10 oz)	277
beef stew soup	1 cup (8.8 oz)	221
bird's nest	1 cup (8.6 oz)	112
black bean turtle soup	1 cup (6.5 oz)	240
broccoli cheese	1 cup	165
brunswick stew soup	1 cup (8.5 oz)	232

FOOD	PORTION	CALS
caldo de res beef soup	1 cup	143
chinese velvet corn	1¼ cups	135
corn & cheese chowder	¾ cup	215
duck soup	1 cup (8.6 oz)	412
egg drop	1 cup	73
gazpacho	1 cup	46
greek lemon	¾ cup	63
hot & sour	1 serv (14 oz)	173
matzo ball soup	1 cup	118
minestrone	1 cup	233
miso w/ tofu	1 cup	84
onion soup gratinee	1 serv	492
oxtail	1 cup	68
pasta e fagioli	1 cup (8.8 oz)	194
ratatouille	1 cup (7.5 oz)	266
shark fin	1 bowl (10 oz)	164
shrimp bisque	1 cup	263
shrimp gumbo	1 cup (8.6 oz)	163
sopa de albondigas	1 cup	171
thai lemon grass	1 bowl	100
vietnamese pho beef noodle	1 serv (7.8 oz)	480
wonton soup	1 cup	183
yookgaejang korean beef	1 cup (8.4 oz)	94
zupa koprowa polish dill soup	1 bowl	54

SOUR CREAM

FOOD	PORTION	CALS
fat free	1 tbsp	12
fat free	½ cup (4.5 oz)	95
reduced fat	1 tbsp (0.5 oz)	29
reduced fat	½ cup (4.4 oz)	224
sour cream	½ cup (4 oz)	222
sour cream	1 tbsp (0.4 oz)	23
Breakstone's		
Sour Cream	2 tbsp (1 oz)	60
Cabot		
Light	2 tbsp	35
No Fat	2 tbsp	20
Sour Cream	2 tbsp	50
Friendship		
All Natural	2 tbsp (1 oz)	60

FOOD	PORTION	CALS
Light	1 tbsp (1 oz)	40
Nonfat	2 tbsp (1 oz)	25
Green Valley		
Sour Cream	2 tbsp	100
Horizon Organic		
Lowfat	2 tbsp	35
Sour Cream	2 tbsp	60
Land O'Lakes		
Fat Free	2 tbsp (1.1 oz)	20
Light	2 tbsp (1.1 oz)	40
Sour Cream	2 tbsp (1.1 oz)	60
Nancy's		
Organic	2 tbsp	60
Organic Valley		
Lowfat	2 tbsp	40
SOUR CREAM SUBSTITUTES		
imitation	½ cup (4 oz)	239
Tofutti		
Better Than Sour Cream	2 tbsp (1 oz)	85
Vegan Gourmet		
Alternative Sour Cream	2 tbsp (1 oz)	50
SOURSOP		
fresh	1	416
fresh cut up	1 cup	150

SOY (*see also* CHEESE SUBSTITUTES, ICE CREAM AND FROZEN DESSERTS, MILK SUBSTITUTES, MISO, SMOOTHIES, SOY SAUCE, SOYBEANS, TEMPEH, TOFU, YOGURT FROZEN)

natto	½ cup (3.1 oz)	187
Bob's Red Mill		
Protein Powder	1 tbsp	20
I.M. Healthy		
SoyNut Butter Chocolate	2 tbsp	190
SoyNut Butter Honey Creamy	2 tbsp	170
SoyNut Butter Original Chunky	2 tbsp	170
SoyNut Butter Original Creamy	2 tbsp	170
SoyNut Butter Unsweetened Creamy	2 tbsp	190
Simple Food		
Soynut Butter Chocolate	2 tbsp	190
Soynut Butter No Sugar No Salt	2 tbsp	200

FOOD	PORTION	CALS
Soy Wonder		
Creamy Spread	2 tbsp	170
SoyButter		
Spread	2 tbsp	200

SOY DRINKS (see MILK SUBSTITUTES, SMOOTHIES)

SOY SAUCE

shoyu	1 tbsp	9
soy sauce	1 tbsp	7
tamari	1 tbsp	11
Angostura		
Lite Soy	1 tbsp (0.5 oz)	10
Soy Sauce	1 tbsp (0.5 oz)	10
Dave's Gourmet		
Soyabi Sauce	1 tbsp (0.6 oz)	30
House Of Tsang		
Ginger Soy Sauce	1 tbsp	20
Less Sodium	1 tbsp	5
Kikkoman		
Less Sodium	1 tbsp (0.5 oz)	10
Ponzu	1 tbsp (0.5 oz)	10
Soy Sauce	1 tbsp (0.5 oz)	10
Sushi Sashimi	1 tbsp (0.5 oz)	15
La Choy		
Lite	1 tbsp (0.5 oz)	15
Lee Kum Kee		
Lite	1 tbsp (0.5 oz)	10
Mitsukan		
Ponzu Citrus Seasoned	1 tbsp (0.5 oz)	10
San-J		
Tamari Organic Gluten Free	2 pkg (0.5 oz)	10
Soy Vay		
Wasabiyaki	1 tbsp	35
Tree Of Life		
Organic Shoyu	1 tbsp (0.5 oz)	15
Organic Tamari Wheat Free	1 tbsp (0.5 oz)	15

SOYBEANS

dried cooked	1 cup	298
dry roasted	½ cup	387
green cooked	½ cup	127

FOOD	PORTION	CALS
roasted	½ cup	405
roasted & toasted	1 cup	490
roasted & toasted salted	1 cup	490
sprouts raw	½ cup	43
sprouts steamed	½ cup	38
sprouts stir fried	1 cup	125
Arrowhead Mills		
Organic Dried not prep	¼ cup	160
C&W		
In the Pod	½ cup	110
Crunchies		
Freeze Dried Edamame	⅜ cup (1 oz)	124
Freeze Dried Edamame Grilled	⅜ cup (0.9 oz)	84
Freeze Dried Edamame Salted	¼ cup (0.9 oz)	90
KooLoos		
Soy Nuts & Flaxseed BBQ	1 pkg (1 oz)	130
Soy Nuts & Flaxseed Original	1 pkg (1 oz)	140
Seapoint Farms		
Edamame Dry Roasted Goji Blend	¼ cup	120
Edamame Dry Roasted Lightly Salted	¼ cup	130
Edamame Dry Roasted Wasabi	¼ cup	130
Edamame In Pods	½ cup	100
Edamame In Pods Lightly Salted	½ cup	100
Edamame Shelled	½ cup	100
Organic Edamame In Pods	½ cup	100
Organic Edamame Shelled	½ cup	100
South Beach		
Soy Nuts Dark Chocolate	1 pkg (0.7 oz)	100
Sunrich Naturals		
Edamame Fiesta Blend frzn	½ cup (3 oz)	90
Edamame In The Shell frzn	½ cup (3 oz)	120
Soy Honey Nutz	1 pkg (1 oz)	130

SPAGHETTI (*see* PASTA, PASTA DINNERS, PASTA SALAD, SPAGHETTI SAUCE)

SPAGHETTI SAUCE
JARRED

marinara sauce	1 cup	171
spaghetti sauce	1 cup	272
Amy's		
Organic Family Marinara	½ cup (4.4 oz)	80
Organic Marinara Low Sodium	½ cup (4.4 oz)	40

FOOD	PORTION	CALS
Barilla		
Arrabbiata Tomato & Spicy Pepper	½ cup	90
Garden Vegetable	½ cup	70
Green & Black Olive	½ cup	80
Italian Baking Sauce	¼ cup (4.4 oz)	60
Mushroom & Garlic	½ cup	70
Toscana Tuscan Herb	½ cup (4.4 oz)	70
Dave's Gourmet		
Pasta Sauce Spicy Heirloom Marinara	½ cup (4.4 oz)	45
Pasta Sauce Wild Mushroom	½ cup (4.4 oz)	60
Dei Fratelli		
Arrabbiata	½ cup (4.2 oz)	50
Pizza Sauce	¼ cup (2.2 oz)	30
Del Monte		
Garlic & Onion	½ cup (4.4 oz)	70
W/ Mushrooms	½ cup (4.4 oz)	70
DelGrosso		
Garden Style	½ cup (4.4 oz)	70
Mushroom	½ cup (4.4 oz)	70
New York Style	¼ cup (2.1 oz)	35
Original Meat Flavored	½ cup (4.4 oz)	80
Pizza Sauce Pepperoni	¼ cup (2.2 oz)	40
Three Cheese	½ cup (4.4 oz)	80
Francesco Rinaldi		
Alfredo	¼ cup (2.1 oz)	80
Chunky Eggplant Parmesan	½ cup (4.4 oz)	90
Chunky Mushroom & Pepper	½ cup (4.4 oz)	80
Hearty Mushroom Pepper & Onion	½ cup (4.4 oz)	80
Hearty Sweet & Tasty Tomato	½ cup (4.4 oz)	100
Hearty Three Cheese	½ cup (4.4 oz)	80
Organic Burgundy Marinara	½ cup (4.3 oz)	100
Premium Vodka	¼ cup (2.1 oz)	60
Traditional Meat Flavored	½ cup (4.4 oz)	80
Traditional No Salt Added	½ cup (4.4 oz)	70
Traditional Original	½ cup (4.4 oz)	80
Hunt's		
Pasta Sauce Four Cheese	½ cup (4.4 oz)	60
Pasta Sauce Garlic & Herb	½ cup (4.4 oz)	40
Pasta Sauce Meat	½ cup (4.4 oz)	60
Pasta Sauce Mushroom	½ cup (4.4 oz)	50

FOOD	PORTION	CALS
Tomato Sauce	¼ cup (2.2 oz)	20
Tomato Sauce No Salt Added	¼ cup (2.2 oz)	20
Traditional Pasta Sauce	½ cup (4.4 oz)	50
Knorr		
W/ Meat	4 oz	110
Lucini		
Spicy Tuscan	½ cup (4.4 oz)	80
Tuscan Marinara w/ Roasted Garlic	½ cup (4.4 oz)	60
Mom's		
Artichoke Heart & Asiago Cheese	½ cup (4.2 oz)	90
Fresh Garlic Basil	½ cup (4.2 oz)	30
Martini	½ cup (4.2 oz)	120
Puttanesca	½ cup (4.2 oz)	90
Muir Glen		
Organic Chunky Tomato	¼ cup	15
Organic Garlic Roasted Garlic	½ cup	60
Organic Pizza Sauce	¼ cup	40
Organic Tomato Sauce No Salt Added	¼ cup	25
Pomi		
Strained	½ cup (4.4 oz)	30
Prego		
Heart Smart Traditional Italian	½ cup	100
Italian	½ cup	70
Italian Marinara	½ cup	100
Italian Meat	½ cup	130
Italian Roasted Red Pepper & Garlic	½ cup	90
Italian Three Cheese	½ cup	80
Italian Tomato Basil & Garlic	½ cup	80
Organic Mushroom	½ cup	90
Veggie Smart	½ cup (4.2 oz)	90
Progresso		
Lobster Sauce	½ cup (4.3 oz)	100
Pesto Arrabiata	2 tbsp (1 oz)	140
Pesto Basil & Roasted Garlic	2 tbsp (1 oz)	130
Red Clam	½ cup (4.4 oz)	60
White Clam	½ cup (4.4 oz)	150
Racconto		
Essentials Heart Health Roasted Garlic	½ cup (4.4 oz)	90
Ragu		
Light Tomato & Basil No Sugar Added	½ cup (4.4 oz)	50

FOOD	PORTION	CALS
Old World Style Margherita	½ cup (4.4 oz)	70
Old World Style Meat	½ cup (4.4 oz)	70
Old World Style Sweet Tomato Basil	½ cup (4.4 oz)	60
Pizza Quick Fresh Italian	2 oz	35
Randazzo's		
Alfredo	¼ cup (2.2 oz)	200
Fra Diavolo	1.2 cup (4.4 oz)	90
Puttanesca	½ cup (4.4 oz)	100
Vodka	½ cup (4.4 oz)	230
Robert Rothchild Farm		
Artichoke	½ cup	80
S&W		
Tomato Sauce	¼ cup (2.1 oz)	20
Two Guys		
Jersey Tomato Sauce	½ cup (4.6 oz)	60
Vino De Milo		
Mediterranean Pinot Grigio	½ cup	90
Portobello Shiraz	½ cup	40
Tuscan Merlot	½ cup	80
Walden Farms		
Alfredo Sauce Calorie Free	3 tbsp (1.6 oz)	0
Walnut Acres		
Organic Garlic Garlic	½ cup	125
Organic Marinara & Zinfandel	½ cup	125
Organic Roasted Garlic	½ cup	125
Organic Tomato & Basil	½ cup	125
MIX		
Loney's		
Carbonara as prep	¼ cup (2.1 oz)	33
Rose as prep	¼ cup (2.1 oz)	29
REFRIGERATED		
Buitoni		
Alfredo	¼ cup (2.1 oz)	140
Alfredo Light	¼ cup (2.1 oz)	90
Marinara	½ cup (4.4 oz)	70
Pesto	¼ cup (2.2 oz)	270
Pesto Basil Reduced Fat	¼ cup (2.2 oz)	230
Vodka Sauce	½ cup (4.2 oz)	90
TAKE-OUT		
bolognese	5 oz	195

FOOD	PORTION	CALS
SPANISH FOOD		
FRESH		
Texas Tamale Company		
Tamales Beef	2 (3 oz)	160
Tamales Chicken	2 (3 oz)	130
Tamales Spinach	2 (3 oz)	140
FROZEN		
Amy's		
Bowl Mexican Casserole	1 pkg (9.4 oz)	470
Burrito Black Bean	1 (6 oz)	280
Burrito Cheddar Cheese	1 (6 oz)	300
Burrito Southwestern	1 (5.5 oz)	300
Enchilada Black Bean Vegetable	1 (4.7 oz)	180
Cedarlane		
Organic Burrito Low Fat Rice & Cheese	1 (6 oz)	260
Organic Enchilada Low Fat Black Bean & Tofu	1 (9 oz)	220
Roasted Chile Relleno	1 pkg (10 oz)	400
Zone Burrito Beans & Cheese	1 (6 oz)	350
Contessa		
Fajitas Shrimp	2 (8 oz)	230
Paella w/ Chicken & Seafood	1½ cups	200
Seafood Veracruz not prep	1¾ cups	180
Dr. Praeger's		
Burrito Bites	2 (2 oz)	130
El Monterey		
Burrito Bean & Cheese	1 (5 oz)	280
Burrito Beef & Bean	1 (5 oz)	370
Burrito Half Pound Spicy Red Hot Beef & Bean	1 (8 oz)	600
Burrito Supreme Breakfast Egg Cheese & Sausage	1 (4.5 oz)	300
Burrito Supreme Shredded Steak & Cheese	1 (5 oz)	290
Burrito XX Large Bean & Cheese	1 (10 oz)	590
Burrito XX Large Beef & Bean	1 (10 oz)	730
Cruncheros Cheese & Beef	3 (4.5 oz)	330
Cruncheros Taco Beef & Cheese	4 (5.6 oz)	460
Enchiladas Cheese w/ Sauce	1 serv (8 oz)	250
Enchiladas Shredded Beef w/ Sauce	1 serv (4 oz)	140
Quesadillas Chicken & Cheese	2 (6 oz)	380
Quesadillas Steak & Cheese	2 (6 oz)	400
Tamales Chicken	1 (4.5 oz)	240

FOOD	PORTION	CALS
Tamales Shredded Beef	1 (4.5 oz)	310
Taquitos Corn Shredded Beef	3 (4.5 oz)	300
Taquitos Flour Char-Broiled Chicken Breast	3 (5 oz)	380
Taquitos Flour Chicken & Cheese	3 (4.5 oz)	350
Taquitos Southwest Chicken In A Seasoned Batter	2 (2.8 oz)	175
Tornados Apple Cinnamon	1 (3 oz)	180
Tornados Sausage Egg & Cheese	1 (3 oz)	230
Tornados Shredded Beef	1 (3 oz)	210
Tornados Steak Egg & Cheese	1 (3 oz)	170
Tornados XXL Southwest Chicken	1 (4.2 oz)	210
Farm Rich		
Quesadillas	2 (3.1 oz)	200
Glutenfreeda		
Burrito Breakfast Beef	1 (3.9 oz)	199
Burrito Vegetarian Bean & Cheese	1 (3.9 oz)	196
Health Is Wealth		
Vegetarian Hot Tamale Munchees	6 (3 oz)	160
Helen's Kitchen		
Cheese Enchiladas w/ Tofu Steaks In Spicy Red Sauce	½ pkg (5 oz)	150
Jose Ole		
Burrito Chicken	1 (5 oz)	270
Burrito Steak & Jalapeno	1 (5 oz)	300
Chimichanga Shredded Beef	1 (5 oz)	350
Lean Cuisine		
Simple Favorites Chicken Enchilada Suiza	1 pkg (9 oz)	290
Meals To Live		
White Chicken Burrito w/ Green Sauce	1 pkg (9 oz)	330
Mom Made		
Fiesta Rice	1 pkg (7 oz)	200
Munchie Bean Burrito	1 (2.5 oz)	140
Patio		
Burrito Bean & Cheese	1	280
Burrito Beef & Bean Mild	1	300
Enchilada & Beef Tamale	1 meal	460
Enchilada Beef	1 meal	380
Enchilada Cheese	1 meal	390
Enchilada Combo Dinner	1 meal	380

FOOD	PORTION	CALS
Stouffer's		
Chicken Enchilada w/ Cheese Sauce & Rice	1 pkg (7.13 oz)	280
Tyson		
Meal Kit Chicken Fajita	1 (3.8 oz)	130
Meal Kit Quesadilla Chicken	1 (4 oz)	250
READY-TO-EAT		
taco shell corn	1 (6.5 inch)	98
taco shell flour	1 (7 inch)	173
TAKE-OUT		
arroz con coco	1 cup	532
burrito w/ beans	1 med (5 oz)	295
burrito w/ beans & rice	1 (3.5 oz)	221
burrito w/ beef	1 sm (3.4 oz)	297
burrito w/ beef & beans	1 med (5 oz)	331
burrito w/ beef beans & cheese	1 med (5 oz)	379
burrito w/ chicken & beans	1 med (5 oz)	295
burrito w/ pork & beans	1 med (5 oz)	320
chiles rellenos meat & cheese filled	1 (5 oz)	213
chimichanga w/ bean cheese lettuce & tomato	1 (4.1 oz)	271
chimichanga w/ beef & rice	1 (10 oz)	634
chimichanga w/ beef beans lettuce & tomato	1 (4.1 oz)	254
chimichanga w/ beef cheese lettuce & tomato	1 (4.1 oz)	337
chimichanga w/ chicken sour cream lettuce & tomato	1 (4 oz)	277
empanada fruit filled	1 (3.8 oz)	452
empanada meat & vegetable	1 (7.8 oz)	881
empanada sweet potato	1 (7.8 oz)	546
enchilada w/ beans	1 (4.1 oz)	179
enchilada w/ beans & cheese	1 (4.6 oz)	233
enchilada w/ beef	1 (4 oz)	214
enchilada w/ beef & beans	1 (4 oz)	195
frijoles	1 cup	278
frijoles w/ cheese	1 cup	225
nachos w/ beans & cheese	1 serv (9.4 oz)	616
nachos w/ beef beans cheese & sour cream	1 serv (19 oz)	1620
paella	1 serv (7 oz)	308
pupusa meat filled	1 (3.6 oz)	187
quesadilla w/ cheese	1 (5 oz)	498
quesadilla w/ meat & cheese	1 (6.5 oz)	605
taco de jueye w/ crab meat	1 (4.2 oz)	266

FOOD	PORTION	CALS
taco w/ beans lettuce tomato & salsa	1 (2.8 oz)	117
taco w/ chicken lettuce tomato & salsa	1 (2.5 oz)	114
taco w/ fish lettuce tomato & salsa	1 (2.7 oz)	101
tostada w/ beef lettuce tomato & salsa	1 (2.7 oz)	143

SPICES (see INDIVIDUAL NAMES, HERBS/SPICES)

SPINACH
CANNED

drained	1 cup	49
Freshlike		
Cut Leaf	½ cup	45
Popeye		
Leaf Spinach	½ cup	30
Leaf Spinach No Salt Added	½ cup	40
S&W		
Leaf	½ cup (4 oz)	30
FRESH		
baby raw	2 cups	20
cooked	1 cup	41
malabar cooked	1 cup	10
mustard cooked	1 cup	29
new zealand cooked	1 cup	22
raw	1 cup	7
Dole		
Baby Spinach	1½ cups (3 oz)	20
Fresh Express		
Baby Spinach	3 cups	20
Organic Baby Spinach	3 cups	35
Ready Pac		
Microwave Spinach as prep	½ cup (3 oz)	20
FROZEN		
chopped cooked	1 cup	30
Birds Eye		
Chopped	⅓ cup	20
Creamed	½ cup (4.4 oz)	90
C&W		
Baby Chopped	1 cup	30
Creamed	½ cup	100
Cascadian Farm		
Organic Cut	⅓ cup	25

FOOD	PORTION	CALS
Cedarlane		
Organic Spanakopita Spinach & Feta Pie	½ pkg (5 oz)	260
Health Is Wealth		
Creamed	½ pkg (4.5 oz)	100
Spinach Munchees	6 (3 oz)	180
Seabrook Farms		
Chopped	⅓ cup (2.9 oz)	20
Creamed	½ cup (4.4 oz)	100
Stouffer's		
Creamed	½ pkg (4.5 oz)	200
Tabatchnick		
Creamed	1 serv (3.7 oz)	40
Tandoor Chef		
Palak Paneer	½ pkg (5 oz)	170
The Fillo Factory		
Spanakopita Spinach & Cheese Fillo Appetizers	3 (3 oz)	190
Veggie Patch		
Spinach Bites	3 (2.6 oz)	150
TAKE-OUT		
indian saag	1 serv	28
spanakopita spinach pie	1 serv (3 oz)	148

SPINACH JUICE

juice	7 oz	14

SPORTS DRINKS (see ENERGY DRINKS)

SPOT

baked	3 oz	134

SPROUTS

kidney bean	½ cup	27
lentil sprouts	½ cup	40
mung bean	½ cup	16
mung bean canned	½ cup	8
mung bean cooked	½ cup	13
pea	½ cup (2.1 oz)	74
radish	½ cup	8
Brassica		
BroccoSprouts	½ cup (1 oz)	16
La Choy		
Bean Sprouts	⅔ cup	15

FOOD	PORTION	CALS
TAKE-OUT		
mung bean stir fried	½ cup	31
SQUAB		
boneless baked	1 (4 oz)	242

SQUASH (see also SQUASH SEEDS, ZUCCHINI)

CANNED		
crookneck sliced	½ cup	14
Sunshine		
Slice Yellow	½ cup	25
FRESH		
acorn cooked mashed	½ cup	41
acorn cubed baked	½ cup	57
butternut baked	½ cup	41
crookneck sliced cooked	½ cup	18
hubbard baked	½ cup	51
hubbard cooked mashed	½ cup	35
scallop sliced cooked	½ cup	14
spaghetti cooked	½ cup	23
Glory		
Yellow Sliced	¾ cup	20
Mann's		
Butternut Cubes	1 serv (3 oz)	40
FROZEN		
butternut cooked mashed	½ cup	47
crookneck sliced cooked	½ cup	24
C&W		
Butternut	½ cup	45
McKenzie's		
Southland Butternut	½ cup	70
TAKE-OUT		
fritter	1 (0.8 oz)	81
squash pie	1 slice (5.4 oz)	291

SQUASH SEEDS		
kernels dried	¼ cup (1.1 oz)	180
kernels roasted	¼ cup (1 oz)	169
kernels roasted w/ salt	¼ cup (1 oz)	169
whole roasted w/ salt	¼ cup (0.5 oz)	71
whole roasted w/o salt	¼ cup (0.5 oz)	71

FOOD	PORTION	CALS
SQUID		
baked	1 cup	192
canned in its own ink	1 can (4 oz)	122
dried	1 sm (1.5 oz)	147
pickled	1 oz	26
steamed	1 cup	147
Contessa		
Calamari + Sauce	13 pieces + 2 tbsp sauce	160
Margaritaville		
Captain's Calamari Rings + Sauce	3 + 2 tbsp sauce	320
Van de Kamp's		
Fried Calamari	15 pieces (4 oz)	270
TAKE-OUT		
arroz con calamares	1 cup	400
calamari breaded & fried	1 cup	296
SQUIRREL		
roasted	3 oz	147
STARFRUIT		
fresh	1	42
STRAWBERRIES		
canned in heavy syrup	½ cup	117
fresh halves	1 cup	49
fresh whole	1 pint	114
fresh whole	1 cup	46
frzn sweetened sliced	½ cup	122
frzn sweetened whole	1 cup	199
frzn whole unsweetened	1 cup	77
organic fresh whole	8 med	45
C&W		
Ultimate Sliced frzn	⅔ cup	50
Chukar Cherries		
Dried	¼ cup	120
Crunchies		
Freeze Dried	¼ cup (6 g)	20
Crunchy N'Yummy		
Organic Freeze Dried	1 pkg (1 oz)	60
Dole		
Sliced frzn	1 pkg (3 oz)	35

FOOD	PORTION	CALS
Squish'ems	1 pkg	70
Whole Fresh	1 cup (5.2 oz)	45
Whole frzn	1 cup (4.9 oz)	50
Emily's		
Dark Chocolate Covered	6 (1.4 oz)	170
LiteHouse		
Glaze Sugar Free	3 tbsp	35
Marie's		
Glaze	2 tbsp	40
Polar		
Strawberries In Syrup	½ cup	90
Stoneridge Orchards		
Dried	⅓ cup (1.4 oz)	140
STUFFING/DRESSING		
Fresh Gourmet		
All Natural Multi-Grain w/ Cranberries not prep	⅓ cup (1 oz)	110
Organic Seasoned not prep	⅓ cup (1 oz)	110
Pepperidge Farm		
Corn Bread	¾ cup	170
Cube	¾ cup	140
Herb Seasoned	¾ cup (1.5 oz)	170
One Step Turkey	½ cup	170
TAKE-OUT		
bread	1 cup	352
cornbread	½ cup	179
kishke stuffed derma	1 piece (1.3 oz)	166
oyster	1 cup	304
sausage	½ cup	292
STURGEON		
broiled	3 oz	115
roe raw	1 oz	59
smoked	1 oz	49
TAKE-OUT		
breaded & fried	4 oz	252
SUCKER		
white baked	3 oz	101
SUGAR (*see also* FRUCTOSE, SUGAR SUBSTITUTES, SYRUP)		
brown organic	1 tsp	17

FOOD	PORTION	CALS
brown packed	1 cup (7.7 oz)	828
brown unpacked	1 cup (5.1 oz)	547
cinnamon sugar	1 tsp	16
cube	1 (2 g)	9
maple	1 piece (1 oz)	99
powdered	1 tbsp (0.3 oz)	31
powdered unsifted	1 cup (4.2 oz)	467
raw	1 pkg (5 g)	19
sugarcane stem	3 oz	54
white	1 tsp (4 g)	15
white	1 tbsp (0.4 oz)	49
white	1 cup (7 oz)	773
white	1 pkg (3 g)	12
Bob's Red Mill		
Date Sugar	1 tsp	11
Turbinado	1 tsp	10
Coconut World		
Coconut Sugar	1 tsp (3 g)	10
Domino		
Dark Brown	1 tsp (4 g)	15
Demerara Raw Cane	1 tsp	15
Equinox		
Organic Maple Flakes	2 tsp	15
Maple Grove Farms		
Granulated Maple	1 tsp (4 g)	15
Sugar In The Raw		
Turbinado Sugar	1 pkg (5 g)	20
Tree Of Life		
Date Sugar	1 tsp (4 g)	10
Organic Cane Juice Dehydrated	1 tsp (3.5 g)	15
Turbinado	1 tsp (4 g)	15
Wholesome Sweeteners		
Organic	1 tsp (4 g)	15
Organic Fair Trade Dark Brown Sugar	1 tsp (4 g)	15
Organic Fair Trade Powdered	¼ cup (1 oz)	120
Organic Fair Trade Sucanat	1 tsp (4 g)	15
Organic Turbinado	1 tsp (4 g)	15

SUGAR SUBSTITUTES
Emerald City

Erythritol	1 tsp (4 g)	0

FOOD	PORTION	CALS
Emerald Forest		
Xylitol	1 tsp (4 g)	10
Equal		
Packet	1 pkg	0
Fibrelle		
Fiber-Rich Sweetener	1 tsp (4 g)	5
Fructevia		
All Natural	1 tsp (4 g)	5
Fruit Sweetness		
Sugar Substitute	1 serv (0.9 oz)	0
Ideal		
Brown	1 tsp (1.5 g)	0
Confectionary	¼ cup (1 oz)	86
Packets	1 (1.5 g)	0
White Granulated	1 tsp (1.5 g)	0
Nature's Family		
Sun Crystals	1 pkg (4.5 g)	4
Nevella		
No Calorie Sweetener	1 tsp (0.5 g)	0
Neway		
Sweet Sensation	¼ tsp	0
PureVia		
All Natural	1 pkg (2 g)	0
Splenda		
Brown Sugar Blend	½ tsp (2 g)	10
Flavors For Coffee	1 pkg (1 g)	0
No Calorie Granulated	1 tsp (0.5 g)	0
No Calorie Sweetener w/ Antioxidants	1 pkg	0
No Calorie Sweetener w/ B Vitamins	1 pkg	0
No Calorie Sweetener w/ Fiber	1 pkg	0
Steel's		
Nature Sweet Brown Crystals	1 tsp (3 g)	6
Nature Sweet Crystals	1 tsp (4 g)	8
Sugar Free Vanilla Flavor	1 tbsp (0.5 oz)	23
Stevia In The Raw		
100% Natural Sweetener	1 pkg (1 g)	0
Steviva		
Blend	1 tbsp (0.4 oz)	2
Sugar Twin		
Granulated Brown	1 tsp (0.4 g)	0

FOOD	PORTION	CALS
Granulated White	1 tsp (0.4 g)	0
Liquid	¼ tsp (1.3 g)	0
Packets	1 (0.8 g)	0
Sun Crystals		
Natural Sweetener	1 pkg (5 g)	5
Susta		
Natural Sweetener	1 pkg (2 g)	5
Suzanne		
Somersweet Baking Blend	1 tsp (4 g)	5
Sweet Fiber		
All Natural	1 pkg	0
Sweete		
Sugar Free	1 pkg	0
Swerve		
Sweetener	1 tsp (5 g)	0
Truvia		
Calorie Free Sweetener	1 pkg (3.5 g)	0
Whey Low		
Gold	1 tsp	4
Granular	1 tsp	4
Maple Buzz	¼ cup	57
Wholesome Sweeteners		
Organic Zero	1 pkg (6 g)	0
ZSweet		
All Natural	1 pkg (1 g)	0
SUGAR-APPLE		
fresh	1	146
fresh cut up	1 cup	236
SUNCHOKE		
fresh raw sliced	½ cup	57
SUNFISH		
pumpkinseed baked	3 oz	97
SUNFLOWER		
seeds dry roasted w/ salt	¼ cup	186
seeds dry roasted w/o salt	¼ cup	186
seeds w/ hulls dried	¼ cup	66
Arrowhead Mills		
Organic Seeds	¼ cup	170

FOOD	PORTION	CALS
Bob's Red Mill		
Seeds Roasted & Salted	3 tbsp	186
Dakota Gourmet		
Seeds Honey Roasted	¼ cup (1 oz)	170
David		
Kernels	¼ cup (1.1 oz)	190
Seeds Reduced Sodium w/o Shell	¼ cup (1.1 oz)	190
Seeds w/o Shell	¼ cup (1.1 oz)	190
Frito Lay		
Seeds	1 oz	190
Kaia Foods		
Seeds Sprouted Cocoa Mole	⅙ pkg (1 oz)	80
Sprouted Seeds Sweet Curry	⅙ pkg (1 oz)	80
Lance		
Shelled Seeds	1 pkg (1.8 oz)	300
Planters		
Kernels	1 oz	160
Seeds Roasted & Salted	¾ cup (1 oz)	160
Spitz		
Seeds Salted	⅓ pkg (1 oz)	180
SunButter		
Creamy	2 tbsp	200
Organic	2 tbsp	203
SunGold		
Seeds Roasted Salted	1 oz	172
Sunrich Naturals		
Kernels Cocoa Sunnies	1 pkg (2 oz)	280
Kernels Honey Roasted	1 pkg (1 oz)	170
Kernels Lightly Salted	1 pkg (1 oz)	170
Tree Of Life		
Seeds Kernels Raw	¼ cup (1.3 oz)	210
SUSHI		
TAKE-OUT		
california roll	1 (1.2 oz)	48
crabmeat mayonnaise	1 (1.2 oz)	60
futomaki roll	1 (1.8 oz)	73
ikura salmon roe & cucumber	1 piece (1.1 oz)	50
inari	1 sm (1.2 oz)	46
kappa cucumber roll	1 (1.1 oz)	43
kim bap	1 (1.2 oz)	56

FOOD	PORTION	CALS
nigiri	1 (0.7 oz)	27
prawn cooked	1 (1.1 oz)	36
preserved radish roll	1 (0.3 oz)	9
saba raw mackerel	1 (0.8 oz)	33
salmon slice	1 (1.2 oz)	59
sashimi ahi	1 slice (0.3 oz)	10
scallop cooked	1 (1.1 oz)	43
seasoned baby octopus	1 (1.2 oz)	55
seasoned jellyfish	1 (1.2 oz)	58
seaweed roll	1 (1.1 oz)	43
sweet beancurd	1 (1.2 oz)	64
tekka tuna maki	1 (0.6 oz)	25
torigai cockle	1 piece (1.1 oz)	41
tuna roll	1 (0.6 oz)	19
unagi grilled eel	1 (1 oz)	54
vegetable roll	1 (1.2 oz)	27
vinegared ginger	⅓ cup (1.6 oz)	48
wasabi	2 tsp (0.3 oz)	5
yellowtail roll	1 (0.6 oz)	25

SWAMP CABBAGE
chopped cooked w/o salt	1 cup	20

SWEET POTATO (see also YAM)
baked w/ skin w/o salt	1 lg (6.3 oz)	162
baked w/ skin w/o salt	1 med (4 oz)	103
canned in syrup	½ cup	106
canned mashed	½ cup	129
leaves cooked w/o salt	1 cup	22
paste dulce de calabaza	1 oz	82
Diner's Choice		
Mashed	⅔ cup	160
Glory		
Casserole	½ cup	180
Cut Fresh	1 serv (5 oz)	140
Sweet Potatoes	⅔ cup	160
Green Giant		
Candied	¾ cup	240
Health Is Wealth		
Southern Style	½ pkg (5 oz)	190

FOOD	PORTION	CALS
Jake & Amos		
Sweet Potato Butter	1 tbsp (0.5 oz)	25
Mann's		
Fresh Cubes	1 serv (3 oz)	60
Fries Fresh	1 serv (3 oz)	60
Mrs. Paul's		
Candied	1 serv (5 oz)	300
Princella		
In Light Syrup	⅔ cup	160
Mashed	⅔ cup	120
Royal Prince		
Candied	½ cup	210
Trappey's		
Sugary Sam Cut Sweet	⅔ cup	160
Tree Of Life		
Organic Puree	½ cup (4.5 oz)	130
TAKE-OUT		
candied	1 serv (3.7 oz)	151
white fried batata blanca frita	1 serv (8 oz)	792
SWEETBREAD (PANCREAS)		
beef braised	3 oz	230
lamb braised	3 oz	199
pork braised	3 oz	186
veal braised	3 oz	218
Rumba		
Beef	4 oz	260
SWISS CHARD		
cooked	½ cup	18
raw chopped	½ cup	3
SWORDFISH		
cooked	3 oz	132
raw	3 oz	103
SYRUP		
corn dark & light	¼ cup	240
date syrup	1 tbsp	63
maple	1 tbsp	52
maple	1 cup (11.1 oz)	824
raspberry	1 oz	76

FOOD	PORTION	CALS
rose hip	1 oz	9
sorghum	1 cup (11.6 oz)	957
sorghum	1 tbsp (0.7 oz)	61
sugar syrup	¼ cup	76
Cary's		
Maple	¼ cup	210
Sugar Free	¼ cup	30
Domino		
Agave Nectar Organic Light or Amber	1 tbsp (0.7 oz)	60
Hershey's		
Caramel	2 tbsp (1.4 oz)	110
Strawberry	2 tbsp (1.4 oz)	100
Strawberry Sugar Free	2 tbsp (1 oz)	10
Lundberg		
Organic Sweet Dreams Brown Rice	2 tbsp	110
Maple Grove Farms		
Apricot	¼ cup (2.1 oz)	170
Butter Flavor Sugar Free	¼ cup (2.1 oz)	30
Red Raspberry	¼ cup (2.1 oz)	230
Monin		
Acai	1 oz	90
Amaretto	1 oz	97
Banana	1 oz	98
Coconut	1 oz	100
Organic Vanilla	1 oz	100
Pure Cane	1 oz	101
Nature's Agave		
Agave Nectar Organic Amber Clear or Raw	1 tbsp (0.7 oz)	60
Navitas Naturals		
Yacon	2 tbsp	90
Nesquik		
Strawberry Calcium Fortified	2 tbsp (1.4 oz)	110
Neway		
Sweet Sensation Luo Han Guo Syrup	1 tsp	8
Smucker's		
Blackberry	¼ cup (2.1 oz)	200
Blueberry Sugar Free	¼ cup (2.1 oz)	25
Plate Scrapers Caramel	2 tbsp (1.4 oz)	100
Plate Scrapers Raspberry	2 tbsp (1.3 oz)	100
Plate Scrapers Vanilla	2 tbsp (1.4 oz)	110

FOOD	PORTION	CALS
Pure Maple	¼ cup (2.1 oz)	210
Red Raspberry	¼ cup (2.1 oz)	200
Steel's		
Maple Flavor No Sugar Added	3 tbsp (1.6 oz)	64
Tree Of Life		
Maple Grade A	¼ cup	200
Wholesome Sweeteners		
Organic Blue Agave	1 tbsp (0.7 oz)	60
Organic Blue Agave Cinnamon	2 tbsp (1 oz)	120
Organic Blue Agave Maple	2 tbsp (1 oz)	120
Organic Corn Syrup	2 tbsp (1 oz)	120

TAHINI (*see* SESAME)

TAMARIND

dried sweetened pulpitas	1 piece (0.8 oz)	56
dried sweetened pulpitas	½ cup	279
fresh	1 (2 g)	5
fresh cut up	1 cup	143

TAMARIND JUICE

nectar	1 cup	143

TANGERINE
CANNED

in light syrup	1 cup	154
juice pack	1 cup	92

FRESH

fresh	1 sm (2.7 oz)	40
fresh	1 med (3.1 oz)	47
fresh	1 lg (4.2 oz)	64
sections	1 cup	103
Noble		
Florida Tangerines	1 (3.8 oz)	50
River Pride		
Sweet	1 (3.8 oz)	50

TANGERINE JUICE

canned sweetened	1 cup	124
fresh	1 cup	106
Italian Volcano		
Organic	8 oz	113

FOOD	PORTION	CALS
Natalie's Orchid Island Juice		
100% Juice	8 oz	106
Odwalla		
100% Juice	8 oz	110
Santa Cruz		
Organic Sparkling	8 oz	110
SSips		
Drink	1 box (7 oz)	120
TAPIOCA		
pearl dry	¼ cup (1.3 oz)	136
starch	1 oz	98
Let's Do Organic		
Granulated	1 tbsp	35
Starch	1 tbsp	0
Mon Chong Loong		
Starch	1 oz	110
TARO		
chips	10 (0.8 oz)	115
leaves cooked	½ cup	18
raw sliced	½ cup	56
shoots sliced cooked	½ cup	10
sliced cooked	½ cup (2.3 oz)	94
tahitian sliced cooked	½ cup	30
TARPON		
fresh	3 oz	87
TARRAGON		
dried crumbled	1 tsp	2
ground	1 tsp	5
TEA/HERBAL TEA (*see also* ICED TEA)		
HERBAL		
chamomile brewed	1 cup	2
Bigelow		
Cozy Chamomile	1 tea bag	0
Celestial Seasonings		
Chamomile Honey Vanilla as prep	1 cup (8 oz)	0
REGULAR		
brewed tea	1 cup (6 oz)	2

FOOD	PORTION	CALS
Daily Detox		
Original	1 tea bag	0
Hansen's		
Tea Stix Blackberry	½ pkg (2 g)	5
Lipton		
Black Tea as prep	8 oz	0
Green Tea as prep	1 cup (8 oz)	0
Green Tea Cranberry Pomegranate	1 tea bag	0
Oregon Chai		
Chai Tea Latte Original Caffeine Free Concentrate	½ cup	78
Chai Tea Latte Original Concentrate	½ cup	78
Chai Tea Latte Spiced Original Mix	1 pkg	100
Chai Tea Latte Vanilla Mix	1 pkg	120
Organic Chai Cider Concentrate	½ cup	110
Organic Chai Nog Concentrate	½ cup	90
Red Rose		
English Breakfast Tea Bag as prep	1 cup	0
Tastefully Simple		
Oh My! Itty Bitty Chai Mix as prep w/ water	1 pkg (1.2 oz)	140
Tetley		
Classic Black as prep	1 teabag	0
TAKE-OUT		
chai spiced latte	1 cup	130
TEMPEH		
tempeh	½ cup (2.9 oz)	160
White Wave		
Five Grain	⅓ block (2.7 oz)	160
WildWood		
Organic Nori Seaweed	3 oz	170
TESTICLES		
prairie oysters cooked	1 pair (6.8 oz)	241
THYME		
dried crumbled	1 tsp	3
fresh	1 tsp	1
ground	1 tsp	4

FOOD	PORTION	CALS
TILAPIA		
Beacon Light		
Boneless Fillet Farm Raised	1 (3 oz)	85
Dr. Praeger's		
Fillets Lightly Breaded	1 (4.5 oz)	220
Gorton's		
Grilled Fillets Roasted Garlic & Butter	1 (3 oz)	80
High Liner		
Loins	1 fillet (4 oz)	110
SeaPak		
Tenders	2 (4 oz)	280
Van de Kamp's		
Lightly Breaded Fillets	1 (4 oz)	240
TAKE-OUT		
battered & fried	1 fillet (4 oz)	206
breaded & fried	1 fillet (4 oz)	300
broiled w/o fat	1 fillet (3.5 oz)	128
TILEFISH		
cooked	3 oz	125
cooked	½ fillet (5.3 oz)	220
raw	3 oz	81
TOFU		
firm	½ cup	183
firm	¼ block (3 oz)	118
fresh fried	1 piece (0.5 oz)	35
fuyu salted & fermented	1 block (⅓ oz)	13
koyadofu dried frozen	1 piece (½ oz)	82
okara	½ cup	47
regular	½ cup	94
regular	¼ block (4 oz)	88
Amy's		
Organic Tofu Scramble w/ Hash Browns & Veggies	1 pkg (8.9 oz)	320
Azumaya		
Extra Firm	3 oz	70
Lite Extra Firm	⅕ pkg (2.8 oz)	60
Silken	⅕ pkg (3.2 oz)	40
House		
Atsu-Age Cutlet	1 (2.5 oz)	100

FOOD	PORTION	CALS
Cut-Age Shredded Fried	1 serv (0.5 oz)	50
Ganmodoki Fritter Small	3 (1.6 oz)	120
Medium Firm	3 oz	60
Organic Extra Firm	3 oz	90
Organic Firm	3 oz	60
Soft Silken	3 oz	50
Steak Cajun	1 (3 oz)	40
Steak Grilled	1 (3 oz)	90
Sukui	3 oz	45
Tokusen Kinugoshi	1 piece (5 oz)	90
Yaki Broiled	3 oz	90
Nasoya		
Extra Firm	⅕ pkg (2.8 oz)	80
Silken	⅕ pkg (3.2 oz)	160
Sprouted	3 oz	160
TofuTown		
Tofu Tenders Havana Black Bean	½ pkg (5 oz)	210
Tofu Tenders Mediterranean Tahini	½ pkg (5 oz)	240
Tofu Tenders Sesame Ginger Teriyaki	½ pkg (5 oz)	240
Tree Of Life		
Organic Firm	½ block (3.2 oz)	110
White Wave		
Baked Garlic Herb Italian	1 piece (2 oz)	90
Baked Sesame Peanut Thai	1 piece (2 oz)	90
Baked Zesty Lemon Pepper	1 piece (2 oz)	90
Extra Firm	⅕ block (3.2 oz)	110
Organic Extra Firm	⅕ block (3.2 oz)	110
Organic Firm	⅓ block (3.2 oz)	110
Organic Soft	⅕ block (3.2 oz)	110
Reduced Fat	⅕ block (3.2 oz)	90
WildWood		
Organic Baked Aloha	1 piece (3.5 oz)	180
Organic Calcium Rich Medium	3 oz	70
Organic Golden Pineapple Teriyaki	3 oz	160
Organic High Protein Super Firm	3 oz	100
Organic Smoked Mild Szechuan	3 oz	150
TAKE-OUT		
breaded deep fried w/ soy sauce japanese style	1 piece (0.4 oz)	15
soy sauce marinated & grilled	1 serv (4 oz)	181
stir-fried w/ vegetables	1 cup (7.6 oz)	186

FOOD	PORTION	CALS
TOMATILLO		
fresh	1 (1.2 oz)	11
fresh chopped	½ cup (2.3 oz)	21
TOMATO		
CANNED		
green pickled	½ cup (2.5 oz)	26
green whole pickled	1 (2.6 oz)	27
paste	1 can (6 oz)	139
paste	¼ cup (2.3 oz)	54
paste no salt added	1 can (6 oz)	139
puree	1 can (28 oz)	312
puree	1 cup (8.8 oz)	95
puree w/o salt	1 can (28 oz)	312
sauce	1 cup (8.6 oz)	59
sauce no salt added	1 cup (8.6 oz)	102
stewed	1 cup (8.9 oz)	66
Cento		
Paste	2 tbsp (1.2 oz)	30
Contadina		
Paste Italian Herbs	2 tbsp	35
Dei Fratelli		
Chopped Italian Tomatoes	½ cup (4.3 oz)	40
Del Monte		
Diced w/ Garlic & Onion	½ cup	40
Organic Tomato Paste	2 tbsp	30
Petite Cut Garlic & Olive Oil	½ cup (4.4 oz)	40
Hunt's		
Crushed	½ cup (4.2 oz)	45
Diced	½ cup (4.2 oz)	30
Diced Fire Roasted	½ cup (4.3 oz)	30
Diced In Sauce	½ cup (4.3 oz)	35
Diced No Salt Added	½ cup (4.2 oz)	30
Diced Petite	½ cup (4.2 oz)	30
Diced w/ Roasted Garlic	½ cup (4.2 oz)	35
Stewed	½ cup (4.2 oz)	45
Stewed No Salt Added	½ cup (4.2 oz)	40
Whole	½ cup (4.2 oz)	25
Whole No Salt Added	½ cup (4.2 oz)	30
Muir Glen		
Organic Chunky Tomato & Herb	½ cup	60

FOOD	PORTION	CALS
Organic Diced Fire Roasted	½ cup	30
Organic Diced w/ Basil & Garlic	½ cup	30
Polar		
Grape	½ cup	50
Pomi		
Chopped	½ cup	20
Progresso		
Crushed w/ Added Puree	¼ cup (2.1 oz)	20
Diced	½ cup (4.4 oz)	25
Puree	¼ cup (2.2 oz)	25
Whole Peeled w/ Basil	½ cup (4.2 oz)	20
Redpack		
Crushed In Puree	¼ cup	20
Crushed w/ Basil Garlic & Oregano	¼ cup (2.1 oz)	20
Diced In Juice	½ cup	25
Petite Diced Onion Celery & Green Pepper	½ cup	45
Rienzi		
Italian Cherry Tomatoes No Salt Added	⅓ can (4.5 oz)	30
S&W		
Crushed	¼ cup (2.1 oz)	20
Paste	2 tbsp (1.2 oz)	30
Petite Cut	½ cup (4.4 oz)	25
Puree	¼ cup (2.2 oz)	30
Ready-Cut Italian Recipe	½ cup (4.2 oz)	25
Ready-Cut No Salt Added	½ cup (4.4 oz)	25
Stewed No Salt Added	½ cup (4.4 oz)	35
Stewed Original	½ cup (4.3 oz)	35
Whole Peeled	½ cup (4.4 oz)	25
DRIED		
sun dried	¼ cup (0.5 oz)	35
sun dried	1 piece (2 g)	5
sun dried in oil drained	¼ cup (1 oz)	59
sun dried in oil drained	1 piece (3 g)	6
tomato powder	1 oz	85
Bella Sun Luci		
Sun Dried w/ Italian Basil	⅐ pkg (0.5 oz)	35
Sun Dried w/ Zesty Peppers	⅐ pkg (0.5 oz)	35
FRESH		
bruschetta	¼ cup	50
cherry	½ cup (2.6 oz)	13

FOOD	PORTION	CALS
cherry	1 (0.6 oz)	3
grape tomatoes	20	30
green	1 sm (3.2 oz)	21
green	1 med (4.3 oz)	28
green	1 lg (6.4 oz)	42
green chopped	1 cup (6.3 oz)	41
orange	1 (4 oz)	18
orange chopped	1 cup (5.5 oz)	25
plum	1 (2.2 oz)	11
red	1 sm (3.2 oz)	16
red	1 med (4.3 oz)	22
red	1 lg (6.4 oz)	33
red chopped	½ cup (3.2 oz)	16
red slice	1 lg (0.9 oz)	5
roma	1 (2.2 oz)	11
yellow	1 (7.4 oz)	32
yellow chopped	½ cup (2.4 oz)	10
Earthbound Farms		
Organic Roma	1 med (5.2 oz)	35
Ready Pac		
Bruchetta	2 tbsp (1.6 oz)	70
TAKE-OUT		
aspic	½ cup (4 oz)	32
broiled slices	2 (2.9 oz)	18
broiled whole	1 med (3.7 oz)	23
bruschetta on toasted italian bread	1 slice	106
fried slices	2 (2.5 oz)	122
scalloped	½ cup (4 oz)	99
stewed	½ cup (1.8 oz)	40
stuffed w/ rice	1 (5.2 oz)	110
stuffed w/ rice & meat	1 (5.2 oz)	142

TOMATO JUICE

FOOD	PORTION	CALS
tomato juice	1 cup (8.5 oz)	41
tomato juice w/o added salt	1 cup (8.5 oz)	41
Campbell's		
Healthy Request	8 oz	50
Low Sodium	8 oz	50
Organic	8 oz	50
Dei Fratelli		
Tomato Juice	8 oz	40

FOOD	PORTION	CALS
Lakewood		
Organic	8 oz	35
Tree Of Life		
Organic 100% Juice	8 oz	50
TONGUE		
beef simmered	3 oz	241
lamb braised	3 oz	234
pork braised	3 oz	230
veal braised	3 oz	172
Rumba		
Beef	4 oz	250
TORTILLA		
corn	1 (6 in diam)	56
corn w/o salt	1 (6 in diam)	56
flour w/o salt	1 (8 in diam)	114
French Meadow Bakery		
Fat Flush	1 (1 oz)	100
Gluten Free	1 (1.5 oz)	120
Hemp	1 (1.1 oz)	90
La Tortilla Factory		
Corn Chipotle	1 (1.4 oz)	90
Smart & Delicious 100 Calorie 100% Whole Wheat	1 (2 oz)	100
Smart & Delicious 100 Calorie Traditional	1 (2 oz)	100
Smart & Delicious Low Carb Whole Wheat	1 (2.2 oz)	80
White Corn	1 (1.4 oz)	90
Rudi's Organic Bakery		
Spelt	1 (2 oz)	140
Salba Smart		
Whole Wheat Omega-3 Enriched	1 (1.5 oz)	120
Tumaro's		
Honey Wheat	1 (8 in)	110
Low In Carbs Garden Vegetable	1 (8 in)	100
Low In Carbs Green Onion	1 (8 in)	100
Low In Carbs Multi Grain	1 (8 in)	100
Low In Carbs Salsa	1 (8 in)	100
Pesto & Garlic	1 (8 in)	110
Premium White	1 (8 in)	120
Soy-full Heart 8 Grain 'N Soy	1 (1.4 oz)	100

FOOD	PORTION	CALS
Soy-full Heart Apple 'N Cinnamon	1 (1.4 oz)	90
Soy-full Heart Wheat Soy & Flax	1 (1.4 oz)	90
Spinach & Vegetables	1 (8 in)	110

TORTILLA CHIPS (see CHIPS)

TRAIL MIX
Back To Nature
Bar Harbor Blend	1 oz	130
Harvest Blend	1 oz	150
Nantucket Blend	1 oz	130
Pacific Heights Blend	1 oz	160

Bear Naked
Peak Chocolate Cherry	½ cup (1.1 oz)	120
Peak Pecan Apple Flax	½ cup (1.1 oz)	140

Craisins
Cranberry & Chocolate	1 pkg (1.75 oz)	230
Fruit & Nuts	1 pkg (1.4 oz)	230

Emerald
Breakfast On The Go Berry Nut Blend	1 pkg (1.5 oz)	180
Breakfast On The Go Breakfast Nut Blend	1 pkg (1.5 oz)	180
Breakfast On The Go Smores Nut Blend	1 pkg (1.5 oz)	200

Enjoy Life
Gluten Free Not Nuts! Beach Bash	1 oz	130
Gluten Free Not Nuts! Mountain Mambo	1 oz	140

Frito Lay
Nut & Fruit	1 oz	150
Original	3 tbsp	160

Kopali
Organic Mix	½ pkg (1 oz)	130

Mrs. May's
Coconut Almond Crunch	1 oz	183

Navitas Naturals
3 Berry Cacao Nibs & Cashews	1 oz	110
Goji Cacao Nibs & Cashews	1 oz	120
Goji Golden Berry & Mulberry	1 oz	90

Planters
Berry Nut & Chocolate	3 tbsp (1 oz)	120
Daybreak Blend Berry & Almond	⅓ pkg (1.5 oz)	180
Energy Go-Paks	1 (1.5 oz)	250
Fruit & Nut	⅙ pkg (1 oz)	140
Sweet & Nutty	⅓ pkg (1.1 oz)	160

FOOD	PORTION	CALS
SunRidge Farms		
Cherry Pecan Vanilla Dream	¼ cup (1.4 oz)	200
Mountain Rainbow Mix	¼ cup (1 oz)	150
Organic Deluxe	¼ cup (1 oz)	140
SunRise		
Honey Coated	3 tbsp (1 oz)	137
W/ Fruit	3 tbsp (1 oz)	130
TREE FERN		
chopped cooked	½ cup	28
TRIPE		
beef simmered	3 oz	80
Rumba		
Beef Tripe	4 oz	110
TAKE-OUT		
mondongo w/ potatoes	1 cup	300
TRITICALE		
dry	½ cup (3.4 oz)	323
TROUT		
baked	3 oz	162
rainbow cooked	3 oz	129
seatrout baked	3 oz	113
TRUFFLES		
fresh	0.5 oz	4
Aux Delices Des Bois		
Black Truffle Butter	0.5 oz	90
TUNA		
CANNED		
light in oil	1 can (6 oz)	399
light in oil	3 oz	169
light in water	3 oz	99
light in water	1 can (5.8 oz)	192
white in oil	1 can (6.2 oz)	331
white in oil	3 oz	158
white in water	3 oz	116
white in water	1 can (6 oz)	234
Arroyabe		
Bonito In Olive Oil	2 oz	109

FOOD	PORTION	CALS
Bumble Bee		
Sensations Lemon & Pepper w/ Crackers	1 pkg (3.6 oz)	200
Solid White Albacore In Water	¼ cup (2 oz)	60
Chicken Of The Sea		
Albacore Chunk White In Water	½ can (2.5 oz)	50
Albacore Solid White In Oil	2 oz	90
Albacore Solid White In Water	2 oz	80
Chunk Light 50% Less Sodium	2 oz	80
Chunk Light In Oil	2 oz	100
Chunk Light In Water	2 oz	50
Chunk White In Water Very Low Sodium	2 oz	50
Genova		
Tonno In Olive Oil	2 oz	110
Polar		
Albacore Solid White In Water	2 oz	70
Chunk Light In Water	2 oz	60
Progresso		
Albacore Solid White Olive Oil	¼ cup (2 oz)	90
Light Olive Oil drained	¼ cup (2 oz)	120
StarKist		
Chunk Light In Water	¼ cup (2 oz)	60
Chunk Light In Water Flavor Pouch	1 pkg (3 oz)	90
Low Sodium Chunk White In Water	¼ cup (2 oz)	60
Solid Light In Water	2 oz	60
Solid White Albacore In Water	2 oz	70
Tuna Creations Hickory Smoked Flavor Pouch	2 oz	60
Tonnino		
Fillets In Olive Oil	2 oz	90
Fillets In Olive Oil w/ Jalapeno	2 oz	80
Fillets In Olive Oil w/ Oregano	2 oz	90
Fillets In Spring Water Wild Caught	2 oz	50
Ventresca In Olive Oil	2 oz	110
Tree Of Life		
Wild Light Tongol Chunk In Spring Water No Salt Added	¼ cup (2.4 oz)	50
Wild Planet		
Albacore Wild	2 oz	120
Albacore Wild Fillet	2 oz	120
Albacore Wild No Salt	2 oz	120
Albacore Wild Smoked Troll Caught	2 oz	90
Skipjack Wild Light	2 oz	69

FOOD	PORTION	CALS
FRESH		
bluefin cooked	3 oz	157
bluefin raw	3 oz	122
skipjack baked	3 oz	112
yellowfin baked	3 oz	118
FROZEN		
SeaPak		
Seasoned Ahi Steaks	1 (4.5 oz)	240
MIX		
StarKist		
Lunch To-Go Chunk Light	1 pkg	310
Tuna Helper		
Creamy Broccoli as prep	1 cup	310
Creamy Pasta as prep	1 cup	320
Tetrazzini as prep	1 cup	290
TAKE-OUT		
tuna salad	1 cup	383
TURBOT		
european baked	3 oz	104
TURKEY (see also JERKY, TURKEY DISHES, TURKEY SUBSTITUTES)		
CANNED		
w/ broth	1 cup	220
Hormel		
Chunk White & Dark	2 oz	70
Premium Chunk White	2 oz	60
FRESH		
breast roasted pre-basted w/ skin	3.5 oz	126
breast roasted w/ skin	4 oz	212
breast roasted w/o skin	4 oz	212
dark meat w/o skin roasted	1 cup (5 oz)	262
dark meat w/o skin roasted	3 oz	170
ground cooked	3 oz	193
leg w/ skin roasted	1 (19 oz)	1136
light meat w/ skin roasted half turkey	2.3 lbs	2069
light meat w/o skin roasted	4 oz	183
neck simmered	1 (5.3 oz)	274
skin roasted	1 oz	141
skin roasted from half turkey	8.7 oz	1096
tail cooked	1 (2 oz)	197

FOOD	PORTION	CALS
w/ skin roasted	½ turkey (4 lbs)	3857
w/ skin roasted	1 serv (4.2 oz)	249
w/o skin roasted	1 serv (3.7 oz)	177
w/o skin roasted	1 cup (5 oz)	238
wing w/ skin roasted	1 (6.5 oz)	426
wing w/o skin roasted	1 (5.2 oz)	237
Butterball		
Burger Patties	1 (4 oz)	150
Cutlets	4 oz	120
Drumstick	4 oz	170
Ground 7% Fat	4 oz	150
Ground White	4 oz	130
Strips	4 oz	120
Thighs	4 oz	170
Wings	1 (6.3 oz)	380
Empire		
Ground White	4 oz	160
Foster Farms		
Breast Cutlets	4 oz	120
Necks	4 oz	150
Tails	4 oz	380
Honeysuckle White		
85% Lean Ground	4 oz	240
93% Lean Patties	1 (4 oz)	160
97% Lean Ground White	4 oz	130
99% Fat Free Breast Cutlets	4 oz	120
99% Fat Free Breast Tenderloin	4 oz	120
Drumettes	4 oz	180
Marinated Strips Asian Grill	4 oz	160
Necks	4 oz	150
Tenderloins Creamy Dijon Mustard	4 oz	140
Tenderloins Homestyle	4 oz	130
Tenderloins Teriyaki	4 oz	140
Thighs	4 oz	190
Whole Honey Roasted	4 oz	180
Wings	4 oz	220
Perdue		
Breast Fillets Boneless Skinless cooked	3 oz	110
Drumsticks roasted	3 oz	140
Ground Breast cooked	3 oz	110

FOOD	PORTION	CALS
Patties cooked	1 (3 oz)	160
Whole Breast Bone-In Seasoned	4 oz	140
Whole Dark Meat cooked	3 oz	190
Whole White Meat roasted	3 oz	150
Shady Brook		
Breast Tenderloin Lemon Garlic	4 oz	130
Breast Tenderloin Rotisserie	4 oz	130
Tenderloin Zesty Italian Herb	4 oz	130
FROZEN		
roast boneless seasoned light & dark meat roasted	3.5 oz	155
sticks breaded fried	1 (2.2 oz)	179
Butterball		
Boneless Roast	4 oz	130
Breast Boneless Roast	4 oz	110
Breast Tenderloin Teriyaki	4 oz	110
Breast Whole	4 oz	110
Breast Whole Smoked Cooked	3 oz	120
Whole Turkey	1 serv (4 oz)	170
Whole Turkey Baked	3 oz	130
Honeysuckle White		
Breast Boneless Roast	4 oz	170
Jennie-O		
Burger	1 (4 oz)	160
Organic Prairie		
Whole Young	4 oz	90
READY-TO-EAT		
bologna	1 slice (1 oz)	59
breast	1 slice (0.7 oz)	22
ham	1 slice (1 oz)	35
pastrami	2 oz	70
salami	1 slice (1 oz)	48
Applegate Farms		
Organic Herb	2 oz	50
Butterball		
Breast Honey Roasted Thick Sliced	1 slice (1 oz)	35
Breast Oven Roasted Extra Thin Slice	7 slices (2 oz)	70
Breast Smoked Thin Sliced	4 slices (1.9 oz)	70
Breast Strips Oven Roasted	½ pkg (3 oz)	90
Deep Fried Original Thick Sliced	1 slice (1 oz)	30

FOOD	PORTION	CALS
Carl Buddig		
Honey Roasted Sliced	2 oz	90
Turkey Sliced	2 oz	90
Foster Farms		
Breast Honey Roasted	1 slice (1 oz)	25
Breast Oven Roasted	1 slice (1 oz)	30
Healthy Ones		
Oven Roasted 97% Fat Free	7 slices (2 oz)	60
Honeysuckle White		
Simply Done Whole Breast	4 oz	160
Hormel		
Natural Choice Deli Turkey Honey	4 slices (2 oz)	60
Natural Choice Deli Turkey Oven Roasted	4 slices (2 oz)	60
Natural Choice Deli Turkey Smoked	4 slices (2 oz)	60
Oscar Mayer		
Breast Smoked Shaved	2 oz	50
Sara Lee		
Breast Cracked Pepper	4 slices (1.8 oz)	50
Breast Hardwood Smoked	4 slices (1.8 oz)	50
Tyson		
Breast Oven Roasted	2 slices (1.6 oz)	40
TURKEY DISHES		
FROZEN		
gravy & turkey	1 cup (8.4 oz)	160
TAKE-OUT		
boneless breast w/ cranberry apple stuffing	1 serv (5 oz)	260
turkey a la king	1 cup (8.5 oz)	465
turkey creole w/o rice	1 cup	189
turkey croquette	1 (2 oz)	158
turkey divan	1 cup	321
turkey fricassee	1 cup	322
turkey meatloaf	1 lg slice (5 oz)	243
turkey salad	1 cup	417
turkey tetrazzini	1 cup	369
TURKEY SUBSTITUTES		
Worthington		
Turkee Slices	3 slices (3.3 oz)	180
Yves		
Meatless Deli Turkey Slices	4 slices	100
Meatless Ground Turkey	⅓ cup	60

FOOD	PORTION	CALS
TURMERIC		
ground	1 tsp	8
TURNIPS		
canned greens	½ cup	17
cooked mashed	½ cup (4.2 oz)	47
cubed cooked	½ cup (3 oz)	33
fresh greens chopped cooked	½ cup	15
frzn greens cooked	½ cup	24
greens raw chopped	½ cup	7
raw cubed	½ cup (2.4 oz)	25
Allens		
Seasoned	½ cup	35
Glory		
Greens Fresh	2 cups	20
Greens Seasoned canned	½ cup	35
Root Cut Fresh	½ cup	20
Sensibly Seasoned Greens	½ cup	20
TURTLE		
raw	3.5 oz	85
TUSK FISH		
raw	3.5 oz	79
VANILLA		
vanilla extract	1 tbsp (0.5 oz)	37
vanilla extract	1 tsp (4.2 g)	12
vanilla extract alcohol free	1 tsp (4.2 g)	2
Bob's Red Mill		
Organic Extract	1 tsp	0
Nielsen-Massey		
Madagascar Bourbon Extract	1 tsp	11
VEAL (see also VEAL DISHES)		
breast braised	3 oz	226
chop breaded fried	1 med (6.5 oz)	290
chop cooked	1 med (6.5 oz)	230
cubed braised	3 oz	160
cutlet cooked	3 oz	141
ground broiled	3 oz	146
leg roasted	3 oz	136

FOOD	PORTION	CALS
loin roasted	3 oz	184
patty breaded fried	1 (2.8 oz)	211
shank braised	3 oz	162

VEAL DISHES
TAKE-OUT

FOOD	PORTION	CALS
cordon bleu	1 serv (8 oz)	490
marengo	1 serv (8.8 oz)	274
marsala	1 slice + sauce (3.4 oz)	268
paprikash	1 serv (8.6 oz)	280
parmigiana	1 serv (6.4 oz)	362
picatta	1 piece + sauce (3.5 oz)	154
scallopini	1 slice + sauce (3.4 oz)	238
stew	1 serv (8.8 oz)	192

VEGETABLE JUICE

FOOD	PORTION	CALS
low sodium tomato & vegetable juice	1 cup	53
vegetable juice cocktail	8 oz	46
Bolthouse Farms		
Vedge Tomato Carrot Celery	8 oz	60
Dei Fratelli		
Vegetable Juice	8 oz	45
Green To Go		
100% Natural Organic as prep	1 pkg (0.3 oz)	32
Lakewood		
Super Veggie	6 oz	40
Mott's		
100% Juice Veggie Blend	1 bottle (14 oz)	90
V8		
100% Vegetable Essential Antioxidants	8 oz	50
Calcium Enriched	8 oz	50
High Fiber	8 oz	60
Low Sodium	8 oz	50
Low Sodium Spicy Hot	8 oz	50
Vegetable Juice	8 oz	50
Walnut Acres		
Organic Incredible Vegetable	8 oz	50

FOOD	PORTION	CALS
VEGETABLES MIXED		
CANNED		
mixed vegetables	½ cup	39
peas & carrots	½ cup (4.5 oz)	48
peas & onions	½ cup (2.1 oz)	31
succotash	½ cup	102
Del Monte		
Savory Sides Homestyle Vegetable Medley	½ cup	70
Savory Sides Rio Grande Vegetables	½ cup	70
McSweet		
Giardiniera	5 pieces (1 oz)	25
S&W		
Mixed	½ cup (4.4 oz)	45
Peas & Pearl Onions	½ cup (4.3 oz)	40
The Gracious Gourmet		
Tapenade Fennel Blood Orange	2 tbsp (1 oz)	50
Veg-All		
Original Mixed	½ cup	40
DRIED		
Crunchies		
Freeze Dried Power Veggies Buttered	½ cup (0.7 oz)	110
Freeze Dried Power Veggies Herb Spiced	½ cup (0.7 oz)	110
Freeze Dried Roasted Veggies	⅝ cup (1 oz)	100
Freeze Dried Roasted Veggies BBQ	½ cup (0.8 oz)	100
Fun-Yums		
Fresh Crispy Mixed Veggies	1 serv (0.9 oz)	114
FRESH		
Dole		
Stir Fry Medley	1 cup (3 oz)	30
Vegetable Medley	3 oz	30
Mann's		
Broccoli & Carrots	1 serv (3 oz)	25
Broccoli & Cauliflower	1 serv (3 oz)	25
California Stir Fry	1 serv (3 oz)	30
Low Mein Stir Fry	1 serv (3 oz)	80
Medley	1 serv (3 oz)	25
Ready Pac		
Carrots & Celery w/ Ranch Dressing	1 pkg (7 oz)	250
Ready Fixin's Chop Suey	1½ cups (3 oz)	15

FOOD	PORTION	CALS
FROZEN		
mixed vegetables cooked	½ cup	54
peas & carrots cooked	½ cup (2.8 oz)	38
peas & carrots creamed	½ cup (4.3 oz)	111
succotash cooked	½ cup	79
Birds Eye		
Asparagus Gold & White Corn & Baby Carrots	⅔ cup	70
Italian Herb Harvest Vegetables	1¼ cups	90
Spring Vegetables In Citrus Sauce	1¼ cups	70
Steamfresh Asian Medley	1 cup (3.3 oz)	50
Steamfresh Broccoli Cauliflower & Carrots	¾ cup	30
Steamfresh Broccoli & Cauliflower	1 cup	30
Steamfresh Broccoli Carrots Sugar Snap Peas & Water Chestnuts	¾ cup (2.9 oz)	35
Steamfresh Mixed Vegetables	⅔ cup (3.2 oz)	40
C&W		
Early Harvest Peas & Baby Carrots	⅔ cup	60
Petite Peas & Pearl Onions	⅔ cup	60
Cascadian Farm		
Organic Peas & Carrots	⅔ cup	50
Organic Mixed Vegetables	⅔ cup	60
French Meadow Bakery		
Vegetarian Sweet N' Spicy Cuban Style Veggies	1 pkg (12 oz)	250
Green Giant		
Garden Vegetable Medley as prep	½ cup	70
Mixed Vegetables as prep	½ cup	50
Southwestern Style as prep	½ cup	90
Steamers Basil Vegetable Medley as prep	¾ cup	45
Szechuan Vegetables as prep	½ cup	50
Health Is Wealth		
Veggie Munchees Vegan	6 (3 oz)	150
La Choy		
Chop Suey Vegetables	½ cup (2.2 oz)	15
Fancy Chinese Mixed Vegetables	½ cup (2.9 oz)	15
Stir Fry Vegetables	½ cup	15
Melrose Made Gourmet		
Vegetable Souffle Fat Free	1 serv (4 oz)	70
Seapoint Farms		
Organic Veggie Blends w/ Edamame Eat Your Greens	¾ cup	60

FOOD	PORTION	CALS
Veggie Blends w/ Edamame Garden	¾ cup	60
Veggie Blends w/ Edamame Oriental	¾ cup	60
TAKE-OUT		
buddha's delight	1 serv (16 oz)	174
fukujinzuke japanese pickled vegetables	1 tbsp (6 g)	8
pakoras	4 (1.7 oz)	57
ratatouille	1 serv (3.5 oz)	96
samosa	1 (2.4 oz)	206
stir fry mixed vegetables	1 serv (4 oz)	66
succotash	½ cup	111
VENISON (see also JERKY)		
cubed stewed	1 cup (5 oz)	266
hamburger grilled	1 (3.3 oz)	174
loin steak lean only broiled	1 (2 oz)	81
shoulder lean only braised	3 oz	162
tenderloin roasted	3 oz	127
top round lean only broiled	3 oz	129
TAKE-OUT		
meatloaf	1 lg slice (5 oz)	238
stew w/ potatoes & vegetables	1 cup (8.8 oz)	179
VINEGAR		
balsamic	1 tbsp	14
cider	1 tbsp	3
coconut	1 tbsp (0.5 oz)	1
red wine	1 tbsp	3
white	1 tbsp	3
Barengo		
Balsamic	1 tbsp (0.5 oz)	15
Red Wine	1 tbsp (0.5 oz)	0
Carapelli		
Balsamic	1 tbsp	15
Red Wine	1 tbsp	5
White Wine	1 tbsp	5
Gedney		
Apple Cider	1 tbsp	3
Distilled White	1 tbsp	3
Gourme Mist		
Balsamic Of Modena	1 sec spray	1
Balsamic Vinegar+ Raspberry	1 sec spray	1

FOOD	PORTION	CALS
Heinz		
Apple Cider	1 tbsp (0.5 oz)	0
Malt	1 (0.5 oz)	0
Red Wine	1 tbsp (1 oz)	0
Tarragon	1 tbsp (0.5 oz)	0
White	1 tbsp (0.5 oz)	0
Holland House		
Malt	1 tbsp (0.5 oz)	0
Red Wine	1 tbsp (0.5 oz)	0
Latino Chef		
Lulo	1 tbsp	35
Passion Fruit	1 tbsp	40
Lucini		
Balsamic 10 Year Gran Reserve	1 tbsp (0.5 oz)	20
Balsamic Dark Cherry Infused	1 tbsp	30
Italian Wine Pinot Noir	1 tbsp (0.5 oz)	<1
Mitsukan		
Rice	1 tbsp (0.5 oz)	0
Rice Seasoned	1 tbsp (0.5 oz)	25
Nakano		
Natural Rice	1 tbsp (0.5 oz)	0
Red Wine Italian Herb Seasoned	1 tbsp (0.5 oz)	20
Rice Pesto Seasoned	1 tbsp (0.5 oz)	20
Rice Red Pepper Seasoned	1 tbsp (0.5 oz)	20
Progresso		
Balsamic	2 tbsp (0.5 oz)	10
Tree Of Life		
Organic Apple Cider Raw Unfiltered	1 tbsp	0

WAFFLES
FROZEN

FOOD	PORTION	CALS
Aunt Jemima		
Blueberry	2 (2.5 oz)	170
Buttermilk	2 (2.5 oz)	190
Homestyle	2 (2.5 oz)	160
Low Fat	2 (2.5 oz)	160
Kashi		
Heart To Heart Honey Oat	2 (3 oz)	160
Lifestream		
Organic Fig + Flax	2 (2.8 oz)	210
Organic Pomegran Plus	2 (2.8 oz)	190

FOOD	PORTION	CALS
Smucker's		
Snack'n Waffles Blueberry	1 (2 oz)	230
Snack'n Waffles Maple	1 (2 oz)	220
Van's		
Belgian Multigrain	2 (2.7 oz)	190
Mini Homestyle	4 (2.8 oz)	210
Organic Flax	2 (2.7 oz)	190
Organic Homestyle	2 (2.7 oz)	200
Original 97% Fat Free	2 (2.7 oz)	140
Original Buttermilk	2 (2.7 oz)	220
Wheat Free Buckwheat	2 (3 oz)	230
Wheat Free Flax	2 (3 oz)	210
MIX		
plain as prep	1 (2.6 oz) 7 in diam	218
READY-TO-EAT		
Kashi		
GoLean Blueberry	2 (3 oz)	170
GoLean Original	2 (3 oz)	170
Unique Belgique		
Imported From Belgium	2 (2.3 oz)	230
TAKE-OUT		
belgian	1 (4.7 oz)	412
blueberry 9 in sq	1 (7 oz)	556
round 10 in diam	1 (6.8 oz)	598
square 9 in	1 (7 oz)	620
whole wheat 9 in sq	1 (7 oz)	534
WALNUTS		
black chopped	¼ cup	193
english chopped	¼ cup	191
english ground	¼ cup	131
english halves	14 (1 oz)	185
english in shell	7 (1 oz)	183
honey roasted	¼ cup	172
Back To Nature		
Unroasted Unsalted	1 oz	190
Diamond		
Chopped	¼ cup	200
Planters		
Halves	1 oz	190

FOOD	PORTION	CALS
NUT-rition Omega-3 Mix	¼ cup (1.1 oz)	160
Recipe Ready Pieces	½ pkg (1 oz)	210
WASABI (see HORSERADISH)		
WATER		
ice cubes	3	0
tap water	8 oz	0
Acquafibre		
Fiber Enhanced All Flavors	1 bottle (11.15 oz)	5
Adirondack		
Sparkling All Flavors	8 oz	0
Aloe Breeze		
Organic All Flavors	8 oz	0
Apple & Eve		
Water Fruits All Flavors	1 bottle (10 oz)	90
Aqua Pacific		
Water	1 liter	0
Aquafina		
Alive Wellness Berry Pomegranate	8 oz	10
Arizona		
Rescue Relax	8 oz	25
Vapor	8 oz	0
Ayala's		
Herbal All Flavors	1 bottle	0
Bot		
Fortified All Flavors	1 bottle (12 oz)	40
Dasani		
Purified Water	8 oz	0
Dox		
Cardio Water	1 bottle (12 oz)	20
Evian		
Spring Water	1 liter	0
EX		
Aqua Vitamins Raspberry	1 bottle (16.9 oz)	110
Fiji		
Natural Artesian	1 liter	0
Gerolsteiner		
Sparkling Mineral	8 oz	0
H 10 O		
Citrus Sport For Men	1 bottle (15.9 oz)	0
Peach Mango Tea For Women	1 bottle (15.9 oz)	0

FOOD	PORTION	CALS
H2Odwalla		
Enhanced Tropical Orange	1 bottle (20 oz)	120
Organic Enhanced Blueberry Tea	1 bottle (20 oz)	120
Organic Enhanced Jasmine Lime	1 bottle (20 oz)	120
Hawaiian Springs		
Naturally Pure	1 liter	0
Highland Spring		
Spring Water	1 liter	0
IQ		
H2O Orange Mango	8 oz	40
Island Chill		
Artesian Water	1 liter	0
Jana		
Natural European Artesian	1 liter	0
Jones Soda		
24C Multi Vitamin Enhanced All Flavors	1 bottle	100
Klear Splash		
Mini Sip	1 pkg (4 oz)	0
Life Water		
B-Strong	1 bottle (20 oz)	100
Enlighten	1 bottle (20 oz)	100
Zingseng	1 bottle (20 oz)	100
Liquid Salvation		
Ultra Hydrating	1 bottle	0
Nui		
All Natural Kid Water	10 oz	90
O Water		
Hydrate Black Raspberry	8 oz	25
Replenish Lemon Lime	8 oz	25
Vitalize Peach Mango	8 oz	25
Propel		
Fitness Water All Flavors	1 bottle (24 oz)	30
R.W. Knudsen		
Organic Sparkling Essence Lemon	1 can (10.5 oz)	0
San Benedetto		
Sparkling Mineral Water	1 liter	0
Skinny Water		
Hi-Energy Acai Grape Blueberry	8 oz	0
Total-V Passionfruit Lemonade	8 oz	0

FOOD	PORTION	CALS
Snapple		
Antioxidant Water Awaken Dragonfruit	8 oz	50
Antioxidant Water Restore Agave Melon	8 oz	60
Lyte Water	8 oz	0
SoNu		
Organic 10 Calories All Flavors	8 oz	10
Organic All Flavors	8 oz	45
Sparkling Ice		
All Flavors	1 bottle (16 oz)	0
Special K2O		
Protein Water All Flavors	1 bottle (16.6 oz)	50
Trim Water		
Purified	1 bottle (20 oz)	10
Twist		
Organics All Flavors	8 oz	10
Victoria's Kitchen		
Almond Water	8 oz	55
Vitamin + Fiber Water		
All Fruit Flavors	8 oz	50
VitaminWater		
XXX Acai Blueberry Pomegranate	8 oz	50
WaterPlus		
Antioxidants Acai Berry	8 oz	50
Electrolytes Fruit Punch	8 oz	50
Extra-C Orange Tangerine	8 oz	50
Vitamins Dragonfruit Kiwi	8 oz	50
WATER CHESTNUTS		
chinese sliced canned	½ cup	35
fresh sliced	½ cup	66
La Choy		
Sliced	½ cup	25
Polar		
Sliced	2 tbsp	10
WATERCRESS		
cooked w/o fat	1 cup	15
raw chopped	1 cup	4
WATERMELON		
cut up	1 cup	46
seeds dried	¼ cup	150

FOOD	PORTION	CALS
wedge	1 sm (2.5 oz)	21
wedge	1 med (10 oz)	86
wedge	1 lg (20 oz)	172
whole melon	1 (9 lb)	1227
Jake & Amos		
Pickled Sweet Rind	2 tbsp (1 oz)	70
Mini Me		
Personal Seedless	2 cups (10 oz)	80

WATERMELON JUICE

juice	8 oz	71
Arizona		
Fruit Juice Cocktail	8 oz	100
EarthWise		
Watermelon Supreme	8 oz	100
Izze		
Esque Sparkling Watermelon	1 bottle (12 oz)	50

WHALE

beluga dried	1 oz	93
beluga raw	3.5 oz	111

WHEAT

sprouted	1 cup (3.8 oz)	214
starch	3.5 oz	348
Amazing Grass		
Organic Wheat Grass	1 tbsp (0.3 oz)	35
Arrowhead Mills		
Whole Grain Wheat	¼ cup (1.6 oz)	150
Bob's Red Mill		
Vital Wheat Gluten	¼ cup	120
Near East		
Taboule Wheat Salad as prep	⅔ cup (3.5 oz)	120
White Wave		
Seitan Chicken Meat Of Wheat	3 oz	130
Seitan Traditional	3 oz	90
Seitan Vegetarian Stir Fry Strips	3 oz	110

WHEAT GERM

plain	¼ cup	108
Bob's Red Mill		
Wheat Germ	2 tbsp	59

FOOD	PORTION	CALS
Kretschmer		
Original Toasted	¼ cup (0.6 oz)	35
Mother's		
Wheat Germ	2 tbsp (0.5 oz)	50
Tree Of Life		
Toasted	3 tbsp (0.8 oz)	100
WHEY		
acid dry	1 tbsp	10
sweet dry	1 tbsp	26
sweet fluid	½ cup	33
whey cheese	1 oz	126
Action Whey		
Dream Shake All Flavors	1 scoop (0.8 oz)	90
Bob's Red Mill		
Protein Concentrate	¼ cup	80
Sweet Dairy	1 tbsp	30
Premier		
100% Whey Isolate	2 scoops (1.5 oz)	160
Wellements		
Whey Protein Chocolate	1 scoop (1 oz)	120
Whey Protein Vanilla	1 scoop (1 oz)	120
WHIPPED TOPPINGS		
dairy fat free pressurized	¼ cup (0.6 oz)	24
nondairy fat free frzn	¼ cup (0.7 oz)	28
nondairy frzn	¼ cup (0.7 oz)	60
nondairy lowfat frzn	¼ cup (0.7 oz)	42
nondairy pressurized	¼ cup (0.6 oz)	46
Cool Whip		
Chocolate	2 tbsp	25
Free	2 tbsp	15
Regular	2 tbsp	25
Strawberry	2 tbsp	25
Soyatoo		
Rice Whip	2 tbsp (6 g)	10
Soy Whip	2 tbsp (6 g)	10
Truwhip		
Whipped Topping	2 tbsp (0.4 oz)	30

FOOD	PORTION	CALS
WHITE BEANS		
canned	1 cup (9.2 oz)	299
dried small cooked w/o salt	1 cup (6.3 oz)	254
WHITEFISH		
baked	3 oz	146
fillet grilled no added fat	1 (5.4 oz)	265
smoked boneless	1 oz	31
WHITING		
broiled w/o fat	3 oz	99
fillet broiled w/o fat	1 (2.5 oz)	84
fillet steamed w/o fat	1 (2.6 oz)	84
hake raw	3.5 oz	84
TAKE-OUT		
fillet battered & fried	1 (3.1 oz)	157
fillet breaded & fried	1 (3.1 oz)	191
WILD RICE		
cooked	1 cup (5.8 oz)	166
Gourmet House		
Cracked as prep	1 cup	170
Quick Cooking not prep	½ cup	170
Thai Jasmine as prep	¾ cup	160
Lundberg		
Organic Quick not prep	¼ cup	150
WINE		
chianti	1 serv (5 oz)	125
chinese cooking	1 bottle (15 oz)	559
cooking	¼ cup (2 oz)	29
haiku	1 serv	93
japanese plum	3 oz	139
japanese sake	2 oz	78
kir	1 serv	78
liebfraumilch	4 oz	86
madeira	3.5 oz	169
marsala	4 oz	80
merlot	4 oz	95
muscat	1 serv (5 oz)	123
nonalcoholic	1 serv (5 oz)	9
port	1 serv (3.5 oz)	165

FOOD	PORTION	CALS
red barbera	1 serv (5 oz)	125
red burgundy	1 serv (5 oz)	127
red cabernet franc	1 serv (5 oz)	122
red claret	1 serv (5 oz)	122
red gamay	1 serv (5 oz)	115
red mouvedre	1 serv (5 oz)	129
red pinot noir	1 serv (5 oz)	121
red syrah	1 serv (5 oz)	122
red zinfandel	1 serv (5 oz)	129
sake screwdriver	1 serv	175
sangria	1 serv	88
sangria blanco	1 serv	155
sherry	2 oz	84
vermouth dry	3.5 oz	105
vermouth sweet	3.5 oz	167
wassail wine	1 serv	142
white	1 serv (5 oz)	121
white fume blanc	1 serv (5 oz)	121
white pinot blanc	1 serv (5 oz)	119
white pinot grigio	1 serv (5 oz)	122
white riesling	1 serv (5 oz)	118
white sauvignon blanc	1 serv (5 oz)	119
wine cooler	1 (7 oz)	116
wine spritzer	1 serv (7 oz)	73
Almaden		
Merlot	5 oz	115
Bartles & Jaymes		
Wine Cooler Classic Original	1 bottle (12 oz)	190
Beringer		
Chardonnay	5 oz	125
Carlo Rossi		
Cabernet Sauvignon	5 oz	125
Franzia Vinter		
Select Merlot	5 oz	105
Holland House		
Cooking Wine Marsala	2 tbsp (1 oz)	45
Cooking Wine Red	2 tbsp (1 oz)	20
Cooking Wine Sherry	2 tbsp (1 oz)	45
Cooking Wine Vermouth	2 tbsp (1 oz)	35
Cooking Wine White	2 tbsp (1 oz)	20

FOOD	PORTION	CALS
Kedem		
Cooking Red	2 tbsp (1 oz)	30
Cooking Sherry	2 tbsp (1 oz)	40
Cooking Wine Marsala	2 tbsp (1 oz)	40
Twin Valley		
Cabernet Sauvignon	5 oz	120

WINGED BEANS

dried cooked w/o salt	1 cup	253

WRAPS (see BREAD, SANDWICHES)

YACON

Navitas Naturals		
Slices Dried	1 oz	90

YAM (see also SWEET POTATO)
CANNED

Glory		
Candied	½ cup	210
S&W		
Candied	½ cup (4.9 oz)	170
FRESH		
mountain yam hawaii cooked w/o salt	1 cup	119
yam cooked w/o salt	1 cup	158
Earthbound Farms		
Organic	1 med (4.6 oz)	130
House		
Black Ita Konnyaku Yam Cake	1 serv (2 oz)	5

YARDLONG BEANS

sliced cooked w/o salt	1 cup	49

YAUTIA (see MALANGA)

YEAST

baker's compressed	1 cake (0.6 oz)	18
baker's dry	1 tbsp	35
baker's dry	1 pkg (7 g)	21
brewer's dry	1 tbsp	35
Bob's Red Mill		
Active Dry	1 tbsp	25

FOOD	PORTION	CALS
YELLOW BEANS		
fresh cooked w/o salt	1 cup	44
fresh raw	1 cup	34
YELLOWTAIL		
baked	4 oz	199
YOGURT (see also YOGURT DRINKS, YOGURT FROZEN)		
plain lowfat	8 oz	143
plain nonfat	8 oz	127
plain whole milk	8 oz	138
tofu yogurt	1 cup	246
Better Whey		
All Fruit Flavors	1 pkg (6 oz)	145
Plain	1 pkg (6 oz)	130
Breyers		
Creme Savers All Flavors	1 pkg (6 oz)	160
Fruit On The Bottom Black Cherry	1 pkg (6 oz)	160
Fruit On The Bottom Chocolate Raspberry	1 pkg (6 oz)	170
Fruit On The Bottom Mixed Berry	1 pkg (6 oz)	160
Fruit On The Bottom Peach Mango Orange	1 pkg (6 oz)	160
Fruit On The Bottom Pineapple	1 pkg (6 oz)	150
Fruit On The Bottom Strawberry	1 pkg (6 oz)	150
Inspirations Cherry Chocolate Chip	1 pkg (4 oz)	140
Inspirations Mint Chocolate Chip	1 pkg (4 oz)	140
Inspirations Vanilla Bean	1 pkg (4 oz)	110
Light Blueberry	1 pkg (4 oz)	50
Smooth & Creamy Peaches 'N Cream	1 pkg (4 oz)	120
Smooth & Creamy Strawberry	1 pkg (4 oz)	110
Cabot		
Greek	1 pkg (6 oz)	210
Greek 2%	1 pkg (6 oz)	160
Non Fat Berry Banana	1 cup	130
Non Fat Black Cherry	1 cup	130
Non Fat French Vanilla	1 cup	130
Non Fat Plain	1 cup	100
Non Fat Raspberry	1 cup	130
Chobani		
Champions Honey-nana	1 pkg (3.5 oz)	100
Greek Yogurt Nonfat Blueberry	1 pkg (6 oz)	140
Greek Yogurt Nonfat Caramel	1 pkg (6 oz)	140

FOOD	PORTION	CALS
Greek Yogurt Nonfat Honey	1 pkg (6 oz)	150
Greek Yogurt Nonfat Peach	1 pkg (6 oz)	140
Greek Yogurt Nonfat Plain	1 pkg (6 oz)	100
Greek Yogurt Nonfat Pomegranate	1 pkg (6 oz)	140
Greek Yogurt Nonfat Raspberry	1 pkg (6 oz)	140
Greek Yogurt Nonfat Strawberry	1 pkg (6 oz)	140
Greek Yogurt Nonfat Vanilla	1 pkg (6 oz)	120
Dannon		
Activia Blueberry	1 pkg (4 oz)	110
Activia Cherry	1 pkg (4 oz)	110
Activia Harvest Picks Strawberry	1 pkg (4 oz)	110
Activia Peach	1 pkg (4 oz)	110
Activia Prune	1 pkg (4 oz)	110
Activia Strawberry	1 pkg (4 oz)	120
Activia Strawberry Banana	1 pkg (4 oz)	110
Activia Vanilla	1 pkg (4 oz)	110
Activia Light Blueberry	1 pkg (4 oz)	70
Activia Light Peach	1 pkg (4 oz)	70
Activia Light Raspberry	1 pkg (4 oz)	70
Activia Light Strawberry	1 pkg (4 oz)	70
Activia Light Vanilla	1 pkg (4 oz)	70
All Natural Coffee	1 pkg (6 oz)	150
All Natural Lemon	1 pkg (6 oz)	150
All Natural Plain	1 pkg (6 oz)	100
All Natural Vanilla	1 pkg (6 oz)	150
Ehrmann		
Bavarian Lowfat Peach	1 pkg	104
Bavarian Lowfat Strawberry	1 pkg	140
Emmi		
Apricot Low-fat	1 pkg (6 oz)	170
Green Apple Low-fat	1 pkg (6 oz)	170
Pink Grapefruit Low-fat	1 pkg (6 oz)	170
Plain Low-fat	1 pkg (6 oz)	170
Fage		
Total Cherry	1 pkg (5.3 oz)	170
Total Peach	1 pkg (5.3 oz)	170
Total Plain	1 pkg (5.3 oz)	190
Total Strawberry	1 pkg (5.3 oz)	170
Total 0% Cherry	1 pkg (5.3 oz)	130
Total 0% Cherry Pomegranate	1 pkg (5.3 oz)	130

FOOD	PORTION	CALS
Total 0% Honey	1 pkg (5.3 oz)	120
Total 0% Mango Guanabana	1 pkg (5.3 oz)	120
Total 0% Peach	1 pkg (5.3 oz)	120
Total 0% Plain	1 pkg (5.3 oz)	100
Total 2% Cherry	1 pkg (5.3 oz)	140
Total 2% Plain	1 pkg (5.3 oz)	150
Total 2% Strawberry	1 pkg (5.3 oz)	140
Fiber One		
Creamy Nonfat Vanilla	1 pkg (4 oz)	80
Friendship		
Plain	1 cup	150
Green Valley		
Organic Lactose Free Blueberry	1 pkg (6 oz)	140
Organic Lactose Free Honey	1 pkg (6 oz)	140
Organic Lactose Free Plain	1 pkg (6 oz)	100
Organic Lactose Free Vanilla	1 pkg (6 oz)	120
Horizon Organic		
Kids Strawberry	1 pkg (4 oz)	110
Lowfat Blended Blueberry	1 pkg (6 oz)	160
Tube Lowfat Blueberry	1 (2 oz)	70
Whole Milk Plain	1 cup	160
Karoun		
Plain Lowfat	1 cup (8 oz)	180
Plain Whole Milk	1 cup (8 oz)	210
La Yogurt		
Lowfat Blueberries 'N' Cream	1 pkg (6 oz)	200
Lowfat Fruit On The Bottom Cherry	1 pkg (8 oz)	230
Lowfat Fruit On The Bottom Probiotic Peach	1 pkg (6 oz)	160
Lowfat Fruit On The Bottom Strawberry	1 pkg (8 oz)	220
Lowfat Peaches 'N' Cream	1 pkg (6 oz)	200
Lowfat Pina Colada	1 pkg (6 oz)	160
Lowfat Probiotic Pina Colada	1 pkg (6 oz)	160
Lowfat Probiotic Plain	1 pkg (6 oz)	100
Lowfat Probiotic Vanilla	1 pkg (6 oz)	150
Lowfat Vanilla 'N' Cream	1 pkg (6 oz)	200
Nonfat Banana Cream	1 pkg (6 oz)	100
Nonfat Probiotic Cherry	1 pkg (6 oz)	100
Nonfat Probiotic Peach	1 pkg (6 oz)	90
Nonfat Probiotic Raspberry	1 pkg (6 oz)	90
Nonfat Probiotic Vanilla	1 pkg (6 oz)	90

FOOD	PORTION	CALS
Sabor Latino Lowfat Dulce De Leche	1 pkg (6 oz)	190
Sabor Latino Lowfat Guava	1 pkg (6 oz)	190
Sabor Latino Lowfat Horchata	1 pkg (6 oz)	210
Sabor Latino Lowfat Papaya	1 pkg (6 oz)	190
Land O'Lakes		
Strawberry Light	1 pkg (8 oz)	80
Strawberry Lowfat	1 pkg (8 oz)	190
Liberte		
Plain Lowfat	1 pkg (6 oz)	110
Six Grains Peach	1 pkg (6 oz)	150
Six Grains Pear	1 pkg (6 oz)	160
Lowell		
Multi Grain Peach & Whole Grain	1 pkg (6 oz)	170
Mountain High		
Black Cherry Classic Lowfat	1 pkg (6 oz)	140
Blueberry Classic Lowfat	1 pkg (6 oz)	140
Lemon Lowfat	1 pkg (8 oz)	190
Mountain Berry Classic Lowfat	1 pkg (6 oz)	150
Plain Fat Free	1 pkg (8 oz)	120
Plain Lowfat	1 pkg (8 oz)	140
Plain Original	1 pkg (8 oz)	180
Strawberry Classic Lowfat	1 pkg (6 oz)	140
Vanilla Fat Free	1 pkg (8 oz)	160
Vanilla Lowfat	1 pkg (8 oz)	180
Vanilla Original	1 pkg (8 oz)	210
Nancy's		
Lowfat Lemon	1 pkg (8 oz)	150
Lowfat Maple	1 pkg (8 oz)	180
Lowfat Peach	1 pkg (8 oz)	170
Lowfat Plain	1 pkg (8 oz)	150
Lowfat Vanilla	1 pkg (8 oz)	140
Organic Soy Kiwi Lime	1 pkg (6 oz)	160
Organic Soy Mango	1 (6 oz)	170
Organic Soy Plain	1 pkg (6 oz)	150
Organic Soy Vanilla	1 pkg (6 oz)	120
Organic Whole Milk Fruit On The Top Blackberry	1 pkg (8 oz)	220
Organic Whole Milk Fruit On The Top Cherry	1 pkg (8 oz)	220
Organic Whole Milk Fruit On The Top Peach	1 pkg (8 oz)	220
Organic Whole Milk Honey	1 pkg (8 oz)	170
Organic Whole Milk Plain	1 pkg (8 oz)	130

FOOD	PORTION	CALS
Oikos		
Blueberry	1 pkg (5.3 oz)	120
Caramel	1 pkg (4 oz)	110
Chocolate	1 pkg (4 oz)	110
Honey	1 pkg (5.3 oz)	120
Plain	1 pkg (5.3 oz)	80
Strawberry	1 pkg (5.3 oz)	110
Super Fruits	1 pkg (5.3 oz)	130
Vanilla	1 pkg (5.3 oz)	110
Olympus		
Greek Strained Strawberry 1% Lowfat	1 pkg (6 oz)	155
Rachel's		
Essence Berry Jasmine w/ Zinc	1 pkg (6 oz)	160
Essence Plum Honey Lavender	1 pkg (6 oz)	160
Essence Pomegranate Acai	1 pkg (6 oz)	170
Exotic Kiwi Passion Fruit Lime	1 pkg (6 oz)	160
Exotic Orange Strawberry Mango	1 pkg (6 oz)	160
Exotic Pomegranate Blueberry	1 pkg (6 oz)	170
Siggi's		
Icelandic Skyr Vanilla 0% Milkfat	1 pkg (6 oz)	120
Silk		
Live! Blueberry	1 pkg (6 oz)	150
Soy Blueberry	1 pkg (6 oz)	150
Soy Key Lime	1 pkg (6 oz)	150
Soy Plain	1 cup (8 oz)	150
Soy Vanilla	1 pkg (6 oz)	150
Strawberry	1 pkg (6 oz)	160
SoDelicious		
Coconut Milk Plain	1 pkg (6 oz)	130
Coconut Milk Vanilla	1 pkg (6 oz)	150
Dairy Free Cinnamon Bun	1 pkg (6 oz)	160
Dairy Free Raspberry	1 pkg (6 oz)	150
Stonyfield Farm		
0% Fat Chocolate Underground	1 pkg (6 oz)	150
0% Fat Fruit On The Bottom Blueberry	1 pkg (6 oz)	120
0% Fat Fruit On The Bottom Pomegranate Raspberry	1 pkg (6 oz)	120
0% Fat Fruit On The Bottom Strawberry	1 pkg (6 oz)	110
0% Fat Smooth & Creamy Black Cherry	1 pkg (6 oz)	100
0% Fat Smooth & Creamy French Vanilla	1 pkg (6 oz)	100

FOOD	PORTION	CALS
0% Fat Smooth & Creamy Key Lime	1 pkg (6 oz)	100
0% Fat Smooth & Creamy Lemon	1 pkg (6 oz)	100
0% Fat Smooth & Creamy Peach	1 pkg (6 oz)	100
0% Fat Smooth & Creamy Plain	1 pkg (6 oz)	80
0% Fat Smooth & Creamy Pomegranate Berry	1 pkg (6 oz)	100
0% Fat Smooth & Creamy Strawberry	1 pkg (6 oz)	100
Lowfat Cherry Vanilla	1 pkg (6 oz)	130
Lowfat Fruit On The Bottom Blueberry	1 pkg (6 oz)	120
Lowfat Fruit On The Bottom Peach	1 pkg (6 oz)	130
Lowfat Fruit On The Bottom Strawberry	1 pkg (6 oz)	120
Lowfat Plain	1 pkg (6 oz)	90
O'Soy Chocolate	1 pkg (6 oz)	160
O'Soy Fruit On The Bottom Peach	1 pkg (6 oz)	170
O'Soy Fruit On The Bottom Strawberry	1 pkg (6 oz)	170
O'Soy Vanilla	1 pkg (6 oz)	150
Whole Milk Cream Top French Vanilla	1 pkg (6 oz)	170
Whole Milk Cream Top White Chocolate Raspberry	1 pkg (6 oz)	170
Straus		
Organic Blueberry Pomegranate	1 cup (8 oz)	220
Organic Cinnamon Nonfat	1 cup (8 oz)	190
Organic Maple Whole Milk	1 cup (8 oz)	210
Organic Plain Lowfat	1 cup (8 oz)	150
Organic Plain Nonfat	1 cup (8 oz)	120
Organic Vanilla Nonfat	1 cup (8 oz)	190
The Greek Gods		
Honey Nonfat	1 pkg (6 oz)	250
Plain	1 pkg (6 oz)	60
Plain Traditional	1 pkg (4 oz)	130
Pomegranate	1 pkg (6 oz)	230
Vanilla Cinnamon Orange Reduced Fat	1 pkg (6 oz)	170
Voskos		
Greek Yogurt Exotic Fig	1 pkg (8 oz)	160
Greek Yogurt Plain Low Fat	1 pkg (8 oz)	160
Greek Yogurt Plain Non Fat	1 pkg (8 oz)	140
Greek Yogurt Plain Original	1 pkg (8 oz)	280
Greek Yogurt Wild Blueberry	1 pkg (8 oz)	120
Organic Vanilla Bean	1 pkg (5.3 oz)	130
Wallaby		
Lowfat Banana Vanilla	1 pkg (6 oz)	140

FOOD	PORTION	CALS
Lowfat Lemon	1 pkg (6 oz)	140
Lowfat Maple	1 pkg (6 oz)	140
Lowfat Plain	1 pkg (8 oz)	140
Lowfat Raspberry	1 pkg (6 oz)	140
Lowfat Vanilla	1 pkg (6 oz)	140
Original Guava	1 pkg (6 oz)	170
Whole Soy & Co.		
Apricot Mango	1 pkg (6 oz)	160
Cherry	1 pkg (6 oz)	170
Lemon	1 pkg (6 oz)	160
Plain	1 pkg (6 oz)	150
Strawberry	1 pkg (6 oz)	160
Vanilla	1 pkg (6 oz)	160
WildWood		
Organic Soyogurt Low Fat Peach	1 pkg (6 oz)	160
Organic Soyogurt Low Fat Vanilla	1 pkg (6 oz)	160
Organic Soyogurt Plain Unsweetened	1 pkg (6 oz)	110
Yofarm		
YoSmooth Apricot	1 pkg	220
YoSmooth Peach	1 pkg	220
YoSmooth Raspberry	1 pkg	230
Yoplait		
Delights Chocolate Raspberry	1 pkg (4 oz)	100
Delights Lemon Torte	1 pkg (4 oz)	100
Delights Triple Berry Creme	1 pkg (4 oz)	100
Light Strawberry	1 pkg (4 oz)	50
Original Coconut Cream	1 pkg (6 oz)	190
Original Lemon Burst	1 pkg (6 oz)	180
Original PassionFruit	1 pkg (6 oz)	170
Original Pina Colada	1 pkg (6 oz)	170
Whips All Chocolate Flavors	1 pkg (6 oz)	160
Whips All Fruit Flavors	1 pkg (4 oz)	140
Yo Plus All Flavors	1 pkg (4 oz)	110
YOGURT DRINKS (*see also* SMOOTHIES)		
lassi	7 oz	78
Dahlicious		
Lassi Green Tea	1 bottle	110
Lassi Mango	1 bottle	130
Lassi Plain	1 bottle	110

FOOD	PORTION	CALS
Dannon		
Activia Mixed Berry	1 bottle (6 oz)	160
Activia Peach	1 bottle (6 oz)	170
Activia Vanilla	1 bottle (6 oz)	160
Danactive Blueberry	1 bottle (3.1 oz)	80
Danactive Strawberry	1 bottle (3.1 oz)	80
Danactive Vanilla	1 bottle (3.1 oz)	80
Danimals Smoothies Rockin' Raspberry	1 bottle (3.1 oz)	70
Danimals Smoothies Strawberry Explosion	1 bottle (3.1 oz)	70
Danimals Smoothies Strikin' Strawberry Kiwi	1 bottle (3.1 oz)	70
Light & Fit Smoothie Mixed Berry & Pomegranate	1 bottle (7 oz)	70
Light & Fit Smoothie Peach	1 bottle (7 oz)	70
Light & Fit Smoothie Strawberry Banana	1 bottle (7 oz)	70
Gopi		
Lassi	8 oz	126
Karoun		
Yogurt Drink	8 oz	126
Lifeway		
Lassi Mango	8 oz	160
Lassi Strawberry	8 oz	160
Promise		
Activ All Flavors	1 bottle (3.5 oz)	70
Yo On The Go		
All Flavors	1 box (8 oz)	180
Yo-Goat		
All Flavors	8 oz	160
Plain	8 oz	150
Yoplait		
Kids All Flavors	1 bottle (3.1 oz)	70
YOGURT FROZEN		
chocolate soft serve	1 cup	230
vanilla soft serve	1 cup	236
Ben & Jerry's		
Greek Banana Peanut Butter	½ cup (3.5 oz)	210
Greek Blueberry Vanilla Graham	½ cup (3.5 oz)	200
Greek Raspberry Fudge Chunk	½ cup (3.4 oz)	200
Greek Strawberry Shortcake	½ cup (3.5 oz)	180
Dippin' Dots		
Strawberry Cheesecake	½ cup	100

FOOD	PORTION	CALS
Haagen-Dazs		
Lowfat Coffee	½ cup (3.7 oz)	200
Lowfat Tart Natural	½ cup (3.6 oz)	180
Lowfat Vanilla	½ cup (3.7 oz)	200
Lowfat Wildberry	½ cup (3.7 oz)	180
Julie's		
Organic Blackberry	½ cup	190
Organic Peanut Butter Fudge	½ cup	260
Organic Strawberry	½ cup	200
Organic Vanilla	½ cup	220
Stonyfield Farm		
Fat Free After Dark Chocolate	1 serv (4 oz)	100
Fat Free Gotta Have Vanilla	1 serv (4 oz)	100
Fat Free Vanilla Fudge Swirl	1 serv (4 oz)	120
Low Fat Creme Caramel	1 serv (4 oz)	130
Lowfat Cookies 'N Cream	1 serv (4 oz)	130
Turkey Hill		
Fudge Ripple	½ cup	100
Neapolitan	½ cup	90
Smoothie Orange Cream Swirl	½ cup	100
Smoothie Peach Mango	½ cup	90
Vanilla Bean	½ cup	100
YOUNGBERRY JUICE		
Ceres		
100% Juice	8 oz	120
ZUCCHINI		
baby raw	1 (0.5 oz)	3
canned italian style	1 cup	66
fresh	1 sm (4.1 oz)	19
pickled	¼ cup	16
raw sliced	1 cup	19
sliced cooked w/o salt	1 cup	29
C&W		
Yellow & Green	⅔ cup	20
TAKE-OUT		
breaded & fried	6 slices (3 oz)	141
indian pakora	1 serv	46
sticks breaded & fried	6 (2 oz)	90

PART TWO

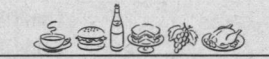

Restaurant Chains

When eating out, remember:

- The larger the portion size you are served and the more variety you are offered, the more likely you are to overeat.
- Go easy on super-sizes.
- Choose wisely at buffets.

  Put no more than 3 foods on your plate at one time.

  This forces you to make choices and return to the buffet for more food.

  This helps you think about what and how much you are eating.

FOOD	PORTION	CALS
A&W		
BEVERAGES		
Coke	1 sm (11 oz)	145
Diet Coke	1 sm (11 oz)	0
Diet Root Beer	1 sm (15 oz)	0
Float Diet Root Beer	1 sm (14 oz)	170
Float Root Beer	1 sm (14 oz)	330
Milkshake Chocolate	1 med	700
Milkshake Strawberry	1 med	670
Milkshake Vanilla	1 med	720
Root Beer	1 sm (15 oz)	220
DESSERTS		
Cone Vanilla	1 med	260
Freeze A&W Root Beer	1 med	480
Polar Swirl M&M	1 med	710
Polar Swirl Oreo	1 med	690
Polar Swirl Reese's	1 med	740
Sundae Caramel	1 med	340
Sundae Chocolate	1 med	320
Sundae Hot Fudge	1 med	350
Sundae Strawberry	1 med	300
Sundae Vanilla	1 med	310
MAIN MENU SELECTIONS		
Cheese Curds	1 serv	570
Cheese Dog	1	320
Cheeseburger Original Bacon	1	570
Cheeseburger Original Bacon Double	1	800
Cheeseburger Original Double	1	720
Chicken Strips	3	500
Chili Bowl	1 serv	190
Coney Chili Dog	1	310
Coney Chili Dog Cheese	1	350
Fries	1 lg	430
Fries Cheese	1 serv	380
Fries Chili	1 serv	370
Fries Chili & Cheese	1 serv	400
Hot Dog Plain	1	280
Onion Rings	1 serv	350
Papa Burger	1	720

FOOD	PORTION	CALS
Sandwich Crispy Chicken	1	590
Sandwich Grilled Chicken	1	440
SAUCES		
Dipping Sauce BBQ	1 serv (1 oz)	40
Dipping Sauce Honey Mustard	1 serv (1 oz)	100
Dipping Sauce Ranch	1 serv (1 oz)	160
Dipping Sauce Sweet & Sour	1 serv (1 oz)	45

ARBY'S
BEVERAGES

FOOD	PORTION	CALS
Dr. Pepper	1 (16 oz)	180
Jamocha Shake	1 reg	498
Pepsi	1 (16 oz)	130
Shake Chocolate	1 reg	507
Shake Orange Cream	1 (17 oz)	637
Shake Strawberry	1 reg	498
Shake Strawberry Banana Swirl	1 (17 oz)	567
Shake Vanilla	1 reg	437
Sierra Mist	1 (16 oz)	100
BREAKFAST SELECTIONS		
Biscuit	1	273
Biscuit Bacon	1	340
Biscuit Bacon Egg & Cheese	1	461
Biscuit Chicken	1	417
Biscuit Ham	1	316
Biscuit Ham Egg & Cheese	1	437
Biscuit Sausage	1	436
Biscuit Sausage Egg & Cheese	1	557
Biscuit Sausage Gravy	1	961
Breakfast Syrup	1 serv (1 oz)	78
Cinnamon Roll Original Gourmet	1	507
Croissant	1	190
Croissant Bacon & Egg	1	337
Croissant Bacon Egg & Cheese	1	378
Croissant Ham & Cheese	1	274
Croissant Ham Egg & Cheese	1	434
Croissant Sausage & Egg	1	433
Croissant Sausage Egg & Cheese	1	475
French Toastix	1 serv	312
Muffin Blueberry	1	320

FOOD	PORTION	CALS
Pecan Sticky Bun	1	688
Sourdough Bacon Egg & Cheese	1	437
Sourdough Egg & Cheese	1	392
Sourdough Ham Egg & Cheese	1	679
Sourdough Sausage Egg & Cheese	1	514
Twist Chocolate	1	250
Twist Cinnamon	1	260
Wrap Bacon Egg & Cheese	1	515
Wrap Ham Egg & Cheese	1	568
Wrap Sausage Egg & Cheese	1	689
CHILDREN'S MENU SELECTIONS		
Kids Meal Chicken Tenders	1 serv	289
Kids Meal Junior Roast Beef Sandwich	1	272
Market Fresh Mini Ham & Cheese Sandwich	1	228
Market Fresh Mini Turkey & Cheese Sandwich	1	235
DESSERTS		
Cookie Chocolate Chip	1 (1.6 oz)	202
Turnover Apple	1	377
Turnover Cherry	1	377
SALAD DRESSINGS AND SAUCES		
Arby's Sauce	1 serv (0.5 oz)	15
Dipping Sauce BBQ	1 pkg (1 oz)	40
Dipping Sauce Bronco Berry	1 serv (2 oz)	122
Dipping Sauce Buffalo	1 serv (1 oz)	10
Dipping Sauce Cool Ranch Sour Cream	1 serv (1.5 oz)	158
Dipping Sauce Honey Mustard	1 serv (1 oz)	129
Dressing Buttermilk Ranch	1 serv (2.2 oz)	325
Dressing Buttermilk Ranch Light	1 serv (2 oz)	112
Dressing Sante Fe Ranch	1 pkg (2.2 oz)	296
Horsey Sauce	1 pkg (0.5 oz)	62
Ketchup	1 pkg	13
Sauce Cheddar Cheese	1 serv (0.7 oz)	30
Sauce Spicy Three Pepper	1 serv (0.5 oz)	22
Sauce Tangy Southwest	1 serv (2 oz)	333
SALADS		
Chicken Club	1 serv	487
Martha's Vineyard	1 serv	277
Santa Fe	1 serv	477
SANDWICHES		
Arby's Melt	1	302

FOOD	PORTION	CALS
Beef'N Cheddar	1	445
Chicken Bacon & Swiss Crispy	1	624
Chicken Bacon & Swiss Grilled	1	462
Chicken Cordon Bleu Crispy	1	650
Chicken Cordon Bleu Grilled	1	488
Chicken Fillet Crispy	1	576
Chicken Fillet Grilled	1	414
Chicken Salad w/ Pecans	1	769
Corned Beef Reuben	1	606
Fish	1	543
French Dip	1	391
French Dip & Swiss	1	473
Ham & Swiss Melt	1	275
Roast Beef Cheddar	1	521
Roast Beef Regular	1	320
Roast Beef Super	1	398
Roast Beef Swiss	1	777
Roast Ham Swiss	1	705
Roast Turkey & Swiss	1	725
Roast Turkey Ranch & Bacon	1	834
Roast Turkey Reuben	1	611
Sourdough Melt Beef	1	355
Sourdough Melt Ham	1	380
Spicy Cajun Fish	1	603
Sub Toasted Classic Italian	1	828
Sub Toasted French Dip & Swiss	1	622
Sub Toasted Philly Beef	1	739
Sub Toasted Turkey Bacon Club	1	619
Swiss Melt	1	303
Ultimate BLT	1	779
Wrap Chicken Salad w/ Pecans	1	638
Wrap Corned Beef Reuben	1	577
Wrap Roast Turkey Ranch & Bacon	1	700
Wrap Roast Turkey Reuben	1	581
Wrap Southwest Chicken	1	567
Wrap Ultimate BLT	1	648
SIDES		
Bites Jalapeno	5	305
Bites Loaded Potato	5	353
Cheddar Fries	1 med	465

FOOD	PORTION	CALS
Chicken Tenders	3 pieces	379
Croutons Cheese & Garlic	1 pkg	77
Curly Fries	1 lg	631
Curly Fries	1 sm	338
Fruit Cup	1 serv	35
Homestyle Fries	1 lg	566
Homestyle Fries	1 sm	302
Mozzarella Sticks	8 pieces	849
Onion Petals	1 reg	331
Popcorn Chicken	1 reg	365
Potato Cakes	2	246
Seasoned Tortilla Strips	1 serv	71

AU BON PAIN
BAKED SELECTIONS

FOOD	PORTION	CALS
Bagel Asiago Cheese	1	360
Bagel Cinnamon Raisin	1	320
Bagel Everything	1	350
Bagel Honey 9 Grain	1	330
Bagel Jalapeno Double Cheddar	1	350
Bagel Onion Dill	1	350
Bagel Plain	1	290
Bagel Poppy Seed	1	290
Bagel Sesame Seed	1	330
Baguette Artisan Honey Multigrain Salad Size	1 (3.5 oz)	240
Baguette Artisan Honey Multigrain Sandwich Size	1 (4.7 oz)	310
Baguette Artisan Salad Size	1 (3.5 oz)	210
Baguette Artisan Sandwich Size	1 (4.7 oz)	290
Blondie	1	330
Bread Artisan Multigrain	1 serv (4 oz)	260
Bread Artisan Sundried Tomato	1 serv (4 oz)	240
Bread Cheese	1 serv (4.8 oz)	290
Bread Country White	1 serv (4 oz)	240
Bread Bowl	1 (9.24 oz)	640
Bread Stick Rosemary Garlic	1 (2.3 oz)	200
Brownie Chocolate Chip	1	380
Brownie Hazelnut Mocha	1	430
Brownie Rocky Road	1	410
Ciabatta	1 sm	180

FOOD	PORTION	CALS
Cinnamon Roll	1	350
Cookie Chocolate Chip	1 (2 oz)	260
Cookie Confetti	1 (2.4 oz)	310
Cookie English Toffee	1 (2 oz)	210
Cookie Gingerbread	1 (2.7 oz)	300
Cookie Hazelnut Fudge	1 (2.25 oz)	290
Cookie Oatmeal Raisin	1 (2 oz)	230
Cookie Shortbread	1 (2.3 oz)	310
Creme De Fleur	1 serv	550
Croissant Almond	1	560
Croissant Apple	1	230
Croissant Chocolate	1	330
Croissant Plain	1 (2.8 oz)	260
Croissant Raspberry Cheese	1	330
Croissant Sweet Cheese	1	320
Danish Cherry	1	370
Danish Sweet Cheese	1	380
Focaccia	1 piece (4.4 oz)	310
Lahvash	1 (4 oz)	320
Macaroon Chocolate Dipped Cranberry Almond	1	320
Mini Loaf Bacon & Cheese	1 (4.8 oz)	540
Muffin Blueberry	1	510
Muffin Carrot Walnut	1	520
Muffin Corn	1	460
Muffin Cranberry Walnut	1	500
Muffin Double Chocolate Chunk	1	590
Muffin Pumpkin	1	490
Muffin Raisin Bran	1	410
Muffin Low Fat Triple Berry	1	290
Pastry Hazelnut Creme	1	540
Poundcake Cappuccino	1 slice (5.2 oz)	530
Poundcake Chocolate	1 slice (4.7 oz)	500
Poundcake Lemon	1 slice (4.9 oz)	520
Poundcake Marble	1 slice (4.7 oz)	490
Roll Pecan	1	630
Roll Soft	1 (4.7 oz)	410
Scone Cinnamon	1	430
Scone Orange	1	410
Shortbread Chocolate Dipped	1	350

FOOD	PORTION	CALS
Toasts Basil Pesto Cheese	3 pieces (2 oz)	140
Tulip Blueberry	1	370
Tulip Chocolate Raspberry	1	430
Tulip Key Lime	1	440
BEVERAGES		
Blast Caramel	1 med (16 oz)	540
Blast Coffee	1 med (16 oz)	440
Blast Mocha	1 med (16 oz)	440
Blast Vanilla	1 med (12 oz)	540
Caffe Americano	1 sm (12 oz)	5
Cappuccino	1 sm (12 oz)	120
Caramel Macchiato	1 sm (12 oz)	350
Chocolate Milk	1 (12 oz)	320
Hot Chocolate	1 sm (12 oz)	350
Iced Caramel Macchiato	1 sm (12 oz)	290
Iced Tea Peach	1 med (22 oz)	120
Latte Caffe	1 sm (12 oz)	200
Latte Chai	1 sm (12 oz)	290
Latte Iced Caffe	1 sm (12 oz)	110
Latte Iced Chai	1 sm (12 oz)	190
Latte Iced Mocha	1 sm (12 oz)	210
Latte Iced Vanilla	1 sm (12 oz)	240
Latte Iced White Chocolate	1 sm (12 oz)	250
Latte Mocha	1 sm (12 oz)	300
Latte Vanilla	1 sm (12 oz)	320
Latte White Chocolate	1 sm (12 oz)	310
Lemonade	1 med (22 oz)	300
Orange Juice	1 (8 oz)	110
Smoothie Peach	1 med (16 oz)	310
Smoothie Strawberry	1 med (16 oz)	310
MAIN MENU SELECTIONS		
Fruit Cup	1 sm (6 oz)	70
Harvest Rice Bowl Cajun Shrimp	1 (20 oz)	520
Harvest Rice Bowl Cajun Shrimp w/ Brown Rice	1 (20 oz)	560
Harvest Rice Bowl Mayan Chicken	1 (19.25 oz)	490
Harvest Rice Bowl Mayan Chicken w/ Brown Rice	1 (19.25 oz)	540
Harvest Rice Bowl Steak Teriyaki	1 (19.25 oz)	530
Harvest Rice Bowl Steak Teriyaki w/ Brown Rice	1 (19.25 oz)	570
Macaroni & Cheese	1 med (12 oz)	440

FOOD	PORTION	CALS
Stew Beef	1 med (12 oz)	300
Stew Chicken Vegetable	1 med (12 oz)	290
SALAD DRESSINGS AND SPREADS		
Artichoke Aioli	1 serv (1 oz)	130
Basil Pesto	1 serv (1 oz)	140
Chili Dijon	1 serv (1 oz)	120
Cream Cheese Honey Pecan	1 serv (2 oz)	120
Cream Cheese Honey Walnut	1 serv (2 oz)	140
Cream Cheese Lite	1 serv (2 oz)	120
Cream Cheese Plain	1 serv (2 oz)	170
Cream Cheese Strawberry	1 serv (2 oz)	180
Cream Cheese Sundried Tomato	1 serv (2 oz)	120
Cream Cheese Vegetable	1 serv (2 oz)	170
Dressing Balsamic Vinaigrette	1 serv (2.25 oz)	190
Dressing Blue Cheese	1 serv (1.75 oz)	230
Dressing Caesar	1 serv (2 oz)	280
Dressing Fat Free Raspberry Vinaigrette	1 serv (2.25 oz)	70
Dressing Light Honey Mustard	1 serv (2.25 oz)	180
Dressing Light Olive Oil Vinaigrette	1 serv (2.25 oz)	130
Dressing Light Ranch	1 serv (2.25 oz)	150
Dressing Thai Peanut	1 serv (2.25 oz)	230
Guacamole	1 serv (1 oz)	60
Honey Mustard	1 serv (2.5 oz)	210
Hummus Roasted Red Pepper	1 serv (2 oz)	80
Mayonnaise	1 serv (1 oz)	200
Mayonnaise Herb	1 serv (1 oz)	210
Mayonnaise Jalapeno	1 serv (1 oz)	140
Mayonnaise Tarragon Sauce	1 serv (2 oz)	420
Mustard	1 tsp	0
Spread Herb Bagel	1 serv (2 oz)	130
Spread Sundried Tomato	1 serv (0.53 oz)	70
SALADS		
Caesar Asiago	1 serv	210
Caesar Asiago Grilled Chicken	1 (8.5 oz)	340
Caesar Asiago Side	1 (3.2 oz)	120
Chef's	1 serv	230
Garden	1 (7 oz)	80
Garden Side	1 (3.6 oz)	50
Mediterranean Chicken	1 (9.75 oz)	330
Riviera	1 (9.5 oz)	260

FOOD	PORTION	CALS
Thai Peanut Chicken	1 (11 oz)	250
Tuna Garden	1 (10.5 oz)	350
Turkey Medallion Cobb	1 (11 oz)	340
Turkey Spinach Sonoma	1 (12.3 oz)	310
SANDWICHES		
Arizona Chicken	1 (12 oz)	750
Baguette Turkey & Swiss	1 (12.3 oz)	770
Baja Turkey	1 (13 oz)	700
Breakfast Asiago Bagel Prosciutto & Egg	1 (9.6 oz)	660
Breakfast Asiago Bagel Sausage Egg & Cheddar	1 (10.2 oz)	770
Breakfast Bagel & Bacon	1 (4.2 oz)	340
Breakfast Egg On A Bagel	1 (6.8 oz)	370
Breakfast Egg On A Bagel w/ Bacon	1 (7.2 oz)	410
Breakfast Egg On A Bagel w/ Bacon Cheese	1 (7.9 oz)	500
Breakfast Egg On A Bagel w/ Cheese	1 (7.6 oz)	450
Breakfast Onion Dill Bagel Smoked Salmon & Wasabi	1 (7.1 oz)	490
Caprese	1 (11.8 oz)	700
Chicken Mozzarella	1 (14.5 oz)	800
Chicken Pesto	1 (12.5 oz)	700
Chicken Tarragon	1 (11 oz)	720
Ciabatta Bacon & Egg Melt	1 (7 oz)	400
Ciabatta Ham & Cheddar	1 (12 oz)	650
Club Smoked Turkey	1 (11.6 oz)	780
Croissant Ham & Cheese	1 (4.2 oz)	350
Croissant Spinach & Cheese	1	250
Hot BBQ Chicken On Farmhouse Roll	1 (14.3 oz)	970
Hot Eggplant & Mozzarella	1 (12.4 oz)	710
Hot Steakhouse On Ciabatta	1 (13 oz)	800
Melt Tuna	1 (12.5 oz)	760
Melt Turkey	1 (12.2 oz)	890
Portobello & Goat Cheese	1 (10 oz)	610
Portobello Egg & Cheddar	1 (8.5 oz)	590
Prosciutto Mozzarella	1 (12.7 oz)	880
Spicy Tuna	1 (10.3 oz)	640
The Montana	1 (12.5 oz)	560
Turkey & Cranberry Chutney	1 (10.9 oz)	680
Wrap Chicken Caesar Asiago	1	700
Wrap Chopped Turkey Club	1 (12 oz)	660
Wrap Hot Cajun Shrimp	1 (14.9 oz)	700

FOOD	PORTION	CALS
Wrap Hot Mayan Chicken	1 (13.5 oz)	630
Wrap Hot Steak Teriyaki	1 (13.5 oz)	660
Wrap Mediterranean	1 (12.8 oz)	670
Wrap Southwest Tuna	1 (14 oz)	900
Wrap Thai Peanut Chicken	1 (14.5 oz)	660
Wrap Turkey Spinach Sonoma	1 (12 oz)	630
SOUPS		
Baked Stuffed Potato	1 med (12 oz)	350
Broccoli Cheddar	1 med (12 oz)	310
Carrot Ginger	1 med (12 oz)	130
Chicken & Dumplings	1 med (12 oz)	210
Chicken Florentine	1 med (12 oz)	240
Chicken Noodle	1 med (12 oz)	130
Clam Chowder	1 med (12 oz)	320
Corn & Green Chili Bisque	1 med (12 oz)	250
Corn Chowder	1 med (12 oz)	350
Curried Rice & Lentil	1 med (12 oz)	150
French Moroccan Tomato Lentil	1 med (12 oz)	180
French Onion	1 med (12 oz)	130
Garden Vegetable	1 med (12 oz)	80
Harvest Pumpkin	1 med (12 oz)	190
Hearty Cabbage	1 med (12 oz)	110
Italian Wedding	1 med (12 oz)	170
Jamaican Black Bean	1 med (12 oz)	180
Mediterranean Pepper	1 med (12 oz)	100
Old Fashioned Tomato Rice	1 med (12 oz)	120
Pasta E Fagioli	1 med (12 oz)	240
Portuguese Kale	1 med (12 oz)	120
Potato Cheese	1 med (12 oz)	250
Potato Leek	1 med (12 oz)	300
Red Beans Italian Sausage & Rice	1 med (12 oz)	200
Southern Black Eyed Pea	1 med (12 oz)	180
Southwest Tortilla	1 med (12 oz)	200
Southwest Vegetable	1 med (12 oz)	160
Split Pea	1 med (12 oz)	210
Thai Coconut Curry	1 med (12 oz)	150
Tomato Basil Bisque	1 med (12 oz)	210
Tomato Cheddar	1 med (12 oz)	240
Tomato Florentine	1 med (12 oz)	120
Tuscan Vegetable	1 med (12 oz)	170

FOOD	PORTION	CALS
Vegetable Beef Barley	1 med (12 oz)	140
Vegetarian Chili	1 med (12 oz)	230
Vegetarian Lentil	1 med (12 oz)	140
Vegetarian Minestrone	1 med (12 oz)	120
Wild Mushroom Bisque	1 med (12 oz)	190
YOGURT		
Blueberry w/ Fruit	1 sm (7.5 oz)	220
Blueberry w/ Granola & Fruit	1 sm (8.5 oz)	310
Strawberry w/ Blueberries	1 sm (7.5 oz)	220
Strawberry w/ Granola & Blueberries	1 sm (8.5 oz)	310
Vanilla w/ Blueberries	1 sm (7.5 oz)	190
Vanilla w/ Granola & Blueberries	1 sm (8.5 oz)	310

AUNTIE ANNE'S
BEVERAGES

FOOD	PORTION	CALS
Dutch Ice Blue Raspberry	1 (14 oz)	165
Dutch Ice Grape	1 (14 oz)	180
Dutch Ice Kiwi Banana	1 (14 oz)	190
Dutch Ice Lemonade	1 (14 oz)	315
Dutch Ice Lemonade Strawberry	1 (14 oz)	330
Dutch Ice Mocha	1 (14 oz)	400
Dutch Ice Orange Creme	1 (14 oz)	280
Dutch Ice Pina Colada	1 (14 oz)	220
Dutch Ice Strawberry	1 (14 oz)	220
Dutch Ice Watermelon	1 (14 oz)	200
Dutch Ice Wild Cherry	1 (14 oz)	210
Dutch Latte Caramel	1 (14 oz)	350
Dutch Latte Coffee	1 (14 oz)	290
Dutch Latte Mocha	1 (14 oz)	160
Dutch Shake Chocolate	1 (14 oz)	580
Dutch Shake Coffee	1 (14 oz)	590
Dutch Shake Strawberry	1 (14 oz)	610
Dutch Shake Vanilla	1 (14 oz)	510
Dutch Smoothie Blue Raspberry	1 (14 oz)	230
Dutch Smoothie Grape	1 (14 oz)	230
Dutch Smoothie Kiwi Banana	1 (14 oz)	240
Dutch Smoothie Lemonade	1 (14 oz)	300
Dutch Smoothie Mocha	1 (14 oz)	330
Dutch Smoothie Orange Creme	1 (14 oz)	280
Dutch Smoothie Pina Colada	1 (14 oz)	260

FOOD	PORTION	CALS
Dutch Smoothie Strawberry	1 (14 oz)	250
Dutch Smoothie Wild Cherry	1 (14 oz)	250
Lemonade	1 (22 oz)	180
Lemonade Strawberry	1 (22 oz)	190
DIPPING SAUCES		
Caramel Dip	1 serv (1.5 oz)	135
Cheese Sauce	1 serv (1.25 oz)	100
Cream Cheese Light	1 serv (1.25 oz)	70
Hot Salsa Cheese	1 serv (1.25 oz)	100
Marinara Sauce	1 serv (1.25 oz)	10
Sweet	1 serv (1.4 oz)	40
Sweet Mustard	1 serv (1.25 oz)	60
PRETZELS		
Almond	1	400
Almond w/o Butter	1	350
Cinnamon Raisin w/o Butter	1	350
Cinnamon Sugar	1	450
Garlic	1	350
Garlic w/o Butter	1	320
Glazin' Raisin	1	510
Glazin' Raisin w/o Butter	1	470
Jalapeno	1	310
Jalapeno w/o Butter	1	270
Original	1	370
Original w/o Butter	1	340
Pretzel Dog	1	290
Sesame	1	410
Sesame w/o Butter	1	350
Sour Cream & Onion	1	340
Sour Cream & Onion w/o Butter	1	310
Stix	6	370
Stix w/o Butter	6	340
Whole Wheat	1	370
Whole Wheat w/o Butter	1	350

BABS DELI
BAGELS

FOOD	PORTION	CALS
Apple Cinnamon	1	332
Banana Nut	1	340
Blueberry	1	330

FOOD	PORTION	CALS
Blueberry Cobbler	1	392
Cheddar Herb	1	352
Cheddar Nacho	1	352
Chocolate Chip	1	348
Cinnamon Apple Pie	1	386
Cinnamon Bun	1	400
Cinnamon Danish	1	396
Cinnamon Raisin	1	336
Cinnamon Sugar	1	350
Cranberry Walnut	1	352
Egg	1	328
Everything	1	336
French Toast	1	372
Garlic	1	330
Honey Oat	1	320
Jalapeno	1	350
Onion	1	336
Plain	1	334
Poppy	1	344
Pumpernickel	1	332
Quiche Lorraine	1	354
Salt	1	324
Sesame	1	358
Spinach	1	356
Strawberry	1	342
Strawberry White Chocolate	1	364
Swiss Melt	1	368
Tomato Basil	1	322
Vegetable	1	318
Wheat	1	330
White Chocolate Swirl	1	396
BEVERAGES		
Americano	1 (16 oz)	12
Cafe Caramello	1 (16 oz)	212
Cappuccino 2% Milk	1 (16 oz)	195
Cappuccino Fat Free Milk	1 (16 oz)	133
Coffee Black Forest	1 (16 oz)	198
Icepresso Caramel Decadence	1 (16 oz)	300
Icepresso Classic	1 (16 oz)	300
Icepresso Java Chip	1 (16 oz)	360

FOOD	PORTION	CALS
Icepresso Latte	1 (16 oz)	300
Icepresso Mocha	1 (16 oz)	300
Icepresso Strawberry	1 (16 oz)	340
Italiano 2% Milk	1 (16 oz)	131
Italiano Fat Free Milk	1 (16 oz)	89
Jittery Monkey 2% Milk	1 (16 oz)	482
Jittery Monkey Fat Free Milk	1 (16 oz)	429
Latte 2% Milk	1 (16 oz)	212
Latte Cinnamon Toast 2% Milk	1 (16 oz)	299
Latte Cinnamon Toast Fat Free Milk	1 (16 oz)	240
Latte Creme Caramel 2% Milk	1 (16 oz)	303
Latte Creme Caramel Fat Free Milk	1 (16 oz)	244
Latte Fat Free Milk	1 (16 oz)	145
Latte Oregon Chai Tea 2% Milk	1 (16 oz)	274
Latte Oregon Chai Tea Fat Free Milk	1 (16 oz)	231
Latte Raspberry Cheesecake 2% Milk	1 (16 oz)	319
Latte Raspberry Cheesecake Fat Free Milk	1 (16 oz)	259
Latte Vanilla Crème 2% Milk	1 (16 oz)	275
Mocha Whipped Cream 2% Milk	1 (16 oz)	454
Mocha Whipped Cream Fat Free Milk	1 (16 oz)	392
Turtle Mocha Fat Free Milk	1 (16 oz)	522
MUFFINS		
My Favorite Banana Nut	2 mini	195
My Favorite Blueberry	2 mini	168
My Favorite Blueberry Cheesecake	2 mini	199
My Favorite Boston Cream Pie	2 mini	176
My Favorite Cherry Cheesecake	2 mini	170
My Favorite Chocolate Cheesecake	2 mini	202
My Favorite Chocolate Chip	2 mini	211
My Favorite Cinnamon Crumb Cake	2 mini	212
My Favorite Cinnamon Swirl Cheesecake	2 mini	214
My Favorite Deep Dish Apple	2 mini	177
My Favorite Double Chocolate	2 mini	210
My Favorite Fat Free Blueberry	2 mini	108
My Favorite Fat Free Cherry Pie	2 mini	109
My Favorite Fat Free Chocolate Marble	2 mini	125
My Favorite Fat Free Cinnamon Bun	2 mini	168
My Favorite Fat Free Raspberry Amaretto	2 mini	127
My Favorite Golden Corn Bread	2 mini	197
My Favorite Lemon Poppyseed	2 mini	201
My Favorite Pumpkin Spice	2 mini	181

FOOD	PORTION	CALS
SALADS		
Calypso Chicken	1 (13.6 oz)	637
Calypso Chicken w/ Lite Italian	1 (13.6 oz)	317
Chicken Caesar	1 (11.5 oz)	524
Chicken Caesar w/ Lite Italian	1 (11.5 oz)	268
Classic Caesar	1 (8.4 oz)	414
Classic Caesar Cafe	1 (4.3 oz)	225
Classic Ceasar w/ Lite Italian	1 (8.4 oz)	158
Garden Mix	1 (12.4 oz)	197
Garden Mix Cafe	1 (6.5 oz)	100
Grilled Chicken Club	1 (17.9 oz)	820
Grilled Chicken Club w/ Lite Italian	1 (17.9 oz)	500
Mediterranean Bread	1 (18.8 oz)	973
Mediterranean Bread w/ Lite Italian	1 (18.8 oz)	626
Tuna Salad Plate Low Carb	1 serv (8.9 oz)	356
SANDWICHES		
Breakfast BLT	1	704
Breakfast Lox & Cream Cheese	1	602
Breakfast Morning Classic	1	486
Breakfast Northern Omelette	1	699
Breakfast So Tradition w/ Bacon	1	566
Breakfast So Tradition w/ Ham	1	547
Breakfast So Tradition w/ Sausage	1	696
Build Your Own Ham	1	495
Build Your Own Roast Beef	1	480
Build Your Own Tuna	1	547
Build Your Own Turkey	1	465
Enchilada Bagellata	1	522
Gourmet Classic Turkey	1	552
Gourmet Holey Guacamole	1	476
Gourmet Kick-N Roast Beef	1	579
Gourmet Mediterranean Veg-Out	1	506
Overstuffed Classic Reuben	1	962
Overstuffed Corned Beef	1	661
Overstuffed Ham & Cheese	1	889
Overstuffed Manhattan Club	1	1122
Overstuffed Pastrami	1	661
Overstuffed TD Classic California	1	759
Overstuffed TD Classic Club	1	1110

FOOD	PORTION	CALS
Overstuffed TD Clubhouse	1	1079
Pizzaah Bruschetta	1 piece	162
Pizzaah Cheese	1 piece	189
Pizzaah Grilled Chicken Bruschetta	1 piece	343
Pizzaah Sausage	1 piece	211
Pizzaah Veggie	1 piece	238
Specialty All American Duo	1	752
Specialty Big Apple Club	1	797
Specialty Chicken Caesar	1	611
Specialty Roma Italian	1	764
Specialty Turkey Club	1	782
Toasted Cafe Chicken Melt	1	815
Toasted Deli Style Turkey	1	732
Toasted Roast Beef Parmesan Grinder	1	583
Toasted Spicy Italian Sub	1	770
Toasted Tuna Melt	1	641
SOUPS		
Beef Barley Mushroom	1 serv (8 oz)	100
Boston Clam Chowder	1 serv (8 oz)	210
Chicken & Wild Rice	1 serv (8 oz)	190
Chicken Gumbo	1 serv (8 oz)	130
Cream Of Potato	1 serv (8 oz)	240
Hearty Vegetable Beef	1 serv (8 oz)	100
New England Clam Chowder	1 serv (8 oz)	220
Split Pea w/ Ham	1 serv (8 oz)	90
Wisconsin Cheese	1 serv (8 oz)	210
SPREADS		
Cream Cheese	2 tbsp	90
Cream Cheese Cheddar Jalapeno	2 tbsp	90
Cream Cheese Garden Vegetable	2 tbsp	90
Cream Cheese Lite	2 tbsp	60
Cream Cheese Onion Chive	2 tbsp	80
Cream Cheese Strawberry	2 tbsp	90
Cream Cheese Whipped	2 tbsp	70
Cream Cheese Whipped Brown Sugar Cinnamon	2 tbsp	70
Cream Cheese Whipped Reduced Fat Spring Veggie	2 tbsp	60

FOOD	PORTION	CALS
BAHAMA BREEZE		
BEVERAGES		
Beer Light	1 serv (12 oz)	103
Beer Regular	1 serv (12 oz)	153
Berries In Paradise	1 serv	110
Captain Berry Island	1 serv	110
Island Refresher	1 serv	370
Lemon Breeze	1 serv	410
Mango Beach	1 serv	300
Mango Mango Man	1 serv	300
Raspberry Surfer	1 serv	210
Shake Banana	1 serv	590
Shake Chocolate	1 serv	700
Shake Chocolate Banana	1 serv	760
Shake Mango	1 serv	450
Shake Raspberry	1 serv	560
Shake Strawberry	1 serv	530
Shake Strawberry Banana	1 serv	600
Shake Vanilla	1 serv	560
Slushies Kiwi	1 serv	120
Slushies Mango	1 serv	180
Slushies Strawberry	1 serv	240
Strawberry Beach	1 serv	370
Virgin Bahama Rita	1 serv	160
Virgin Ultimate Pina Colada	1 serv	340
Wine	1 serv (5 oz)	122
CHILDREN'S MENU SELECTIONS		
Bowtie Mac N' Cheese	1 serv	790
Cheese Pizza	1 sm	750
Crispy Chicken	1 serv	420
French Fries	1 serv	265
Fresh Fruit Salad	1 serv	40
DESSERTS		
Bananas Supreme	1 serv	940
Chocolate Island	1 serv	1380
Dulce De Leche Cheesecake	1 serv	940
Rebecca's Key Lime Pie	1 serv	990
Warm Chocolate Pineapple Upside Down Cake	1 serv	1140

FOOD	PORTION	CALS
MAIN MENU SELECTIONS		
Bahamian Grilled Chicken Kabobs w/ Yellow Rice	1 serv	770
Breeze Wood Grilled Chicken Breast w/ Citrus Butter Sauce	1 serv	680
Breeze Wood Grilled Chicken Breast w/ Citrus Butter Sauce Lighter Portion	1 serv	390
Broccoli	1 serv	120
Burger Wood Grilled Angus	1 serv	680
Chicken Santiago	1 serv	1180
Chicken Santiago Lighter Portion	1 serv	1020
Cinnamon Mashed Sweet Potatoes	1 serv	260
Coconut Shrimp Dinner	1 serv	794
Crab Claws St. Thomas	1 serv	710
Crab Shrimp & Avocado Stack w/ Honey Red Pepper Drizzle	1 serv	250
Creole Baked Goat Cheese	1 serv	380
Crispy Yuca	1 serv	620
Filet Mignon w/ Onion Rings	1 serv	450
Fire Roasted Jerk Shrimp	1 serv	260
French Fries	1 serv	530
Garlic Mashed Potatoes	1 serv	290
Herb Cheese Toast	1 slice	120
Island Flatbread Grilled Chicken	1	515
Island Flatbread Shrimp	1	480
Island Flatbread Vine Ripened Tomato	1	430
Island Onion Rings	1 serv	1910
Jamaican Grilled Chicken Breast	1 serv	310
Jamaican Grilled Chicken Breast Lighter Portion	1 serv	160
Linguine Calypso Shrimp Lighter Portion	1 serv	790
Margarita Chicken w/ Roasted Corn Salsa	1 serv	470
Margarita Chicken w/ Roasted Corn Salsa Lighter Portion	1 serv	310
Pasta Jerk Chicken	1 serv	1430
Pasta Jerk Chicken Lighter Portion	1 serv	780
Pasta Lobster & Shrimp	1 serv	1080
Pasta Pan-Seared Salmon	1 serv	1550
Pasta Pan-Seared Salmon Lighter Portion	1 serv	910
Plantains	1 serv	270

FOOD	PORTION	CALS
Quesadilla Fresh Vegetable	1	435
Quesadilla Fresh Vegetable & Chicken	1	480
Roasted Cuban Bread	1 serv	590
Sandwich Cuban	1	1130
Sandwich Oak Grilled Chicken	1	530
Sandwich Sun Drenched Portobello & Veg	1	670
Seafood Paella	1 serv	800
Smothered Pork Tenderloin w/ Lemon Butter	1 serv	900
Spinach Dip w/ Island Chips	1 serv	680
Tacos Key West Fish	1 serv	550
Tostones w/ Chicken	1 serv	1250
West Indies Patties	1 serv	1150
West Indies Ribs	1 serv	810
Wings Habanero	1 serv	920
Wings Jamaican Grilled	1 serv	960
Wood Grilled Top Sirloin w/ Cheese & Peppers	1 serv	440
Yellow Rice	1 serv	220
Yellow Rice & Black Beans	1 serv	280
SALAD DRESSINGS AND TOPPINGS		
Citrus Mustard	1 serv	95
Dip Cilantro Vinaigrette	1 serv	110
Dipping Sauce Tangy	1 serv	50
Dressing Blue Cheese	1 serv	175
Dressing Caesar	1 serv	200
Dressing Ranch	1 serv	130
Dressing Tropical Island Vinaigrette	1 serv	60
Guava BBQ Sauce	1 serv	50
Homemade Croutons	12	500
Salsa Apple Mango	1 serv	20
Salsa Black Bean & Corn	1 serv	70
Salsa Mango Pineapple	1 serv	60
Salsa Tomato	1 serv	30
Sauce Chili Horseradish	1 serv	130
Sour Cream	1 serv	90
Sour Cream Ancho Chili	1 serv	70
SALADS		
Breeze No Dressing	1 serv	90
Caesar No Dressing	1 serv	70
Crispy Chicken Club w/ BBQ Drizzle	1 serv	880
Fresh Fruit	1 serv	130

FOOD	PORTION	CALS
Grilled Chicken Ceasar w/ Croutons w/o Dressing	1 serv	490
Grilled Chicken Cobb	1 serv	600
Grilled Fresh Salmon Tostada w/ Chimichurri Sauce w/o Dressing	1 serv	1045
Tropical Fruit & Grilled Chicken On Greens w/o Dressing	1 serv	430
Vine Ripened Tomato	1 serv	60
SOUPS		
Bahamian Seafood Chowder	1 serv	600
Chicken Tortilla	1 serv	290
Cuban Black Bean	1 serv	320

BAJA FRESH
CHILDREN'S MENU SELECTIONS

Kid's Mini Burrito Bean & Cheese	1 serv	540
Kid's Mini Burrito Bean & Cheese w/ Chicken	1 serv	590
Kid's Mini Quesadilla Cheese	1 serv	610
Kid's Mini Quesadilla Cheese w/ Chicken	1 serv	650
Kid's Taquitos Chicken	1 serv	630
MAIN MENU SELECTIONS		
Black Beans	1 serv	360
Burrito Baja Breaded Fish	1 serv	850
Burrito Baja Carnitas	1 serv	830
Burrito Baja Chicken	1 serv	790
Burrito Baja Mahi Mahi	1 serv	780
Burrito Baja Shrimp	1 serv	760
Burrito Baja Steak	1 serv	850
Burrito Bare Carnitas	1 serv	600
Burrito Bare Chicken	1 serv	640
Burrito Bare Steak	1 serv	700
Burrito Bare Veggie & Cheese	1 serv	580
Burrito Bean & Cheese Breaded Fish	1 serv	1030
Burrito Bean & Cheese Carnitas	1 serv	1010
Burrito Bean & Cheese Chicken	1 serv	970
Burrito Bean & Cheese Mahi Mahi	1 serv	960
Burrito Bean & Cheese No Meat	1 serv	840
Burrito Bean & Cheese Shrimp	1 serv	950
Burrito Bean & Cheese Steak	1 serv	1030
Burrito Dos Manos Breaded Fish	1 serv	890

FOOD	PORTION	CALS
Burrito Dos Manos Carnitas	1 serv	780
Burrito Dos Manos Chicken	1 serv	760
Burrito Dos Manos Mahi Mahi	1 serv	780
Burrito Dos Manos Shrimp	1 serv	780
Burrito Dos Manos Steak	1 serv	795
Burrito Grilled Veggie	1 serv	506
Burrito Mexicano Breaded Fish	1 serv	850
Burrito Mexicano Carnitas	1 serv	830
Burrito Mexicano Chicken	1 serv	790
Burrito Mexicano Mahi Mahi	1 serv	790
Burrito Mexicano Shrimp	1 serv	770
Burrito Mexicano Steak	1 serv	860
Burrito Ultimo Breaded Fish	1 serv	940
Burrito Ultimo Carnitas	1 serv	920
Burrito Ultimo Chicken	1 serv	880
Burrito Ultimo Mahi Mahi	1 serv	880
Burrito Ultimo Shrimp	1 serv	860
Burrito Ultimo Steak	1 serv	950
Chips & Guacamole	1 serv	1340
Chips & Salsa Baja	1 serv	810
Fajitas Corn Tortillas Breaded Fish	1 serv	1060
Fajitas Corn Tortillas Carnitas	1 serv	920
Fajitas Corn Tortillas Chicken	1 serv	860
Fajitas Corn Tortillas Mahi Mahi	1 serv	840
Fajitas Corn Tortillas Shrimp	1 serv	840
Fajitas Corn Tortillas Steak	1 serv	960
Fajitas Flour Tortillas Breaded Fish	1 serv	1340
Fajitas Flour Tortillas Carnitas	1 serv	1190
Fajitas Flour Tortillas Chicken	1 serv	1140
Fajitas Flour Tortillas Mahi Mahi	1 serv	1120
Fajitas Flour Tortillas Shrimp	1 serv	1120
Fajitas Flour Tortillas Steak	1 serv	960
Guacamole Side	1 (3 oz)	110
Nachos Breaded Fish	1 serv	2090
Nachos Carnitas	1 serv	2060
Nachos Cheese	1 serv	1890
Nachos Chicken	1 serv	2020
Nachos Mahi Mahi	1 serv	2020
Nachos Shrimp	1 serv	2000
Nachos Steak	1 serv	2120

FOOD	PORTION	CALS
Pico De Gallo Side	1 serv (8 oz)	50
Pinto Beans	1 serv	320
Pronto Guacamole Side	1 serv (6 oz)	560
Quesadilla Breaded Fish	1 serv	1400
Quesadilla Carnitas	1 serv	1370
Quesadilla Cheese	1 serv	1200
Quesadilla Chicken	1 serv	1330
Quesadilla Mahi Mahi	1 serv	1330
Quesadilla Shrimp	1 serv	1310
Quesadilla Steak	1 serv	1430
Quesadilla Veggie	1 serv	1260
Rice	1 serv	280
Rice & Beans Plate	1 serv	420
Salsa Baja Side	1 serv (8 oz)	70
Salsa Roja Side	1 serv (8 oz)	70
Salsa Verde Side	1 serv (8 oz)	50
Soup Tortilla w/ Chicken	1 serv (13.6 oz)	320
Soup Tortilla w/o Chicken	1 serv (12.4 oz)	270
Taco Baja Breaded Fish	1 serv	250
Taco Baja Chicken	1 serv	210
Taco Baja Shrimp	1 serv	200
Taco Baja Steak	1 serv	230
Taco Grilled Mahi Mahi	1 serv	230
Taco Soft Breaded Fish	1 serv	240
Taco Soft Carnitas	1 serv	250
Taco Soft Chicken	1 serv	230
Taco Soft Mahi Mahi	1 serv	240
Taco Soft Shrimp	1 serv	230
Taco Soft Steak	1 serv	260
Taquitos Chicken w/ Beans	3	780
Taquitos Chicken w/ Rice	3	740
Veggie Mix	1 serv	110
SALAD DRESSINGS		
Chipotle Vinaigrette	1 serv (2.5 oz)	110
Fat Free Salsa Verde	1 serv (2.5 oz)	15
Olive Oil Vinaigrette	1 serv (2.5 oz)	290
Ranch	1 serv (2.5 oz)	260
SALADS		
Baja Ensalada Chicken	1 serv	310
Baja Ensalada Shrimp	1 serv	230

FOOD	PORTION	CALS
Baja Ensalada Steak	1 serv	450
Chipotle w/ Carnitas	1 serv	640
Chipotle w/ Chicken	1 serv	590
Chipotle w/ Steak	1 serv	700
Side By Side Carnitas	1 serv	570
Side By Side Chicken	1 serv	500
Side By Side Steak	1 serv	620
Side Salad	1 (6.5 oz)	130
Tostada Breaded Fish	1 serv	1200
Tostada Carnitas	1 serv	1180
Tostada Chicken	1 serv	1140
Tostada Mahi Mahi	1 serv	1130
Tostada No Meat	1 serv	1010
Tostada Shrimp	1 serv	1120
Tostada Steak	1 serv	1230

BASKIN-ROBBINS
BEVERAGES

FOOD	PORTION	CALS
Cappuccino Blast w/ Whipped Cream	1 sm (16 oz)	330
Shake Chocolate Chip	1 sm (16 oz)	660
Shake Chocolate Chip Cookie Dough	1 sm (16 oz)	750
Shake Mint Chocolate Chip	1 sm (16 oz)	680
Shake Vanilla	1 sm (16 oz)	670

FROZEN YOGURT

FOOD	PORTION	CALS
Cherries Jubilee	1 scoop (4 oz)	240
Vanilla Fat Free	1 scoop (4 oz)	150

ICE CREAM

FOOD	PORTION	CALS
Butter Almond Crunch Reduced Fat No Sugar Added	1 scoop (4 oz)	220
Butter Pecan	1 scoop (4 oz)	280
Cabana Berry Banana Reduced Fat No Sugar Added	1 scoop (4 oz)	150
Chocolate	1 scoop (4 oz)	260
Chocolate Chip	1 scoop (4 oz)	270
Chocolate Chip Cookie Dough	1 scoop (4 oz)	310
Chocolate Overload Reduced Fat No Sugar Added	1 scoop (4 oz)	190
Gold Medal Ribbon	1 scoop (4 oz)	260
Mint Chocolate Chip	1 scoop (4 oz)	270
Nutty Coconut	1 scoop (4 oz)	300

FOOD	PORTION	CALS
Oreo Cookies 'N Cream	1 scoop (4 oz)	280
Peanut Butter 'N Chocolate	1 scoop (4 oz)	320
Pistachio Almond	1 scoop (4 oz)	290
Pralines 'N Cream	1 scoop (4 oz)	280
Reese's Peanut Butter Cup	1 scoop (4 oz)	300
Rocky Road	1 scoop (4 oz)	290
Sundae Caramel Soft Serve	1 (10 oz)	580
Sundae Hot Fudge Soft Serve	1 (10 oz)	610
Sundae Strawberry Soft Serve	1 (10 oz)	450
Tax Crunch	1 scoop (4 oz)	330
Vanilla	1 scoop (4 oz)	260
Vanilla Soft Serve	1 serv (6 oz)	280
Very Berry Strawberry	1 scoop (4 oz)	320
ICES		
Sherbet Rainbow	1 scoop (4 oz)	160
Sorbet Lemon	1 scoop (4 oz)	130
Sorbet Mango	1 scoop (4 oz)	120
Sorbet Strawberry	1 scoop (4 oz)	130

BEAR ROCK CAFE
SANDWICHES

FOOD	PORTION	CALS
Colorado Turkey Club	1	855
Coop's Chicken Salad Croissant	1	439
Garden Grill Ciabatta	1	406
Giant Panda Wrap	1	556
Hoot Owl	1	641
Rising Sunflower	1	596
Roast Turkey & Bacon	1	522
Rockslide Focaccia	1	958
The Moose	1	976

BEN & JERRY'S
FROZEN YOGURT

FOOD	PORTION	CALS
Low Fat Cherry Garcia	½ cup	170
Low Fat Chocolate Fudge Brownie	½ cup	190
Low Fat Half Baked	½ cup	190
Phish Food	½ cup	220
ICE CREAM		
Bar Cherry Garcia	1	270
Bar Half Baked	1	340
Bar Vanilla	1	300

FOOD	PORTION	CALS
Bar Vanilla Almond	1	340
Black & Tan	½ cup	230
Brownie Batter	½ cup	310
Butter Pecan	½ cup	280
Cherry Garcia	½ cup	250
Chocolate	½ cup	260
Chocolate Chip Cookie Dough	½ cup	270
Chocolate Fudge Brownie	½ cup	260
Chubby Hubby	½ cup	330
Chunky Monkey	½ cup	300
Coffee	½ cup	240
Coffee Heath Bar Crunch	½ cup	290
Dave Matthews Band Magic Brownies	½ cup	250
Dublin Mudslide	½ cup	270
Everything But The	½ cup	310
Fossil Fuel	½ cup	280
Fudge Central	½ cup	300
Half Baked	½ cup	280
In A Crunch	½ cup	350
Karamel Sutra	½ cup	280
Marsha Marsha Marshmallow	½ cup	300
Mint Chocolate Cookie	½ cup	260
Neapolitan Dynamite	½ cup	250
New York Super Fudge Chunk	½ cup	310
Oatmeal Cookie Chunk	½ cup	270
Organic Chocolate Fudge Brownie	½ cup	270
Organic Strawberry	½ cup	210
Organic Sweet Cream & Cookies	½ cup	250
Organic Vanilla	½ cup	220
Peanut Butter Cup	½ cup	360
Phish Food	½ cup	280
Pistachio Pistachio	½ cup	260
Sandwich Wich Ice Cream Cookie	1	350
Strawberry	½ cup	230
The Godfather	½ cup	270
Turtle Soup	½ cup	280
Uncanny Cashew	½ cup	290
Vanilla Caramel Fudge	½ cup	280
Vanilla Heath Bar Crunch	½ cup	290
Vermonty Python	½ cup	310

FOOD	PORTION	CALS
SORBETS		
Berried Treasure	½ cup	110
Jamaican Me Crazy	½ cup	130
Strawberry Kiwi Swirl	½ cup	110
BILLY'S BURGER HUT		
BEVERAGES		
Shake Chocolate	1 (20 oz)	420
Shake Vanilla	1 (20 oz)	320
MAIN MENU SELECTIONS		
Big Billy's Roast Beef Sub	1	843
Billyburger	1	426
Billyburger w/ Cheese	1	498
Billy's Best Red Potato Salad	1 serv	190
Billy's Biggest Burger ½ Pounder w/ Everything	1	852
Billy's Famous 7 Layer Salad	1 serv	558
Billy's Seafood Sandwich	1	399
Caesar Side Salad	1 serv	360
Chili w/ Cheese & Onion	1 serv	380
Cowboy Cobb Salad	1 serv	735
Cowboy Coleslaw	1 serv	180
French Fries	1 reg	230
Onion Rings	1 serv	250
Super Billy Burger w/ Bacon	1	663
BLIMPIE		
DESSERTS		
Cookie Chocolate Chunk	1 (1.5 oz)	200
Cookie Oatmeal Raisin	1 (1.5 oz)	180
Cookie Peanut Butter	1 (1.5 oz)	210
Cookie Sugar	1 (2.5 oz)	320
Cookie White Chocolate Macadamia Nut	1 (1.5 oz)	200
SALAD DRESSINGS AND SAUCES		
Dressing Blue Cheese	1 serv (1.5 oz)	230
Dressing Buttermilk Ranch	1 serv (1.5 oz)	230
Dressing Buttermilk Ranch Light	1 serv (1.5 oz)	70
Dressing Creamy Caesar	1 serv (1.5 oz)	210
Dressing Creamy Italian	1 serv (1.5 oz)	180
Dressing Dijon Honey Mustard	1 serv (1.5 oz)	180
Dressing Italian Fat Free	1 serv (1.5 oz)	25
Dressing Italian Light	1 serv (1.5 oz)	20

FOOD	PORTION	CALS
Dressing Peppercorn	1 serv (1.5 oz)	240
Dressing Thousand Island	1 serv (1.5 oz)	210
Guacamole	1 serv (1 oz)	45
Mayonnaise	1 serv (1 oz)	200
Mustard Yellow Deli	1 serv (0.5 oz)	15
Oil Blend	1 serv (0.5 oz)	130
Sauce Blimpie Special	1 serv (0.5 oz)	40
Sauce Red Hot Original	1 serv (1 oz)	10
SALADS		
Antipasto	1 serv (11.6 oz)	254
Buffalo Chicken	1 serv (7.7 oz)	220
Chicken Caesar	1 serv (9.4 oz)	190
Cole Slaw	1 side (4 oz)	160
Garden	1 serv (6.5 oz)	30
Macaroni	1 side (5 oz)	330
Northwest Potato	1 side (5 oz)	260
Potato	1 side (4.7 oz)	230
Tuna	1 serv (9.4 oz)	270
Ultimate Club	1 serv (10.1 oz)	280
SANDWICHES		
6 Inch Sub Blimpie Best	1 (10.4 oz)	450
6 Inch Sub Blimpie Best Super Stacked	1 (12.8 oz)	550
6 Inch Sub Blimpie Trio Super Stacked	1 (13.5 oz)	510
6 Inch Sub BLT	1 (7.2 oz)	430
6 Inch Sub BLT Super Stacked	1 (8.4 oz)	640
6 Inch Sub Chicken Cheddar Bacon Ranch	1 (12.1 oz)	600
6 Inch Sub Chicken Teriyaki	1 (8.7 oz)	450
6 Inch Sub Club	1 (10.2 oz)	410
6 Inch Sub Cuban	1 (8.2 oz)	410
6 Inch Sub French Dip	1 (13.4 oz)	410
6 Inch Sub Ham & Swiss	1 (10 oz)	420
6 Inch Sub Hot Pastrami	1 (7.2 oz)	430
6 Inch Sub Hot Pastrami Super Stacked	1 (10.1 oz)	570
6 Inch Sub Meatball	1 (10 oz)	580
6 Inch Sub Reuben	1 (9.2 oz)	530
6 Inch Sub Roast Beef & Provolone	1 (10.8 oz)	430
6 Inch Sub Roast Beef & Provolone On Wheat	1 (11.3 oz)	430
6 Inch Sub Tuna	1 (8.9 oz)	470
6 Inch Sub Turkey & Provolone	1 (10.8 oz)	410
6 Inch Sub Turkey & Provolone On Wheat	1 (11.3 oz)	420

FOOD	PORTION	CALS
6 Inch Sub VegiMax	1 (10.2 oz)	520
Blimpie Burger	1 (6 oz)	460
Blimpie Dog	1 (6.3 oz)	510
Ciabatta Buffalo Chicken	1 (11.3 oz)	540
Ciabatta French Dip	1 (13.8 oz)	430
Ciabatta Grilled Chicken Caesar	1 (10.1 oz)	580
Ciabatta Mediterranean	1 (10.1 oz)	450
Ciabatta Roast Beef Turkey & Cheddar	1 (10 oz)	520
Ciabatta Sicilian	1 (10 oz)	590
Ciabatta Spicy Chicken & Pepperoni	1 (10.1 oz)	710
Ciabatta Tuscan	1 (9.9 oz)	570
Ciabatta Ultimate Club	1 (7.4 oz)	520
Wrap Chicken Caesar	1 (9.7 oz)	220
Wrap Southwestern	1 (10 oz)	530
SOUPS		
Bean w/ Ham	1 serv (8.6 oz)	140
Chicken Noodle	1 serv (8.6 oz)	130
Chicken w/ White & Wild Rice	1 serv (8.6 oz)	250
Cream Of Broccoli w/ Cheese	1 serv (8.6 oz)	250
Cream Of Potato	1 serv (8.6 oz)	190
Garden Vegetable	1 serv (8.6 oz)	80
Grande Chili w/ Bean & Beef	1 serv (8.6 oz)	310
Tomato Basil w/ Raviolini	1 serv (8.6 oz)	110
Vegetable Beef	1 serv (8.6 oz)	80

BOB EVANS
BREAKFAST SELECTIONS

FOOD	PORTION	CALS
Bacon	1 piece	36
Benedict Ham & Cheese	1 serv	826
Country Benedict Sausage	1 serv	936
Country Benedict Spinach Bacon & Tomato	1 serv	729
Country Biscuit Breakfast	1 serv	659
Egg Hardcooked	1	60
Egg Over Easy	1	101
Egg Scrambled	1 serv	255
Egg Beaters	1 serv	173
French Toast	1 slice	131
French Toast Stuffed Plain	1 serv	599
Fruit & Yogurt Plate	1 serv	403
Grits	1 serv	178

FOOD	PORTION	CALS
Ham Smoked	1 slice	87
Hotcake Blueberry	1	328
Hotcake Buttermilk	1	318
Hotcake Cinnamon	1	417
Hotcake Multigrain	1	322
Mush	1 serv	79
Oatmeal	1 serv	172
Omelette Bacon & Cheese	1 serv	825
Omelette Border Scramble	1	756
Omelette Egg Beaters Bacon & Cheese	1 serv	615
Omelette Egg Beaters Border Scramble	1 serv	517
Omelette Egg Beaters Farmer's Market	1 serv	569
Omelette Egg Beaters Garden Harvest	1 serv	444
Omelette Egg Beaters Ham & Cheddar	1 serv	426
Omelette Egg Beaters Sausage & Cheddar	1 serv	502
Omelette Egg Beaters Three Cheese	1 serv	435
Omelette Farmer's Market	1	778
Omelette Garden Harvest	1 serv	654
Omelette Ham & Cheddar	1 serv	634
Omelette Sausage & Cheddar	1 serv	741
Omelette Three Cheese	1 serv	645
Omelette Western	1 serv	654
Pot Roast Hash	1 serv	652
Sausage Gravy Bowl	1 serv	268
Sausage Link	1	125
Skillet Sunshine	1 serv	842
Waffles Sweet Cream	1 serv	598
CHILDREN'S MENU SELECTIONS		
Hotcakes	1 serv	501
Kid's Macaroni & Cheese	1 serv	320
Kid's Pasta	1 serv	113
Mini Cheeseburgers	1 serv	306
Smiley Face Potatoes	1 serv	524
Sundae Reese's I'm Smiling	1 serv	330
MAIN MENU SELECTIONS		
Seniors Chicken Parmesan	1 serv	522
Seniors Garden Vegetable Alfredo	1 serv	363
Seniors Garden Vegetable Alfredo Chicken	1 serv	452
Seniors Steak Tips & Noodles	1 serv	422
Seniors Stir-Fry Chicken	1 serv	368

FOOD	PORTION	CALS
SOUPS		
Bean	1 cup	144
Cheddar Baked Potato	1 cup	294
Sausage Chili	1 cup	268
Vegetable Beef	1 cup	135
BOJANGLES		
Biscuit	1	243
Biscuit Sandwich Bacon	1	290
Biscuit Sandwich Bacon Egg Cheese	1	550
Biscuit Sandwich Cajun Filet	1	454
Biscuit Sandwich Country Ham	1	270
Biscuit Sandwich Egg	1	400
Biscuit Sandwich Sausage	1	350
Biscuit Sandwich Smoked Sausage	1	380
Biscuit Sandwich Steak	1	649
Botato Rounds	1 serv	235
Buffalo Bites	1 serv	180
Cajun Pintos	1 serv	110
Cajun Spiced Breast	1 serv	278
Cajun Spiced Leg	1 serv	264
Cajun Spiced Thigh	1 serv	310
Cajun Spiced Wing	1 serv	355
Chicken Supremes	1 serv	337
Corn On The Cob	1 serv	140
Dirty Rice	1 serv	166
Green Beans	1 serv	25
Macaroni & Cheese	1 serv	198
Marinated Cole Slaw	1 serv	136
Potatoes w/o Gravy	1 serv	80
Sandwich Cajun Filet w/ Mayo	1	437
Sandwich Cajun Filet w/o Mayo	1	337
Sandwich Grilled Filet w/ Mayo	1	335
Sandwich Grilled Filet w/o Mayo	1	235
Seasoned Fries	1 serv	344
Southern Style Breast	1 serv	261
Southern Style Leg	1 serv	254
Southern Style Thigh	1 serv	308
Southern Style Wing	1 serv	337
Sweet Biscuit Bo Berry	1	320
Sweet Biscuit Cinnamon	1	320

FOOD	PORTION	CALS
BOSTON MARKET		
DESSERTS		
Apple Pie	1 slice	420
Brownie Chocolate Chip Fudge	1	580
Chocolate Cake	1 serv	600
Cookie Chocolate Chip	1	370
Cornbread	1 piece	180
MAIN MENU SELECTIONS		
Broccoli w/ Garlic Butter	1 serv	80
Butternut Squash	1 serv	140
Carver Boston Chicken	1	700
Carver Boston Meatloaf	1	940
Carver Boston Sirloin Dip	1	1000
Carver Boston Turkey	1	770
Carver Boston Turkey Dip	1	770
Cinnamon Apples	1 serv	210
Cranberry Walnut Relish	1 serv	140
Creamed Spinach	1 serv	280
Dip Spinach Artichoke	1 serv	100
Family Meals Boneless Turkey Breast	1 serv (5 oz)	180
Family Meals Roasted Turkey	1 serv (5 oz)	180
Family Meals Rotisserie Chicken	1 serv (6 oz)	290
Family Meals Spiral Sliced Ham	1 serv (8 oz)	450
Family Meals Whole Turkey	1 serv (6.7 oz)	310
Fresh Vegetable Stuffing	1 serv	190
Garden Fresh Coleslaw	1 serv	170
Garlic Dill New Potatoes	1 serv	140
Green Bean Casserole	1 serv	60
Green Beans	1 serv	60
Individual Meals 1 Thigh & 1 Drumstick	1 serv	300
Individual Meals ¼ White Rotisserie Chicken	1 serv	290
Individual Meals ¼ White Rotisserie Chicken No Skin	1 serv	210
Individual Meals 3 Piece Dark	1 serv	380
Individual Meals 3 Piece Dark Skinless	1 serv	240
Individual Meals Award Winning Roasted Sirloin	1 serv	290
Individual Meals Meatloaf	1	480
Individual Meals Roasted Turkey	1 serv	180
Macaroni & Cheese	1 serv	330

FOOD	PORTION	CALS
Mashed Potatoes	1 serv	210
Pot Pie Pastry Topped Chicken	1	780
Poultry Gravy	1 serv (4 oz)	15
Seasonal Fresh Fruit Salad	1 serv	60
Spinach w/ Garlic Butter Sauce	1 serv	130
Squash Casserole	1 serv	320
Steamed Fresh Vegetables	1 serv	60
Sweet Corn	1 serv	170
Sweet Potato Casserole	1 serv	460
SALADS		
Entree Caesar	1	500
Entree Caesar w/o Dressing	1	140
Entree Market Chopped	1	580
Entree Market Chopped w/o Dressing	1	210
Side Caesar	1	400
Side Caesar w/o Dressing	1	40
Side Market Chopped	1	440
Side Market Chopped w/o Dressing	1	80
SOUPS		
Chicken Noodle	1 serv	170
Chicken Tortilla w/ Toppings	1 serv	340
Tortilla Soup w/o Toppings	1 serv	80

BOSTON PIZZA
CHILDREN'S MENU SELECTIONS

Baked Salmon w/ Caesar Salad	1 serv	330
Bug N' Cheese	1 serv	500
Chicken Fingers w/ Fries	1 serv	390
Pizza Pint Size	1	390
Quesadilla Bacon Double Cheeseburger w/ Caesar Salad	1 serv	540
Reduced Size Fruit Cup	1 serv	80
Sandwich Grilled Chicken w/ Garden Greens	1 serv	600
Super Spaghetti	1 serv	440
Wrap Ham & Cheese w/ Fries	1 serv	550
DESSERTS		
Blondie Maple	1	850
Blondie Maple Bite Size	1	430
Brownie Chocolate Addiction	1	490
Brownie Chocolate Addiction Bite Size	1	200

FOOD	PORTION	CALS
Cheesecake New York	1 slice	620
Cheesecake Vanilla Bean	1 slice	770
Chocolate Explosion	1 serv	890
Tarte Au Sucre	1 serv	310
MAIN MENU SELECTIONS		
Angus Beef Sirloin Steak w/ Spaghetti	1 serv	1260
Baked 3 Cheese Penne	1 half order	460
Baked Seven Cheese Ravioli	1 half order	310
Baked Shrimp & Feta Penne	1 half order	480
Boston's Lasagne	1 half order	340
Boston's Smokey Mountain Spaghetti	1 order	1290
Chicken & Mushroom Fettuccini	1 half order	710
Chicken Parmesan w/ Seasonal Vegetables	1 serv	1060
Fries	1 serv	430
Garlic Mashed Potatoes	1 serv	730
Garlic Toast	1 slice	150
Homestyle Lasagna	1 order	590
Jambalaya Fettuccini	1 half order	860
Lemon Baked Salmon w/ Fries	1 serv	1150
Mama Meata Penne	1 half order	940
Mushroom Chicken w/ Garlic Mashed Potatoes	1 serv	1030
Pad Thai w/ Chicken	1 serv	2110
Pad Thai w/ Shrimp	1 serv	2090
Pollo Pomodoro Spaghetti	1 serv	520
Salmon Filet Lemon Baked	1 serv	430
Scallop & Prawn Fettuccini	1 half order	710
Seasoned Vegetables	1 serv	70
Shrimp Skewers Lime & Parmesan	1 serv	190
Sicilian Penne	1 half order	720
Sirloin Steak w/ Prawns & Fries	1 serv	1480
Slow Roasted Pork Back Ribs w/ Fries	1 serv	1680
Spaghetti w/ Alfredo Sauce	1 half order	440
Spaghetti w/ Bolognese	1 half order	400
Spaghetti w/ Creamy Tomato Sauce	1 half order	410
Spaghetti w/ Pomodoro Sauce	1 half order	450
Spicy Italian Penne	1 half order	980
Starter Baked Raviolo Bites	1 serv	450
Starter Basket Garlic Twist	1 serv	1140
Starter Basket Three Cheese Toast	1 serv	730
Starter Boston's Poutine	1 serv	740

FOOD	PORTION	CALS
Starter Bruschetta Sun Dried Tomato	1 serv	470
Starter Cactus Cuts Potatoes & Dip	1 serv	1150
Starter Chicken Fingers	1 serv	360
Starter Chicken Fingers Buffalo Style	1 serv	370
Starter Cracked Pepper Dry Ribs	1 serv	380
Starter Nachos Cactus w/ Cactus Dip	1 serv	1830
Starter Nachos Spicy Chicken w/ Sour Cream & Salsa	1 serv	1430
Starter Nachos Taco Beef w/ Sour Cream & Salsa	1 serv	1560
Starter Nachos w/ Sour Cream & Salsa	1 serv	1320
Starter Panzerotti Roll	1	820
Starter Pizza Bread Bandera w/ Santa Fe Ranch Dip	1 serv	960
Starter Pizza Bread w/o Sauce	1 serv	500
Starter Potato Skins	1 serv	650
Starter Quesadilla Oven Roasted Chicken	1 serv	900
Starter Quesadilla Southwest w/ Sour Cream & Salsa	1 serv	770
Starter Shrimp Stuffed Mushroom Caps	1 serv	490
Starter Team Platter w/ Dips & Sauces	1 serv	3030
Starter Thai Chicken Bites	1 serv	540
Starter Wings Breaded BBQ	1 serv	930
Starter Wings Breaded Honey Garlic	1 serv	940
Starter Wings Breaded Mild	1 serv	880
Starter Wings Breaded Teriyaki	1 serv	940
Starter Wings Breaded Thai	1 serv	1110
Starter Wings Oven Roasted BBQ	1 serv	670
Starter Wings Oven Roasted Honey Garlic	1 serv	700
Starter Wings Oven Roasted Hot	1 serv	620
Starter Wings Oven Roasted Teriyaki	1 serv	670
Starter Wings Oven Roasted Thai Chili	1 serv	770
The Ribber w/ Spaghetti	1 serv	970
Tortellini w/ Alfredo Sauce	1 half order	340
Tortellini w/ Bolognese	1 half order	300
Tortellini w/ Creamy Tomato Sauce	1 half order	310
Tortellini w/ Pomodoro Sauce	1 half order	340
Veal Parmesan w/ Spaghetti	1 serv	1020
PIZZA		
Bacon Double Cheeseburger Individual	1 pie	1140

FOOD	PORTION	CALS
Bacon Double Cheeseburger Slice	1 med	280
BBQ Chicken Individual	1 pie	730
BBQ Chicken Slice	1 med	190
Boston Royal Individual	1 pie	840
Boston Royal Slice	1 med	210
Californian Slice	1 med	280
Clubhouse Individual	1 pie	1040
Deluxe Individual	1 pie	850
Deluxe Slice	1 med	220
Great White North Slice	1 med	240
Hawaiian Individual	1 pie	780
Hawaiian Slice	1 med	210
Indy California	1 (11.3 oz)	440
La Quebecoise Individual	1 pie	770
La Quebecoise Slice	1 med	200
Meateor Individual	1 pie	950
Meateor Slice	1 med	260
Pepperoni Individual	1 pie	750
Pepperoni Slice	1 med	200
Pepperoni & Mushroom Individual	1 pie	750
Pepperoni & Mushroom Slice	1 med	200
Popeye Individual	1 pie	720
Popeye Slice	1 med	200
Rustic Italian Individual	1 pie	950
Rustic Italian Slice	1 med	260
Spicy Perogy Individual	1 pie	980
Spicy Perogy Slice	1 med	280
Szechuan Individual	1 pie	750
Szechuan Slice	1 med	200
Tandoori Individual	1 pie	730
Tandoori Slice	1 med	200
Thai Chicken Individual	1 pie	840
Thai Chicken Slice	1 med	240
The Basic Individual	1 pie	620
The Basic Slice	1 med	160
Tropical Chicken Individual	1 pie	970
Tropical Chicken Slice	1 med	260
Tuscan Individual	1 pie	940
Tuscan Slice	1 med	250
Ultimate Pepperoni Individual	1 pie	870

FOOD	PORTION	CALS
Ultimate Pepperoni Slice	1 med	230
Vegetarian Individual	1 pie	680
Vegetarian Slice	1 med	180
Zorba The Greek Individual	1 pie	800
Zorba The Greek Slice	1 med	210
SALAD DRESSINGS AND TOPPINGS		
House Dressing	1 serv (2 oz)	270
Ketchup	1 serv (2 oz)	60
Salsa	1 serv (2 oz)	20
Sour Cream	1 serv (2 oz)	100
SALADS		
Chipotle Chicken & Bacon	1 serv	630
Crispy Chicken Pecan	1 serv	1100
Entree Caesar	1 serv	500
Entree Spinach	1 serv	450
Garden Greens w/ House Dressing	1 serv	310
Garden Greens w/ Low Fat Raspberry Vinaigrette	1 serv	130
Side Caesar	1 serv	170
Starter Spinach	1 serv	250
Taco Salad Beef w/o Sour Cream & Salsa	1 serv	610
Taco Salad Chicken w/o Sour Cream & Salsa	1 serv	480
Thai Chicken Salad	1 serv	1060
SANDWICHES		
Beef Dip w/ Fries & Au Jus	1 serv	1340
Boston Brute w/ Caesar Salad & Au Jus	1 serv	820
Boston Cheesesteak w/ Caesar Salad & Au Jus	1 serv	1300
Buffalo Chicken w/ Fries	1 serv	1220
Chicken Parmesan w/ Fries	1 serv	1370
Ciabatta Chicken w/ Caesar Salad	1 serv	920
New York Steak w/ Garden Greens & Au Jus	1 serv	660
Stromboli Bacon Double Cheeseburger w/ Caesar Salad	1 serv	910
Stromboli Chicken Santa Fe w/ Caesar Salad	1 serv	750
Stromboli Smoked Ham & Chicken w/ Caesar Salad	1 serv	880
Wrap Thai Chicken	1	570
SOUPS		
Baked French Onion	1 serv	330
Clam Chowder	1 serv	260

FOOD	PORTION	CALS

BRUEGGER'S BAGELS
BAGELS

FOOD	PORTION	CALS
Asiago Parmesan	1	330
Baked Apple	1	370
Blueberry	1	330
Chocolate Chip	1	350
Cinnamon Sugar	1	330
Cranberry Orange	1	330
Everything	1	320
Garlic	1	320
Honey Grain	1	330
Jalapeno Bagel	1	320
Multi-Grain	1	350
Onion	1	320
Plain	1	320
Poppy	1	320
Pumpernickel	1	330
Pumpkin	1	330
Rosemary Olive Oil	1	350
Salt	1	320
Sesame	1	360
Sourdough	1	340
Square Asiago Parmesan	1	360
Square Everything	1	320
Square Plain	1	350
Square Sesame	1	360
Sun Dried Tomato	1	320
Whole Wheat	1	390

DESSERTS

FOOD	PORTION	CALS
Brownie Chocolate Chunk	1	330
Cake Lemon Pound	1 slice	320
Cookie Chocolate Chip	1	500
Cookie Oatmeal Raisin	1	460
Cookie Peanut Butter	1	480
Cookie Triple Chocolate Chunk	1	560
Cookie White Chocolate Macadamia	1	580
Luscious Lemon Bar	1	300
Marshmallow Chew	1	280
Muffin Blueberry	1	450
Muffin Chocolate	1	460

FOOD	PORTION	CALS
Oreo Dream Bar	1	470
Pecan Chocolate Chunk	1 slice	310
Raspberry Sammies	1 slice	340
Seven Layer Bar	1	650
Toffee Almond Bar	1	400
SALADS		
Caesar w/ Dressing	1 serv	270
Tossed Chicken Caesar w/ Dressing	1 serv	370
Tossed Mandarin Medley	1 serv	340
Tossed Sesame Chicken	1 serv	480
SANDWICHES		
BLT w/ Mayo	1	570
Chicken Breast	1	660
Chicken Fajita	1	530
Chicken Salad w/ Mayo	1	630
Cranberry Gobbler	1	620
Cuban Chicken	1	680
Denver Egg	1	460
Egg Cheese	1	420
Egg Cheese Bacon	1	460
Egg Cheese Ham	1	460
Egg Cheese Sausage	1	640
Ham	1	460
Herby Turkey	1	560
Leonardo Da Veggie	1	480
Radishy Roast Beef	1	560
Roadhouse Chicken	1	710
Roast Beef	1	730
Santa Fe Turkey	1	490
Smoked Salmon	1	490
Softwich BLT w/ Mayo	1	600
Softwich Chicken Breast	1	630
Softwich Chicken Fajita	1	570
Softwich Chicken Salad	1	670
Softwich Cranberry Gobbler	1	730
Softwich Cuban Chicken	1	810
Softwich Garden Veggie	1	380
Softwich Ham	1	510
Softwich Herby Turkey	1	580
Softwich Hummus	1	540

FOOD	PORTION	CALS
Softwich Leonardo De Veggie	1	550
Softwich Mediterranean	1	790
Softwich Peanut Chicken	1	590
Softwich Radishy Roast Beef	1	670
Softwich Roadhouse Chicken	1	670
Softwich Roast Beef	1	750
Softwich Roasted Turkey	1	550
Softwich Smoked Salmon	1	520
Softwich Supreme Club w/o Mayo	1	880
Softwich Tuna Salad	1	720
Softwich Western Wheat	1	820
Supreme Club w/o Mayo	1	470
Tuna Salad	1	620
Turkey	1	510
Wrap Classic w/ Bacon	1	520
Wrap Classic w/ Ham	1	510
Wrap Classic w/ Sausage	1	660
Wrap Rio Grande Bacon	1	560
Wrap Rio Grande Ham	1	630
Wrap Rio Grande Sausage	1	510
Wrap Sesame Chicken Salad	1	770
Wrap Tossed Chicken Caesar	1	660
Wrap Tossed Mandarin Medley Salad	1	630
SOUPS		
Chicken Pot Pie	1 cup	250
Chicken Spaetzle	1 cup	120
Chicken Wild Rice	1 cup	260
Creamy Tomato	1 cup	150
Hearty Mushroom Barley	1 cup	110
Italian Wedding	1 cup	160
Minestrone	1 cup	120
Moroccan Stew	1 cup	140
New England Clam	1 cup	300
Sweet Potato Cheddar	1 cup	200
SPREADS		
Cream Cheese Bacon Scallion	1 scoop (1.5 oz)	140
Cream Cheese Cucumber Dill	1 scoop (1.5 oz)	140
Cream Cheese Garden Veggie	1 scoop (1.5 oz)	130
Cream Cheese Honey Walnut	1 scoop (1.5 oz)	150
Cream Cheese Jalapeno	1 scoop (1.5 oz)	140

FOOD	PORTION	CALS
Cream Cheese Light Garden Veggie	1 scoop (1.5 oz)	90
Cream Cheese Light Herb Garlic	1 scoop (1.5 oz)	100
Cream Cheese Light Plain	1 scoop (1.5 oz)	100
Cream Cheese Olive Pimento	1 scoop (1.5 oz)	140
Cream Cheese Onion & Chive	1 scoop (1.5 oz)	140
Cream Cheese Plain	1 scoop (1.5 oz)	130
Cream Cheese Pumpkin	1 scoop (1.5 oz)	120
Cream Cheese Strawberry	1 scoop (1.5 oz)	140
Cream Cheese Wildberry	1 scoop (1.5 oz)	140
Hummus	1 scoop (2 oz)	110

BURGER KING
BEVERAGES

FOOD	PORTION	CALS
Apple Juice	1 (6.67 oz)	90
BK Joe Regular	1 sm	5
BK Joe Turbo	1 sm (12 oz)	10
Chocolate Milk 1% Low Fat	1 (9 oz)	180
Coke Classic	1 sm (16 oz)	140
Diet Coke	1 sm (16 oz)	0
Dr Pepper	1 sm (16 oz)	140
Iced Coffee Mocha BK Joe	1 (16 oz)	380
Icee Coco Cola	1 sm (16 oz)	110
Icee Minute Maid Cherry	1 sm (16 oz)	110
Milk 1% Low Fat	1	110
Minute Maid Orange Juice	8 oz	140
Shake Chocolate	1 sm (16 oz)	470
Shake Oreo Sundae Chocolate	1 sm (16 oz)	680
Shake Oreo Sundae Strawberry	1 sm (16 oz)	660
Shake Oreo Sundae Vanilla	1 sm (16 oz)	610
Shake Strawberry	1 sm (16 oz)	460
Shake Vanilla	1 sm (16 oz)	400
Sprite	1 sm (16 oz)	140
Water Nestle Pure Life	1 bottle (16 oz)	0

BREAKFAST SELECTIONS

FOOD	PORTION	CALS
Biscuit Bacon Egg & Cheese	1	410
Biscuit Ham Egg & Cheese	1	390
Biscuit Sausage	1	390
Biscuit Sausage Egg & Cheese	1	530
Croissan'wich Bacon Egg & Cheese	1	340
Croissan'wich Double w/ Bacon Egg & Cheese	1	430

FOOD	PORTION	CALS
Croissan'wich Double w/ Ham Bacon Egg & Cheese	1	420
Croissan'wich Double w/ Ham Egg & Cheese	1	420
Croissan'wich Double w/ Ham Sausage Egg & Cheese	1	550
Croissan'wich Double w/ Sausage Bacon Egg & Cheese	1	550
Croissan'wich Double w/ Sausage Egg & Cheese	1	680
Croissan'wich Egg & Cheese	1	300
Croissan'wich Ham Egg & Cheese	1	340
Croissan'wich Sausage & Cheese	1	370
Croissan'wich Sausage Egg & Cheese	1	470
French Toast Sticks	3 pieces	240
Hash Browns	1 sm	260
Hash Browns	1 lg	620
Omelet Sandwich Enormous	1	730
Omelet Sandwich Ham	1	290
DESSERTS		
Cini-minis	1 serv	390
Dutch Apple Pie	1 serv	300
Hershey Sundae Pie	1	310
MAIN MENU SELECTIONS		
BK Chicken Fries	6 pieces	260
BK Stacker Double	1	610
BK Stacker Quad	1	1000
BK Stacker Triple	1	800
BK Veggie Burger	1	420
Cheeseburger	1	330
Cheeseburger Double	1	500
Chicken Sandwich Original	1	660
Chicken Sandwich Tendercrisp	1	790
Chicken Sandwich Tendergrill	1	510
Chicken Tenders	5 pieces	210
Chick'n Crisp Spicy Sandwich	1	480
Double Cheeseburger	1	410
French Fries No Salt Added	1 sm	230
French Fries Salted	1 sm	230
French Fries Salted	1 lg	500
Hamburger	1	290

FOOD	PORTION	CALS
Onion Rings	1 sm	140
Onion Rings	1 lg	440
Sandwich BK Big Fish	1	640
The Angus Steak Burger	1	640
Whopper	1	670
Whopper w/ Cheese	1	760
Whopper Double	1	900
Whopper Double w/ Cheese	1	990
Whopper Jr.	1	370
Whopper Jr. w/ Cheese	1	410
Whopper Triple	1	1130
Whopper Triple w/ Cheese	1	1230
SALAD DRESSINGS AND TOPPINGS		
Breakfast Syrup	1 serv (1 oz)	80
Croutons Garlic Parmesan	1 serv	60
Dipping Sauce Barbecue	1 serv (1 oz)	40
Dipping Sauce Honey Mustard	1 serv (1 oz)	90
Dipping Sauce Ranch	1 serv (1 oz)	140
Dipping Sauce Sweet And Sour	1 serv (1 oz)	40
Dressing Ken's Creamy Caesar	1 serv (2 oz)	210
Dressing Ken's Fat Free Ranch	1 serv (2 oz)	60
Dressing Ken's Honey Mustard	1 serv (2 oz)	270
Dressing Ken's Ranch	1 serv (2 oz)	190
Jam Grape	1 serv	30
Jam Strawberry	1 serv	30
Ketchup	1 pkg	10
Mayonnaise	1 pkg	80
SALADS		
Chicken Garden Tendercrisp	1	410
Chicken Garden Tendergrill w/o Dressing or Croutons	1	240
Side Garden w/o Dressing	1	15

BURGERVILLE
BEVERAGES

FOOD	PORTION	CALS
Barq's Root Beer	1 (20 oz)	180
Coca-Cola	1 (20 oz)	161
Diet Coke	1 (20 oz)	0
Hot Chocolate Ghirardelli	1 (12 oz)	230
House Coffee	1 (10 oz)	5

FOOD	PORTION	CALS
Iced Tea	1 (20 oz)	0
Iced Tea Nestea Raspberry	1 (20 oz)	127
Lemonade Odwalla	1 (20 oz)	240
Milk 2%	1 (8 oz)	121
Orange Juice Odwalla	1 (10 oz)	138
Pibb Xtra	1 (20 oz)	163
Sprite	1 (20 oz)	158
BREAKFAST SELECTIONS		
Bagel	1	310
Bagel Bacon And Egg	1	490
Bagel Ham And Egg	1	490
Bagel Sausage And Egg	1	640
Breakfast Platter w/ Bacon	1 serv	730
Breakfast Platter w/ Ham	1 serv	725
Breakfast Platter w/ Sausage	1 serv	880
Hash Browns	1 serv	230
Toaster Biscuit	1	320
Toaster Biscuit Bacon And Egg	1	450
Toaster Biscuit Ham And Egg	1	440
Toaster Biscuit Sausage And Egg	1	600
DESSERTS		
Cone Vanilla	1	250
Cone YoCream Frozen Yogurt	1	190
Cookie Chocolate Chunk	1	320
Cookie Oatmeal Raisin	1	290
Cookie Sugar	1	305
Cookie White Chocolate Macadamia	1	340
Strawberry Shortcake	1 serv	440
Sundae Caramel	1	380
Sundae Fresh Strawberry	1	340
Sundae Hot Fudge	1	380
Sundae Triple Berry	1	340
Sundae YoCream Caramel	1	260
Sundae YoCream Hot Fudge	1	260
Sundae YoCream Strawberry	1	220
Sundae YoCream Triple Berry	1	200
MAIN MENU SELECTIONS		
Apple Slices	1 serv	29
Cheeseburger	1	350
Cheeseburger Colossal	1	520

FOOD	PORTION	CALS
Cheeseburger Double Beef	1	430
Cheeseburger Tillamook	1	630
Cheeseburger Tillamook Pepper Bacon	1	690
Chicken Strips	5	320
French Fries	1 serv	410
Gardenburger Spicy Black Bean	1	550
Gardenburger The Original	1	450
Halibut	3 pieces	320
Hamburger	1	300
Hamburger Burgerville Classic	1	510
Onion Rings Walla Walla	1 serv	810
Sandwich Crispy Chicken	1	490
Sandwich Deluxe Crispy Chicken	1	590
Sandwich Halibut	1	480
Sandwich Low Fat Grilled Chicken	1	320
Sandwich Nine Grain Turkey Club	1	550
Sweet Potato Fries	1 serv	530
Turkey Burger Seasoned	1	540
Yukon Golds	1 serv	450
SALAD DRESSINGS AND TOPPINGS		
Burgerville Spread Cup	1	280
Cream Cheese	1 serv	100
Cream Cheese Light	1 serv	70
Dip BBQ Sauce	1 serv	60
Dressing Blue Cheese	1 serv	240
Dressing Caesar	1 serv	220
Dressing Honey Mustard	1 serv	210
Dressing Ranch	1 serv	195
Sauce Sweet And Sour	1 serv	90
Tartar Cup	1	260
Vinaigrette Honey Lime	1 serv	250
Vinaigrette Raspberry	1 serv	45
SALADS		
Grilled Chicken	1	430
Rogue River Smokey Blue	1	290
Side Salad	1	50
Wild Smoked Salmon & Hazelnuts	1	440

FOOD	PORTION	CALS
CARL'S JR.		
BEVERAGES		
Malt Chocolate	1 (15 oz)	780
Malt Oreo Cookie	1 (15 oz)	790
Malt Strawberry	1 (15 oz)	770
Malt Vanilla	1 (15 oz)	760
Shake Chocolate	1 (14 oz)	710
Shake Oreo Cookie	1 (14 oz)	720
Shake Strawberry	1 (14 oz)	700
Shake Vanilla	1 (14 oz)	710
BREAKFAST SELECTIONS		
Breakfast Burger	1	830
Burrito Bacon & Egg	1	570
Burrito Loaded Breakfast	1	820
Burrito Steak & Egg	1	660
French Toast Dips w/o Syrup	5	430
Hash Brown Nuggets	1 serv	330
Sandwich Sourdough Breakfast	1 serv	460
Sunrise Croissant Sandwich	1	560
DESSERTS		
Cheesecake Strawberry Swirl	1 serv	290
Chocolate Cake	1 serv	300
Cookie Chocolate Chip	1	350
MAIN MENU SELECTIONS		
Burger Jalapeno	1	720
Burger Teriyaki	1	660
Cheeseburger Double Western Bacon	1	970
Cheeseburger Western Bacon	1	710
Chicken Breast Strips	3	420
Chicken Stars	4	170
CrissCut Fries	1 serv	410
Famous Star w/ Cheese	1	660
Fish & Chips	1 serv	630
French Fries	1 sm	290
Fried Zucchini	1 serv	320
Hamburger Big	1	470
Hamburger Kid's	1	460
Onion Rings	1 serv	430
Sandwich Bacon Swiss Crispy Chicken	1	720
Sandwich Carl's Catch Fish	1	660

FOOD	PORTION	CALS
Sandwich Charbroiled BBQ Chicken	1	360
Sandwich Charbroiled Chicken Club	1	550
Sandwich Charbroiled Santa Fe Chicken	1	610
Sandwich Spicy Chicken	1	560
Six Dollar Burger The Bacon Cheese	1	1070
Six Dollar Burger The Guacamole Bacon	1	1140
Six Dollar Burger The Jalapeno	1	1030
Six Dollar Burger The Low Carb	1	490
Six Dollar Burger The Original	1	1010
Six Dollar Burger The Western Bacon	1	1130
Super Star w/ Cheese	1	930
SALAD DRESSINGS		
Balsamic Low Fat	1 serv (2 oz)	35
Blue Cheese	1 serv (2 oz)	320
House	1 serv (2 oz)	220
Italian Fat Free	1 serv (2 oz)	15
Thousand Island	1 serv (2 oz)	240
SALADS		
Charbroiled Chicken	1	260
Side	1	50

CARVEL

FOOD	PORTION	CALS
Brown Bonnet	1	370
Cake Ice Cream	1 slice	270
Carvelanche Cake Mix	1 reg (16 oz)	720
Carvelanche Cookies & Cream	1 reg (16 oz)	550
Carvelanche Triple Fudge Cake Mix	1 reg (16 oz)	900
Chipsters	1	330
Cone Cake Chocolate	1 sm	260
Cone Cake Chocolate	1 lg	600
Cone Cake Vanilla	1 sm	280
Cone Cake Vanilla	1 lg	650
Cone Sugar Chocolate	1 sm	300
Cone Sugar Vanilla	1 sm	320
Cone Waffle Chocolate	1 sm	330
Cone Waffle Chocolate	1 lg	660
Cone Waffle Vanilla	1 sm	350
Cone Waffle Vanilla	1 lg	710
Dashers Banana Barge	1	940
Dashers Bananas Foster	1	600

FOOD	PORTION	CALS
Dashers Fudge Brownie	1	810
Dashers Mint Chocolate Chip	1	720
Dashers Peanut Butter Cup	1	1090
Dashers Strawberry Shortcake	1	590
Flying Saucer 98% Fat Free Chocolate	1	180
Flying Saucer 98% Fat Free Vanilla	1	180
Flying Saucer Chocolate	1	230
Flying Saucer Deluxe Sprinkles	1	330
Flying Saucer Vanilla	1	240
Ice Cream Chocolate	1 sm (4 oz)	250
Ice Cream Vanilla	1 sm (4 oz)	240
Ice Cream No Fat Chocolate	1 sm (4 oz)	160
Ice Cream No Fat Vanilla	1 sm (4 oz)	160
Sherbet All Flavors	1 sm (4 oz)	180
Sinful Love Bar	1	460
Sprinkle Cup	1	230
Sundae Bittersweet Fudge	1 reg	690
Sundae Caramel	1 reg	670
Sundae Hot Fudge	1 reg	670
Sundae Mini Chocolate Syrup	1	200
Sundae Strawberry	1 reg	580
Thick Shake Chocolate	1 reg (16 oz)	650
Thick Shake Vanilla	1 reg (16 oz)	610
Thinny Thin Classic Sundae No Fat Fudge	1 reg	380
Thinny Thin Classic Sundae No Fat Strawberry	1 reg	320
Thinny Thin Miniature Sundae No Fat	1	190
Thinny Thin Miniature Sundae No Sugar Added	1	200
Thinny Thin No Fat Carvelanche Strawberry	1 (16 oz)	430
Thinny Thin No Fat Chocolate	1 sm	160
Thinny Thin No Fat Vanilla	1 sm	160
Thinny Thin No Sugar Added Vanilla	1 sm	180
Thinny Thin Parfait No Fat	1	190
Thinny Thin Shake No Fat Chocolate	1 (16 oz)	440
Thinny Thin Shake No Fat Mocha	1 (16 oz)	440
Thinny Thin Shake No Fat Vanilla	1 (16 oz)	300

CHICKEN OUT ROTISSERIE
MAIN MENU SELECTIONS

¼ Dark Chicken w/ Skin	1 serv	337
¼ Dark Chicken w/o Skin	1 serv	223

FOOD	PORTION	CALS
Apple Cornbread Stuffing	1 serv (7 oz)	453
Baked Potato Wedges	1 serv (8 oz)	220
Chunky Cinnamon Applesauce	1 serv (7 oz)	241
Cranberry Relish	1 serv (7 oz)	285
Creamed Spinach	1 serv (6 oz)	320
Edamame Beans In Sweet Pepper Sauce	1 serv (7 oz)	200
Farm Fresh Cole Slaw	1 serv (7 oz)	226
Fresh Fruit Salad	1 serv (7 oz)	110
Grilled Chicken Filet Skinless	1 (6 oz)	290
Half Sandwich BBQ & Cole Slaw	1	340
Half Sandwich Classic Grilled Chicken	1	405
Half Sandwich Signature Chicken Salad	1	305
Just The Turkey Burger	1 (7 oz)	360
Macaroni & Cheese	1 serv (7 oz)	290
Mashed Sweet Potatoes	1 serv (7 oz)	423
Pulled BBQ Chicken	1 serv (6 oz)	380
Pulled Rotisserie Chicken Breast	1 serv (6 oz)	290
Red Skin Mashed Potatoes	1 serv (7 oz)	334
Sandwich Hot Openfaced Pulled Chicken On Biscuit	1	1180
Steamed Vegetable Medley	1 serv (7 oz)	30
Wrap Apricot Chicken Salad	½	412
Wrap Asian Chicken Salad	½	341
Wrap BBQ Chicken w/ Cole Slaw	½	395
Wrap Chopped Veggie	½	315
Wrap Cobb Salad	½	430
Wrap Freshly Roasted Turkey w/ Cucumber Sauce	½	325
Wrap Garden Veggie & Cheese	½	352
Wrap Grilled Chicken	½	359
Wrap Grilled Chicken Caesar	½	386
Wrap Santa Fe	½	371
Wrap Spinach & Milan Cutlet	½	315
SALAD DRESSINGS		
Buttermilk Ranch	1 oz	110
Creamy Caesar	1 oz	181
Creamy Cole Slaw	1 oz	125
Honey Balsamic Vinaigrette	1 oz	161
Honey Mustard Fat Free	1 oz	50
Southwest	1 oz	146

FOOD	PORTION	CALS
SALADS		
Apricot Chicken Salad	1 serv (6 oz)	610
Asian Chicken w/o Dressing or Wontons	1 serv	325
Caesar Grilled Chicken w/o Dressing or Croutons	1 serv	310
Caesar w/o Dressing Croutons or Roll	1 serv	90
Chicken Cobb	1 serv	720
Chopped Veggie & Chicken w/o Dressing or Croutons	1 serv	300
Freshly Roasted Turkey Breast	1 serv	320
Garden Grilled Chicken w/o Dressing or Croutons	1 serv	269
Green Leaf Fruit & Granola	1 serv	380
Milan Chicken Cutlet	1 serv	348
Santa Fe Chicken w/o Dressing or Tortilla Strips	1 serv	399
Signature Chicken Salad	1 serv (6 oz)	790
Spinach w/ Milan Cutlet	1 serv	550
SOUPS		
Chicken Noodle	1 serv (13 oz)	211
Vegetable Primavera	1 serv (13 oz)	330
CHICK-FIL-A		
BEVERAGES		
Coca-Cola	1 med	170
Coffee 100% Colombian	1 med	5
Diet Coke	1 med	0
Dr Pepper	1 med	180
Ice Tea Sweetened	1 med	130
Iced Tea Unsweetened	1 med	0
Lemonade	1 med	240
Lemonade Diet	1 med	20
Milkshake Chocolate	1 sm	600
Milkshake Peach	1 sm	780
Milkshake Strawberry	1 sm	610
BREAKFAST SELECTIONS		
Bagel Multigrain Chicken Egg & Cheese	1	490
Biscuit Bacon Egg & Cheese	1	500
Biscuit Chicken	1	440
Biscuit Plain	1	310
Biscuit Sausage	1	590

FOOD	PORTION	CALS
Biscuit Spicy Chicken	1	450
Breakfast Burrito Chicken	1	450
Breakfast Burrito Sausage	1	510
Chick-N-Minis	3	280
Cinnamon Cluster	1 serv	430
Hashbrowns	1 serv	270
Yogurt Parfait	1	230
Yogurt Parfait w/ Chocolate Cookie Crumbs	1	240
Yogurt Parfait w/ Granola	1	290
DESSERTS		
Cheesecake	1 slice	310
Fudge Nut Brownie	1	370
Icedream	1 cup	290
Icedream Cone	1	170
Lemon Pie	1 slice	360
MAIN MENU SELECTIONS		
Chick-N-Strips	3	360
Cool Wrap Chargrilled Chicken	1	410
Cool Wrap Chicken Caesar	1	460
Cool Wrap Spicy Chicken	1	410
Hearty Breast of Chicken Soup	1 med	140
Nuggets	8	260
Sandwich Chargrilled Chicken	1	290
Sandwich Chargrilled Chicken Club	1	410
Sandwich Chicken	1	430
Sandwich Chicken Deluxe	1	490
Sandwich Chicken Salad On Wheat Bread	1	490
Sandwich Spicy Chicken	1	480
Sandwich Spicy Chicken Deluxe	1	570
Waffle Potato Fries	1 med	360
SALAD DRESSINGS AND SAUCES		
Dressing Berry Balsamic Vinaigrette Reduced Fat	½ pkg (1.25 oz)	70
Dressing Blue Cheese	½ pkg (1.25 oz)	160
Dressing Buttermilk Ranch	½ pkg (1.25 oz)	160
Dressing Caesar	½ pkg (1.25 oz)	160
Dressing Honey Mustard Fat Free	½ pkg (1.25 oz)	60
Dressing Italian Light	½ pkg (1.25 oz)	15
Dressing Spicy	½ pkg (1.25 oz)	140
Dressing Thousand Island	½ pkg (1.25 oz)	150

FOOD	PORTION	CALS
Sauce Barbecue	½ pkg (0.5 oz)	45
Sauce Buffalo	½ pkg (0.4 oz)	10
Sauce Buttermilk Ranch	½ pkg (0.4 oz)	110
Sauce Chick-fil-A	½ pkg (0.5 oz)	140
Sauce Honey Mustard	½ pkg (1.25 oz)	45
Sauce Honey Roasted BBQ	½ pkg	60
Sauce Polynesian	½ pkg (0.5 oz)	110
SALADS		
Carrot & Raisin Salad	1 med	260
Chargrilled Chicken Garden Salad	1 serv	180
Chargrilled & Fruit	1 serv	220
Chicken Salad Bacon & Egg	1 cup	350
Chick-N-Strips Salad	1 serv	460
Cole Slaw	1 med	360
Croutons Garlic & Butter	1 pkg	60
Fruit Cup	1 serv	70
Harvest Nut Granola	1 pkg	60
Honey Roasted Sunflower Kernels	1 pkg	90
Side Salad	1 serv	70
Southwest Chargrilled Salad	1 serv	240
Tortilla Strips	1 pkg	80

CHIPOTLE

FOOD	PORTION	CALS
Barbacoa	1 serv (4 oz)	228
Black Beans	1 serv (4 oz)	130
Carnitas	1 serv (4 oz)	227
Cheese	1 serv (1 oz)	110
Chicken	1 serv (4 oz)	219
Chips	1 serv (4 oz)	490
Crispy Taco Shells	3	180
Fajita Vegetables	1 serv (3 oz)	100
Flour Tortilla	1 (6 inch)	300
Flour Tortilla	1 (13 inch)	330
Guacamole	1 serv (4 oz)	170
Lettuce	1 serv (1 oz)	5
Pinto Beans	1 serv (4 oz)	138
Rice	1 serv (3.5 oz)	168
Salsa Corn	1 serv (4 oz)	100
Salsa Tomato	1 serv (4 oz)	25
Sour Cream	1 serv (2 oz)	120

FOOD	PORTION	CALS
Steak	1 serv (4 oz)	230
Tomatillo Green	1 serv (2 oz)	15
Tomatillo Red	1 serv (2 oz)	28
Vinaigrette	1 serv (2 oz)	282

CHURCH'S CHICKEN
DESSERTS

Pie Apple	1 pie (3 oz)	280
Pie Edward's Double Lemon	1 pie (3 oz)	300
Pie Edward's Strawberry Cream Cheese	1 pie (2.8 oz)	280

MAIN MENU SELECTIONS

Biscuit Honey Butter	1	240
Cajun Rice	1 reg	130
Chicken Fried Steak w/ White Gravy	1 serv (7.5 oz)	610
Cole Slaw	1 reg	150
Corn On The Cob	1 ear	140
Country Fried Steak w/ White Gravy	1 serv (5.8 oz)	470
Crunchy Tenders	1 (2 oz)	120
French Fries	1 reg	290
Jalapeno Cheese Bombers	4 (4 oz)	240
Macaroni & Cheese	1 reg	210
Mashed Potatoes & Gravy	1 reg	70
Okra	1 reg	350
Original Breast	1	200
Original Leg	1	110
Original Thigh	1	330
Original Wing	1	300
Sandwich Bigger Better Chicken w/ Cheese	1	510
Sandwich Country Fried Steak	1	490
Sandwich Spicy Fish	1	320
Spicy Breast	1	320
Spicy Crunchy Tenders	1 (2 oz)	135
Spicy Fish Fillet	1 piece (2.3 oz)	160
Spicy Leg	1	180
Spicy Thigh	1	480
Spicy Wing	1	430
Sweet Corn Nuggets	1 reg	600
Whole Jalapeno Peppers	2	10

SAUCES

BBQ	1 pkg	30

FOOD	PORTION	CALS
Creamy Jalapeno	1 pkg	100
Honey	1 pkg	27
Honey Mustard	1 pkg	110
Hot Sauce	1 pkg	0
Ketchup	1 pkg	18
Purple Pepper	1 pkg	45
Ranch	1 pkg	130
Sweet & Sour	1 pkg	30

CICI'S
EXTRAS

FOOD	PORTION	CALS
Apple Pizza	1 slice	149
Brownie	1	143
Cinnamon Roll	1	139
Garlic Bread	1 slice	99

PIZZA

FOOD	PORTION	CALS
Buffet 12 Inch Alfredo	1 slice	139
Buffet 12 Inch Bacon Cheddar	1 slice	145
Buffet 12 Inch Bar-B-Que	1 slice	172
Buffet 12 Inch Beef	1 slice	170
Buffet 12 Inch Cheese	1 slice	152
Buffet 12 Inch Ham & Pineapple	1 slice	141
Buffet 12 Inch Ole	1 slice	108
Buffet 12 Inch Pepperoni	1 slice	175
Buffet 12 Inch Pepperoni & Jalapeno	1 slice	163
Buffet 12 Inch Sausage	1 slice	197
Buffet 12 Inch Spinach Alfredo	1 slice	151
Buffet 12 Inch Zesty Ham & Cheese	1 slice	153
Buffet 12 Inch Zesty Pepperoni	1 slice	157
Buffet 12 Inch Zesty Tomato Alfredo	1 slice	136
Buffet 12 Inch Zesty Veggie	1 slice	124
To-Go 15 Inch Bar-B-Que	1 slice	289
To-Go 15 Inch Cheese	1 slice	223
To-Go 15 Inch Ham & Pineapple	1 slice	225
To-Go 15 Inch Ole	1 slice	169
To-Go 15 Inch Pepperoni	1 slice	240
To-Go 15 Inch Spinach Alfredo	1 slice	243
To-Go 15 Inch Zesty Pepperoni	1 slice	246
To-Go 15 Inch Zesty Veggie	1 slice	213

FOOD	PORTION	CALS
CINNABON		
BAKED SELECTIONS		
Caramel Pecanbon	1	1100
Cinnabon Bites	6	520
Cinnabon Classic	1	813
Cinnabon Stix	1	379
Cinnamon Filled Churro	1	281
Minibon	1	339
BEVERAGES		
Caramelatta Chill	1 (16 oz)	520
Chillatta Cappuccino	1 (16 oz)	330
Chillatta Caramel	1 (16 oz)	480
Chillatta Chocolate Mocha	1 (16 oz)	460
Chillatta Mango	1 (16 oz)	340
Chillatta Strawberry	1 (16 oz)	330
Chillatta Strawberry Banana	1 (16 oz)	350
Chillatta Tropical Blast	1 (16 oz)	330
Mochalatta Chill	1 (16 oz)	450
CORNER BAKERY		
BREAKFAST SELECTIONS		
Baked French Toast	1 serv	570
Buckhead Cheese Grits	1 serv	350
Fresh Berry Parfait	1 serv	330
Oatmeal	1 serv	280
Oatmeal Crunchy Honey Banana	1 serv	380
Oatmeal Swiss	1 serv	330
Panini Ham & Cheddar	1	720
Panini Smoked Bacon & Cheddar	1	680
Scrambler All American w/o Potatoes & Bread	1 serv	310
Scrambler Anaheim w/o Potatoes & Bread	1 serv	490
Scrambler Farmer's w/o Potatoes & Bread	1 serv	430
The Commuter Croissant	1	720
PASTA		
Chicken Carbonara	1 serv	740
Half Moon Cheese Ravioli	1 serv	550
Penne w/ Marinara	1 serv	550
Pesto Cavatappi	1 serv	930
SALAD DRESSINGS		
Caesar	1 serv	310

FOOD	PORTION	CALS
House	1 serv	280
Ranch	1 serv	160
Vinaigrette Balsamic	1 serv	300
SALADS		
Caesar	1 serv	520
Caesar w/ Roasted Chicken & Croutons	1 serv	640
Chopped w/o Bread	1 serv	810
Harvest	1 serv	860
Harvest w/ Roasted Chicken	1 serv	980
Santa Fe Ranch	1 serv	680
Santa Fe Ranch w/ Roasted Chicken	1 serv	800
Side Cucumber Tomato	1 (6 oz)	120
Side Egg	1 (6 oz)	570
Side Roasted Potato Bacon	1 (6 oz)	370
Side Seasonal Fruit Medley	1 (6 oz)	90
Side Tomato Mozzarella Pasta	1 (6 oz)	205
Side Tuna	1 (6 oz)	310
SANDWICHES		
Bavarian w/ Ham	1	720
Bavarian w/ Turkey	1	690
Chicken Pesto	1	840
Panini California Grille	1	700
Panini Chicken Pomodori	1	890
Panini Club	1	900
Panini Corned Beef Reuben	1	930
Panini Grilled Ham & Swiss	1	880
Southwest Roast Beef	1	840
Tomato Mozzarella	1	670
Tuna Salad On Olive Bread	1	450
Turkey Derby	1	650
Turkey Frisco	1	850
Uptown Turkey	1	660
SOUPS		
Big Al's Chili w/ Cheddar Cheese	1 (10 oz)	380
Bread Bowl	1	420
Cheddar	1 (10 oz)	310
Chicken Wild Mushroom Brie Stew	1 (10 oz)	260
Loaded Baked Potato w/ Garnish	1 (10 oz)	420
Mom's Chicken Noodle	1 (10 oz)	170
Old Fashioned Beef Stew	1 (10 oz)	260

FOOD	PORTION	CALS
Roasted Poblano Corn Chowder	1 (10 oz)	330
Roasted Tomato Basil w/o Garnish	1 (10 oz)	170
Zesty Chicken Tortilla w/ Tortilla Strips	1 (10 oz)	230

D'ANGELO'S
CHILDREN'S MENU SELECTIONS
D'Lite Turkey	1	217
Sub Cheeseburger	1	294
Sub Ham & Cheese	1	227
Sub Kidz Tuna	1	438
Sub Meatball	1	330

SALAD DRESSINGS
Bleu Cheese	1 serv	152
Caesar	1 serv	397
Caesar Fat Free	1 serv	57
Creamy Italian	1 serv	340
Greek w/ Feta Cheese	1 serv	227
Honey Mustard	1 serv	150
Olive Oil Vinaigrette	1 serv	170
Ranch Lite	1 serv	240

SALADS
Antipasto	1 serv	284
Caesar w/ Dressing	1 serv	474
Chicken Caesar w/ Dressing	1 serv	533
Chicken Stir Fry w/o Dressing	1 serv	168
Cobb w/o Dressing	1 serv	292
Greek	1 serv	290
Lobster w/o Dressing	1 serv	376
Roast Beef w/o Dressing	1 serv	131
Steak Tip Caesar	1 serv	661
Tossed Garden w/o Dressing	1 serv	49
Turkey w/o Dressing	1 serv	157

SANDWICHES
D'Lite Chicken Caesar Salad	1	374
D'Lite Chicken Stir Fry	1	426
D'Lite Classic Veggie	1	362
D'Lite Fresh Veggie	1	348
D'Lite Grilled Chicken Breast	1	388
D'Lite Roast Beef	1	338
D'Lite Turkey	1	347

FOOD	PORTION	CALS
D'Lite Turkey Cranberry	1	444
Pokket Big Papi	1	469
Pokket BLT & Cheese	1	397
Pokket Caesar Salad	1	616
Pokket Capicola & Cheese	1	362
Pokket Cheese	1	519
Pokket Cheeseburger	1	459
Pokket Chicken Caesar Salad	1	674
Pokket Chicken Club	1	526
Pokket Chicken Honey Dijon	1	508
Pokket Chicken Salad	1	623
Pokket Chicken Stir Fry	1	380
Pokket Classic Vegetable	1	368
Pokket Classic Veggie No Cheese	1	212
Pokket Greek	1	790
Pokket Grilled Chicken	1	303
Pokket Ham	1	229
Pokket Ham & Cheese	1	326
Pokket Ham & Salami	1	386
Pokket Hamburger	1	399
Pokket Italian	1	525
Pokket Lobster	1	530
Pokket Meatball	1	574
Pokket Mortadella & Cheese	1	410
Pokket Number 9	1	407
Pokket Pastrami	1	438
Pokket Pepperoni	1	407
Pokket Roast Beef	1	247
Pokket Salad	1	196
Pokket Salami & Cheese	1	509
Pokket Seafood Salad	1	449
Pokket Steak	1	305
Pokket Steak & Cheese	1	377
Pokket Steak Bomb	1	631
Pokket Steak Tip	1	452
Pokket Tuna	1	664
Pokket Turkey	1	256
Pokket Turkey Club	1	332
Sub Big Papi	1 sm	525
Sub BLT & Cheese	1 sm	463

FOOD	PORTION	CALS
Sub Capicola & Cheese	1 sm	408
Sub Cheese	1 sm	589
Sub Cheeseburger	1 sm	526
Sub Chicken Club	1	593
Sub Chicken Honey Dijon	1	575
Sub Chicken Salad	1 sm	692
Sub Chicken Stir Fry	1 sm	449
Sub Classic Veggie	1 sm	462
Sub Grilled Chicken	1 sm	369
Sub Ham	1 sm	302
Sub Ham & Cheese	1 sm	395
Sub Ham & Salami	1 sm	456
Sub Hamburger	1 sm	466
Sub Italian	1 sm	614
Sub Lobster	1 sm	598
Sub Meatball	1 sm	644
Sub Meatballs & Cheese	1 sm	750
Sub Mortadella & Cheese	1 sm	479
Sub Number 9	1 sm	450
Sub Pastrami	1 sm	613
Sub Pepperoni	1 sm	603
Sub Roast Beef	1 sm	320
Sub Salad	1 sm	281
Sub Salami & Cheese	1 sm	579
Sub Seafood Salad	1 sm	498
Sub Steak	1 sm	373
Sub Steak & Cheese	1 sm	446
Sub Steak Bomb	1 sm	670
Sub Steak Tip	1 sm	545
Sub Tuna	1	685
Sub Turkey Club	1 sm	401
Sub Toasted Italian Bistro	1 sm	585
Sub Toasted Pastrami Reuben	1 sm	750
Sub Toasted Roast Beef & Cheddar	1 sm	564
Sub Toasted Spicy Meatball	1 sm	933
Sub Toasted Tuna & Swiss	1 sm	796
Sub Toasted Turkey & Ham	1 sm	532
Sub Toasted Turkey Thanksgiving	1 sm	705
Wrap Big Papi	1	593
Wrap BLT & Cheese	1	544

FOOD	PORTION	CALS
Wrap Buffalo Chicken Salad	1	823
Wrap Caesar Salad	1	711
Wrap Capicola & Cheese	1	494
Wrap Cheese	1	675
Wrap Cheeseburger	1	609
Wrap Chicken Caesar Salad	1	830
Wrap Chicken Cobb	1	931
Wrap Chicken Filet & Bacon	1	639
Wrap Chicken Honey Dijon	1	672
Wrap Chicken Salad	1	782
Wrap Chicken Stir Fry	1	535
Wrap Classic Veggie	1	486
Wrap Greek	1	765
Wrap Grilled Chicken	1	422
Wrap Ham & Cheese	1	435
Wrap Ham & Salami	1	513
Wrap Hamburger	1	509
Wrap Italian	1	631
Wrap Lobster	1	749
Wrap Meatball	1	687
Wrap Mortadella & Cheese	1	522
Wrap Number 9	1	517
Wrap Pastrami	1	550
Wrap Peppercorn Steak	1	702
Wrap Pepperoni	1	519
Wrap Roast Beef	1	448
Wrap Salad	1	324
Wrap Salami & Cheese	1	605
Wrap Seafood Salad	1	541
Wrap Steak	1	392
Wrap Steak & Cheese	1	464
Wrap Steak Bomb	1	670
Wrap Steak Tip	1	432
Wrap Tuna	1	731
Wrap Turkey	1	369
Wrap Turkey Club	1	415
SOUPS		
Beef Stew	1 sm	220
Broccoli & Cheddar Cheese	1 sm	270
Chicken Noodle	1 sm	110

FOOD	PORTION	CALS
Hearty Vegetable	1 sm	40
Italian Wedding	1 sm	120
Lobster Bisque	1 sm	360
New England Clam Chowder	1 sm	320
Portuguese Kale	1 sm	130

DENNY'S
BEVERAGES

FOOD	PORTION	CALS
Apple Juice	1 sm (10 oz)	141
Cappuccino	1 (8 oz)	100
Chocolate Milk	1 sm (10 oz)	160
Hot Chocolate	1 (8 oz)	100
Iced Tea Raspberry	1 serv (16 oz)	78
Lemonade	1 serv (15 oz)	150
Milk	1 sm (10 oz)	130
Orange Juice	1 sm (10 oz)	140
Ruby Red Grapefruit	1 sm (10 oz)	164
Tomato Juice	1 sm (10 oz)	56

BREAKFAST SELECTIONS

FOOD	PORTION	CALS
All American Slam w/o Choices	1 serv (10 oz)	800
Bacon Turkey	4 slices	150
Bacon Strips	4	140
Banana	1	110
Egg	1 (2 oz)	120
Eggs White	1 serv (4 oz)	50
English Muffin w/o Margarine	1	130
Grand Slam Slugger w/o Choices	1 serv (13 oz)	780
Grapes	1 serv (3 oz)	55
Grits w/ Margarine	1 serv (12 oz)	220
Ham Slice Grilled Honey	1 (3 oz)	120
Hash Browns	1 serv	210
Hash Browns Cheddar Cheese	1 serv (5 oz)	300
Hash Browns Everything	1 serv (8 oz)	340
Lumberjack Slam w/o Choices	1 serv (15 oz)	940
Moon Over My Hammy Omelette w/ Hash Browns w/o Choices	1 serv (16 oz)	770
Oatmeal w/ Milk	1 serv (16 oz)	290
Omelette Southern w/ Hash Browns w/o Bread	1 serv (18 oz)	1070
Omelette Veggie Cheese w/o Choices	1 serv (13 oz)	460
Omelette w/ Hash Browns w/o Choices	1 serv (16 oz)	700

FOOD	PORTION	CALS
Pancakes Buttermilk	2	330
Platter Chocolate Chip Pancakes w/o Meat	1 serv (13 oz)	640
Sausage Links	4 (3 oz)	370
Senior Omelette w/o Choices	1 serv (9 oz)	470
Senior Scrambled Eggs & Cheddar	1 serv (13 oz)	870
Senior Slam Belgian Waffle w/ Egg w/o Choices	1 serv (8 oz)	450
Skillet Bananas Foster French Toast w/o Meat	1 serv (15 oz)	860
Slam Belgian Waffle w/ Margarine w/o Syrup	1 serv (13 oz)	1030
Slam Everyday Value w/ Bacon	1 serv (12 oz)	650
Slam Everyday Value w/ Sausage	1 serv (13 oz)	760
Slam French Toast	1 serv (15 oz)	940
Ultimate Omelette w/o Choices	1 serv (12 oz)	620
CHILDREN'S MENU SELECTIONS		
Blender Blaster Oreo	1 serv (12 oz)	680
Jr Grand Slam	1 serv (5 oz)	380
Pancake Softball w/ Meat	1 serv (4 oz)	250
Pancakes Chocolate Chip-In	1 serv (7 oz)	450
Pit Stop Pizza w/o Side	1 serv (8 oz)	590
Slam Dribblers	1 serv (6 oz)	410
Slap Shot Slider w/o Side	1 (4 oz)	310
Spaghetti Set Go w/o Side	1 serv (6 oz)	260
Track & Cheese w/o Side	1 serv (7 oz)	340
DESSERTS		
Apple Crisp A La Mode	1 serv (13 oz)	740
Blender Blaster Oreo	1 serv (14 oz)	890
Cake Carrot	1 serv (8 oz)	820
Cake Hershey's Chocolate	1 serv (5 oz)	580
Cheesecake New York Style	1 serv (7 oz)	640
Float Rootbeer or Cola	1 (16 oz)	430
Hot Fudge Brownie A La Mode	1 serv (9 oz)	830
Milkshake	1 (12 oz)	560
Pie Apple	1 serv (7 oz)	480
Pie Chocolate Peanut Butter Silk	1 serv (6 oz)	680
Pie Coconut Cream	1 serv (7 oz)	630
Pie Cookies & Cream	1 serv (7 oz)	630
Pie French Silk	1 serv (5 oz)	770
Pie Key Lime	1 serv (7 oz)	560
Pie Lemon Meringue	1 serv (7 oz)	500
Pie Pecan	1 serv (7 oz)	730
Pie Pumpkin	1 serv (7 oz)	500

FOOD	PORTION	CALS
Sundae Oreo	1 (9 oz)	760
Sundae Single Scoop	1 (4 oz)	300
Topping Cherry	1 serv (2 oz)	57
Topping Chocolate	1 serv (2 oz)	133
Topping Fudge	1 serv (2 oz)	201
Topping Strawberry	1 serv (2 oz)	77
MAIN MENU SELECTIONS		
Basket Of Puppies w/o Syrup	10 pieces	520
Burger Bacon Cheddar w/o Choices	1 (15 oz)	900
Burger Classic & Fries	1 serv (19 oz)	1190
Burger Fit Fare Veggie w/o Choice	1 (10 oz)	460
Burger Mushroom Swiss w/o Choices	1 (18 oz)	880
Burger Veggie w/ Dressing w/o Choices	1 (11 oz)	520
Burger Western w/o Choice	1 (17 oz)	1120
Cheeseburger Double w/o Choices	1 serv (23 oz)	1420
Chicken Strips Sweet & Tangy BBQ w/o Dipping Sauce	1 serv (13 oz)	820
Chicken Strips w/ Buffalo Sauce	1 serv (13 oz)	720
Chicken Wings Sweet & Tangy BBQ	1 serv (8 oz)	450
Chicken Wings w/ Buffalo Sauce	1 serv (8 oz)	330
Chopped Steak Mushroom Swiss w/o Choices	1 serv (13 oz)	900
Chopped Steak Spicy Cowboy w/o Choices	1 serv (15 oz)	1050
Club Sandwich w/o Choices	1 (10 oz)	550
Coleslaw	1 serv (5 oz)	260
Corn	1 serv (4 oz)	130
Cottage Cheese	1 serv (3 oz)	70
Country Fried Steak w/ Gravy	1 serv (13 oz)	990
Dippable Veggies w/o Dressing	1 serv (2.5 oz)	30
Fiesta Corn	1 serv (4 oz)	100
Fit Fare Grilled Tilapia	1 serv (17 oz)	600
Fit Fare Sweet & Tangy BBQ Chicken w/ Vegetables & Tomatoes	1 serv (13 oz)	640
French Fries Salted	1 serv (5 oz)	430
Fried Shrimp Platter w/ Fries	1 serv (18 oz)	1050
Garlic Dinner Bread	2 pieces	170
Green Beans	1 serv (3 oz)	25
Haddock Fillet w/o Bread	1 serv (20 oz)	1330
Homestyle Meatloaf w/ Gravy	1 serv (7 oz)	600
Lemon Pepper Tilapia w/o Choices	1 serv (13 oz)	640
Mashed Potatoes Plain	1 serv (5 oz)	170

FOOD	PORTION	CALS
Mashed Potatoes Smoked Cheddar	1 serv (4 oz)	120
Mozzarella Sticks w/o Sauce	1 serv (8 oz)	560
Onion Rings	1 serv (5 oz)	520
Quesadilla Cheese	1 (8 oz)	690
Ranchero Tilapia w/o Bread	1 serv (19 oz)	450
Sampler w/o Sauce	1 serv (17 oz)	1380
Sandwich Bacon Lettuce & Tomato w/o Choices	1 (7 oz)	520
Sandwich Chicken Ranch Melt w/o Choices	1 serv (12 oz)	790
Sandwich Fried Cheese Melt w/ Marinara Sauce w/o Choices	1 (12 oz)	830
Sandwich Hickory Grilled Chicken w/o Choices	1 (15 oz)	1020
Sandwich Patty Melt w/o Choices	1 (13 oz)	1040
Sandwich Philly Melt Prime Rib w/o Choices	1 serv (13 oz)	670
Sandwich Pulled BBQ Chicken w/ Coleslaw	1 serv (14 oz)	670
Sandwich Smoked Chicken Melt w/o Choices	1 (12 oz)	840
Sandwich Spicy Buffalo Chicken Melt w/o Choices	1 (15 oz)	860
Sandwich The Super Bird w/o Choices	1 (11 oz)	620
Seasoned Fries Senior Country Fried Steak w/o Choices	1 serv (5 oz)	510
Senior Grilled Chicken w/o Choices	1 serv (5 oz)	200
Senior Grilled Shrimp Skewer w/o Choices	1 serv (8 oz)	280
Senior Homestyle Meatloaf w/o Choices	1 serv (4 oz)	290
Senior Mini Burgers Bacon Cheddar w/o Choice	1 (11 oz)	720
Senior Sandwich Club w/o Choices	1 (10 oz)	570
Senior Sandwich Grilled Cheese Deluxe w/o Choices	1 (7 oz)	520
Senior Slam French Toast w/ Egg	1 serv (5 oz)	300
Senior Starter w/o Choices	1 serv (3 oz)	210
Shrimp Breaded	6	190
Shrimp Grilled Skewer	1	90
Skillet Bacon Chipotle Chicken w/o Sides	1 serv (7 oz)	360
Skillet Prime Rib Premium	1 serv (21 oz)	850
Skillet Santa Fe	1 serv (14 oz)	710
Skillet Ultimate	1 serv (15 oz)	740
Slamburger Bacon w/ Fries	1 serv (15 oz)	1030
Smothered Cheese Fries	1 serv (10 oz)	860
Spinach Sauteed	1 serv (2 oz)	70

FOOD	PORTION	CALS
Spinach w/ Pico De Gallo	1 serv (3 oz)	110
T-Bone Steak w/o Choices	1 serv (12 oz)	640
T-Bone Steak & Breaded Shrimp	1 serv (13 oz)	830
T-Bone Steak & Shrimp Skewer	1 serv (12 oz)	730
The Big Dipper w/ Salsa w/o Dipping Sauce	10 pieces	1230
Three Dip & Chips	1 serv (12 oz)	560
Tomatoes Slices	2	10
Tsing Tsing Chicken	1 serv (14 oz)	900
Vegetable Rice Pilaf	1 serv (5 oz)	190
Wrap Buffalo Chicken	1 (14 oz)	830
Zesty Nachos	1 serv (22 oz)	1340
SALAD DRESSINGS AND TOPPINGS		
BBQ Sweet & Spicy	1 serv (1.5 oz)	110
Cherry Topping	1 serv (3 oz)	86
Croutons	1 serv (0.25 oz)	90
Dressing Bleu Cheese	1 serv (1 oz)	110
Dressing Caesar	1 serv (1 oz)	100
Dressing French	1 serv (1 oz)	74
Dressing Honey Mustard	1 serv (1 oz)	160
Dressing Italian Fat Free	1 serv (1 oz)	9
Dressing Ranch	1 serv (1 oz)	130
Dressing Ranch Fat Free	1 serv(1 oz)	25
Dressing Thousand Island	1 serv (1 oz)	107
Pico De Gallo	1 serv (3 oz)	21
Sour Cream	1 serv (1.5 oz)	91
Syrup Maple Flavored	3 tbsp (1.5 oz)	143
Syrup Sugar Free Maple	1 serv (1.5 oz)	23
Vinaigrette Balsamic Low Fat	1 serv (1 oz)	35
Whipped Margarine	1 tbsp	50
SALADS		
Cranberry Apple w/ Chicken w/o Dressing	1 serv (11 oz)	320
Deluxe Salad w/ Chicken Strips w/o Choices	1 serv (18 oz)	590
Deluxe Salad w/ Grilled Chicken Breast w/o Choices	1 serv (17 oz)	340
Nacho	1 serv (20 oz)	850
SOUPS		
Broccoli & Cheddar	1 serv (12 oz)	370
Chicken Noodle	1 serv (12 oz)	140
Clam Chowder	1 serv (12 oz)	270

FOOD	PORTION	CALS
Loaded Baked Potato	1 serv (12 oz)	310
Vegetable Beef	1 serv (12 oz)	140

DOMINO'S PIZZA
OTHER MENU SELECTIONS

FOOD	PORTION	CALS
Breadsticks	8	870
Buffalo Chicken Kickers	1 serv	510
Cheesy Bread	1 serv	930
Chocolate Lava Crunch Cakes	2	690
Cinna Stix	8	940

PIZZA MEDIUM

FOOD	PORTION	CALS
Deep Dish Marinara Cheese	⅛ pie	219
Hand Tossed Marinara Cheese	⅛ pie	190
Thin Crust Marinara Cheese	⅛ pie	141

TOPPINGS FOR 1 MEDIUM PIZZA

FOOD	PORTION	CALS
Anchovies	1 serv	110
Bacon	1 serv	340
Banana Peppers	1 serv	15
Beef	1 serv	300
Cheddar Cheese	1 serv	230
Cheese American	1 serv	310
Cheese Provolone	1 serv	200
Chicken	1 serv	140
Chorizo	1 serv	90
Feta Cheese	1 serv	90
Garlic	1 serv	40
Green Chile Pepper	1 serv	10
Green Pepper	1 serv	10
Ham	1 serv	90
Jalapenos	1 serv	15
Mushroom	1 serv	20
Olives Black	1 serv	100
Olives Green	1 serv	100
Onion	1 serv	15
Parmesan Shredded	1 serv	170
Pepperoni	1 serv	240
Philly Steak	1 serv	90
Pineapple	1 serv	60
Red Pepper Roasted	1 serv	10
Salami	1 serv	220

FOOD	PORTION	CALS
Sausage Italian	1 serv	350
Spinach	1 serv	10
Tomato	1 serv	20
Wing Sauce	1 serv	10

DONATOS PIZZA
PIZZA

FOOD	PORTION	CALS
Hand Tossed Chicken Bacon Club	2 slices	780
Hand Tossed Chicken Spinach Mozzarella	2 slices	587
Hand Tossed Chicken Vegy Medley	2 slices	517
Hand Tossed Classic Trio	2 slices	640
Hand Tossed Founder's Favorite	2 slices	678
Hand Tossed Fresh Mozzarella Trio	2 slices	690
Hand Tossed Hawaiian	2 slices	578
Hand Tossed Margherita	2 slices	583
Hand Tossed Mariachi Beef	2 slices	591
Hand Tossed Mariachi Chicken	2 slices	617
Hand Tossed Pepperoni	2 slices	499
Hand Tossed Pepperoni Zinger	2 slices	645
Hand Tossed Serious Cheese	2 slices	597
Hand Tossed Serious Meat	2 slices	735
Hand Tossed Vegy	2 slices	550
Hand Tossed Works	2 slices	669
Thicker Crust Chicken Vegy Medley Large	¼ pie	580
Thicker Crust Founder's Favorite Large	¼ pie	780
Thicker Crust Hawaiian Large	¼ pie	680
Thicker Crust Mariachi Beef Large	¼ pie	710
Thicker Crust Mariachi Chicken Large	¼ pie	710
Thicker Crust Serious Meat Large	¼ pie	850
Thicker Crust The Works Large	¼ pie	770
Thicker Crust Vegy Large	¼ pie	630
Thin Crust Chicken Medley Vegy Large	¼ pie	497
Thin Crust Classic Trio Large	¼ pie	674
Thin Crust Founder's Favorite Large	¼ pie	702
Thin Crust Hawaiian Large	¼ pie	588
Thin Crust Mariachi Beef Large	¼ pie	630
Thin Crust Mariachi Chicken Large	¼ pie	639
Thin Crust Pepperoni Large	¼ pie	627
Thin Crust Serious Cheese Large	¼ pie	710
Thin Crust Serious Meat Large	¼ pie	736

FOOD	PORTION	CALS
Thin Crust The Works	¼ pie	689
Thin Crust Vegy Large	¼ pie	544
SALAD DRESSINGS		
House Italian	1 serv (1.5 oz)	230
Italian Light	1 serv (1.5 oz)	20
Pizza Dip Chicken Bacon Ranch	1 serv (3 oz)	450
SALADS		
Chicken Harvest w/o Dressing Entree	1	540
Harvest Side	1 serv	81
Italian Chef w/o Dressing Entree	1	290
Italian Side w/o Dressing	1	110
SIDES AND SUBS		
3 Cheese Garlic Bread	2 pieces	174
Big Don White Italian	1	717
Breadsticks w/ Pizza Sauce	2	261
Buffalo Wings Hot	5	597
Buffalo Wings Mild	5	618
Fresh Vegy Wheat	1	532
Stromboli 3 Meat	1	689
Stromboli Cheese	1	693
Stromboli Deluxe	1	613
Stromboli Pepperoni	1	716
Stromboli Vegy	1	606

DUNKIN' DONUTS
BAGELS

Blueberry	1	330
Cinnamon Raisin	1	330
Everything	1	350
Garlic	1	340
Multigrain	1	390
Onion	1	310
Plain	1	320
Poppy Seed	1	350
Salt	1	320
Sesame	1	360
Wheat	1	320
BAKED SELECTIONS		
Apple Fritter	1	400
Biscuit	1	280

FOOD	PORTION	CALS
Bismark Chocolate Iced	1	350
Brownie	1	430
Coffee Roll	1	370
Coffee Roll Chocolate Frosted	1	380
Coffee Roll Maple Frosted	1	380
Coffee Roll Vanilla Frosted	1	380
Cookie Chocolate Chunk	1	540
Cookie Oatmeal Raisin	1	480
Croissant Plain	1	310
Danish Apple Cheese	1	330
Danish Cheese	1	330
Danish Strawberry Cheese	1	320
Donut Apple Crumb	1	460
Donut Apple N' Spice	1	240
Donut Bavarian Kreme	1	250
Donut Blueberry Cake	1	330
Donut Blueberry Crumb	1	470
Donut Boston Kreme	1	280
Donut Bow Tie	1	310
Donut Chocolate Coconut	1	340
Donut Chocolate Frosted	1	340
Donut Chocolate Glazed Cake	1	280
Donut Chocolate Kreme Filled	1	310
Donut Cinnamon	1	290
Donut Double Chocolate Cake	1	290
Donut Glazed	1	220
Donut Glazed Cake	1	320
Donut Jelly Filled	1	260
Donut Maple Frosted	1	230
Donut Marble Frosted	1	230
Donut Old Fashioned	1	280
Donut Powdered	1	300
Donut Strawberry Frosted	1	230
Donut Sugar Raised	1	190
Donut Triple Chocolate	1	420
Donut Vanilla Kreme Filled	1	320
Eclair	1	350
English Muffin	1	160
French Cruller	1	250
Fritter Glazed	1	400

FOOD	PORTION	CALS
Muffin Blueberry	1	510
Muffin Blueberry Reduced Fat	1	450
Muffin Chocolate Chip	1	630
Muffin Coffee Cake	1	660
Muffin Corn	1	510
Muffin Cranberry Orange Low Fat	1	390
Muffin Honey Bran Raisin	1	500
Muffin Triple Chocolate	1	660
Munchkins Cinnamon Cake	1	60
Munchkins Glazed Cake	1	60
Munchkins Glazed Chocolate Cake	1	60
Munchkins Jelly Filled	1	60
Munchkins Plain Cake	1	50
Munchkins Powdered Cake	1	60
Munchkins Sugar Raised	1	40
Stick Cinnamon Cake	1	310
Stick Glazed Cake	1	340
Stick Glazed Chocolate Cake	1	390
Stick Jelly	1	400
Stick Plain Cake	1	300
Stick Powdered Cake	1	320
BEVERAGES		
Cappuccino	1 sm (10 oz)	80
Cappuccino Frozen w/ Skim Milk	1 sm (16 oz)	280
Cappuccino Frozen w/ Whole Milk	1 sm (16 oz)	300
Cappuccino w/ Sugar	1 sm (10 oz)	140
Coffee Blueberry	1 sm (10 oz)	15
Coffee Caramel	1 sm (10 oz)	10
Coffee Cinnamon	1 sm (10 oz)	15
Coffee Coconut	1 sm (10 oz)	10
Coffee French Vanilla	1 sm (10 oz)	10
Coffee Hazelunt	1 sm (10 oz)	10
Coffee Mocha	1 sm (10 oz)	110
Coffee Mocha w/ Cream	1 sm (10 oz)	170
Coffee Raspberry	1 sm (10 oz)	15
Coffee Regular	1 sm (10 oz)	5
Coffee Regular	1 med (14 oz)	10
Coffee Regular	1 lg (20 oz)	10
Coffee Regular	1 extra lg	15
Coffee Toasted Almond	1 sm (10 oz)	10

FOOD	PORTION	CALS
Coffee White Chocolate	1 sm (10 oz)	110
Coffee White Chocolate w/ Cream	1 sm (10 oz)	160
Coffee w/ Cream	1 sm (10 oz)	60
Coffee w/ Milk	1 sm (10 oz)	25
Coffee w/ Milk & Sugar	1 sm (10 oz)	80
Coffee w/ Skim Milk	1 sm (10 oz)	15
Coffee w/ Skim Milk & Splenda	1 sm (10 oz)	25
Coffee w/ Skim Milk & Sugar	1 sm (10 oz)	70
Coffee w/ Splenda	1 sm (10 oz)	15
Coffee w/ Sugar	1 sm (10 oz)	60
Coolatta Coffee w/ Cream	1 sm (16 oz)	400
Coolatta Coffee w/ Milk	1 sm (16 oz)	240
Coolatta Coffee w/ Skim Milk	1 sm (16 oz)	210
Coolatta Strawberry Fruit	1 sm (16 oz)	300
Coolatta Tropicana Orange	1 sm (16 oz)	220
Coolatta Vanilla Bean	1 sm (16 oz)	430
Dunkaccino	1 sm (10 oz)	230
Espresso	1 (1.75 oz)	0
Espresso w/ Sugar	1 (1.75 oz)	30
Hot Chocolate	1 sm (10 oz)	210
Iced Coffee	1 sm (16 oz)	10
Iced Coffee Mocha w/ Cream	1 sm (16 oz)	180
Iced Coffee White Chocolate w/ Cream	1 sm (16 oz)	170
Iced Coffee w/ Cream	1 sm (16 oz)	70
Iced Coffee w/ Cream & Sugar	1 sm (16 oz)	120
Iced Coffee w/ Milk	1 sm (16 oz)	30
Iced Coffee w/ Milk & Sugar	1 sm (16 oz)	90
Iced Coffee w/ Skim Milk	1 sm (16 oz)	20
Iced Coffee w/ Skim Milk & Sugar	1 sm (16 oz)	80
Iced Coffee w/ Sugar	1 sm (16 oz)	70
Iced Latte	1 sm (16 oz)	120
Iced Latte Caramel Swirl	1 sm (16 oz)	220
Iced Latte Caramel Swirl w/ Skim Milk	1 sm (16 oz)	180
Iced Latte Lite	1 med (24 oz)	120
Iced Latte Mocha Swirl	1 sm (16 oz)	220
Iced Latte Mocha Swirl w/ Skim Milk	1 sm (16 oz)	180
Iced Latte w/ Skim Milk	1 sm (16 oz)	70
Iced Latte w/ Skim Milk & Sugar	1 sm (16 oz)	130
Iced Latte w/ Sugar	1 sm (16 oz)	170
Latte	1 sm (10 oz)	120

FOOD	PORTION	CALS
Latte Caramel Swirl	1 sm (10 oz)	220
Latte Lite	1 sm (10 oz)	80
Latte Lite Vanilla	1 sm (10 oz)	90
Latte Mocha Raspberry	1 med (16 oz)	340
Latte Mocha Spice	1 med (16 oz)	330
Latte Mocha Swirl	1 sm (10 oz)	220
Latte w/ Sugar	1 sm (10 oz)	170
Latte White Chocolate	1 med (16 oz)	320
Tea Regular Or Decaffeinated	1 (10 oz)	0
Tea w/ Milk	1 (10 oz)	20
Tea w/ Milk & Sugar	1 (10 oz)	80
Tea w/ Skim Milk	1 (10 oz)	10
Tea w/ Skim Milk & Sugar	1 (10 oz)	70
Tea w/ Sugar	1 (10 oz)	60
Turbo Shot	1 sm (1.75 oz)	0
CREAM CHEESE		
Blueberry Reduced Fat	1 serv (1.75 oz)	150
Onion & Chive Reduced Fat	1 serv (1.75 oz)	130
Plain	1 serv (1.75 oz)	150
Plain Reduced Fat	1 serv (1.75 oz)	100
Salmon Reduced Fat	1 serv (1.75 oz)	140
Strawberry Reduced Fat	1 serv (1.75 oz)	150
Veggie Reduced Fat	1 serv (1.75 oz)	120
SANDWICHES		
Bagel Bacon Egg Cheese	1	510
Bagel Egg Cheese	1	470
Bagel Ham Egg Cheese	1	510
Bagel Sausage Egg Cheese	1	640
Biscuit Egg Cheese	1	430
Biscuit Sausage Egg Cheese	1	610
Croissant Bacon Egg Cheese	1	510
Croissant Egg Cheese	1	470
Croissant Ham Egg Cheese	1	510
Croissant Original Chicken	1	640
English Muffin Bacon Egg Cheese	1	360
English Muffin Egg Cheese	1	320
English Muffin Egg White & Cheese	1	270
English Muffin Ham Egg Cheese	1	360
English Muffin Ham Egg White & Cheese	1	310
English Muffin Sausage Egg Cheese	1	490

FOOD	PORTION	CALS
English Muffin Wheat Egg White & Cheese	1	260
English Muffin Wheat Ham Egg White & Cheese	1	300
Flatbread Egg White Turkey	1	280
Flatbread Egg White Veggie	1	290
Flatbread Grilled Cheese	1	380
Flatbread Ham & Cheese	1	320
Flatbread Turkey Cheddar & Bacon	1	410
Pressed Cuban	1	680
SOUPS		
Broccoli Cheddar	1 serv (8 oz)	190
Chicken Noodle	1 serv (8 oz)	130

EINSTEIN BROS BAGELS
BAGELS AND BREADS

FOOD	PORTION	CALS
Bagel Asiago Cheese	1 (4 oz)	310
Bagel Black Russian	1 (3.9 oz)	280
Bagel Blueberry	1 (3.8 oz)	300
Bagel Chocolate Chip	1 (3.8 oz)	290
Bagel Cinnamon Raisin	1 (3.8 oz)	290
Bagel Cinnamon Sugar	1 (3.9 oz)	290
Bagel Cranberry	1 (3.8 oz)	270
Bagel Croutons	1 serv (1 oz)	90
Bagel Egg	1 (3.5 oz)	300
Bagel Everything	1 (3.7 oz)	270
Bagel Garlic	1 (3.7 oz)	270
Bagel Green Chili	1 (5.4 oz)	350
Bagel Honey Whole Wheat	1 (3.6 oz)	260
Bagel Onion	1 (3.7 oz)	270
Bagel Plain	1 (3.5 oz)	260
Bagel Poppy	1 (3.7 oz)	280
Bagel Potato	1 (3.5 oz)	270
Bagel Power	1 (4 oz)	310
Bagel Pumpernickel	1 (3.5 oz)	240
Bagel Salt	1 (3.7 oz)	260
Bagel Sesame	1 (3.7 oz)	280
Bagel Six Cheese	1 (4.3 oz)	330
Bagel Spinach Florentine	1 (4.7 oz)	340
Bagel Poppers Cinnamon Sugar	1 (5 oz)	450
Bagel Poppers Pretzel w/ Nacho Cheese	1 (5 oz)	320

FOOD	PORTION	CALS
Bagel Poppers Sweet Cream Cheese	1 (6 oz)	440
Bagel Thin Singles Everything	1 (2 oz)	150
Bagel Thin Singles Honey Whole Wheat	1 (2 oz)	140
Bagel Thin Singles Plain	1 (2 oz)	140
Bread Ciabatta	1 serv (4.25 oz)	300
Pizza Bagel Pepperoni	1 (6 oz)	450
Roll Challah	1 (2.75 oz)	210
BEVERAGES		
Americano	1 reg (12 oz)	0
Barq's Root Beer	1 reg (20 oz)	260
Cafe Latte Nonfat Milk	1 reg (12 oz)	100
Cafe Latte Reduced Fat Milk	1 reg (12 oz)	150
Cappuccino	1 reg (12 oz)	140
Cappuccino Nonfat Milk	1 reg (12 oz)	70
Cappuccino Reduced Fat Milk	1 reg (12 oz)	90
Chai Tea Latte	1 reg (12 oz)	230
Chai Tea Latte Nonfat Milk	1 reg (12 oz)	210
Chai Tea Latte Reduced Fat Milk	1 reg (12 oz)	220
Coca-Cola	1 reg (20 oz)	230
Coca-Cola Cherry	1 reg (20 oz)	250
Coffee Black All Sizes	1	0
Diet Coke	1 reg (20 oz)	0
Espresso Single	1 (2 oz)	0
Fanta Orange	1 (20 oz)	270
Frozen Blended Cafe Caramel	1 (18 oz)	520
Frozen Blended Cafe Mocha	1 (18 oz)	510
Frozen Blended Strawberry	1 (18 oz)	450
Frozen Blended Wild Berry	1 (18 oz)	350
Half & Half	1 oz	40
Hi-C Fruit Punch	1 (20 oz)	270
Hot Chocolate	1 reg (12 oz)	270
Hot Chocolate Nonfat Milk	1 reg (12 oz)	220
Iced Americano	1 med	0
Iced Coffee	1 med	0
Iced Latte	1 med (12 oz)	110
Iced Latte Nonfat Milk	1 med (16 oz)	60
Iced Latte Reduced Fat Milk	1 med (16 oz)	90
Iced Mocha	1 med (16 oz)	220
Iced Mocha Nonfat Milk	1 med (16 oz)	180
Iced Mocha Reduced Fat Milk	1 med (16 oz)	200

FOOD	PORTION	CALS
Macchiato Caramel	1 reg (12 oz)	300
Macchiato Caramel Nonfat Milk	1 reg (12 oz)	260
Macchiato Caramel Reduced Fat Milk	1 reg (12 oz)	290
Minute Maid Lemonade Lite	1 reg (20 oz)	40
Mocha	1 reg (12 oz)	260
Mocha Nonfat Milk	1 reg (12 oz)	180
Mocha Reduced Fat Milk	1 reg (12 oz)	220
Nestea Iced Tea Unsweetened	1 reg (20 oz)	0
Pibb Xtra	1 reg (20 oz)	250
Skim Milk	8 oz	80
Sprite	1 reg (20 oz)	230
Whole Milk	8 oz	150
DESSERTS		
Cinnamon Twist	1 (4 oz)	370
Coffee Cake Apple Cinnamon	1 serv (7 oz)	700
Coffee Cake Chocolate Chip	1 serv (6.4 oz)	800
Coffee Cake Mixed Berry	1 serv (7 oz)	710
Cookie Chocolate Chip	1 (2.75 oz)	360
Cookie Chocolate Mudslide	1 (2.8 oz)	320
Cookie Iced Sugar	1 (3.7 oz)	480
Cookie Oatmeal Raisin	1 (3 oz)	320
Marshmallow Crispy Treat	1 (4 oz)	410
Muffin Blueberry	1 (5 oz)	480
Muffin Double Chocolate	1 (5 oz)	440
Muffin Strawberry White Chocolate	1 (6 oz)	500
Strudel Cinnamon Walnut	1 piece (6 oz)	640
SALAD DRESSINGS		
Caesar	1 serv (3 oz)	410
Vinaigrette Chipotle	1 serv (3 oz)	290
Vinaigrette Raspberry	1 serv (3 oz)	410
SALADS		
Bros Bistro	1 (10.5 oz)	820
Bros Bistro Half	1 serv (5.3 oz)	410
Bros Bistro w/ Chicken	1 (14.5 oz)	950
Bros Bistro w/ Chicken Half	1 serv (7.3 oz)	470
Caesar	1 (9.5 oz)	600
Caesar Half	1 serv (4.5 oz)	280
Caesar w/ Chicken	1 (14 oz)	730
Caesar w/ Chicken Half	1 (6.5 oz)	340
Chipotle	1 (11.7 oz)	590

FOOD	PORTION	CALS
Chipotle Half	1 serv (5.8 oz)	290
Chipotle w/ Chicken Half	1 serv (7.8 oz)	360
Chipotle w/ Chicken	1 (15.7 oz)	720
Fruit	1 (11 oz)	140
Fruit Cup	1 (5 oz)	60
Potato	1 serv (3 oz)	160
SANDWICHES		
Bagel Asiago Tasty Turkey	1 (13 oz)	540
Bagel Dogs Asiago	1 (7 oz)	550
Bagel Dogs Chicken Apple	1 (5 oz)	290
Bagel Dogs Original	1 (7 oz)	540
Bagel Thin Asparagus Mushroom & Swiss	1 (6 oz)	290
Bagel Thin BLT w/ Avocado	1 (7 oz)	400
Bagel Thin Panini Bacon & Cheese	1 (6 oz)	400
Bagel Thin Tuna	1 (8 oz)	320
Bagel Thin Turkey	1 (8 oz)	270
Bagel Thin Turkey Sausage w/ Salsa	1 (6 oz)	240
Breakfast Wraps Sante Fe	1 (12 oz)	720
Breakfast Wraps Spicy Elmo	1 (11 oz)	720
Challah Club Mex	1 (11 oz)	740
Deli Albacore Tuna Salad	1 (9 oz)	390
Deli Chicken Salad	1 (10 oz)	480
Deli Ham	1 (11 oz)	610
Deli Open Face Melts Ham & Swiss	1 (9 oz)	480
Deli Open Face Melts Turkey & Cheddar	1 (9 oz)	490
Deli Turkey Breast	1 (11 oz)	590
Egg Bacon & Cheddar	1 (9 oz)	590
Egg Cheese Only	1 (8 oz)	510
Egg Ham & Swiss	1 (10 oz)	550
Egg Nova Lox & Bagel	1 (9 oz)	480
Egg Spinach Mushroom & Swiss	1 (10 oz)	560
Egg Turkey Sausage & Cheddar	1 (10 oz)	580
Egg Paninis Southwest Turkey Sausage	1 (12 oz)	680
Egg Paninis Spinach & Bacon	1 (12 oz)	830
Nova Lox & Bagel	1 (9 oz)	480
Panini Italian Chicken	1 (13 oz)	820
Panini Turkey Club	1 (13 oz)	790
Wrap California Chicken	1 (16 oz)	720
Wrap Chipotle Turkey	1 (13 oz)	750
Wrap Turkey Tornado	1 (7 oz)	270

FOOD	PORTION	CALS
SOUPS		
Broccoli Cheese	1 cup (8.75 oz)	290
Chicken Noodle	1 cup (8.75 oz)	120
Turkey Chili	1 cup (8.75 oz)	170
SPREADS		
Butter Blend	1 serv (1 oz)	170
Cream Cheese Light Whipped Plain	1 serv (1.25 oz)	80
Cream Cheese Onion & Chive	1 serv (1.25 oz)	120
Cream Cheese Plain	1 serv (1.25 oz)	120
Cream Cheese Reduced Fat Blueberry	1 serv (1.25 oz)	120
Cream Cheese Reduced Fat Garden Vegetable	1 serv (1.25 oz)	110
Cream Cheese Reduced Fat Garlic Herb	1 serv (1.25 oz)	110
Cream Cheese Reduced Fat Honey Almond	1 serv (1.25 oz)	120
Cream Cheese Reduced Fat Jalapeno Salsa	1 serv (1.25 oz)	110
Cream Cheese Reduced Fat Plain	1 serv (1.25 oz)	110
Cream Cheese Reduced Fat Strawberry	1 serv (1.25 oz)	120
Cream Cheese Reduced Fat Sundried Tomato Basil	1 serv (1.25 oz)	110
Cream Cheese Smoked Salmon	1 serv (1.25 oz)	110
Honey Butter	1 serv (1 oz)	140
Hummus	1 serv (1 oz)	70
Mayo Ancho	1 serv (1.5 oz)	310
Mustard Creamy	1 serv (1.5 oz)	270
Mustard Deli	1 tsp (5 g)	5
Mustard Yellow	1 tbsp (5 g)	0
Peanut Butter Creamy	1 serv (2 oz)	330
Salsa Ancho Lime	1 serv (1.5 oz)	20
Spicy Roasted Tomato	1 serv (1.5 oz)	210
EL POLLO LOCO		
DESSERTS		
Caramel Flan	1 serv (5.5 oz)	290
Churros	2	300
Cone Vanilla	1	330
Soft Serve Vanilla	1 cup (5 oz)	300
MAIN MENU SELECTIONS		
BBQ Black Beans	1 serv (6 oz)	200
Bowl The Original Pollo	1 serv	540
Burrito BRC	1 (7.5 oz)	390
Burrito Classic Chicken	1 (10.3 oz)	500

FOOD	PORTION	CALS
Burrito Twice Grilled	1 (15 oz)	830
Burrito Ultimate Grilled	1 (13.6 oz)	650
Chicken Breast	1 (4.3 oz)	220
Chicken Breast Skinless	1 (4 oz)	180
Chicken Leg	1 (1.8 oz)	90
Chicken Thigh	1 (3.1 oz)	220
Chicken Wing	1 (1.3 oz)	90
Cole Slaw	1 serv (6 oz)	120
Corn Cobbette	1 (5 oz)	90
French Fries	1 serv (5.5 oz)	440
Fresh Vegetables w/ Margarine	1 serv (4.1 oz)	60
Fresh Vegetables w/o Margarine	1 serv (4 oz)	35
Gravy	1 serv (1 oz)	10
Loco Nachos	1 serv	170
Macaroni & Cheese	1 serv (5.5 oz)	280
Mashed Potatoes	1 serv (5 oz)	100
Pinto Beans	1 serv (6 oz)	140
Quesadilla Cheese	1 (4.5 oz)	420
Refried Beans w/ Cheese	1 serv (6.3 oz)	270
Skinless Breast Meal	1 serv	310
Soup Chicken Tortilla w/o Tortilla Strips	1 serv (10 oz)	140
Spanish Rice	1 serv (4.5 oz)	160
Taco Al Carbon	1 (3.1 oz)	150
Taco Soft Chicken	1 (4.5 oz)	270
Taquito Chicken	1	190
Tortilla Chips	1 serv (1.5 oz)	210
Tortilla Corn 6 Inches	2	120
Tortilla Flour 6.5 Inches	2	210
SALAD DRESSINGS AND TOPPINGS		
Creamy Cilantro	1 serv (1.5 oz)	220
Creamy Cilantro Light	1 pkg	70
Guacamole	1 serv (1 oz)	45
Hot Sauce Jalapeno	1 pkg	5
Jack & Poblano Queso	1 serv (1.8 oz)	100
Ketchup	1 pkg	10
Light Italian	1 pkg	20
Pico De Gallo Medium	1 serv (1 oz)	10
Ranch	1 pkg	230
Salsa Avocado Hot	1 serv (1 oz)	30
Salsa Chipotle Hot	1 serv (1 oz)	5

FOOD	PORTION	CALS
Salsa House Mild	1 serv (1 oz)	5
Sour Cream	1 serv (1 oz)	60
Thousand Island	1 pkg	220
SALADS		
Caesar Pollo	1 (11.4 oz)	520
Caesar Pollo w/o Dressing	1 (9.4 oz)	220
Garden	1 (4.8 oz)	120
Tostada Chicken	1 (17.3 oz)	840
Tostada Chicken w/o Shell	1 (14.7 oz)	410

EMERALD CITY SMOOTHIE

FOOD	PORTION	CALS
Apple Andie	1 (11 oz)	230
Berry Berry	1 (13 oz)	350
Blueberry Blast	1 (13 oz)	380
Coconut Passion	1 (11 oz)	600
Cranberry Delight	1 (10 oz)	550
Energizer	1 (10 oz)	350
Fruity Supreme	1 (9 oz)	280
Grape Escape	1 (10 oz)	480
Guava Sunrise	1 (13 oz)	366
Kiwi Kic	1 (11 oz)	400
Lean Body	1 (11 oz)	330
Lean Out	1 (11 oz)	600
Low Carb	1 (10 oz)	350
Mango Mania	1 (8 oz)	370
Marionberry Fuel	1 (13 oz)	380
Mega Mass	1 (14 oz)	610
Mini Mass	1 (13 oz)	520
Mocha Bliss	1 (10 oz)	550
Nutty Banana	1 (11 oz)	720
Orange Twister	1 (10 oz)	140
Pacific Splash	1 (12 oz)	240
PB&J	1 (14 oz)	630
Peach Pleasure	1 (12 oz)	270
Peanut Passion	1 (11 oz)	580
Pineapple Bliss	1 (12 oz)	210
Power Fuel	1 (11 oz)	450
Quick Start	1 (10 oz)	280
Raspberry Dream	1 (13 oz)	410
Rejuvenator	1 (10 oz)	340

FOOD	PORTION	CALS
Sambazon	1 (15 oz)	410
Slim N Fit	1 (10 oz)	350
The Builder	1 (18 oz)	1270
Zesty Lemon	1 (14 oz)	430
Zip Zip	1 (10 oz)	240
Zone Zinger	1 (14 oz)	430

EVOS
BEVERAGES
Shake Mango Guava	1 reg (16 oz)	180
Shake Multi-Berry	1 reg (20 oz)	200
Shake Strawberry Banana	1 reg (16 oz)	190
Shake Organic Cappuccino	1 reg (16 oz)	230
Shake Organic Vanilla	1 reg (16 oz)	180

CHILDREN'S MENU SELECTIONS
Kids Champion Burger	1	400
Kids Chicken Strips	1 serv	130
Kids Freerange Steakburger	1	390
Kids Good Corn Dog	1	150

MAIN MENU SELECTIONS
Airbaked Chicken Strips	1 serv	260
Airfries	1 reg	230
American Champion	1	420
American DeLite	1	330
Burger Bun	1	190
Cheddar Cheese Slice	1	80
Crispy Mesquite Chicken	1 serv	330
Freerange Steakburger	1	400
Fresh Fruit Bowl	1 serv	200
Good Corn Dog	1	150
Herb Crusted Trout	1 serv	440
Honey Mesquite Chicken	1 serv	290
Spicy Chipotle Turkey	1 serv	370
Veggie Chili	1 reg	110
Veggie Garden Grill Italian	1	350
Wraps Avocado Turkey	1	480
Wraps Crispy Buffalo Chicken	1	440
Wraps Crispy Thai Trout	1	660
Wraps Freerange Beef Taco	1	600
Wraps Honey Wheat	1	300

FOOD	PORTION	CALS
Wraps Southwest Soy Taco	1	500
Wraps Spicy Thai Chicken	1	510
Wraps Spinach Herb	1	310
Wraps Tomato Basil Chicken	1	520
SALAD DRESSINGS AND TOPPINGS		
Balsamic Vinegar	1 serv (0.5 oz)	5
Crispy Noodles	1 serv (7 g)	35
Croutons Multi-Grain	1 serv (7 g)	30
Dressing Avocado	1 serv (3 oz)	190
Dressing Caesar	1 serv (1.7 oz)	300
Dressing Fat Free Vinaigrette	1 serv (1 oz)	5
Dressing Raspberry	1 serv (2 oz)	50
Dressing Spicy Thai	1 serv (1.4 oz)	150
Extra Virgin Olive Oil	1 serv (1 oz)	250
Herb Spread	1 serv (0.7 oz)	30
Ketchup Cayenne Firewalker	1 serv (1.2 oz)	35
Ketchup Garlic Gravity	1 serv (1.2 oz)	35
Ketchup Mesquite Magic	1 serv (1.2 oz)	35
Mustard	1 serv (0.5 oz)	10
Mustard Mesquite Honey	1 serv (0.7 oz)	80
Southwest Sour Cream	1 serv (1.4 oz)	60
Spicy Chipotle Mayo	1 serv (0.7 oz)	30
Tomato Basil Sauce	1 serv (1.4 oz)	150
SALADS		
Bordeaux Bistro w/o Dressing	1	260
For Salads Chicken Strips	1 serv (3 oz)	130
For Salads Grilled Chicken	1 serv (3 oz)	90
Mediterranean Summer w/o Dressing	1	200
Santa Ana Caesar w/o Dressing	1	20
Side Salad w/o Dressing	1	35
Spicy Thai w/o Dressing	1	35
SUPPLEMENTS		
Fat Burner	1 serv (5 g)	16
Go Energy	1 serv (5 g)	15
Mega Protein	1 serv (0.5 oz)	45
Multi-Vitamin	1 serv (5 g)	10

FOOD	PORTION	CALS
FAZOLI'S		
BEVERAGES		
Lemon Ice All Flavors Original	1	360
Lemon Ice	1 reg	180
CHILDREN'S MENU SELECTIONS		
Fettuccine Alfredo	1 serv	290
Meat Lasagna	1 serv	260
Ravioli w/ Marinara	1 serv	290
Spaghetti w/ Meatballs	1 serv	350
Ziti w/ Meat Sauce	1 serv	190
DESSERTS		
Cheesecake Original	1 slice	290
Cheesecake Turtle	1 slice	450
Cookie Chocolate Chunk	1	510
MAIN MENU SELECTIONS		
Breadstick	1	100
Breadstick Garlic	1	150
Fettuccine Alfredo	1 sm	520
Fettuccine w/ Marinara	1 serv	450
Fettuccine w/ Meat Sauce	1 serv	500
Oven Baked Chicken Parmesan	1 serv	960
Oven Baked Meat Lasagna	1 serv	510
Oven Baked Rigatoni Romano	1 serv	1090
Oven Baked Spaghetti	1 serv	680
Oven Baked Spaghetti w/ Meatballs	1 serv	940
Panini Four Cheese & Tomato	1	510
Panini Grilled Chicken	1	540
Panini Smoked Turkey	1	620
Penne w/ Alfredo	1 serv	520
Penne w/ Marinara	1 serv	450
Penne w/ Meat Sauce	1 serv	500
Pizza Slice Cheese	1	270
Pizza Slice Pepperoni	1	310
Platter Classic Sampler	1	810
Platter Ultimate Sampler	1	980
Ravioli w/ Marinara	1 serv	500
Ravioli w/ Meat Sauce	1 serv	550
Spaghetti w/ Alfredo	1 serv	520
Spaghetti w/ Marinara	1 sm	450
Spaghetti w/ Meat Sauce	1 sm	500

FOOD	PORTION	CALS
Submarinos Club	half	973
Submarinos Ham n'Swiss	1	680
Submarinos Italian Beef	half	660
Submarinos Original	half	940
Topping Broccoli	1 serv	25
Topping Broccoli & Tomatoes	1 serv	30
Topping Garlic Shrimp	1 serv	160
Topping Italian Sausage	1 serv	240
Topping Meatballs	1 serv	160
Topping Peppery Chicken	1 serv	70
Ziti w/ Meat Sauce	1 serv	480
SALAD DRESSINGS		
Caesar	1 serv	220
Fat Free Honey Mustard	1 serv	60
Fat Free Italian	1 serv	25
Honey French	1 serv	220
Italian	1 serv	160
Ranch	1 serv	220
Ranch Lite	1 serv	120
SALADS		
Chicken & Fruit	1	220
Chicken & Pasta Caesar	1	440
Chicken BLT Ranch	1	270
Parmesan Chicken	1	360
Side Caesar	1	40
Side Garden	1	25
Side Pasta	1	320

FIVE GUYS BURGERS AND FRIES
MAIN MENU SELECTIONS

FOOD	PORTION	CALS
Bacon Burger	1 (9.8 oz)	780
Bacon Cheese Dog	1 (7 oz)	695
Bacon Dog	1 (6.4 oz)	625
Cheese Dog	1 (6.5 oz)	615
Cheeseburger Bacon	1 (10.6 oz)	840
Cheeseburger	1 (11 oz)	920
Fries	1 lg (16 oz)	1464
Fries	1 reg (8.6 oz)	620
Grilled Cheese	1 (4 oz)	430
Hamburger	1 (9.3 oz)	700

FOOD	PORTION	CALS
Hot Dog	1 (5.9 oz)	545
Little Burgers Bacon Burger	1 (6.5 oz)	560
Little Burgers Cheeseburger	1 (6.7 oz)	550
Little Burgers Cheeseburger Bacon	1 (7.2 oz)	630
Little Burgers Hamburger	1 (6 oz)	480
Veggie Sandwich	1 (7.3 oz)	440
TOPPINGS		
A1 Steak Sauce	1 tbsp (0.6 oz)	15
Bacon	2 slices (0.5 oz)	80
BBQ Sauce	1 tbsp (0.6 oz)	60
Cheese	1 slice (0.7 oz)	70
Green Peppers	1 serv (0.8 oz)	5
Hot Sauce	1 tsp (5 g)	0
Jalapenos	1 serv (0.4 oz)	3
Ketchup	1 tbsp (0.6 oz)	15
Lettuce	1 serv (1 oz)	4
Mayonnaise	1 serv (0.5 oz)	100
Mushrooms	1 serv (0.9 oz)	10
Mustard	1 tbsp (0.6 oz)	0
Onions	1 serv (0.9 oz)	10
Pickle Chips	6 (1 oz)	5
Relish	1 serv (0.5 oz)	15
Tomatoes	1 serv (1.8 oz)	9

FRIENDLY'S
BEVERAGES

Milkshake Double Thick Vanilla	1	770
MAIN MENU SELECTIONS		
Apple Slices	1 serv	100
Applesauce	1 serv	110
Broccoli	1 serv	80
Burger All American	1	1190
Burger BBQ Fronion	1	1560
Burger Mushroom Swiss Bacon	1	1570
Burger Soft Pretzel Bacon	1	1420
Burger The Vermonter	1	1420
Burger Ultimate Bacon Cheese	1	1400
Burgermelt Deluxe Cheese Set-Up	1	1180
Burgermelt Swiss Patty	1	1360
Burgermelt Ultimate Grilled Cheese	1	1500

FOOD	PORTION	CALS
Burgermelt Zesty Questo	1	1380
Carrot & Celery Sticks w/ Ranch Dressing	1 serv	100
Chicken Strips Basket w/o Dipping Sauce	5 pieces	1030
Chicken Strips Honey BBQ w/o Dipping Sauce	5 pieces	1560
Chicken Strips Kickin' Buffalo w/o Dipping Sauce	5 pieces	1530
Clamboat Basket	1 serv	1710
Coleslaw	1 serv	160
Corn	1 serv	160
Fishamajig	1	970
Friendly Frank	1	750
Friendly's BTL	1	990
Fronions Jumbo	1 serv	1430
Garlic Bread	1 serv	330
Grilled Cheese	1	790
Grilled Flounder	1 serv	980
Mandarin Oranges	1 serv	80
Mashed Potatoes Homestyle	1 serv	240
Mini Mozzarella Cheese Sticks	1 serv	680
Mixed Vegetables	1 serv	110
New England Fish 'N Chips	1 serv	1150
Quesadillas Chicken	1 serv	1330
Quesadillas Chicken Fajita	1 serv	1540
Rice	1 serv	210
Shrimp Basket	1 serv	1090
Sirloin Steak Tips	1 serv	1140
Sliders Cheeseburger	1 serv	500
Sliders Chicken	1 serv	740
Spanish Rice	1 serv	330
Supermelt Bruschetta Mozzarella	1	1140
Supermelt Cheddar Jack Chicken	1	1070
Supermelt Grilled Chicken Pesto	1	1360
Supermelt Honey BBQ Chicken	1	1400
Supermelt Kickin Buffalo Chicken	1	1430
Supermelt Reuben	1	1130
Supermelt Steak 'N Mushroom	1	1150
Supermelt Tuna	1	1140
Supermelt Turkey Club	1	990
Tuna Roll	1	920
Waffle Fries	1 serv	590

FOOD	PORTION	CALS
Waffle Fries Loaded	1 serv	920
Wrap Buffalo Chicken	1	1510
Wrap Crispy Chicken	1	1140
Wrap Crispy Chicken Caesar	1	1500
Wrap Grilled Chicken Deluxe	1	1000
SALAD DRESSINGS AND TOPPINGS		
Dressing Bleu Cheese	1 serv	470
Dressing Honey Mustard	1 serv	360
Dressing Italian	1 serv	410
Dressing Italian Fat Free	1 serv	30
Dressing Peppercorn Parmesan Lite	1 serv	230
Dressing Ranch	1 serv	330
Dressing Salsa Ranch	1 serv	170
Dressing Sesame Oriental	1 serv	270
Dressing Thousand Island	1 serv	390
Dressing Vinegarette Dijon Low Fat	1 serv	110
Sauce BBQ	1 serv	90
Sauce Honey Mustard	1 serv	180
Vinegarette Balsamic	1 serv	180
SALADS		
Apple Walnut Chicken w/o Dressing	1 serv	390
Asian Chicken w/o Dressing	1 serv	490
Chicken Caesar	1 serv	1030
Chipotle Chicken w/o Dressing	1 serv	550
Crispy Chicken w/o Dressing	1 serv	630
Kickin Buffalo Chicken w/o Dressing	1 serv	710
Side w/o Dressing	1 serv	60
Steak & Bleu Cheese w/o Dressing	1 serv	640
SOUPS		
Broccoli Cheddar	1 cup	200
Chili	1 cup	270
Chunky Chicken Noodle	1 cup	280
Homestyle Clam Chowder	1 cup	270
Minestrone	1 cup	90

FRUITFULL
BREADS

Almond Cherry	½ slice (2 oz)	226
Apple Spice	½ slice (2 oz)	186
Banana	½ slice (2 oz)	165

FOOD	PORTION	CALS
Cappuccino Chocolate Chip	½ slice (2 oz)	229
Carrot	½ slice (2 oz)	190
Chocolate	½ slice (2 oz)	120
Old Fashion Pound Cake	½ slice (2 oz)	227
Orange Cranberry	½ slice (2 oz)	130
Pumpkin	½ slice (2 oz)	130
Sweet Potato	½ slice (2 oz)	176
Zucchini	½ slice (2 oz)	190
FROZEN BARS		
Cream Banana	1 (4 oz)	110
Cream Coconut	1 (4 oz)	130
Cream Horchata	1 (4 oz)	240
Cream Mango Cream	1 (4 oz)	170
Cream Pina Colada	1 (4 oz)	90
Cream Raspberry Cream	1 (4 oz)	110
Cream Sapote Lucuma	1 (4 oz)	180
Cream Strawberry Cream	1 (4 oz)	110
Juice Fuzzy Navel	1 (4 oz)	70
Juice Green Tea Melon	1 (4 oz)	90
Juice Guava	1 (4 oz)	70
Juice Lemon	1 (4 oz)	90
Juice Lime	1 (4 oz)	80
Juice Passionate Cherry	1 (4 oz)	80
Juice Pineapple	1 (4 oz)	80
Juice Raspberry	1 (4 oz)	70
Juice Strawberry	1 (4 oz)	70
Juice Tamarind	1 (4 oz)	90
Juice Tropical Splash	1 (4 oz)	80
Juice Watermelon	1 (4 oz)	60
Mamey Sapote Lucuma	1 (4 oz)	180
SNACKS		
All About Almonds	1 pkg (1 oz)	170
Blueberry Thrill	1 pkg (1 oz)	150
Buzzworthy Banana	1 pkg (1.1 oz)	140
Calypso Cashews	1 pkg (1.1 oz)	170
Chocolate Covered Nuts	1 pkg (1.5 oz)	230
Chocolate Twisted Bliss	1 pkg (1.4 oz)	190
Cin-sational Apple Crunch	1 pkg (1 oz)	160
Dark Chocolate Covered Almonds	1 pkg (1.4 oz)	210
Dark Chocolate Covered Cashews	1 pkg (1.4 oz)	220

FOOD	PORTION	CALS
Dark Chocolate Covered Cranberries	1 pkg (1.4 oz)	180
Debbie Loves Fruit	1 pkg (1 oz)	110
Eat Your Veggies	1 pkg (1.5 oz)	180
Got Nuts?	1 pkg (1.1 oz)	180
Hit The Road Jack	1 pkg (1.1 oz)	130
Honey I Ate The Peanuts	1 pkg (1 oz)	160
Just Peachy	1 pkg (1.4 oz)	140
Mammoth Malts	1 pkg (1 oz)	150
Nice Catch Swedish Fish	1 pkg (1.4 oz)	140
Off The Hook Gummy Worms	1 pkg (1.5 oz)	130
PB Pretzel Poppers	1 pkg (1 oz)	140
Power Pistachios	1 pkg (1.5 oz)	260
Pumpkin Seeds	1 pkg (1 oz)	180
Reggae Rice Crackers	1 pkg (1.1 oz)	110
Rockin' Raisins	1 pkg (1.4 oz)	170
Rocky Mountain Munch	1 pkg (1.1 oz)	120
Smokin' Nuts	1 pkg (1.3 oz)	170
Soft Twisters Green Apple	1 pkg (1 oz)	120
Soft Twisters Watermelon	1 pkg (1.3 oz)	120
Sour Wiggle Giggle	1 pkg (1.5 oz)	150
Strawberry Fields	1 pkg (1 oz)	140
Sunflower Seeds Tummy	1 pkg (1.1 oz)	190
Swinging Sesame Stix	1 pkg (1.1 oz)	180
Whassup Wasabi	1 pkg (1.1 oz)	150

GREAT STEAK & POTATO
BEVERAGES

Great Steak Lemonade	1 sm (12 oz)	180
Orange Juice	1 (12 oz)	118

BREAKFAST SELECTIONS

Potatoes Deluxe Home	1 serv (12 oz)	390
Potatoes Fresh Cut Home	1 serv (10.6 oz)	380
Sandwich Bacon Egg Cheese	1 (7.6 oz)	600
Sandwich Egg Cheese	1 (7 oz)	500
Sandwich Ham Cheese	1 (5.5 oz)	430
Sandwich Ham Egg Cheese	1 (9 oz)	570
Sandwich Sausage Egg Cheese	1 (9 oz)	700
Sandwich Steak Egg Cheese	1 (10 oz)	600

CHILDREN'S MENU SELECTIONS

Grilled Cheese w/ Fry	1 serv (8.8 oz)	530

FOOD	PORTION	CALS
Kid's Great Fry	1 (6.1 oz)	270
Kids Nuggets	1 serv (2.7 oz)	165
Slider Chicken w/ Fry	1 serv (11.5 oz)	570
Slider Steak w/ Fry	1 serv (11.8 oz)	580
MAIN MENU SELECTIONS		
Baked Potato Broccoli & Cheese	1 (8.9 oz)	400
Baked Potato Cheese & Bacon	1 (7.8 oz)	530
Baked Potato Plain	1 (6 oz)	160
Baked Potato Sour Cream & Chive	1 (7.3 oz)	350
Baked Potato The King	1 (8.8 oz)	590
Cheeseburger	1 (10.2 oz)	640
Chicagoland Cheesesteak 7 Inch	1 (13.3 oz)	680
Coney Island Fry	1 reg (12.7 oz)	570
Great Fry	1 reg (10.2 oz)	440
Great Steak Cheesesteak 7 Inch	1 (13.6 oz)	740
Great Steak Cheesesteak Wrap	1 (13.7 oz)	820
Gyro	1 (12 oz)	580
Ham Delight 7 Inch	1 (13.1 oz)	710
Ham Explosion 7 Inch	1 (14 oz)	710
Hamburger	1 (9.7 oz)	590
Kansas City BBQ Cheesesteak 7 Inch	1 (12 oz)	680
King Fry	1 reg (11.4 oz)	630
Nacho Fry	1 reg (11.8 oz)	510
Pastrami 7 Inch	1 (13.3 oz)	790
Philly Buffalo Chicken 7 Inch	1 (13.8 oz)	660
Philly Burger	1 (14.2 oz)	820
Philly Chicken Slider	1 (5.4 oz)	300
Philly Original Cheesesteak 7 Inch	1 (11.8 oz)	650
Philly Original Chicken 7 Inch	1 (11 oz)	620
Philly Original Chicken Wrap	1 (11.3 oz)	700
Philly Steak Slider	1 (5.6 oz)	310
Philly Teriyaki Chicken	1 (14 oz)	290
Philly Turkey 7 Inch	1 (13 oz)	670
Philly Ultimate Chicken	1 (14.6 oz)	730
Philly Ultimate Chicken Wrap	1 (14.7 oz)	810
Potato Skins	1 serv (6.4 oz)	390
Reuben 7 Inch	1 (12 oz)	690
Super Steak Wrap Cheesesteak	1 (15.7 oz)	930
The Great Potato Chicken	1 (13 oz)	600
The Great Potato Ham	1 (12.8 oz)	520

FOOD	PORTION	CALS
The Great Potato Steak	1 (13.5 oz)	620
The Great Potato Turkey	1 (12.8 oz)	490
Veggi Delight 7 Inch	1 (12.2 oz)	610
Wacker Fry	1 reg (9.8 oz)	490
Wisconsin Inside-Out 7 Inch	1 (6.2 oz)	560
SALAD DRESSINGS AND SAUCES		
Dressing Ranch	1 oz	170
Dressing Thousand Island	1 oz	130
Mayonnaise	1 oz	200
Mayonnaise Dijon	1 oz	110
Oil	1 serv (0.3 oz)	60
Sauce Buffalo	1 oz	10
Sauce Marinara Dipping	2 oz	15
Sauce Teriyaki	1 oz	25
Sauce Tzatziki	1 oz	50
SALADS		
Chef w/o Dressing	1 (16.1 oz)	260
Garden w/o Dressing	1 (12 oz)	60
Great Salad Grilled Chicken	1 (18.8 oz)	380
Great Salad Grilled Ham	1 (18.8 oz)	360
Great Salad Grilled Steak	1 (19.3 oz)	400
Great Salad Grilled Turkey	1 (18.8 oz)	330
Side w/o Dressing	1 (6 oz)	30
Wedge Grilled Chicken	1 (14.8 oz)	270
Wedge Grilled Steak	1 (15.3 oz)	290

HUNGRY HOWIE'S PIZZA
OTHER MENU SELECTIONS

Cajun Bread	¼ bread	300
Chicken Tenders	2	140
Cinnamon Bread	¼ bread	313
Howie Bread	¼ bread	300
Howie Wings	5	180
Sub Deluxe Italian	½ sub	506
Sub Ham & Cheese	½ sub	475
Sub Pizza	½ sub	689
Sub Pizza Special	½ sub	606
Sub Steak & Cheese	½ sub	491
Sub Turkey	½ sub	466
Sub Turkey Club	½ sub	556

FOOD	PORTION	CALS
Sub Vegetarian	½ sub	530
Three Cheeser Bread	¼ bread	370
PIZZA		
Cheese Slice	1 sm	161
Cheese Slice	1 med	191
Cheese Slice	1 lg	208
Cheese Slice	1 extra lg	395
Cheese Slice Thin	1 med	111
Cheese Slice Thin	1 lg	124
Medium Topping Anchovies	1 serv	44
Medium Topping Bacon	1 serv	32
Medium Topping Banana Peppers	1 serv	6
Medium Topping Beef	1 serv	30
Medium Topping Black Olives	1 serv	7
Medium Topping Ham	1 serv	7
Medium Topping Mushrooms	1 serv	2
Medium Topping Pepperoni	1 serv	22
Medium Topping Pineapple	1 serv	5
Medium Topping Sausage	1 serv	27
SALAD DRESSINGS AND SAUCES		
Dressing Blue Cheese	1 serv (1 oz)	150
Dressing Creamy Italian	1 serv (1 oz)	120
Dressing Fat Free Italian	1 serv (1.5 oz)	25
Dressing Fat Free Ranch	1 serv (1.5 oz)	45
Dressing French Style	1 serv (1 oz)	30
Dressing Greek	1 serv (1 oz)	110
Dressing Italian	1 serv (1 oz)	80
Dressing Ranch	1 serv (1 oz)	180
Dressing Thousand Island	1 serv (1 oz)	140
Sauce Dipping	1 serv (3 oz)	45
SALADS		
Antipasto	1 sm	115
Chef	1 sm	114
Garden	1 sm	20
Greek	1 sm	126

IHOP

Pancake Buttermilk	5	770
Pancake Buttermilk Short Stack	3	490
Pancake Chocolate Chip	4	720

FOOD	PORTION	CALS
Pancake Double Blueberry	4	800
Pancake Harvest Grain'N Nut	4	920
Pancake New York Cheesecake	4	1100
Pancake Strawberry Banana	4	760

IVAR'S SEAFOOD BARS
Chicken	3 pieces (4.5 oz)	250
Chowder Salmon	1 cup	220
Chowder White	1 cup	330
Clams	1 serv (5 oz)	400
Cocktail Sauce	¼ cup	50
Fish	3 pieces	220
French Fries	1 serv (3.5 oz)	300
Oysters	5	290
Prawns	1 serv (5 oz)	290
Salmon Fried	3 pieces (4.5 oz)	210
Scallops	1 serv (5 oz)	240
Tartar Sauce	2 tbsp	140

JACK IN THE BOX
BEVERAGES
Barq's Root Beer	1 (20 oz)	180
Chug Chocolate Milk Low Fat	1 (3.5 oz)	200
Chug Reduced Fat Milk	1 (3.5 oz)	130
Coca-Cola Classic	1 (20 oz)	170
Coffee Regular & Decaf	1 (11 oz)	5
Diet Coke	1 (20 oz)	0
Dr Pepper	1 (20 oz)	150
Fanta Orange	1 (20 oz)	150
Fanta Strawberry	1 (20 oz)	150
Iced Tea	1 (20 oz)	5
Lemonade	1 (20 oz)	160
Orange Juice	1 (10 oz)	140
Shake Chocolate	1 (16 oz)	880
Shake Oreo	1 (16 oz)	910
Shake Strawberry	1 (16 oz)	880
Shake Vanilla	1 (16 oz)	790
Sprite	1 (20 oz)	160

BREAKFAST SELECTIONS
Biscuit Bacon Egg Cheese	1	430
Biscuit Chicken	1	450

FOOD	PORTION	CALS
Biscuit Sausage	1	440
Biscuit Sausage Egg Cheese	1	740
Biscuit Spicy Chicken	1	460
Breakfast Sandwich Ciabatta	1	710
Breakfast Sandwich Ultimate	1	570
Breakfast Jack	1	290
Breakfast Jack Bacon	1	300
Breakfast Jack Sausage	1	450
Burrito Hearty Breakfast	1	480
Burrito Sirloin Steak & Egg w/o Salsa	1	790
Croissant Sausage	1	580
Croissant Supreme	1	450
French Toast Sticks	4 (4.2 oz)	470
French Toast Sticks Blueberry	4	450
Hash Browns	1 serv	150
Sandwich Extreme Sausage	1	670
DESSERTS		
Cake Chocolate Overload	1 serv (3.2 oz)	300
Cheesecake	1 serv (3.6 oz)	310
MAIN MENU SELECTIONS		
Bacon Cheddar Potato Wedges	1 serv (9 oz)	720
Cheeseburger Bacon Ultimate	1	1090
Cheeseburger Junior Bacon	1	430
Cheeseburger Sourdough Ultimate	1	950
Cheeseburger Ultimate	1	1010
Chicken Fajita Pita	1	280
Chicken Sandwich	1	400
Chicken Strips Crispy	4	500
Chicken Strips Grilled	4 (5 oz)	180
Ciabatta Burger Bacon 'N' Cheese	1	1120
Ciabatta Burger Single Bacon 'N' Cheese	1	870
Ciabatta Chipotle w/ Grilled Chicken	1	690
Ciabatta Chipotle w/ Spicy Crispy Chicken	1	750
Ciabatta Sirloin Steak 'N' Cheddar	1	770
Club Sourdough Grilled Chicken	1	530
Curly Fries Seasoned	1 sm (3 oz)	270
Egg Rolls	1	130
Fish & Chips	1 serv (7.6 oz)	570
Fries Natural Cut	1 sm	340
Fruit Cup	1 serv	90

FOOD	PORTION	CALS
Hamburger	1	310
Hamburger Deluxe	1	370
Hamburger Deluxe w/ Cheese	1	460
Hamburger w/ Cheese	1	350
Jack's Spicy Chicken	1 serv	620
Jack's Spicy Chicken w/ Cheese	1	700
Jumbo Jack	1	600
Jumbo Jack w/ Cheese	1	690
Mozzarella Cheese Sticks	3	240
Onion Rings	8 (4.2 oz)	500
Sampler Trio	1 serv	750
Sandwich Bacon Chicken	1	440
Sirloin Burger w/ American Cheese & Red Onion	1	1120
Sirloin Burger w/ Swiss & Grilled Onions	1	1070
Sirloin Steak Melt	1	640
Sourdough Jack	1	710
Spicy Chicken Bites	1 serv	290
Stuffed Jalapeno	3 (2.5 oz)	230
Taco Monster Beef	1	240
Taco Regular Beef	1	160
SALAD DRESSINGS AND TOPPINGS		
Asian Sesame	1 serv (2.5 oz)	230
Bacon Ranch	1 serv (2.5 oz)	320
Creamy Southwest	1 serv (2.5 oz)	270
Dipping Sauce Barbeque	1 serv (1 oz)	45
Dipping Sauce Buttermilk House	1 serv (0.9 oz)	130
Dipping Sauce Frank's Red Hot Buffalo	1 serv (1 oz)	10
Dipping Sauce Sweet & Sour	1 serv (1 oz)	45
Dipping Sauce Teriyaki	1 serv (1 oz)	60
Dipping Sauce Zesty Marinara	1 serv (0.8 oz)	15
Low Fat Balsamic	1 serv (2.5 oz)	40
Mayo Onion Sauce	1 serv (0.5 oz)	90
Ranch	1 serv (2.5 oz)	390
Ranch Lite	1 serv (2.5 oz)	190
Soy Sauce	1 serv (0.3 oz)	5
Syrup Log Cabin	1 serv (2 oz)	190
Taco Sauce	1 serv (0.3 oz)	0
Tartar Sauce	1 serv (1.5 oz)	210

FOOD	PORTION	CALS
SALADS		
Asian w/ Crispy Chicken w/o Dressing	1 (13.8 oz)	330
Asian w/ Grilled Chicken w/o Dressing	1 (12.8 oz)	160
Chicken Club w/ Crispy Chicken w/o Dressing	1 (14 oz)	480
Chicken Club w/ Grilled Chicken w/o Dressing	1 (13 oz)	320
Side w/o Dressing	1 (4.3 oz)	50
Southwest w/ Crispy Chicken w/o Dressing	1 (16 oz)	480
Southwest w/ Grilled Chicken w/o Dressing	1 (15 oz)	320
JAMBA JUICE		
BEVERAGES		
Acai Super Antioxidant	1 (16 oz)	290
Acai Topper	1 (12 oz)	440
Aloha Pineapple	1 (16 oz)	300
Banana Berry	1 (16 oz)	300
Berry Fulfilling	1 (16 oz)	160
Berry Topper	1 (12 oz)	420
Blackberry Bliss	1 (16 oz)	260
Boost3G Charger Super	1 (3 g)	5
Boost Antioxidant Power Super	1 (2.8 g)	0
Boost Calcium	1	0
Boost Daily Vitamin	1 (4.36 g)	0
Boost Energy	½ tsp (1.1 g)	0
Boost Flax & Fiber	1 (0.4 oz)	30
Boost Heart Happy	1 (0.75 g)	0
Boost Immunity	1 tsp (2.5 g)	0
Boost Soy Protein	1 (8.9 g)	30
Boost Weight Burner Super	1 (3.5 g)	30
Boost Whey Protein Super	1 (12 g)	45
Caribbean Passion	1 (16 oz)	270
Carrot Juice	1 (16 oz)	100
Chocolate Moo'd	1 (16 oz)	460
Chunky Strawberry Topper	1 (12 oz)	480
Coldbuster	1 (16 oz)	270
Mango Mantra	1 (16 oz)	170
Mango Metabolizer	1 (16 oz)	290
Mango Peach Topper	1 (12 oz)	450
Mango-A-Go-Go	1 (16 oz)	310
Matcha Green Tea Blast	1 (16 oz)	290
Mega Mango	1 (16 oz)	250

FOOD	PORTION	CALS
Orange Dream Machine	1 (16 oz)	350
Orange Juice	1 (16 oz)	220
Peach Perfection	1 (16 oz)	230
Peach Pleasure	1 (16 oz)	290
Peanut Butter Moo'd	1 (16 oz)	490
Pomegranate Heart Happy	1 (16 oz)	300
Pomegranate Paradise	1 (16 oz)	260
Pomegranate Pick-Me-Up	1 (16 oz)	280
Protein Berry Workout w/ Soy Protein	1 (16 oz)	290
Protein Berry Workout w/ Whey	1 (16 oz)	300
Razzmatazz	1 (16 oz)	300
Shot Matcha Energy Orange Juice	1 (4 oz)	60
Shot Matcha Energy Soymilk	1 (4 oz)	70
Shot Wheatgrass Detox	1 oz	5
Strawberries Wild	1 (16 oz)	280
Strawberry Energizer	1 (16 oz)	300
Strawberry Nirvana	1 (16 oz)	170
Strawberry Surf Rider	1 (16 oz)	330
Strawberry Whirl	1 (16 oz)	240
FOOD		
Cheddar Tomato Twist	1 (3.2 oz)	240
Cookie Omega-3 Chocolate Brownie	1 (1.5 oz)	150
Cookie Omega-3 Oatmeal	1 (1.5 oz)	150
Loaf Reduced Fat Blueberry Lemon	1 (3 oz)	290
Loaf Reduced Fat Cranberry Orange	1 (3 oz)	310
Loaf Zucchini Walnut	1 (3 oz)	270
Oatcake Blueberry	1 (3.25 oz)	280
Oatmeal Apple Cinnamon	1 serv (9.1 oz)	290
Oatmeal Blueberry & Blackberry	1 serv (8.9 oz)	290
Oatmeal Fresh Banana	1 serv (9.6 oz)	280
Oatmeal w/ Brown Sugar	1 serv (7.6 oz)	220
Pretzel Apple Cinnamon	1 (5.2 oz)	380
Pretzel Sourdough Parmesan	1 (5 oz)	410

JERSEY MIKE'S
SANDWICHES

#05 Super Sub In A Tub	1 (11.9 oz)	290
#05 Super Sub Wheat	1 (16 oz)	280
#05 Super Sub White	1 (16 oz)	580
#06 Roast Beef & Provolone In A Tub	1 (12.2 oz)	430

FOOD	PORTION	CALS
#06 Roast Beef & Provolone Wheat	1 reg (16.2 oz)	720
#06 Roast Beef & Provolone White	1 reg (16.2 oz)	730
#07 Turkey Breast & Provolone In A Tub	1 (11.4 oz)	250
#07 Turkey Breast & Provolone Wheat	1 reg (15.4 oz)	540
#07 Turkey Breast & Provolone White	1 (15.4 oz)	550
#08 Club Sub w/ Mayonnaise In A Tub	1 (13.2 oz)	600
#08 Club Sub w/ Mayonnaise Wheat	1 (17.2 oz)	890
#08 Club Sub w/ Mayonnaise White	1 (17.2 oz)	890
#09 Club Sub Supreme w/ Mayonnaise In A Tub	1 (13.2 oz)	650
#09 Club Supreme w/ Mayonnaise Wheat	1 reg (17.2 oz)	940
#09 Club Supreme w/ Mayonnaise White	1 (17.2 oz)	940
#10 Albacore Tuna In A Tub	1 (12.2 oz)	620
#10 Albacore Tuna Wheat	1 (16.2 oz)	910
#10 Albacore Tuna White	1 (16.2 oz)	910
#13 Original Italian In A Tub	1 (12.9 oz)	390
#13 Original Italian Wheat	1 reg (16.9 oz)	680
#13 Original Italian White	1 reg (16.9 oz)	680
#14 Veggie White	1 reg (15.7 oz)	750
American Classic In A Tub	1 (11.4 oz)	270
American Classic Wheat	1 reg (15.4 oz)	560
American Classic White	1 reg (15.4 oz)	560
BLT In A Tub	1 (8.2 oz)	280
BLT Wheat	1 reg (12.2 oz)	570
BLT White	1 reg (12.2 oz)	570
Hot Sub #15 Meatball & Cheese Wheat	1 reg (13.5 oz)	890
Hot Sub #15 Meatball & Cheese White	1 reg (13.5 oz)	890
Hot Sub #17 Chicken Philly Wheat	1 reg (13 oz)	630
Hot Sub BBQ Beef Wheat	1 reg (11.2 oz)	710
Hot Sub BBQ Beef White	1 reg (11.2 oz)	720
Hot Sub Big Kahuna Chicken Wheat	1 reg (14.2 oz)	680
Hot Sub Big Kahuna Chicken White	1 reg (14.2 oz)	690
Hot Sub Big Kahuna Wheat	1 reg (14.2 oz)	670
Hot Sub Big Kahuna White	1 reg (14.2 oz)	680
Hot Sub Cheese Steak Buffalo Chicken Wheat	1 reg (20.2 oz)	940
Hot Sub Cheese Steak Buffalo Chicken White	1 reg (20.2 oz)	940
Hot Sub Cheese Steak California Chicken Wheat	1 reg (17.4 oz)	890
Hot Sub Cheese Steak California Chicken White	1 reg (17.4 oz)	890
Hot Sub Cheese Steak California Wheat	1 reg (17.4 oz)	870

FOOD	PORTION	CALS
Hot Sub Cheese Steak California White	1 reg (17.4 oz)	880
Hot Sub Cheese Steak Teriyaki Chicken Wheat	1 reg (14.9 oz)	680
Hot Sub Cheese Steak Teriyaki Chicken White	1 reg (14.9 oz)	680
Hot Sub Chicka Phila Roni Wheat	1 reg (12.5 oz)	620
Hot Sub Chicka Phila Roni White	1 reg (12.5 oz)	605
Hot Sub Chicken Parmesan Wheat	1 reg (11 oz)	650
Hot Sub Chicken Philly White	1 reg (13 oz)	630
Hot Sub Chipotle Chicken Wheat	1 reg (14.4 oz)	910
Hot Sub Chipotle Chicken White	1 reg (14.4 oz)	920
Hot Sub Chipotle Steak Wheat	1 reg (14.4 oz)	900
Hot Sub Chipotle Steak White	1 reg (14.4 oz)	910
Hot Sub Chipotle Turkey Wheat	1 reg (17.4 oz)	865
Hot Sub Chipotle Turkey White	1 reg (17.4 oz)	870
Hot Sub Grilled Chicken Wheat	1 reg (12.7 oz)	670
Hot Sub Grilled Chicken White	1 reg (12.7 oz)	670
Hot Sub Pastrami & Swiss Wheat	1 reg (10.7 oz)	580
Hot Sub Pastrami & Swiss White	1 reg (10.7 oz)	590
Hot Sub Reuben Wheat	1 reg (12.2 oz)	700
Hot Sub Reuben White	1 reg (12.2 oz)	710
Hot Sub Sausage Wheat	1 reg (11.5 oz)	600
Hot Sub Sausage White	1 reg (11.4 oz)	600
Hot Sub Steak Philly Wheat	1 reg (13 oz)	620
Hot Sub Steak Philly White	1 reg (13 oz)	620
Jersey Shore Favorite In A Tub	1 (11.4 oz)	270
Jersey Shore Favorite Wheat	1 reg (15.4 oz)	560
Jersey Shore Favorite White	1 reg (15.4 oz)	570
Veggie In A Tub	1 (11.7 oz)	460
Veggie Wheat	1 reg (15.72 oz)	720
Wrap Baja Chicken	1 (15.6 oz)	610
Wrap Buffalo Chicken	1 (14.6 oz)	740
Wrap Chicken Caesar	1 (12 oz)	580
Wrap Grilled Ham & Cheese	1 (14 oz)	740
Wrap Grilled Roast Beef & Cheese	1 (15 oz)	830
Wrap Grilled Veggie	1 (17 oz)	910
Wrap Turkey w/ Honey Mustard Sauce	1 (13 oz)	540
SOUPS		
Beef Steak & Black Bean	1 cup (8.7 oz)	140
Boston Clam Chowder	1 cup (8.5 oz)	130
Broccoli Cheese	1 cup (8.7 oz)	140
Cape Cod Clam Chowder	1 cup (8.7 oz)	140

FOOD	PORTION	CALS
Chicken & Dumplings	1 cup (8.7 oz)	250
Chicken Gumbo	1 cup (9 oz)	100
Chicken Noodle	1 cup (8.7 oz)	90
Chicken Pot Pie	1 cup (8.7 oz)	230
Chicken Tortilla	1 cup (8.7 oz)	140
Cream Of Broccoli	1 cup (8.7 oz)	90
Cream Of Potato	1 cup (8.7 oz)	180
Creamy Tomato Bisque	1 cup (8.5 oz)	90
French Onion	1 cup (8.7 oz)	80
Italian Wedding	1 cup (8.5 oz)	120
Lumberjack Vegetable	1 cup (8.5 oz)	120
Maryland Crab	1 cup (8.7 oz)	70
Minestrone	1 cup (8.7 oz)	70
Potato w/ Bacon	1 cup (8.5 oz)	130
Spicy Chili w/ Beans	1 cup (9.6 oz)	240
Split Pea w/ Ham	1 cup (8.5 oz)	150
Timberline Chili w/ Beans	1 cup (8.7 oz)	280
Tomato Florentine	1 cup (8.7 oz)	90
Vegetable Beef & Barley	1 cup (8.7 oz)	90
Vegetarian Vegetable	1 cup (8.7 oz)	80
Wild & Brown Rice w/ Chicken	1 cup (8.7 oz)	310
Wisconsin Cheese	1 cup (8.5 oz)	220

JIMMY JOHN'S
BEVERAGES

Coke	1 sm	248
Diet Coke	1 sm	0
Iced Tea	1 sm	3
Iced Tea Raspberry	1 sm	195
Lemonade	1 sm	243
Lemonade Light	1 sm	13
Sprite	1 sm	243

SANDWICHES

Giant Club Beach	1	798
Giant Club Billy	1	867
Giant Club Bootlegger	1	720
Giant Club Country	1	840
Giant Club Gourmet Smoked Ham	1	851
Giant Club Gourmet Veggie	1	856
Giant Club Hunter's	1	854

FOOD	PORTION	CALS
Giant Club Italian Night	1	975
Giant Club Lulu	1	790
Giant Club Tuna	1	719
Giant Club Ultimate Porker	1	843
Slim Double Provolone	1	588
Slim Ham & Cheese	1	534
Slim Salami Capicola Cheese	1	624
Slim Tuna Salad	1	577
Slim Turkey Breast	1	407
Sub Big John	1	564
Sub J.J.B.L.T.	1	662
Sub Pepe	1	684
Sub Totally Tuna	1	502
Sub Turkey Tom	1	555
Sub Vegetarian	1	640
Sub Vito	1	579
The J.J. Gargantuan	1	1008
Unwich Hunter's Club	1	520
Unwich The J.J. Gargantuan	1	769
SIDES		
Cookie Chocolate Chunk	1	421
Cookie Raisin Oatmeal	1	421
Jimmy Chips	1 pkg	160
Jimmy Chips BBQ	1 pkg	160
Jimmy Chips Jalapeno	1 pkg	150
Jimmy Chips Sea Salt & Vinegar	1 pkg	140
Pickle Spear	1	4
Pickle Whole	1	15

KENTUCKY FRIED CHICKEN
BEVERAGES

FOOD	PORTION	CALS
Diet Pepsi	1 med (14 oz)	0
Mt. Dew	1 med (14 oz)	190
Pepsi	1 med (14 oz)	180
DESSERTS		
Cake Double Chocolate Chip	1 slice	330
Cookie Sweet Life Chocolate Chip	1 (1.2 oz)	160
Cookie Sweet Life Oatmeal Raisin	1 (1.2 oz)	150
Cookie Sweet Life Sugar	1 (1.2 oz)	160
Lil' Bucket Chocolate Cream	1	280

FOOD	PORTION	CALS
Lil' Bucket Lemon Creme	1 serv	410
Lil' Bucket Strawberry Short Cake	1 serv	210
Pie Mini's Apple	3 (4 oz)	370
Teddy Graham Cinnamon Snacks	1 serv	90
MAIN MENU SELECTIONS		
Baked Beans	1 serv	220
Biscuit	1 (2 oz)	220
Bowl Chicken & Biscuit	1	870
Bowl Mashed Potato w/ Gravy	1	740
Bowl Rice w/ Gravy	1	620
Chicken Pot Pie	1 (15 oz)	770
Cole Slaw	1 serv	180
Corn On The Cob	1 ear (3 inch)	70
Crispy Strips	2 (3.5 oz)	240
Extra Crispy Breast	1 (5.7 oz)	440
Extra Crispy Drumstick	1 (2 oz)	160
Extra Crispy Thigh	1 (4 oz)	370
Extra Crispy Whole Wing	1 (1.8 oz)	170
Green Beans	1 serv	50
KFC Snacker	1	290
KFC Snacker Buffalo	1	260
KFC Snacker Fish	1	330
KFC Snacker Fish w/o Sauce	1	290
KFC Snacker Honey BBQ	1	210
KFC Snacker Ultimate Cheese	1	280
Macaroni & Cheese	1 serv	180
Mashed Potatoes w/ Gravy	1 serv	140
Mashed Potatoes w/o Gravy	1 serv	110
Original Recipe Breast	1 (5.6 oz)	360
Original Recipe Breast w/o Skin Or Breading	1 (3.8 oz)	140
Original Recipe Drumstick	1 (2 oz)	130
Original Recipe Thigh	1 (4.4 oz)	330
Original Recipe Whole Wing	1 (1.6 oz)	130
Popcorn Chicken	1 reg (4 oz)	400
Potato Salad	1 serv	180
Potato Wedges	1 serv	260
Sandwich Crispy Twister	1	550
Sandwich Double Crunch	1	470
Sandwich Honey BBQ	1	280
Sandwich Tender Roast	1	380

FOOD	PORTION	CALS
Sandwich Tender Roast w/o Sauce	1	300
Seasoned Rice	1 serv	180
Twister Oven Roasted	1	420
Twister Oven Roasted w/o Sauce	1	330
Wings Boneless Fiery Buffalo	5	420
Wings Boneless Honey BBQ	5	450
Wings Boneless Sweet & Spicy	5	440
Wings Boneless Teriyaki	5	500
Wings Fiery Buffalo	5	380
Wings Honey BBQ	5	390
Wings Hot	5	350
Wings Hot & Spicy	5	400
Wings Teriyaki	5	480
SALAD DRESSINGS		
Creamy Parmesan Caesar	1 serv (2 oz)	260
Golden Italian Light	1 serv (1.5 oz)	45
Ranch	1 serv (2 oz)	200
Ranch Fat Free	1 serv (1.5 oz)	35
SALADS		
Crispy BLT w/o Dressing	1 (12 oz)	330
Crispy Caesar w/o Dressing & Croutons	1 (11 oz)	350
Croutons Parmesan Garlic	1 pkg	60
Roasted BLT w/o Dressing	1 (12 oz)	200
Roasted Caesar w/o Dressing & Croutons	1 (11 oz)	220
Side Caesar w/o Dressing & Croutons	1 (3 oz)	50
Side House w/o Dressing	1 (3 oz)	15

KOO-KOO-ROO
MAIN MENU SELECTIONS

Baked Yam	1 serv (6 oz)	197
Black Beans	1 serv (6 oz)	125
Buffalo Wings	6	606
Burrito California Chicken	1	810
Burrito Fajita Chicken	1	750
Burrito Original Chicken	1	709
Butternut Squash	1 serv (6 oz)	66
Chicken Bowl Chargrilled w/o Sauce	1	569
Chicken Bowl Spicy Garlic Ginger w/o Sauce	1	485
Creamed Spinach	1 serv (8 oz)	100
Italian Vegetable	1 serv (5.5 oz)	47

FOOD	PORTION	CALS
Kernel Corn	1 serv (4.5 oz)	105
Mashed Potatoes	1 serv (6.5 oz)	188
Original Breast	1 (4.1 oz)	187
Original Chicken Dark	3 pieces (5 oz)	320
Roasted Garlic Potatoes	1 serv (5 oz)	133
Rotisserie Chicken Breast & Wing	1 serv (6.5 oz)	355
Rotisserie Chicken Leg & Thigh	1 serv (4.8 oz)	300
Rotisserie Half Chicken	1 serv (11.3 oz)	655
Sandwich BBQ Chicken	1	562
Sandwich Chicken Caesar	1	781
Sandwich Original Chicken	1	661
Sandwich Turkey Hand Carved	1	599
Southwestern Bowl w/o Sauce	1	570
Tostada Bowl w/o Sauce w/o Shell	1	528
Traditional Turkey Dinner	1 serv	692
Turkey Breast Sliced	1 serv	182
Turkey Pot Pie	1	883
Wrap Caesar Chicken	1	757
Wrap Chipotle Chicken	1	924
SALADS		
BBQ Chicken w/o Dressing	1	365
Cantaloupe & Honeydew	1 serv (5 oz)	50
Chicken Caesar w/o Dressing	1	286
Chinese Chicken w/o Dressing	1	550
Creamy Coleslaw	1 serv (5 oz)	238
Cucumber	1 serv (4.5 oz)	41
House	1	113
Tangy Tomato	1 serv (4.5 oz)	60
Tossed w/ Dressing	1 serv (3 oz)	16
SOUPS		
Chicken Noodle	1 serv (5 oz)	71
Chicken Tortilla	1 serv (5 oz)	112
Ten Vegetable	1 serv (5 oz)	94

KRISPY KREME
BEVERAGES

FOOD	PORTION	CALS
Chillers Fruity Orange You Glad	1 (12 oz)	180
Chillers Fruity Very Berry	1 (12 oz)	170
Chillers Kremey Berries & Kreme	1 (12 oz)	620
Chillers Kremey Chocolate Chocolate	1 (12 oz)	970

FOOD	PORTION	CALS
Chillers Kremey Lemon Sherbert	1 (12 oz)	630
Chillers Kremey Lotta Latte	1 (12 oz)	670
Chillers Kremey Mocha Dream	1 (12 oz)	670
Chillers Kremey Oranges & Kreme	1 (12 oz)	630
DOUGHNUTS		
Apple Fritter	1	380
Caramel Kreme Crunch	1	380
Chocolate Iced Cake	1	280
Chocolate Iced Custard Filled	1	300
Chocolate Iced Glazed	1	250
Chocolate Iced Kreme Filled	1	350
Chocolate Iced w/ Sprinkles	1	270
Cinnamon Apple Filled	1	290
Cinnamon Bun	1	260
Cinnamon Twist	1	240
Dulce De Leche	1	300
Glazed Chocolate Cake	1	300
Glazed Cinnamon	1	210
Glazed Creme Filled	1	340
Glazed Cruller	1	240
Glazed Cruller Chocolate	1	290
Glazed Lemon Filled	1	290
Glazed Maple Iced	1	240
Glazed Original Spice	1	200
Glazed Pumpkin	1	300
Glazed Raspberry Filled	1	300
Glazed Sour Cream	1	300
Holes Glazed Blueberry	4	220
Holes Glazed Cake	4	210
Holes Glazed Chocolate Cake	4	210
Holes Glazed Original	4	200
Holes Glazed Pumpkin Spice	4	210
New York Cheesecake	1	340
Powdered Cake	1	290
Powdered Strawberry Filled	1	290
Sugar	1	200
Traditional Cake	1	230

FOOD	PORTION	CALS
KRYSTAL		
BEVERAGES		
Coca-Cola Classic	1 sm (16 oz)	129
Coca-Cola Classic frzn	1 (16 oz)	130
Diet Coke	1 sm (16 oz)	<1
Sprite	1 sm (16 oz)	126
BREAKFAST SELECTIONS		
4 Carb Scrambler Bacon	1 serv	370
4 Carb Scrambler Sausage	1 serv	600
Biscuit & Gravy	1	280
Biscuit Bacon Egg Cheese	1	390
Biscuit Chik	1	360
Biscuit Plain	1	270
Biscuit Sausage	1	480
Country Breakfast	1 serv	660
Kryspers	1 serv	190
Krystal Sunriser	1	240
Scrambler	1 serv	440
DESSERTS		
Fried Apple Turnover	1	220
Lemon Icebox Pie	1 serv	260
MAIN MENU SELECTIONS		
BA Burger	1	470
BA Burger Cheese	1	530
BA Burger Double Bacon Cheese	1	800
Chik'n Bites	1 sm	310
Chik'n Bites Salad	1 serv	290
Fries	1 reg	470
Fries Chili Cheese	1 serv	540
Krystal	1	160
Krystal Bacon Cheese	1	190
Krystal Cheese	1	180
Krystal Chik	1	240
Krystal Chili	1 serv	200
Krystal Double	1	260
Krystal Double Cheese	1	310
Pup Chili Cheese	1	210
Pup Corn	1	260
Pup Plain	1	170

FOOD	PORTION	CALS

LITTLE CAESARS
DIPS AND SAUCES
Crazy Sauce	1 serv (4 oz)	45
Dip Buffalo	1 serv (1.5 oz)	130
Dip Buffalo Ranch	1 serv (1.5 oz)	220
Dip Buttery Garlic	1 serv (1.5 oz)	380
Dip Cheezy	1 serv (1.5 oz)	210
Dip Chipotle	1 serv (1.5 oz)	220
Dip Ranch	1 serv (1.5 oz)	250

MAIN MENU SELECTIONS
Cheese Bread Italian	1 (1.6 oz)	130
Cheese Bread Pepperoni	1 (1.7 oz)	150
Crazy Bread	1 (1.3 oz)	100
Pizza 3 Meat Treat	⅛ pie (4.8 oz)	350
Pizza Baby Pan!Pan! Cheese & Pepperoni	1 pie (4.9 oz)	360
Pizza Baby Pan!Pan! Just Cheese	1 pie (4.7 oz)	320
Pizza Deep Dish Just Cheese	⅛ pie (4.8 oz)	320
Pizza Deep Dish Pepperoni	⅛ pie (5 oz)	360
Pizza Hot-N-Ready Just Cheese	⅛ pie (4 oz)	240
Pizza Hot-N-Ready Pepperoni	⅛ pie (4.2 oz)	280
Pizza Hulu Hawaiian Pineapple & Canadian Bacon	⅛ pie (5.2 oz)	280
Pizza Hulu Hawaiian Pineapple & Ham	⅛ pie (5.3 oz)	270
Pizza Ultimate Supreme	⅛ pie (5.3 oz)	310
Pizza Ultimate Supreme Vegetarian	⅛ pie (5.4 oz)	270
Wings Barbecue	1 (1.2 oz)	70
Wings Hot	1 (1.2 oz)	60
Wings Mild	1 (1 oz)	60
Wings Oven Roasted	1 (0.9 oz)	50

LONG JOHN SILVER'S
BEVERAGES
Diet Mountain Dew	1 med (32 oz)	0
Diet Pepsi	1 med (32 oz)	0
Dr Pepper	1 med (32 oz)	400
Iced Tea Unsweetened	1 med (32 oz)	0
Iceflow Lemonade	1 sm (16 oz)	190
Iceflow Strawberry Lemonade	1 sm (16 oz)	240
Lipton Raspberry Tea	1 med (32 oz)	320
Mountain Dew	1 med (32 oz)	440

FOOD	PORTION	CALS
Pepsi	1 med (32 oz)	400
Pepsi Wild Cherry	1 med (32 oz)	400
Sierra Mist	1 med (32 oz)	400
Tropicana Fruit Punch	1 med (32 oz)	440
Tropicana Lemonade	1 med (32 oz)	400
DESSERTS		
Pie Chocolate Cream	1 slice (2.6 oz)	280
Pie Pineapple Cream	1 slice (3.1 oz)	300
MAIN MENU SELECTIONS		
Battered Alaskan Pollock	1 piece (3.2 oz)	140
Battered Shrimp	3 (1.5 oz)	130
Bites Broccoli Cheddar	5 (3.3 oz)	230
Bites Jalapeno Cheddar	5 (2.9 oz)	240
Breaded Mozzarella Sticks	3 (1.8 oz)	150
Breaded Clams Strips	1 box (3 oz)	320
Breadstick	1 (2 oz)	170
Buttered Langostino Lobster Bites	1 box (3.2 oz)	230
Chicken Strip	1 (1.8 oz)	140
Cole Slaw	1 serv (4 oz)	200
Corn Cobbette w/ Butter	1 (3.6 oz)	150
Corn Cobbette w/o Butter	1 (3.3 oz)	90
Crumblies	1 serv (1 oz)	170
Freshside Grille Salmon Entree	1 serv (10.7 oz)	280
Freshside Grille Shrimp Scampi Entree	1 serv (10.7 oz)	330
Freshside Grille Tilapia Entree	1 serv (10.2 oz)	250
Fries Basket Portion	1 serv (4 oz)	310
Fries Platter Portion	1 serv (3 oz)	230
Grilled Pacific Salmon Filets	2 (4.5 oz)	150
Grilled Tilapia Filet	1 (4 oz)	110
Hushpuppy	1 (0.8 oz)	60
Jalapeno Peppers	1 (1.3 oz)	15
Longostino Lobster Stuffed Crab Cake	1 (2.2 oz)	170
Popcorn Shrimp	1 box (2.9 oz)	270
Rice	1 serv (5 oz)	180
Sandwich Alaskan Pollock	1 (6.6 oz)	470
Sandwich Chicken Strip	1 (6.6 oz)	440
Sandwich Ultimate Alaskan Pollock	1 (7.2 oz)	240
Sandwich Zesty Chicken Strip	1 (4.5 oz)	380
Shrimp Scampi	8 pieces (4.6 oz)	200
Soup Broccoli Cheese	1 bowl (7.4 oz)	220

FOOD	PORTION	CALS
Taco Baja Chicken Strip	1 (4.3 oz)	370
Taco Baja Fish	1 (4 oz)	360
Vegetable Medley	1 serv (4 oz)	50
SAUCES		
BBQ	1 serv (1 oz)	40
Cocktail	1 serv (1 oz)	25
Honey Mustard	1 serv (1 oz)	100
Ketchup	1 pkg (0.3 oz)	10
Lemon Juice	1 serv (4 g)	0
Louisiana Hot Sauce	1 tsp (5 g)	0
Malt Vinegar	1 serv (0.5 oz)	0
Marinara	1 serv (1 oz)	15
Ranch	1 serv (1 oz)	160
Sweet & Sour	1 serv (1 oz)	45
Tartar	1 serv (1 oz)	100

MAGGIE MOO'S
BEVERAGES

FOOD	PORTION	CALS
Shake Caramel Cowpuccino	1 (15 oz)	740
Shake Cinnamoo Swirl	1 (16 oz)	780
Shake Cookies 'N' Cream	1 (15 oz)	740
Shake Moocha Cowpuccino	1 (15 oz)	710
Shake Peanut Butter S'Moo	1 (16 oz)	780
Shake Strawberries 'N' Cream	1 (15 oz)	620
Zoomer Caramel Coffee	1 (15 oz)	380
Zoomer Creamy Mango	1 (17 oz)	400
Zoomer Mocha Coffee	1 (17 oz)	460
Zoomer Raspberry Pomegranate	1 (17 oz)	460
Zoomer Strawberry Banana	1 (18 oz)	350
Zoomer Triple Berry Pomegranate	1 (17 oz)	460
CONES		
Dark Chocolate	1 (1.5 oz)	200
Dark Chocolate w/ Butterfinger	1 (2 oz)	260
Dark Chocolate w/ Heath Bar	1 (2 oz)	280
Dark Chocolate w/ Peanuts	1 (2 oz)	280
Plain	1 (1 oz)	120
White Chocolate	1 (1.5 oz)	200
White Chocolate w/ Sprinkles	1 (2 oz)	210
ICE CREAM		
Amooretto Cream	1 serv (6 oz)	380

FOOD	PORTION	CALS
Apple Strudel	1 serv (6 oz)	380
Banana Pudding	1 serv (6 oz)	330
Black Cherry	1 serv (6 oz)	380
Blueberry Muffin	1 serv (6 oz)	390
Brownie Batter	1 serv (6 oz)	420
Butter Pecan	1 serv (6 oz)	380
Cake 6 inch Better Batter	1/8 cake (5.7 oz)	480
Cake 6 inch Chocolate Cream	1/8 cake (6.4 oz)	580
Cake 8 inch Caramel Drizzle	1/14 cake (6 oz)	530
Cake 8 inch Chocolate Espresso	1/14 cake (5.6 oz)	460
Cake 8 inch Chocolate Heaven	1/14 cake (5 oz)	400
Cake 8 inch Cookie Dreams	1/14 cake (5.3 oz)	440
Cake 8 inch Cookies 'N' Cream	1/14 cake (5.3 oz)	430
Cake 8 inch Cotton Candy Carnival	1/14 cake (5.9 oz)	490
Cake 8 inch Fudge Fantasy	1/14 cake (5.4 oz)	410
Cake 8 inch Maggie S'Mores	1/14 cake (7 oz)	610
Cake 8 inch Maggie's Mud	1/14 cake (5.3 oz)	440
Cake 8 inch Pecan Perfection	1/14 cake (5.6 oz)	500
Cake 8 inch Sprinkle	1/14 cake (5.7 oz)	370
Cake 8 inch Strawberry Cheesecream	1/14 cake (6.3 oz)	530
Cake 8 inch Truffle Dream	1/14 cake (5.8 oz)	500
Cake 8 inch Turtle	1/14 cake (6.3 oz)	590
Cappuccino	1 serv (6 oz)	380
Caramel Apple	1 serv (6 oz)	400
Carrot Cake	1 serv (6 oz)	420
Cheesecake	1 serv (6 oz)	380
Choco Mallo	1 serv (6 oz)	360
Chocolate	1 serv (6 oz)	390
Chocolate Banana	1 serv (6 oz)	370
Chocolate Better Batter	1 serv (6 oz)	420
Chocolate Peanut Butter	1 serv (6 oz)	450
Chocolate Raspberry	1 serv (6 oz)	380
Cinnamoo	1 serv (6 oz)	380
Cinnamoo Bun	1 serv (6 oz)	530
Cocoa Amooretto	1 serv (6 oz)	390
Cool Mint	1 serv (6 oz)	380
Cotton Candy	1 serv (6 oz)	380
Creamy Coconut	1 serv (6 oz)	380
Cupcake Better Batter	1	430
Cupcake Caramel Pumpkin Pie	1	500

FOOD	PORTION	CALS
Cupcake Cherry Chocolate	1	280
Cupcake Chocolate	1	400
Cupcake Chocolate Heaven	1	340
Cupcake Cool Swirl	1	370
Cupcake Cotton Candy Carnival	1	330
Cupcake Maggie O	1	360
Cupcake Pecan Pie	1	440
Cupcake Snowcap Blush	1	360
Cupcake Sprinkle	1	340
Dark Chocolate	1 serv	390
Egg Nog	1 serv (6 oz)	390
Espresso Bean	1 serv (6 oz)	380
French Vanilla	1 serv	390
Fresh Banana	1 serv (6 oz)	340
Key Lime	1 serv	380
Maggie's Fudge	1 serv	630
Mint Chocolate	1 serv (6 oz)	390
Mocha	1 serv (6 oz)	390
Peanut Butter	1 serv (6 oz)	480
Pina Cowlada	1 serv (6 oz)	360
Pink Bubblegum	1 serv (6 oz)	380
Pink Peppermint Stick	1 serv (6 oz)	420
Pistachio	1 serv (6 oz)	380
Pizza 10 inch Cheese	1/10 pie (5.4 oz)	340
Pizza 10 inch Chocolate Lover's	1/10 pie	390
Pizza 10 inch Supreme	1/10 pie (6.1 oz)	450
Pumpkin Pie	1 serv (6 oz)	370
Raspberry	1 serv (6 oz)	370
Red Velvet Cake	1 serv (6 oz)	420
Rum Raisin	1 serv (6 oz)	380
Southern Peaches	1 serv (6 oz)	330
Strawberry	1 serv	350
Strawberry Banana No Sugar Added	1 serv (6 oz)	170
Udderly Cream	1 serv (6 oz)	380
Vanilla	1 serv (6 oz)	380
Vanilla Low Fat Lactose Free	1 serv (6 oz)	130
Very Yellow Marshmallow	1 serv (6 oz)	350

FOOD	PORTION	CALS
MANHATTAN BAGEL		
BAGELS AND BAKED GOODS		
Bagel Blueberry	1 (3.8 oz)	300
Bagel Blueberry Glaze	1 (4.5 oz)	360
Bagel Cheddar	1 (4 oz)	320
Bagel Chocolate Chip	1 (3.8 oz)	290
Bagel Cinnamon Raisin	1 (4 oz)	330
Bagel Egg	1 (4 oz)	320
Bagel Everything	1 (4.3 oz)	350
Bagel French Toast	1 (3.5 oz)	300
Bagel Garlic	1 (4.3 oz)	340
Bagel Honey Whole Wheat	1 (3.5 oz)	250
Bagel Honey Whole Wheat Everything	1 (3.8 oz)	280
Bagel Jalapeno Cheddar	1 (4 oz)	320
Bagel Onion	1 (4.3 oz)	340
Bagel Plain	1 (4 oz)	320
Bagel Poppy	1 (4.3 oz)	360
Bagel Pumpernickel	1 (3.5 oz)	240
Bagel Rye	1 (4 oz)	310
Bagel Salt	1 (4.3 oz)	320
Bagel Sesame Seed	1 (4.5 oz)	360
Bagel Mini Plain	1 (1.8 oz)	130
Bagel Thin Honey Whole Wheat	1 (2 oz)	120
Bagel Thin Plain	1 (2 oz)	120
MARBLE SLAB CREAMERY		
Cone Honey Wheat	1	130
Cone Sugar	1	130
Cone Vanilla Cinnamon	1	130
Frozen Yogurt Nonfat	½ cup	100
Frozen Yogurt Nonfat No Sugar Added	½ cup	90
Ice Cream Reduced Fat	1 serv (6.75 oz)	390
Ice Cream Superpremium	1 serv (6.75 oz)	450
Sorbet	½ cup	90
MARCO'S PIZZA		
OTHER MENU SELECTIONS		
Cheezybread Bran	1 piece	80
Chicken Tumblers BBQ	1	67
Chicken Tumblers Hot & Spicy	1	57
Chicken Tumblers Naked	1	57

FOOD	PORTION	CALS
Chicken Wings BBQ	1	71
Chicken Wings Hot & Spicy	1	60
Chicken Wings Naked	1	60
Cinnasquares	1 piece	60
Salad Chicken Ranch	1 serv	240
Salad Italian	1 serv	230
Sub Chicken Club	½	385
Sub Ham & Cheese	½	400
Sub Italian	½	430
Sub Steak & Cheese	½	380
Sub Veggie	½	355
PIZZA		
Cheese Large	1 slice	280
Cheese Medium	1 slice	210
Cheese Small	1 slice	200
Chicken Fresco Large	1 slice	350
Chicken Fresco Medium	1 slice	260
Chicken Fresco Small	1 slice	180
Deep Pan Cheese	1 slice	290
Deep Pan Pepperoni	1 slice	330
Deluxe Uno Large	1 slice	380
Deluxe Uno Medium	1 slice	280
Deluxe Uno Small	1 slice	200
Garden Large	1 slice	310
Garden Medium	1 slice	230
Garden Small	1 slice	160
Hawaiian Chicken Large	1 slice	380
Hawaiian Chicken Medium	1 slice	260
Hawaiian Chicken Small	1 slice	180
Meat Supremo Large	1 slice	430
Meat Supremo Medium	1 slice	300
Meat Supremo Small	1 slice	210
Pepperoni Large	1 slice	310
Pepperoni Medium	1 slice	230
Pepperoni Small	1 slice	210
White Cheezy Large	1 slice	340
White Cheezy Medium	1 slice	260
White Cheezy Small	1 slice	170

FOOD	PORTION	CALS
MAUI WOWI		
SMOOTHIES		
Fresh Fruit Banana Banana	1 (12 oz)	210
Fresh Fruit Black Raspberry	1 (12 oz)	240
Fresh Fruit Kiwi Lemon Lime	1 (12 oz)	180
Fresh Fruit Lemon Wave	1 (12 oz)	415
Fresh Fruit Mango Orange Banana	1 (12 oz)	240
Fresh Fruit Passion Papaya	1 (12 oz)	220
Fresh Fruit Pina Colada	1 (12 oz)	240
MAX & ERMA'S		
Black Bean Roll Up	1 serv	577
Caribbean Chicken Lunch Portion	1 serv	536
Fruit Smoothie	1	124
Garlic Breadstick	1	156
Hula Bowl w/ Fat Free Honey Mustard Dressing w/o Breadstick	1 serv	823
Salad Baby Greens w/o Breadstick	1 serv	119
Salad Shrimp Stack	1 serv	322
Salad Dressing Bleu Cheese	2 tbsp	201
Salad Dressing French Fat Free	2 tbsp	126
Salad Dressing Honey Mustard Fat Free	2 tbsp	60
Salad Dressing Italian	2 tbsp	110
Salad Dressing Ranch	2 tbsp	120
Salad Dressing Tex Mex Low Fat	2 tbsp	23
MCALISTER'S DELI		
CHILDREN'S MENU SELECTIONS		
Kid's Nacho	1 serv	734
Mac's Dog	1	307
Pita Pizza	1	503
Sandwich Ham & Cheese	1	455
Sandwich PB&J	1	714
Sandwich Toasted Cheese	1	620
Sandwich Turkey & Cheese	1	451
DESSERTS		
Brownie Chocolate	1 (3.5 oz)	424
Brownie Delight	1 (11 oz)	917
Chocolate Loving Spoon Cake	1 (4 oz)	538
Ice Cream Vanilla Bean	1 scoop (5 oz)	160
Kentucky Pie	1 slice (12 oz)	807

FOOD	PORTION	CALS
New York Cheesecake	1 slice (5 oz)	505
Sundae Topping Caramel	2 tbsp	100
Sundae Topping Chocolate	1 tbsp	110
MAIN MENU SELECTIONS		
Appetizers Chips & Salsa	1 serv (5 oz)	87
Appetizers Dip Cheese & Chili	1 serv (5 oz)	572
Appetizers Dip Cheese & Veggie Chili	1 serv (5 oz)	552
Appetizers Nacho Basket	1 serv (6 oz)	579
Appetizers Nacho Chili	1 serv (6 oz)	564
Appetizers Nacho Veggie Chili	1 serv (6 oz)	537
Chicken Cordon Bleu	1 serv	810
Chili Vegetarian	1 serv (8 oz)	133
Cole Slaw	1 serv (4 oz)	190
Fruit Cup	1 serv (4 oz)	98
Giant Spud Cheese	1 (27 oz)	930
Giant Spud Grilled Chicken	1 (27 oz)	839
Giant Spud Just A Spud	1 (26 oz)	604
Giant Spud Ole	1 (30 oz)	1252
Giant Spud Ole w/ Chili	1 (33 oz)	1512
Giant Spud Ole w/ Veggie Chili	1 (33 oz)	1457
Giant Spud Veggie	1 (28 oz)	668
Macaroni & Cheese	1 serv (4 oz)	200
Mashed Potatoes	1 serv (4 oz)	136
Meatloaf w/ Gravy	1 serv	340
Open-Faced Roast Beef	1 serv	751
Pot Roast Spud	1 serv	906
Potato Salad	1 serv (4 oz)	200
Salmon Filet	1 serv	235
Steamed Vegetables	1 serv (4 oz)	43
SALAD DRESSINGS AND SAUCES		
Au Jus	1 serv (4 oz)	10
Comeback Gravy	1 serv (4 oz)	37
Dressing Blue Cheese	2 tbsp	140
Dressing Greek	2 tbsp	90
Dressing Lite Olive Oil Vinaigrette	2 tbsp	60
Dressing Lite Ranch	2 tbsp	100
Dressing Low Calorie Italian	2 tbsp	25
Dressing Parmesan Peppercorn	2 tbsp	150
Dressing Ranch	2 tbsp	100
Dressing Tomato Basil	2 tbsp	30

FOOD	PORTION	CALS
SALADS		
Caesar w/ Salmon	1 (17 oz)	800
Chicken Fiesta	1 (20 oz)	493
Chicken Grill	1 (21 oz)	840
Garden	1 (15 oz)	264
Garden w/ Chicken Salad	1 (18 oz)	537
Garden w/ Salmon	1 (17 oz)	315
Garden w/ Tuna Salad	1 (18 oz)	373
Greek Chicken	1 (19 oz)	584
Side Caesar	1 (6 oz)	328
Side Garden	1 (8 oz)	138
Taco	1 (26 oz)	641
Taco w/ Veggie Chili	1 (26 oz)	641
SANDWICHES		
BLT	1	654
Chicken Salad	1	677
Deli Corned Beef On Wheat	1	369
Deli Ham On Wheat	1	350
Deli Pastrami On Wheat	1	371
Deli Roast Beef On Wheat	1	398
Deli Salami On Wheat	1	565
Deli Turkey On Wheat	1	342
French Dip	1	676
Grilled Chicken Breast	1	751
Grilled Chicken Club	1	1234
Ham Melt	1	700
McAlisters Club	1	1225
Meatloaf Parmesan	1	708
Memphian	1	585
Muffuletta	¼ (8 oz)	615
New Yorker	1	628
Orange Cranberry Club	1	954
Reuben On Rye	1	492
Roast Beef Melt	1	635
Salmon	1	608
Submarine	1	833
Sweetberry Chicken On Wheatberry	1	701
Tuna Salad On Wheat	1	452
Turkey Melt	1	700
Veggie On Pita	1	522

FOOD	PORTION	CALS
Wrap Greek Chicken	1	630
Wrap Grilled Chicken Caesar	1	533
SOUPS		
Asiago Cheese Bisque	1 (8 oz)	240
Broccoli Cheddar	1 (8 oz)	213
Cheddar Potato	1 (8 oz)	213
Cheesy Chicken Tortilla	1 (8 oz)	150
Chicken & Sausage Gumbo	1 (8 oz)	150
Clam Chowder	1 (8 oz)	200
Country Potato	1 (8 oz)	173
Country Vegetable	1 (8 oz)	93
French Onion	1 (8 oz)	80
Red Beans & Rice	1 (8 oz)	107
Southwest Roasted Corn	1 (8 oz)	90

MCDONALD'S
BEVERAGES

FOOD	PORTION	CALS
Apple Juice	1 box (6.8 oz)	90
Chocolate Milk 1% Low Fat	8 oz	170
Coca-Cola Classic	1 sm (16 oz)	150
Coffee	1 sm (12 oz)	0
Diet Coke	1 sm (16 oz)	0
Half & Half Creamer	1 pkg	20
Hi-C Orange Lavaburst	1 sm (16 oz)	160
Iced Coffee Caramel	1 sm (16 oz)	130
Iced Coffee Hazelnut	1 sm (16 oz)	130
Iced Coffee Regular	1 sm (16 oz)	140
Iced Coffee Vanilla	1 sm (16 oz)	130
Iced Tea	1 sm (16 oz)	0
Milk Lowfat 1%	1 pkg	100
Orange Juice	1 sm (12 oz)	140
Powerade Mountain Blast	1 sm (16 oz)	100
Shake Triple Thick Chocolate	1 sm (12 oz)	440
Shake Triple Thick Strawberry	1 sm (12 oz)	420
Shake Triple Thick Vanilla	1 sm (16 oz)	420
Sprite	1 sm (16 oz)	150
BREAKFAST SELECTIONS		
Big Breakfast Regular Biscuit	1 serv	720
Biscuit Regular	1	250
Biscuit Regular Bacon Egg Cheese	1	450

FOOD	PORTION	CALS
Biscuit Regular Sausage	1	410
Biscuit Regular Sausage w/ Egg	1	500
Burrito Sausage	1	300
Deluxe Breakfast Regular Biscuit w/o Syrup & Margarine	1 serv	1070
English Muffin	1	160
Hash Browns	1 serv	140
Hotcake Syrup	1 pkg (2 oz)	180
Hotcakes w/o Syrup & Margarine	1 serv	350
Hotcakes & Sausage w/o Syrup & Margarine	1 serv	520
McGriddles Bacon Egg Cheese	1	460
McGriddles Sausage	1	420
McGriddles Sausage Egg & Cheese	1	560
McMuffin Sausage	1	370
McMuffin Sausage w/ Egg	1	250
McSkillet Burrito w/ Sausage	1	610
McSkillet Burrito w/ Steak	1	570
Sausage Patty	1	170
Scrambled Eggs	2	170
DESSERTS		
Apple Dippers	1 pkg	35
Apple Pie Baked	1	270
Cinnamon Melts	1 serv	460
Cookie Chocolate Chip	1	180
Cookie Oatmeal	1 (1.1 oz)	150
Cookie Sugar	1 (1.1 oz)	150
Cookies McDonaldland	1 pkg (2 oz)	250
Cookies McDonaldland Chocolate Chip	1 pkg	270
Fruit 'n Yogurt Parfait	1 serv	160
Ice Cream Cone Reduced Fat Vanilla	1	150
Kiddie Cone	1	45
McFlurry M&M's	1 (12 oz)	620
McFlurry Oreo	1 (12 oz)	560
Peanuts For Sundae	1 serv	45
Sundae Hot Caramel	1	340
Sundae Hot Fudge	1	330
Sundae Strawberry	1	280
MAIN MENU SELECTIONS		
Apple Sauce Strawberry	1 serv	90
Big Mac	1	540

FOOD	PORTION	CALS
Big N' Tasty	1	460
Big N' Tasty w/ Cheese	1	510
Cheeseburger	1	300
Cheeseburger Double	1	440
Cheesy Tots	6 pieces	210
Chicken McNuggets	4 pieces	170
Chicken Selects	3 pieces	380
Filet-O-Fish	1	380
French Fries	1 sm	250
French Fries	1 lg	570
Hamburger	1	250
McChicken	1	360
McRib	1	500
Onion Rings	1 sm	140
Quarter Pounder	1	410
Quarter Pounder Double w/ Cheese	1	740
Quarter Pounder w/ Cheese	1	510
Sandwich Chicken Classic Crispy	1	500
Sandwich Chicken Classic Grilled	1	420
Sandwich Club Chicken Crispy	1	660
Sandwich Club Chicken Grilled	1	570
Sandwich Ranch BLT Chicken Crispy	1	600
Sandwich Ranch BLT Chicken Grilled	1	520
Snack Wrap Grilled w/ Chipotle BBQ	1	260
Snack Wrap Grilled w/ Honey Mustard	1	260
Snack Wrap Grilled w/ Ranch	1	270
Snack Wrap w/ Chipotle BBQ	1	320
Snack Wrap w/ Honey Mustard	1	320
Snack Wrap w/ Ranch	1	140
SALAD DRESSINGS AND SAUCES		
Caramel Dip Low Fat	1 pkg	70
Dipping Sauce Buffalo	1 serv (1 oz)	80
Dipping Sauce Zesty Onion Ring	1 serv (1 oz)	150
Dressing Ken's Light Italian	1 pkg (2 oz)	120
Dressing Newman's Own Creamy Caesar	1 pkg (2 oz)	170
Dressing Newman's Own Creamy Southwest	1 pkg (1.5 oz)	100
Dressing Newman's Own Low Fat Balsamic Vinaigrette	1 pkg (1.5 oz)	40
Dressing Newman's Own Low Fat Family Recipe Italian	1 pkg (1.5 oz)	60

FOOD	PORTION	CALS
Dressing Newman's Own Low Fat Sesame Ginger	1 pkg (1.5 oz)	90
Dressing Newman's Own Ranch	1 pkg (2 oz)	170
Honey	1 pkg (0.5 oz)	50
Ketchup	1 pkg	15
Sauce Barbecue	1 pkg (1 oz)	50
Sauce Creamy Ranch	1 pkg (1.5 oz)	200
Sauce Hot Mustard	1 pkg (1 oz)	60
Sauce Southwestern Chipotle Barbeque	1 pkg (1.5 oz)	70
Sauce Spicy Buffalo	1 pkg (1.5 oz)	60
Sauce Sweet'N Sour	1 pkg (1 oz)	50
Sauce Tangy Honey Mustard	1 pkg (1.5 oz)	70
SALADS		
Asian w/ Crispy Chicken w/o Dressing	1 serv	380
Asian w/ Grilled Chicken w/o Dressing	1 serv	300
Asian w/o Chicken & Dressing	1 serv	150
Bacon Ranch w/ Crispy Chicken	1 serv	350
Bacon Ranch w/ Grilled Chicken w/o Dressing	1 serv	260
Bacon Ranch w/o Chicken	1 serv	140
Caesar w/ Crispy Chicken	1 serv	300
Caesar w/ Grilled Chicken	1 serv	220
Caesar w/o Chicken	1 serv	90
Croutons Butter Garlic	1 pkg	60
Fruit & Walnut Snack Size	1 serv	210
Side Salad Southwest w/ Crispy Chicken w/o Dressing	1 serv	20
Southwest w/ Grilled Chicken w/o Dressing	1 serv	320
Southwest w/o Chicken & Dressing	1 serv	140

MIMI'S CAFE
BEVERAGES

FOOD	PORTION	CALS
Cappuccino	1 serv	86
Cappuccino Iced	1 serv	86
Espresso	1 serv	8
Hot Chocolate w/ Whipped Cream	1 serv	986
Mocha Iced	1 serv	376
Mocha Latte	1 serv	376
CHILDREN'S MENU SELECTIONS		
Chicken Fingers	1 serv	408
Grilled Cheese	1 serv	273

FOOD	PORTION	CALS
Macaroni & Cheese	1 serv	353
Mini Burger	1 serv	554
Mini Corn Dogs	1 serv	460
Pancakes Chocolate Chip	1 serv	563
Pancakes Mimi Mouse	1 serv	477
PB&J Soldiers	1 serv	730
Pepperoni Pizzadillas	1 serv	617
Scrambled Eggs& Bacon	1 serv	216
Spaghetti	1 serv	343
Turkey Dinner	1 serv	337
DESSERTS		
Apple Crisp Cinnamon	1 serv	898
Bread Pudding	1 serv	819
Brownie Triple Chocolate	1 serv	1950
Cheesecake New York Style	1 serv	1075
Pie Banana Foster Mud	1 serv	1245
Pie Pecan Chocolate Chip	1 serv	1879
MAIN MENU SELECTIONS		
Appetizer Dip Spinach & Artichoke	1 serv	2459
Appetizer Fried Chicken Tenders	1 serv	800
Appetizer Fried Dill Pickles	1 serv	972
Appetizer Jazz Fest	1 serv	1252
Appetizer Zucchini Parmesan	1 serv	626
Blackened Sole w/ Shrimp Creole	1 serv	852
Broiled Flat Iron Steak	1 serv	1026
Burger Half Pound	1	684
Cafe Fish & Chips	1 serv	1290
Cajun Blackened Salmon	1 serv	919
Cheeseburger BBQ Ranch	1	999
Cheeseburger Half Pound	1	855
Chicken Cordon Bleu	1 serv	1360
Chicken Feta Penne	1 serv	1879
Ciabatta Chicken	1	1251
Ciabatta Meatloaf	1	1036
Ciabatta Turkey Pesto	1	1248
Club Cafe	1	1132
Country Fried Steak	1 serv	1061
Crab Cake Dinner	1 serv	1662
Diablo Center Cut Pork Chops	1 serv	1094
Dip Classic Beef	1	521

FOOD	PORTION	CALS
Fillet Of Soul	1 serv	636
French Quarter	1	1480
Garlic Shrimp Spaghettini	1 serv	860
Grilled Beef Liver	1 serv	1003
Grilled Chicken Tuscan Style	1 serv	880
Hibachi Salmon	1 serv	846
Mimi's Meatloaf	1 serv	910
Mimi's Pot Roast	1 serv	1291
Original Patty Melt	1	976
Parmesan Crusted Chicken Breast	1 serv	1820
Pasta Jambalaya	1 serv	1223
Pot Pie Chicken	1 serv	1403
Reuben West Coast	1	2015
Sandwich 5 Way Grilled Cheese	1	703
Sandwich Albacore & Avocado	1	993
Sandwich Bacon Lettuce & Tomato	1	586
Sandwich Fresh Roasted Turkey Breast	1	532
Sandwich Turkey Walnut Salad On Raisin Bread	1	549
Sandwich Veggie Stack	1	836
Slow Roasted Turkey Breast	1 serv	851
Small Bites Black & Blue Quesadilla	1 serv	1241
Small Bites Chicken & Fruit	1 serv	460
Small Bites Citrus Salmon	1 serv	699
Small Bites Crab Cakes	1 serv	412
Small Bites Smokey Chicken Enchiladas	1 serv	1154
Small Bites Sweet & Sour Coconut Shrimp	1 serv	608
Small Bites Thai Chicken Wrap	1 serv	1004
Top Sirloin	1 serv (12 oz)	947
SALAD DRESSINGS		
Balsamic Vinaigrette	1 serv	316
Blue Cheese	1 serv	298
Caesar	1 serv	273
Chinese Sesame	1 serv	263
Dijon Vinaigrette	1 serv	296
Honey Mustard	1 serv	243
Non Fat French	1 serv	65
Ranch	1 serv	194
Thousand Island	1 serv	232
SALADS		
Asian Chopped	1 serv	751

FOOD	PORTION	CALS
Blue Cheese & Walnut	1 serv	728
Caesar Blackened Chicken	1 serv	570
Chopped Cobb	1 serv	524
Fried Chicken	1 serv	764
Zesty Chicken Tostada	1 serv	1046
SOUPS		
Broccoli Cheddar	1 serv	270
Chicken Gumbo	1 serv	235
Clam Chowder	1 serv	240
Corn Chowder	1 serv	196
Cream Of Chicken	1 serv	337
French Market Onion	1 serv	207
Red Bean & Andouille Sausage	1 serv	256
Split Pea	1 serv	194
Vegetarian Vegetable	1 serv	60

MR. HERO
DESSERTS

FOOD	PORTION	CALS
Eli's Cheesecake Oreo Cookie	1 slice (2.5 oz)	260
Eli's Cheesecake Original Plain	1 slice (2.6 oz)	280
Eli's Cheesecake Snickers	1 slice (2.3 oz)	270
Eli's Cheesecake Strawberry Swirl	1 slice (2.6 oz)	280
SALADS		
Garden Side	1 serv (7.3 oz)	32
Grilled Chicken	1 serv (13.4 oz)	166
Tuna Delight	1 serv (14.4 oz)	403
SANDWICHES		
Cheeseburger	1 (10.4 oz)	776
Cheesesteak Hot Buttered	1 (9.4 oz)	669
Chicken Grilled Philly	1 (9.1 oz)	421
Deli Subs Original Italian	1 (9.5 oz)	641
Deli Subs Tuna 'N Cheese	1 (9.7 oz)	724
Deli Subs Turkey	1 (9.8 oz)	468
Deli Subs Ultimate Italian	1 (10.3 oz)	675
Romanburger	1 (11.3 oz)	861
Steak Tuscan	1 (10.6 oz)	625
Steak Zesty Bacon & Swiss	1 (9.8 oz)	616
Subs Meatball	1 (9.3 oz)	724
Taste Buddies Cheeseburger Bacon	1 (5.9 oz)	264
Taste Buddies Grilled Italiano	1 (5.3 oz)	440

FOOD	PORTION	CALS
Taste Buddies Italian Sausage	1 (5.4 oz)	368
Taste Buddies Tuna 'N Cheese	1 (6 oz)	483
SIDES		
Breadsticks	2 (6 oz)	446
Jalapeno Poppers	1 serv (4.5 oz)	432
Mozzarella Sticks	1 serv (8.7 oz)	565
Onion Petals	1 serv (5.7 oz)	597
Potato Babycakes	1 serv (5.9 oz)	477
Potato Waffle Fries w/ Cheese Sauce	1 serv (7.2 oz)	482

MRS. FIELDS

FOOD	PORTION	CALS
Bites Double Fudge	3 (1.6 oz)	200
Brownie Butterscotch Blondie	1 (2.1 oz)	260
Brownie Double Fudge	1 (2.1 oz)	260
Brownie Pecan Fudge	1 (2.1 oz)	270
Brownie Special Walnut Fudge & Blondie	1 (2.2 oz)	260
Brownie Toffee Fudge	1 (2.1 oz)	260
Brownie Walnut Fudge	1 (2.1 oz)	270
Cake Chocolate Chip	1 piece (2.9 oz)	350
Coffee Cake Chocolate Chip	1 lg (2.4 oz)	250
Coffee Cake Chocolate Chip	1 sm (2.2 oz)	240
Cookie Butter	1 (1.5 oz)	200
Cookie Chocolate Covered Peanut Butter	1 (2.5 oz)	340
Cookie Chocolate Covered Semi-Sweet	1 (2.5 oz)	380
Cookie Chocolate Covered White Chunk Macadamia	1 (2.4 oz)	330
Cookie Cinnamon Sugar	1 (1.8 oz)	210
Cookie Cut Out	1 (2.4 oz)	280
Cookie Frosted Cinnamon Sugar	1 (2.1 oz)	270
Cookie Oatmeal Raisins & Walnuts	1 (1.7 oz)	200
Cookie Semi-Sweet Chocolate	1 (1.7 oz)	210
Cookie Semi-Sweet Chocolate w/ Walnuts	1 (1.7 oz)	220
Cookie Triple Chocolate	1 (1.7 oz)	210
Cookie White Chunk Macadamia	1 (1.7 oz)	230
Jelly Bellys	1 pkg (1.4 oz)	140
Mixed Nuts	1 pkg (2 oz)	350
Muffin Blueberry	1 (1.9 oz)	190
Muffin Chocolate Chip	1 (1.9 oz)	200
Nibbler Cinnamon Sugar	3 (1.4 oz)	180
Nibbler Debra's Special	3 (1.3 oz)	160

FOOD	PORTION	CALS
Nibbler Peanut Butter	3 (1.8 oz)	170
Nibbler Semi-Sweet Chocolate	3 (1.8 oz)	170
Nibbler Triple Chocolate	3 (1.8 oz)	160
Nibbler White Chunk Macadamia	3 (1.8 oz)	180
Taffy	1 pkg (2.4 oz)	160

NAKED PIZZA

FOOD	PORTION	CALS
10 Inch Pie Original Crust	1 slice	81
10 Inch Pie Thin Crust	1 slice	64
12 Inch Pie Original Crust	1 slice	132
12 Inch Pie Thin Crust	1 slice	91
14 Inch Pie Original Crust	1 slice	161
14 Inch Pie Thin Crust	1 slice	114

NATHAN'S

FOOD	PORTION	CALS
Apple Pie	1 (3.49 oz)	314
Bacon Cheeseburger	1 (10.7 oz)	783
Cheese Dog	1 (5.05 oz)	390
Cheese Fries	1 reg (8 oz)	564
Cheesesteak	1 (12.31 oz)	849
Cheesesteak Supreme	1 (16.29 oz)	879
Cheesesteak Supreme Chicken	1 (13.81 oz)	601
Chicken Tender Pita	1 (11.94 oz)	823
Chicken Tender Platter	1 (17.69 oz)	1245
Chicken Tenders	3 (6.19 oz)	526
Chicken Wings	5 (6.65 oz)	400
Chili Dog	1 (5.05 oz)	400
Corn Dog On A Stick	1 (2.89 oz)	380
Corn On The Cob w/ Butter	1 (5.05 oz)	140
Double Burger w/ Cheese	1 (15.61 oz)	1178
Famous Hot Dog	1 (3.53 oz)	297
French Fries	1 reg (6.5 oz)	464
Funnel Cake	1 (4.21 oz)	580
Hot Dog Nuggets	6 (3.49 oz)	348
Mozzarella Sticks + Sauce	3 (5.64 oz)	390
Onion Rings	1 sm (5.6 oz)	544
Platter Grilled Chicken	1 (15 oz)	504
Pretzel Dog	1 (4.02 oz)	390
Pretzel King Size	1 (2.28 oz)	180
Sandwich Chicken Tender	1 (9.65 oz)	706
Sandwich Grilled Chicken	1 (9.03 oz)	554

FOOD	PORTION	CALS
Wrap Grilled Chicken Caesar	1 (10.34 oz)	700
Wrap Krispy Southwest Chipotle	1 (11.71 oz)	750

NOAH'S BAGELS
BAGELS AND BREADS

FOOD	PORTION	CALS
Bagel Asiago Cheese Topped	1 (4.2 oz)	330
Bagel Blueberry	1 (3.7 oz)	270
Bagel Candy Cane	1 (3.7 oz)	270
Bagel Cheddar Stick	1 (4.2 oz)	330
Bagel Chocolate Chip	1 (3.7 oz)	290
Bagel Chopped Garlic	1 (3.9 oz)	290
Bagel Cinnamon Raisin	1 (3.7 oz)	270
Bagel Cinnamon Sugar	1 (4.1 oz)	310
Bagel Cracked Pepper	1 (3.7 oz)	280
Bagel Cranberry Orange	1 (3.5 oz)	250
Bagel Dutch Apple	1 (5 oz)	340
Bagel Egg	1 (3.7 oz)	290
Bagel Everything	1 (3.9 oz)	280
Bagel Good Grains	1 (3.9 oz)	280
Bagel Jalapeno Cheddar	1 (4.9 oz)	350
Bagel Onion	1 (3.7 oz)	270
Bagel Plain	1 (3.7 oz)	270
Bagel Poppyseed	1 (3.9 oz)	290
Bagel Power	1 (4 oz)	310
Bagel Pumpernickel	1 (3.7 oz)	260
Bagel Sesame Seed	1 (3.9 oz)	290
Bagel Six Cheese	1 (4.5 oz)	340
Bagel Spinach Florentine	1 (4.9 oz)	350
Bagel Sun Dried Tomato	1 (3.7 oz)	270
Bagel Whole Wheat	1 (3.7 oz)	260
Bagel Whole Wheat Sesame & Sunflower Seeds	1 (4.4 oz)	370
Bialy	1 (5.3 oz)	380
Bread Ciabatta	1 serv (4.25 oz)	290
Bread Corn Meal Rye	1 slice (2 oz)	150
Bread Harvest Grain	1 slice (2.3 oz)	180
Bread Marble Rye	1 slice (1.7 oz)	160
Bread Potato	1 slice (1.7 oz)	140
Challah Braided	1 serv (2 oz)	160
Challah Roll	1 (3 oz)	230
Pizza Bagel Artichoke Tomato & Red Onion	1 (11.1 oz)	550

FOOD	PORTION	CALS
Pizza Bagel Artichoke & Spinach	1 (12 oz)	670
Pizza Bagel Cheese	1 (6.2 oz)	420
Pizza Bagel Cheesy Garlic & Herb	1 (6.2 oz)	500
Pizza Bagel Pepperoni	1 (6.8 oz)	500
Pizza Bagel Spinach & Mushroom	1 (9.5 oz)	580
Pizza Bagel Tomato & Rosemary	1 (8.7 oz)	540
BEVERAGES AND EXTRAS		
Cafe Latte Low Fat	1 reg (12 oz)	160
Cafe Latte Nonfat	1 reg (12 oz)	110
Cafe Latte Whole	1 reg (12 oz)	200
Cappuccino Low Fat	1 reg (12 oz)	120
Cappuccino Nonfat	1 reg (12 oz)	90
Cappuccino Whole	1 reg (12 oz)	150
Chai Tea Low Fat Milk	1 reg (12 oz)	220
Chai Tea Nonfat Milk	1 reg (12 oz)	210
Chai Tea Whole Milk	1 reg (12 oz)	230
Coca-Cola	8 oz	99
Coca-Cola Cherry	8 oz	104
Coffee Iced Americano	8 oz	0
Coffee Regular & Decaf	1 (12 oz)	0
Diet Coke	8 oz	1
Espresso	1 reg (2 oz)	0
Fanta Orange	8 oz	106
Frozen Drinks Cafe Caramel	1 (18 oz)	620
Frozen Drinks Cafe Mocha	1 (18 oz)	510
Frozen Drinks Strawberry Cream	1 (18 oz)	450
Frozen Drinks Wild Berry Fat Free	1 (18 oz)	270
Half & Half Creamer	1 oz	40
Hi-C Fruit Punch	8 oz	104
Hot Chocolate Nonfat	1 reg (12 oz)	220
Hot Chocolate Whole	1 reg (12 oz)	290
Iced Cappuccino Nonfat	1 reg (12 oz)	90
Iced Mocha Low Fat	1 reg (12 oz)	230
Iced Tea Raspberry	8 oz	78
Iced Tea Unsweetened	8 oz	1
Lemonade	1 (16 oz)	200
Lemonade Blackberry	1 (16 oz)	310
Macchiato Nonfat	1 reg (12 oz)	230
Macchiato Whole	1 reg (12 oz)	290
Milk Low Fat	8 oz	120

FOOD	PORTION	CALS
Milk Skim	8 oz	80
Milk Whole	8 oz	150
Mocha Low Fat	1 reg (12 oz)	230
Mocha Nonfat	1 reg (12 oz)	190
Mocha Whole	1 reg (12 oz)	270
Mr. Pibb	8 oz	97
On Top Reduced Fat Topping	2 tbsp (0.3 oz)	20
Orange Juice	1 (10 oz)	143
Sprite	8 oz	97
Syrup Blackberry	2 tbsp (1 oz)	100
Syrup Caramel	2 tbsp (1 oz)	70
Syrup Hazelnut	2 tbsp (1 oz)	100
Syrup Vanilla	2 tbsp (1 oz)	100
Syrup Vanilla Sugar Free	2 tbsp (1 oz)	116
Tea Hamey & Sons All Flavors	8 oz	0
Whipped Cream Light	2 tbsp (1 oz)	36
CREAM CHEESE AND SPREADS		
Butter	1 tbsp (0.5 oz)	110
Cream Cheese Whipped Onion & Chive	2 tbsp (.07 oz)	70
Cream Cheese Whipped Plain	2 tbsp (.07 oz)	70
Cream Cheese Whipped Reduced Fat Blueberry	2 tbsp (.07 oz)	70
Cream Cheese Whipped Reduced Fat Garden Vegetable	2 tbsp (.07 oz)	60
Cream Cheese Whipped Reduced Fat Garlic Herb	2 tbsp (.07 oz)	60
Cream Cheese Whipped Reduced Fat Honey Almond	2 tbsp (.07 oz)	70
Cream Cheese Whipped Reduced Fat Jalapeno Salsa	2 tbsp (.07 oz)	60
Cream Cheese Whipped Reduced Fat Plain	2 tbsp (.07 oz)	60
Cream Cheese Whipped Reduced Fat Strawberry	2 tbsp (.07 oz)	60
Cream Cheese Whipped Reduced Fat Sun Dried Tomato & Basil	2 tbsp (.07 oz)	60
Cream Cheese Whipped Smoked Salmon	2 tbsp (.07 oz)	60
Deli Mustard	1 tsp (5 g)	0
Garlic Mayo	1 serv (1.5 oz)	270
Grape Jam	1 serv (1 oz)	110
Honey	1 serv (1 oz)	90

FOOD	PORTION	CALS
Hummus	1 serv (2 oz)	90
Mayo	1 tbsp (0.5 oz)	110
DESSERTS		
Cinnamon Twists	1 serv (3.8 oz)	370
Coffee Cake Apple Cinnamon	1 serv (6.6 oz)	700
Coffee Cake Chocolate Chip	1 serv (6.1 oz)	760
Coffee Cake Mixed Berry	1 serv (6.9 oz)	710
Cookie Chocolate Chip	1 (2.8 oz)	360
Cookie Chocolate Mudslide	1 (2.75 oz)	320
Cookie Iced Sugar	1 (3.7 oz)	480
Cookie Oatmeal Raisin	1 (2.8 oz)	320
Cookie Snickerdoodle	1 (2.8 oz)	400
Cookie Mini Chocolate Chip	1 (1.38 oz)	180
Cookie Mini Chocolate Mudslide	1 (1.38 oz)	160
Cookie Mini Iced Sugar	1 (1.87 oz)	230
Cookie Mini Oatmeal Raisin	1 (1.38 oz)	160
Marshmallow Crispy Treat	1 (3.9 oz)	410
Muffin Blueberry	1 (5 oz)	480
Muffin Cranberry Orange	1 (4.6 oz)	460
Muffin Strawberry White Chocolate	1 (5.5 oz)	550
Strudel Cinnamon Walnut	1 serv (5.4 oz)	630
SALAD DRESSINGS		
Caesar	2 tbsp (1 oz)	150
Harvest Chicken Salad	2 tbsp (1 oz)	90
Raspberry Vinaigrette	2 tbsp	160
SALADS		
Caesar	1 (10.5 oz)	600
Caesar Chicken	1 (14 oz)	720
Caesar Side	1 (4.5 oz)	280
City	1 (11.5 oz)	830
City w/ Chicken	1 (15 oz)	950
Southwestern Chicken	1 (15.2 oz)	710
SANDWICHES		
Bagel & Lox	1 (11.2 oz)	520
Bagel Dog Asiago	1 (7.1 oz)	510
Bagel Dog Everything	1 (7.1 oz)	510
Bagel Dog Original	1 (6.9 oz)	490
Bagel Plain w/ Peanut Butter & Jelly	1 (6.2 oz)	550
Breakfast Wrap Santa Fe	1 (14.5 oz)	750
Breakfast Wrap Veggie	1 (15.6 oz)	810

FOOD	PORTION	CALS
California Chicken	1 (9.9 oz)	360
Club Blackened Chicken	1 (10.4 oz)	630
Club Deli Pesto Turkey	1 (10.9 oz)	670
Deli Chicken Salad	1 (11 oz)	1150
Deli Cornbeef	1 (14 oz)	740
Deli Egg Salad Kosher	1 (11.5 oz)	650
Deli Pastrami	1 (14 oz)	750
Deli Roast Beef	1 (14 oz)	730
Deli Tuna Salad	1 (13 oz)	740
Deli Turkey	1 (14.5 oz)	720
Deli Whitefish	1 (12.2 oz)	850
Deli Melts Hummus	1 (10.2 oz)	570
Deli Melts Pastrami	1 (9.6 oz)	530
Deli Melts Roast Beef	1 (9.6 oz)	530
Deli Melts Tuna	1 (11.6 oz)	700
Deli Melts Turkey	1 (9.6 oz)	500
Deli Melts Veggie	1 (12.3 oz)	590
Egg Mit Artichoke & Tomato	1 (12 oz)	620
Egg Mit Bacon & Cheddar	1 (9.2 oz)	620
Egg Mit Cheese	1 (8.5 oz)	520
Egg Mit Cheese & Tomato	1 (10 oz)	530
Egg Mit Lox & Chives	1 (8.8 oz)	490
Egg Mit Plain	1 (7.9 oz)	450
Egg Mit Spinach Mushroom & Swiss	1 (9.8 oz)	530
Egg Mit Turkey Sausage	1 (9.9 oz)	590
Kosher Vegetarian On Plain Bagel	1 (13.9 oz)	860
Panini Albacore Tuna	1 (13.6 oz)	750
Panini Egg Spinach Bacon	1 (11.8 oz)	790
Panini Egg Vegetarian Omelet	1 (13.8 oz)	670
Panini Italian Chicken	1 (12.5 oz)	810
Panini Mediterranean	1 (10.6 oz)	550
Panini Tomato Mozzarella	1 (7.9 oz)	440
Panini Turkey Club	1 (12.3 oz)	610
Sandwich Rachel	1 (13.9 oz)	1030
Sandwich Reuben	1 (13.9 oz)	770
Sandwich Veg Out	1 (10.1 oz)	490
Wrap Albacore Tuna	1 (12.3 oz)	600
Wrap Chicken Caesar	1 (12.6 oz)	790
Wrap Southwestern Turkey	1 (13.5 oz)	750
Wrap Veggie	1 (9.8 oz)	460

FOOD	PORTION	CALS
SIDES		
Cole Slaw	1 serv (3 oz)	120
Egg Salad	1 serv (5 oz)	330
Fresh Fruit Cup	1 (11 oz)	140
Fruit & Yogurt Parfait	1 (12 oz)	220
Kosher Pickle	1	5
Macaroni & Cheese	1 serv (6 oz)	340
Redskin Potato Salad	1 serv (3 oz)	160
Tuna Salad	1 serv (5 oz)	280
SOUPS		
Broccoli Cheese	1 cup (8.7 oz)	290
Chicken Noodle	1 cup (8.7 oz)	110
Italian Wedding	1 cup (8.7 oz)	160
Tortilla	1 cup (8.7 oz)	300
Turkey Chili	1 cup (8.7 oz)	220

NOODLES & COMPANY
MAIN MENU SELECTIONS

FOOD	PORTION	CALS
Bangkok Curry	1 sm	250
Bangkok Curry	1 reg	490
Beef Braised	1 serv	190
Beef Sauteed	1 serv	210
Buttered Noodles	1 sm	310
Buttered Noodles	1 reg	620
Chicken Breast Seasoned	1 serv	130
Chicken Parmesan Crusted	1 serv	190
Ciabatta Roll	1	160
Flatbread	1 serv	210
House Marinara	1 reg	650
House Marinara	1 sm	330
Mushroom Stroganoff	1 reg	780
Mushroom Stroganoff	1 sm	390
Organic Tofu	1 serv	180
Pad Thai	1 reg	700
Pad Thai	1 sm	350
Pasta Fresca	1 sm	420
Pasta Fresca	1 reg	780
Penne Rosa	1 reg	810
Penne Rosa	1 sm	420
Pesto Cavatappi	1 sm	510

FOOD	PORTION	CALS
Pesto Cavatappi	1 reg	910
Potstickers	3	200
Shrimp Sauteed	1 serv	35
Whole Grain Tuscan Linguine	1 sm	450
Whole Grain Tuscan Linguine	1 reg	770
Wisconsin Mac & Cheese	1 sm	450
Wisconsin Mac & Cheese	1 reg	900
SALADS		
Caesar	1 sm	160
Caesar	1 reg	320
Chinese Chopped	1 reg	310
Chinese Chopped	1 sm	150
Cucumber Tomato Side Salad	1	80
The Med	1 reg	310
The Med	1 sm	150
Tossed Green	1	60
SOUPS		
Chicken Noodle	1 reg	300
Chicken Noodle	1 sm	150
Thai Curry	1 sm	240
Thai Curry	1 reg	480
Tomato Basil	1 sm	210
Tomato Basil	1 reg	420

OLD SPAGHETTI FACTORY
BEVERAGES

FOOD	PORTION	CALS
Cherry Coke	1 (12 oz)	140
Coffee Black	1 (8 oz)	0
Coke	1 (12 oz)	130
Diet Coke	1 (12 oz)	0
Hot Tea	1 (8 oz)	0
Iced Tea Strawberry	1 (12 oz)	100
Italian Cream Soda	1 (7.5 oz)	140
Kid's Juice Bar	1 serv (2.4 oz)	60
Lemonade	1 (12 oz)	140
Lemonade Strawberry	1 (12 oz)	200
Masterpiece Shake	1 (8.5 oz)	700
Milk 2%	1 (13 oz)	180
Milk Skim	1 (13 oz)	130
Root Beer	1 (12 oz)	150
Sprite	1 (12 oz)	140

FOOD	PORTION	CALS
CHILDREN'S MENU SELECTIONS		
Fettuccine Alfredo	1 serv (10.3 oz)	770
Macaroni & Cheese	1 serv (8 oz)	390
Ravioli	1 serv (10 oz)	420
Ravioli Spinach & Cheese	1 serv (6.6 oz)	310
Sandwich Grilled Cheese	1 (4.5 oz)	480
Spaghetti Marinara w/ Sicilian Meatballs	1 serv (13 oz)	570
Spaghetti w/ Brown Butter & Mizithra Cheese	1 serv (8.7 oz)	660
Spaghetti w/ Clam Sauce	1 serv (10 oz)	440
Spaghetti w/ Marinara Sauce	1 serv (15 oz)	560
Spaghetti w/ Meat Sauce	1 serv (10 oz)	410
Spinach Tortellini w/ Alfredo Sauce	1 serv (6.8 oz)	530
DESSERTS		
Cake Chocolate Truffle Mousse	1 serv (9 oz)	850
Ice Cream Spumoni	1 serv (3 oz)	180
Ice Cream Vanilla	1 serv (3 oz)	170
Mud Pie	1 serv (6 oz)	490
MAIN MENU SELECTIONS		
Angel Hair	1 serv (8 oz)	420
Appetizer Bay Shrimp Crostini	1 serv (9.3 oz)	720
Appetizer Garlic Fries	1 serv (18.4 oz)	1410
Appetizer Portuguese Linguica	1 serv (17.5 oz)	1080
Baked Chicken	1 serv (18.3 oz)	1030
Baked Lasagna	1 serv (17.5 oz)	800
Bread Sicilian Garlic Cheese	4 serv (16 oz)	1310
Broccoli	1 sm (7.5 oz)	340
Burger Sliders	1 serv (23.6 oz)	1770
Cheese Manicotti w/ Marinara Sauce	1 serv (12 oz)	490
Chicken Marsala	1 serv (17.4 oz)	1050
Chicken Penne	1 serv (14.8 oz)	830
Dip Shrimp Spinach & Artichoke	4 serv (9.3 oz)	590
Factory Burger w/ Chips	1 serv (16.6 oz)	1370
Fettuccine Alfredo	1 serv (14.2 oz)	1080
Fettuccine or Penne	1 serv (8 oz)	420
Garlic Mizithra	1 serv (15 oz)	1240
Hearty Meal Clam Sauce	1 serv (25 oz)	1110
Hearty Meal Italian Sausage w/ Meat Sauce	1 serv (29 oz)	1350
Hearty Meal Marinara Sauce	1 serv (25 oz)	940
Hearty Meal Meat Sauce	1 serv (25 oz)	1020
Hearty Meal Mizithra Cheese & Brown Butter	1 serv (22.4 oz)	1750

FOOD	PORTION	CALS
Hearty Meal Pot Pourri	1 serv (26 oz)	1280
Hearty Meal Sauteed Mushroom Sauce	1 serv (30 oz)	1120
Hearty Meal Sicilian Meatballs	1 serv (31 oz)	1350
Lasagna Vegetariano	1 serv (20.6 oz)	830
Meatloaf Italian	1 serv (18.5 oz)	1180
Olive Tapenade	4 serv (7.4 oz)	800
Panini Chicken Smoked Mozzarella w/ Chips	1 serv (14.4 oz)	1280
Parmigiana Chicken	1 serv (19.2 oz)	810
Pasta Gluten Free	1 serv (9 oz)	470
Pasta Whole Wheat	1 serv (8 oz)	390
Platter #1 Lasagna & Chicken Marsala	1 (27.5 oz)	1090
Platter #2 Ravioli & Spaghetti w/ Meat Sauce	1 (21 oz)	880
Platter #3 Spaghetti w/ Meat Sauce Sausage & Meatballs	1 (25 oz)	1360
Ravioli Crab	1 serv (11 oz)	810
Ravioli Spinach & Cheese	1 serv (11 oz)	480
Ravioli Toasted Beef	4 serv (4 oz)	200
Ravioli Toasted Cheese	4 serv (4 oz)	210
Sandwich Sicilian Style Meatball w/ Chips	1 serv (16.4 oz)	1200
Sandwich Sicilian Style Sausage w/ Chips	1 serv (14.4 oz)	1140
Senior Meal Italian Sausage w/ Meat Sauce	1 serv (14 oz)	740
Senior Meal Pot Pourri	1 serv (10 oz)	520
Senior Meal Spaghetti Marinara	1 serv (10 oz)	370
Senior Meal Spaghetti Marinara w/ Sicilian Meatballs	1 serv (16 oz)	770
Senior Meal Spaghetti Mizithra & Brown Butter	1 serv (10 oz)	660
Senior Meal Spaghetti w/ Clam Sauce	1 serv (10 oz)	440
Senior Meal Spaghetti w/ Meat Sauce	1 serv (10 oz)	410
Senior Meal Spaghetti w/ Mushroom Sauce	1 serv (12 oz)	450
Side Alfredo Sauce	6 oz	640
Side Clam Sauce	6 oz	190
Side Marinara Sauce	6 oz	90
Side Marsala Sauce	6 oz	70
Side Meat Sauce	6 oz	140
Side Sausage	1 serv (4.5 oz)	340
Side Sauteed Mushroom Sauce	9 oz	200
Side Sicilian Meatballs	2 (6 oz)	420
Spaghetti	1 serv (9 oz)	460
Spaghetti Vesuvius	1 serv (15 oz)	710
Spaghetti Squash	1 serv (20.7 oz)	540

FOOD	PORTION	CALS
Spaghetti w/ Clam Sauce	1 serv (15 oz)	660
Spaghetti w/ Italian Sausage w/ Meat Sauce	1 serv (19 oz)	940
Spaghetti w/ Meat Sauce	1 serv (15 oz)	610
Spaghetti w/ Mizithra Cheese & Brown Butter	1 serv (13.4 oz)	1040
Spaghetti w/ Pot Pourri	1 serv (16 oz)	780
Spaghetti w/ Sauteed Mushroom Sauce	1 serv (18 oz)	670
Spaghetti w/ Sicilian Meatballs	1 serv (21 oz)	960
Spinach Tortellini w/ Alfredo Sauce	1 serv (12 oz)	930
SALADS		
BLT	1 (15.4 oz)	1000
Caesar Entree Chicken	1 (21.2 oz)	1130
Caesar Entree w/o Chicken	1 (14.5 oz)	820
Caesar Upgrade	1 (7 oz)	440
House w/ 1000 Island	1 (5 oz)	230
House w/ Balsamic	1 (4.5 oz)	260
House w/ Blue Cheese	1 (5 oz)	280
House w/ Caesar	1 (5 oz)	330
House w/ Creamy Pesto	1 (5 oz)	280
House w/ Fat Free Honey Mustard	1 (4.5 oz)	120
Senior Meal Caesar Chicken	1 serv (17 oz)	870
Senior Meal Caesar w/o Chicken	1 serv (10.2 oz)	560
SOUPS		
Chicken Mulligatawny	1 serv (9 oz)	260
Clam Chowder	1 serv (9 oz)	370
Cream Of Broccoli	1 serv (9 oz)	240
Minestrone	1 serv (9 oz)	60

PACIUGO GELATO

Milk Base Amarena Black Cherry Swirl	1 scoop (3.5 oz)	160
Milk Base Banana Creme Pie	1 scoop (3.5 oz)	80
Milk Base Cheesecake	1 scoop (3.5 oz)	90
Milk Base Chocolate	1 scoop (3.5 oz)	80
Milk Base Chocolate Cookies'N Milk	1 scoop (3.5 oz)	90
Milk Base Coconut	1 scoop (3.5 oz)	80
Milk Base Coffee	1 scoop (3.5 oz)	75
Milk Base Fiordilatte	1 scoop (3.5 oz)	75
Milk Base French Vanilla Bean	1 scoop (3.5 oz)	80
Milk Base Green Tea	1 scoop (3.5 oz)	70
Milk Base Hazelnut	1 scoop (3.5 oz)	85
Milk Base Lemon Custard	1 scoop (3.5 oz)	75

FOOD	PORTION	CALS
Milk Base Mascarpone Chocolate Rum	1 scoop (3.5 oz)	95
Milk Base Pannacotta Wedding Cake	1 scoop (3.5 oz)	75
Milk Base Peppermint	1 scoop (3.5 oz)	75
Milk Base Rose	1 scoop (3.5 oz)	70
Milk Base Tiramisu	1 scoop (3.5 oz)	80
Milk Base Zabajone	1 scoop (3.5 oz)	80
No Sugar Added Chocolate	1 scoop (3.5 oz)	28
No Sugar Added Mint	1 scoop (3.5 oz)	25
No Sugar Added Mocha	1 scoop (3.5 oz)	28
No Sugar Added Strawberry Milk	1 scoop (3.5 oz)	23
Soy Banana	1 scoop (3.5 oz)	40
Soy Blueberry	1 scoop (3.5 oz)	40
Soy Chocolate	1 scoop (3.5 oz)	38
Soy Coffee	1 scoop (3.5 oz)	35
Soy Hazelnut	1 scoop (3.5 oz)	35
Soy Strawberry	1 scoop (3.5 oz)	38
Soy Wild Berries	1 scoop (3.5 oz)	40
Water Base Blackberry	1 scoop (3.5 oz)	28
Water Base Ginger Lemon	1 scoop (3.5 oz)	25
Water Base Green Apple	1 scoop (3.5 oz)	28
Water Base Lemon Sage	1 scoop (3.5 oz)	25
Water Base Lychee	1 scoop (3.5 oz)	25
Water Base Orange Vidalia	1 scoop (3.5 oz)	25
Water Base Passion Fruit	1 scoop (3.5 oz)	23
Water Base Pineapple	1 scoop (3.5 oz)	28
Water Base Strawberry Port	1 scoop (3.5 oz)	25
Water Base Watermelon	1 scoop (3.5 oz)	25

PANERA BREAD
BAKERY

FOOD	PORTION	CALS
Asiago Cheese Loaf	1 slice (2 oz)	160
Bagel Asiago Cheese	1	330
Bagel Blueberry	1	330
Bagel Chocolate Chip	1	370
Bagel Cinnamon Crunch	1	430
Bagel Cinnamon Swirl & Raisin	1	320
Bagel Everything	1	300
Bagel French Toast	1	350
Bagel Jalapeno & Cheddar	1	310
Bagel Plain	1	290

FOOD	PORTION	CALS
Bagel Sesame	1	310
Bagel Sweet Onion & Poppyseed	1	390
Bagel Whole Wheat	1	340
Baguette Whole Grain	1 slice (2 oz)	140
Bear Claw	1	550
Brownie Double Fudge w/ Icing	1	480
Cake Cinnamon Coffee Crumb	1 slice	470
Ciabatta	1 (6.25 oz)	460
Cinnamon Raisin	1 slice (2 oz)	180
Cinnamon Roll	1	620
Cobblestone	1	650
Cookie Candy	1	420
Cookie Chocolate Chipper	1 mini	110
Cookie Chocolate Chipper	1	440
Cookie Chocolate Duet w/ Walnuts	1	450
Cookie Easter Egg	1	480
Cookie Oatmeal Raisin	1	370
Cookie Shortbread	1	350
Cookie Toffee Nut	1	460
Country Loaf	1 slice (2 oz)	140
Croissant French	1	310
Focaccia	1 serv (2 oz)	180
Focaccia w/ Asiago Cheese	1 slice (2 oz)	160
French Baguette	1 slice (2 oz)	150
Honey Wheat Loaf	1 slice (2 oz)	170
Hot Cross Bun	1	220
Muffie Chocolate Chip	1	320
Muffie Pumpkin	1	290
Muffin Apple Crunch	1	450
Muffin Carrot Walnut	1	500
Muffin Pumpkin	1	580
Muffin Wild Blueberry	1	440
Pastry Cheese	1	400
Pastry Cherry	1	500
Pastry Chocolate	1	410
Pastry Fresh Apple	1	380
Pastry Ring Apple Cherry Cheese	1 slice	230
Pecan Braid	1	470
Pecan Roll	1	730
Scone Cinnamon Chip	1	600

FOOD	PORTION	CALS
Scone Orange	1 lg	470
Scone Strawberries & Cream	1	420
Scone Strawberries & Cream	1 mini	140
Scone Wild Blueberry	1	440
Scone Wild Blueberry	1 mini	160
Scones Orange	1 mini	160
Sesame Semolina Loaf	1 slice (2 oz)	140
Sourdough Roll	1 (2.5 oz)	200
Sourdough Round Loaf	1 slice (2 oz)	140
Sourdough Soup Bowl	1 (8 oz)	590
Spring Petites	1 mini	230
Stone Milled Rye Loaf	1 slice (2 oz)	140
Three Cheese Loaf	1 slice (2 oz)	140
Tomato Basil XL Loaf	1 slice (2 oz)	140
White Whole Grain Loaf	1 slice (2 oz)	140
Whole Grain Loaf	1 slice (2 oz)	130
BEVERAGES		
Apple Juice Organic	8 oz	120
Caffe Mocha	1 (11.5 oz)	380
Caramel Frozen	1 (16 oz)	600
Chocolate Milk Organic	8 oz	170
Hot Chocolate	1 (11 oz)	380
Iced Green Tea	1 (16 oz)	90
Iced Latte Chai Tea	1 (16 oz)	160
Latte Caffe	1 (8.5 oz)	120
Latte Caramel	1 (11.5 oz)	420
Latte Chai Tea	1 (10 oz)	200
Lemonade	1 (16 oz)	100
Mango Frozen	1 (16 oz)	330
Milk Organic	8 oz	120
Mocha Frozen	1 (16 oz)	570
Orange Juice	1 sm (8 oz)	110
Smoothie Black Cherry Low Fat	1 (16 oz)	290
Smoothie Mango Low Fat	1 (16 oz)	230
Smoothie Strawberry w/ Ginseng Low Fat	1 (16 oz)	260
Smoothie Wild Berry Low Fat	1 (16 oz)	290
CHILDREN'S MENU SELECTIONS		
Deli Sandwich Roast Beef	1	320
Deli Sandwich Smoked Ham	1	300
Deli Sandwich Smoked Turkey	1	290

FOOD	PORTION	CALS
Mac & Cheese	1 serv	490
Organic Yogurt All Flavors	1 tube	60
Sandwich Grilled Cheese	1	360
Sandwich Peanut Butter & Jelly	1	410
CREAM CHEESE		
Chive & Onion	1 oz	70
Hazelnut Reduced Fat	1 oz	80
Honey Walnut Reduced Fat	1 oz	80
Plain	1 oz	100
Plain Reduced Fat	1 oz	70
Raspberry Reduced Fat	1 oz	70
Veggie Reduced Fat	1 oz	60
SALAD DRESSINGS		
BBQ Ranch	3 tbsp	140
Buttermilk Ranch Light	3 tbsp	80
Caesar	3 tbsp	150
Vinaigrette Asian Sesame Reduced Sugar	3 tbsp	90
Vinaigrette Balsamic Reduced Fat	3 tbsp	130
Vinaigrette Blue Cheese	3 tbsp	180
Vinaigrette Greek Herb	3 tbsp	220
Vinaigrette Thai Chili Low Fat	3 tbsp	60
Vinaigrette White Balsamic Apple	3 tbsp	150
SALADS		
Asian Sesame Chicken	1 full serv	410
BBQ Chopped Chicken	1	500
Caesar	1	390
Caesar Chicken	1	510
Chopped Chicken Cobb	1	500
Chopped Steak & Blue Cheese	1	850
Classic Cafe	1 full serv	170
Fruit Cup	1	60
Fuji Apple w/ Chicken	1	520
Greek	1 full serv	380
Thai Chopped Chicken	1	390
SANDWICHES		
Asiago Roast Beef On Asiago Cheese	1	700
Bacon Turkey Bravo On XL Tomato Basil	1	800
Breakfast Asiago Cheese Bagel w/ Bacon	1	610
Breakfast Asiago Cheese Bagel w/ Egg & Cheese	1	480

FOOD	PORTION	CALS
Breakfast Asiago Cheese Bagel w/ Sausage	1	640
Breakfast Bacon Egg & Cheese On Ciabatta	1	510
Breakfast Egg & Cheese On Ciabatta	1	390
Breakfast French Toast Bagel w/ Sausage	1	670
Breakfast Jalapeno & Cheddar Bagel w/ Bacon	1	590
Breakfast Jalapeno & Cheddar Bagel w/ Egg & Cheese	1	470
Breakfast Jalapeno & Cheddar Bagel w/ Sausage	1	630
Breakfast Power	1	340
Breakfast Sausage Egg & Cheese On Ciabatta	1	550
Breakfast Sweet Onion & Poppyseed Bagel w/ Steak	1	660
Chicken Caesar On Three Cheese	1	720
Italian Combo On Ciabatta	1	980
Jalapeno & Cheddar Bagel w/ Smoked Ham	1	500
Mediterranean Veggie On XL Tomato Basil	1	600
Napa Almond Chicken Salad On Sesame Semolina	1	690
Panini Chipotle Chicken On Artisan French	1	830
Panini Cuban Chicken	1	860
Panini Frontega Chicken On Focaccia	1	850
Panini Smokehouse Turkey On Three Cheese	1	690
Panini Steak & White Cheddar On French Baguette	1	950
Panini Tomato & Mozzarella On Ciabatta	1	770
Panini Turkey Artichoke On Focaccia	1	740
Sierra Turkey w/ Asiago Cheese On Focaccia	1	920
Smoked Ham & Swiss On Stone Milled Rye	1	590
Smoked Turkey Breast On Country	1	420
Tuna Salad On Honey Wheat	1	470
SOUPS		
Baked Potato	1 serv (12 oz)	350
Broccoli Cheddar	1 serv (12 oz)	290
Chicken Noodle Low Fat	1 serv (12 oz)	140
Cream Of Chicken & Wild Rice	1 serv (12 oz)	310
Creamy Tomato	1 serv (12 oz)	380
French Onion	1 serv (12 oz)	250
Garden Vegetable w/ Pesto Low Fat	1 serv (12 oz)	160

FOOD	PORTION	CALS
New England Clam Chowder	1 serv (12 oz)	450
Vegetarian Black Bean Low Fat	1 serv (12 oz)	170

PAPA JOHNS
DESSERTS

Applepie	4 (6.7 oz)	480
Cinnamon Sweetsticks	4 (6.7 oz)	580
Cinnapie	4 (5.9 oz)	560

OTHER MENU SELECTIONS

Breadsticks	2 (4 oz)	290
Breadsticks Garlic Parmesan	2 (4.4 oz)	340
Cheesesticks	4 (4.8 oz)	370
Chickenstrips	2 (2.3 oz)	130
Wings BBQ	2 (2.8 oz)	190
Wings Buffalo	2 (2.8 oz)	170
Wings Honey Chipotle	2 (2.8 oz)	190

PIZZA

BBQ Chicken & Bacon 12 inch	⅛ pie (3.8 oz)	250
BBQ Chicken & Bacon 16 inch	⅒ pie (5.6 oz)	370
BBQ Chicken & Bacon 8 inch	¼ pie (3.5 oz)	230
Cheese 12 inch	⅛ pie (3.2 oz)	210
Garden Fresh 12 inch	⅛ pie (3.9 oz)	200
Garden Fresh 16 inch	⅒ pie (6 oz)	300
Garden Fresh 8 inch	¼ pie (3.6 oz)	180
Hawaiian BBQ Chicken 12 inch	⅛ pie (4.1 oz)	250
Hawaiian BBQ Chicken 16 inch	⅒ pie (6 oz)	370
Original 16 inch	⅒ pie (4.6 oz)	300
Pepperoni 12 inch	⅛ pie (3.2 oz)	230
Pepperoni 16 inch	⅒ pie (4.8 oz)	340
Pepperoni 8 inch	¼ pie (3 oz)	210
Sausage 12 inch	⅛ pie (3.3 oz)	240
Sausage 16 inch	⅒ pie (4.9 oz)	350
Sausage 8 inch	¼ pie (3.1 oz)	220
Spicy Italian 12 inch	⅛ pie (3.6 oz)	270
Spicy Italian 16 inch	⅒ pie (5.5 oz)	400
Spicy Italian 8 inch	¼ pie (3.4 oz)	240
Spinach Alfredo 12 inch	⅛ pie (2.9 oz)	210
Spinach Alfredo 16 inch	⅒ pie (4.4 oz)	310
Spinach Alfredo 8 inch	¼ pie (2.8 oz)	190
The Meats 12 inch	⅛ pie (3.6 oz)	250

FOOD	PORTION	CALS
The Meats 16 inch	1/10 pie (5.5 oz)	400
The Meats 8 inch	1/4 pie (3.4 oz)	240
The Works 12 inch	1/8 pie (3.9 oz)	230
The Works 16 inch	1/10 pie (5.9 oz)	350
The Works 8 inch	1/4 pie (3.6 oz)	210
Tuscan Six Cheese 12 inch	1/8 pie (3.3 oz)	230
Tuscan Six Cheese 16 inch	1/10 pie (4.9 oz)	340
Tuscan Six Cheese 8 inch	1/4 pie (3 oz)	210
SAUCES AND SEASONINGS		
Crushed Red Pepper	1 pkg (1 g)	5
Parmesan Cheese	1 pkg (3.5 g)	15
Sauce Barbeque	1 serv (1 oz)	45
Sauce Blue Cheese	1 serv (1 oz)	160
Sauce Buffalo	1 serv (1 oz)	15
Sauce Cheese	1 serv (1 oz)	40
Sauce Honey Mustard	1 serv (1 oz)	150
Sauce Pizza	1 serv (1 oz)	20
Sauce Ranch	1 serv (1 oz)	100
Sauce Special Garlic	1 serv (1 oz)	150
Special Seasoning	1 pkg (3 g)	5

PAPA MURPHY'S
PIZZA

FOOD	PORTION	CALS
DeLite Thin Crust Large All Meat	1/10 pie	190
DeLite Thin Crust Large Cheese	1/10 pie	140
DeLite Thin Crust Large Hawaiian	1/10 pie	160
DeLite Thin Crust Large Pepperoni	1/10 pie	170
DeLite Thin Crust Large Veggie	1/10 pie	160
Original Crust Family Size All Meat	1/12 pie	360
Original Crust Family Size Cheese	1/12 pie	270
Original Crust Family Size Cowboy	1/12 pie	350
Original Crust Family Size Hawaiian	1/12 pie	290
Original Crust Family Size Murphy's Combo	1/12 pie	360
Original Crust Family Size Papa's Favorite	1/12 pie	360
Original Crust Family Size Pepperoni	1/12 pie	320
Original Crust Family Size Rancher	1/12 pie	330
Original Crust Family Size Specialty Of The House	1/12 pie	320
Original Crust Family Size Veggie Mediterranean	1/12 pie	310

FOOD	PORTION	CALS
Original Crust Family Size Veggie Combo	1/12 pie	300
Original Crust Medium Cheese	1/8 pie	230
Stuffed Family Size 5 Meat	1/16 pie	370
Stuffed Family Size Big Murphy	1/16 pie	370
Stuffed Family Size Chicago Style	1/16 pie	370
Stuffed Family Size Chicken & Bacon	1/16 pie	370
Stuffed Large 5 Meat	1/12 pie	370
Stuffed Large Big Murphy	1/12 pie	360
SALADS		
Club w/o Dressing & Croutons	1/2 serv (6.6 oz)	140
Garden w/o Dressing & Croutons	1 serv (7.2 oz)	100
Italian w/o Dressing & Croutons	1/2 serv (6.5 oz)	140

PEI WEI ASIAN DINER
CHILDREN'S MENU SELECTIONS

FOOD	PORTION	CALS
Kid's Wei Honey Seared Chicken w/o Noodles Or Rice	1 serv	290
Kid's Wei Lo Mein Chicken w/o Noodles Or Rice	1 serv	180
Kid's Wei Teriyaki Chicken w/o Noodles Or Rice	1 serv	240
DESSERTS		
Cookie Chocolate Chip	1	342
Cookie Fortune	1	30
MAIN MENU SELECTIONS		
Bowl w/ Brown Rice Japanese Teriyaki Beef	1 serv	580
Bowl w/ Brown Rice Japanese Teriyaki Chicken	1 serv	460
Bowl w/ Brown Rice Japanese Teriyaki Shrimp	1 serv	410
Bowl w/ Brown Rice Japanese Teriyaki Vegetables & Tofu	1 serv	410
Bowl w/ White Rice Japanese Teriyaki Beef	1 serv	560
Bowl w/ White Rice Japanese Teriyaki Chicken	1 serv	440
Bowl w/ White Rice Japanese Teriyaki Shrimp	1 serv	390
Bowl w/ White Rice Japanese Teriyaki Vegetables & Tofu	1 serv	390
Crispy Potstickers	4	130
Edamame	1 serv	156
Fried Rice Beef	1 serv	630
Fried Rice Chicken	1 serv	525
Fried Rice Shrimp	1 serv	475

FOOD	PORTION	CALS
Fried Rice Vegetables & Tofu	1 serv	440
Ginger Broccoli Beef	1 serv	450
Ginger Broccoli Chicken	1 serv	300
Ginger Broccoli Shrimp	1 serv	230
Ginger Broccoli Vegetables & Tofu	] serv	170
Honey Seared Chicken	1 serv	420
Honey Seared Shrimp	1 serv	370
Hot & Sour Soup	1 cup	150
Lemon Pepper Beef	1 serv	550
Lemon Pepper Chicken	1 serv	440
Lemon Pepper Shrimp	1 serv	380
Lemon Pepper Vegetables & Tofu	1 serv	230
Mandarin Kung Pao Beef	1 serv	610
Mandarin Kung Pao Chicken	1 serv	450
Mandarin Kung Pao Shrimp	1 serv	400
Mandarin Kung Pao Vegetables & Tofu	1 serv	290
Minced Chicken w/ Cool Lettuce Wraps w/o Rice Sticks	1 serv	250
Mongolian Beef	1 serv	420
Mongolian Chicken	1 serv	280
Mongolian Shrimp	1 serv	210
Mongolian Vegetables & Tofu	1 serv	180
Noodles Dan Dan Chicken	1 serv	390
Noodles Lo Mein Beef	1 serv	570
Noodles Lo Mein Chicken	1 serv	460
Noodles Lo Mein Shrimp	1 serv	400
Noodles Lo Mein Vegetables & Tofu	1 serv	400
Noodles Thai Blazing Beef	1 serv	630
Noodles Thai Blazing Chicken	1 serv	520
Noodles Thai Blazing Shrimp	1 serv	482
Noodles Thai Blazing Vegetables & Tofu	1 serv	430
Noodles Egg	1 serv	210
Noodles Rice	1 serv	130
Orange Peel Beef	1 serv	660
Orange Peel Chicken	1 serv	520
Orange Peel Shrimp	1 serv	460
Orange Peel Vegetables & Tofu	1 serv	330
Pad Thai Beef	1 serv	670
Pad Thai Chicken	1 serv	560
Pad Thai Shrimp	1 serv	490

FOOD	PORTION	CALS
Pei Wei Spicy Beef	1 serv	480
Pei Wei Spicy Chicken	1 serv	330
Pei Wei Spicy Shrimp	1 serv	300
Rice Brown	1 serv	170
Rice Fried	1 serv	260
Rice Sticks	1 cup	130
Rice White	1 serv	200
Spicy Korean Beef	1 serv	490
Spicy Korean Chicken	1 serv	350
Spicy Korean Shrimp	1 serv	280
Spicy Korean Vegetables & Tofu	1 serv	240
Spring Rolls	2	90
Sweet & Sour Chicken	1 serv	440
Sweet & Sour Shrimp	1 serv	390
Thai Coconut Curry Beef	1 serv	550
Thai Coconut Curry Chicken	1 serv	380
Thai Coconut Curry Shrimp	1 serv	300
Thai Coconut Curry Vegetables & Tofu	1 serv	220
Thai Dynamite Chicken	1 serv	390
Thai Dynamite Shrimp	1 serv	280
Thai Dynamite Vegetables & Tofu	1 serv	220
Wontons Crab	4	190
SALAD DRESSINGS AND SAUCES		
Dressing Sesame Ginger	1 serv (2 oz)	170
Lime Vinaigrette	1 serv (2 oz)	230
Sauce Lettuce Wrap	1 serv (2 oz)	70
Sauce Sweet Chili	1 serv (2 oz)	140
Sauce Thai Peanut	1 serv (2 oz)	168
SALADS		
Asian Chopped Chicken w/ Dressing	1 serv	280
Asian Chopped Chicken w/o Dressing	1 serv	200
Pei Wei Spicy Chicken w/ Dressing	1 serv	350
Pei Wei Spicy Chicken w/o Dressing	1 serv	210
Vietnamese Chicken Salad Rolls	3	53

P.F. CHANG'S CHINA BISTRO
DESSERTS

	PORTION	CALS
Banana Spring Rolls	¼ serv (4 oz)	240
Flourless Chocolate Dome	½ serv (4 oz)	270
Flourless Chocolate Dome Gluten Free	½ serv (4 oz)	270

FOOD	PORTION	CALS
Mini Cheesecake	1 serv	210
Mini Great Wall	1 serv	160
Mini Red Velvet Cake	1 serv	220
Mini Dessert Apple Pie	1 serv	190
Mini Dessert Carrot Cake	1 serv	210
Mini Dessert Tiramisu	1 serv	180
Mini Dessert Tres Leche Lemon Dream	1 serv	180
Mini Dessert Triple Chocolate Mousse	1 serv	300
Mini Dessert Triple Chocolate Mousse Gluten Free	1	300
The Great Wall Of Chocolate	¼ serv (5 oz)	360
MAIN MENU SELECTIONS		
Almond & Cashew Chicken	⅓ serv (10 oz)	373
Asian Grilled Norwegian Salmon	½ serv (9 oz)	345
Asian Street Taco Mahi Mahi	½ serv (4 oz)	230
Asian Street Taco Red Cooked Pork	½ serv (3 oz)	140
Asian Street Taco Spicy Shrimp	½ serv (3 oz)	180
Asian Street Taco Traditional Beef	½ serv (3 oz)	170
Beef A La Sichuan	⅓ serv (7 oz)	293
Beef w/ Broccoli	⅓ serv (7 oz)	290
Beef w/ Broccoli Gluten Free	⅓ serv (6 oz)	290
Buddha's Feast Steamed	½ serv (6 oz)	55
Buddha's Feast Steamed Gluten Free	½ serv (6 oz)	55
Buddha's Feast Stir Fried	½ serv (11 oz)	220
Buddha's Feast Stir Fried w/ White Rice	½ serv (11 oz)	310
Calamari Salt & Pepper	¼ serv (2 oz)	160
Chang's Spicy Chicken	⅓ serv (6 oz)	323
Chang's Spicy Chicken Gluten Free	⅓ serv (6 oz)	323
Chengdu Spiced Lamb	⅓ serv (5 oz)	237
Chicken w/ Black Bean Sauce	⅓ serv (7 oz)	300
Chopped Chicken w/ Ginger Dressing	1 (8 oz)	365
Coconut Curry Vegetables	½ serv (13 oz)	510
Crispy Green Beans w/o Sauce	¼ serv (4 oz)	260
Crispy Honey Chicken	⅓ serv (6 oz)	477
Crispy Honey Shrimp	½ serv (6 oz)	460
Crispy Wontons	2 (1 oz)	90
Double Pan Fried Noodles Combo	¼ serv (9 oz)	455
Double Pan Fried Noodles w/ Beef	¼ serv (8 oz)	395
Double Pan Fried Noodles w/ Chicken	¼ serv (8 oz)	393
Double Pan Fried Noodles w/ Pork	¼ serv (8 oz)	413

FOOD	PORTION	CALS
Double Pan Fried Noodles w/ Shrimp	¼ serv (8 oz)	363
Double Pan Fried Noodles w/ Vegetable	¼ serv (8 oz)	190
Dumplings Pork Pan Fried	⅙ serv (1 oz)	70
Dumplings Pork Steamed	⅙ serv (1 oz)	60
Dumplings Shrimp Pan Fried	1 (1 oz)	60
Dumplings Shrimp Steamed	1 (1 oz)	45
Dumplings Steamed Edamame	⅓ serv (1 oz)	45
Dumplings Steamed Lemongrass Chicken	⅓ serv (1 oz)	40
Dumplings Steamed Pork & Leek	⅓ serv (1 oz)	50
Dumplings Steamed Shrimp & Pork	⅓ serv (1 oz)	40
Dumplings Vegetable Pan Fried	1 (1 oz)	60
Dumplings Vegetable Steamed	1 (1 oz)	45
Dynamite Shrimp	½ serv (4 oz)	290
Edamame w/ Kosher Salt	1 serv (3 oz)	130
Egg Rolls	1 (3 oz)	215
Eggplant Stir Fried	¼ serv (6 oz)	270
Flaming Red Wontons	⅙ serv (2 oz)	80
Fried Rice Beef	¼ serv (7 oz)	303
Fried Rice Beef Gluten Free	¼ serv (7 oz)	293
Fried Rice Chicken	¼ serv (7 oz)	303
Fried Rice Combo	¼ serv (8 oz)	363
Fried Rice Pork	¼ serv (7 oz)	320
Fried Rice Pork Gluten Free	¼ serv (7 oz)	320
Fried Rice Shrimp	¼ serv (7 oz)	273
Fried Rice Vegetable	¼ serv (7 oz)	230
Garlic Noodles	¼ serv (5 oz)	178
Garlic Snap Peas	⅓ lg serv (3 oz)	64
Garlic Snap Peas Gluten Free	⅓ lg serv (3 oz)	63
Ginger Chicken w/ Broccoli	⅓ serv (9 oz)	273
Ginger Chicken w/ Broccoli Gluten Free	⅓ serv (8 oz)	270
Hunan Hot Fish	⅓ serv (8 oz)	340
Kung Pao Chicken	⅓ serv (5 oz)	383
Kung Pao Scallops	⅓ serv (5 oz)	307
Kung Pao Shrimp	⅓ serv (5 oz)	208
Lettuce Wraps Chicken	¼ serv (5 oz)	160
Lettuce Wraps Chicken Gluten Free	¼ serv (5 oz)	158
Lettuce Wraps Vegetarian	¼ serv (5 oz)	140
Lo Mein Beef	1 serv (7 oz)	270
Lo Mein Chicken	1 serv (7 oz)	267
Lo Mein Combo	⅓ serv (9 oz)	347

FOOD	PORTION	CALS
Lo Mein Pork	1 serv (7 oz)	290
Lo Mein Shrimp	1 serv (7 oz)	227
Lo Mein Vegetable	⅓ serv (7 oz)	420
Lunch Bowl Buddha's Feast Steamed w/ Brown Rice	½ serv (9 oz)	210
Lunch Bowl Buddha's Feast Steamed w/ White Rice	½ serv (9 oz)	235
Ma Po Tofu	⅓ serv (10 oz)	350
Mahi Mahi	½ serv (10 oz)	420
Mandarin Chicken	½ serv (10 oz)	360
Mongolian Beef	⅓ serv (6 oz)	337
Mongolian Beef Gluten Free	⅓ serv (6 oz)	337
Moo Goo Gai Pan	⅓ serv (9 oz)	247
Mu Shu Chicken	½ serv (10 oz)	285
Mu Shu Pork	½ serv (10 oz)	320
Mu Shu Pork Pancake	1	90
Noodles Dan Dan	¼ serv (9 oz)	270
Norwegian Salmon Steamed w/ Ginger Gluten Free	½ serv (10 oz)	330
Norwegian Salmon w/ Ginger	½ serv (10 oz)	330
Oolong Marinated Sea Bass	½ serv (9 oz)	315
Orange Peel Beef	⅓ serv (5 oz)	283
Orange Peel Chicken	⅓ serv (5 oz)	333
Orange Peel Shrimp	⅓ serv (5 oz)	187
Pepper Steak	⅓ serv (8 oz)	297
Pepper Steak Gluten Free	⅓ serv (8 oz)	300
Rice Brown Steamed	1 serv (6 oz)	190
Rice White Steamed	1 serv (6 oz)	220
Salt & Pepper Prawns	⅓ serv (6 oz)	197
Shanghai Cucumbers	⅓ lg serv (4 oz)	40
Shanghai Cucumbers Gluten Free	⅓ lg serv (4 oz)	40
Shanghai Shrimp w/ Garlic Sauce	½ serv (9 oz)	195
Shrimp w/ Candied Walnuts	⅓ serv (7 oz)	377
Shrimp w/ Lobster Sauce	½ serv (10 oz)	250
Shrimp w/ Lobster Sauce Gluten Free	½ serv (10 oz)	255
Sichuan Asparagus	⅓ lg serv (5 oz)	100
Sichuan Scallops	⅓ serv (7 oz)	295
Sichuan Shrimp	⅓ serv (5 oz)	173
Singapore Street Noodles	⅓ serv (6 oz)	300
Singapore Street Noodles Gluten Free	⅓ serv (7 oz)	300

FOOD	PORTION	CALS
Siu Mai Steamed Bacon & Egg	⅓ serv (1 oz)	70
Siu Mai Steamed Pork & Rice	⅓ serv (1 oz)	50
Spare Ribs Chang's	¼ serv (4 oz)	344
Spare Ribs Northern Style	¼ serv (4 oz)	343
Spicy Green Beans	⅓ lg serv (5 oz)	110
Spinach Stir-Fried w/ Garlic	⅓ lg serv (5 oz)	53
Spinach Stir-Fried w/ Garlic Gluten Free	⅓ lg serv (3 oz)	53
Spring Roll	1 (1.5 oz)	156
Starters Seared Ahi Tuna	½ serv (4 oz)	160
Street Dumplings Shanghai	½ serv (2 oz)	140
Sweet & Sour Chicken	⅓ serv (5 oz)	370
Sweet & Sour Pork	½ serv (10 oz)	460
Tuna Tataki Crisp	⅓ serv (1 oz)	60
VIP Duck	½ serv (12 oz)	650
Wok Charred Beef	⅓ serv (8 oz)	317
Wok Seared Lamb	⅓ serv (7 oz)	283
Wontons Crab	2	163
SALAD DRESSINGS AND SAUCES		
Sauce Crispy Green Bean	1 serv (2 oz)	310
Sauce Plum	1 serv (2 oz)	200
Sauce Potsticker	1 serv (2 oz)	50
Sauce Shrimp Dumpling	1 serv (2 oz)	15
Sauce Sweet & Sour	1 serv (2 oz)	80
Sauce Sweet & Sour Mustard	1 serv (2 oz)	90
SOUPS		
Chicken Noodle	1 bowl (7 oz)	120
Egg Drop	1 cup (7 oz)	60
Egg Drop Gluten Free	1 cup (7 oz)	60
Hot & Sour	1 bowl (7 oz)	80
Wonton	1 bowl (7 oz)	92

PINKBERRY

Frozen Yogurt Coffee	½ cup	90
Frozen Yogurt Green Tea	½ cup	50
Frozen Yogurt Original	½ cup	70

PIZZA FUSION
DESSERTS

Brownies Gluten Free	½ serv	232
Calzone Chocolate	½	209

FOOD	PORTION	CALS
Cookies Chocolate Chip	⅓ serv	250
Pastry Strawberry Cheese	1 serv	338
PIZZA		
BBQ Chicken	1 slice	181
Big Kahuna	1 slice	236
Bruschetta	1 slice	159
Cheese	1 slice	167
Eggplant & Mozzarella	1 slice	181
Farmer's Market	1 slice	190
Founder's Pie	1 slice	201
Four Cheese & Sundried Tomato	1 slice	175
Greek	1 slice	204
Pepperoni	1 slice	220
Personal BBQ Chicken	½ pie	272
Personal Big Kahuna	½ pie	365
Personal Bruschetta	½ pie	234
Personal Cheese	½ pie	233
Personal Eggplant & Mozzarella	½ pie	304
Personal Farmer's Market	½ pie	279
Personal Founder's Pie	½ pie	347
Personal Four Cheese & Sundried Tomato	½ pie	262
Personal Greek	½ pie	299
Personal Pepperoni	½ pie	359
Personal Philly Steak	½ pie	358
Personal Sausage & Tri-Peppers	½ pie	323
Personal Spinach & Artichoke	½ pie	270
Personal Very Vegan	½ pie	321
Philly Steak	1 slice	220
Sausage & Tri-Peppers	1 slice	212
Spinach & Artichoke	1 slice	184
Very Vegan	1 slice	195
SALADS		
Caesar & Roasted Chicken	½ serv	358
Chicken Bruschetta	½ serv	331
Fusion	½ serv	244
Pan Roasted Steak	½ serv	388
Pear & Gorgonzola	½ serv	380
Roasted Beet & Feta	½ serv	320
Side Salad Arugula	1 serv	48

FOOD	PORTION	CALS
SANDWICHES		
Philly Phusion	½	473
Portabello Grill	½	380
Roasted Chicken	½	357
Roasted Turkey	½	417
STARTERS		
Flatbread	1 (2 serv)	198
Stuffed Portabello Mushroom	½ serv	140
Trio Of Dips	⅓ serv	191
PIZZA HUT		
BEVERAGES		
Diet Pepsi	1 (16 oz)	0
Mountain Dew	1 (16 oz)	220
Pepsi	1 (16 oz)	200
Sierra Mist	1 (16 oz)	200
OTHER MENU SELECTIONS		
Breadstick	1 (1.5 oz)	140
Breadstick Cheese	1 (2 oz)	170
Dipping Sauce Marinara	1 serv (3 oz)	60
Dipping Sauce Ranch	1 serv (1.5 oz)	220
Dipping Sauce Wing Blue Cheese	1 serv (1.5 oz)	230
Dipping Sauce Wing Ranch	1 serv (1.5 oz)	220
Fried Cheese Sticks	4 (4.2 oz)	380
Tuscani Pasta Chicken Alfredo	1 serv (10 oz)	580
Tuscani Pasta Meaty Marinara	1 serv (9.5 oz)	450
Wedge Fries	1 serv (4.3 oz)	320
Wings Crispy Bone In All American	2 (1.9 oz)	200
Wings Crispy Bone In Buffalo Burnin Hot	2 (2.6 oz)	230
Wings Crispy Bone In Buffalo Medium	2 (2.6 oz)	230
Wings Crispy Bone In Buffalo Mild	2 (2.6 oz)	230
Wings Crispy Bone In Garlic Parmesan	2 (2.5 oz)	300
Wings Crispy Bone In Honey BBQ	2 (2.9 oz)	260
Wings Crispy Bone In Lemon Pepper	2 (2.6 oz)	270
Wings Crispy Bone In Spicy Asian	2 (2.9 oz)	250
Wings Crispy Bone In Spicy BBQ	2 (2.9 oz)	240
Wings Traditional All American	2 (1.4 oz)	80
Wings Traditional Buffalo Medium	2 (2 oz)	110
Wings Traditional Buffalo Mild	2 (2 oz)	110
Wings Traditional Burnin Hot	2 (2 oz)	110

FOOD	PORTION	CALS
Wings Traditional Garlic Parmesan	2 (2 oz)	180
Wings Traditional Honey BBQ	2 (2.4 oz)	140
Wings Traditional Lemon Pepper	2 (2 oz)	150
Wings Traditional Spicy Asian	2 (2.3 oz)	130
Wings Traditional Spicy BBQ	2 (2.3 oz)	120
PIZZA		
Fit 'N Delicious 12 Inch Chicken Mushrooms & Jalapeno	1 slice (3.3 oz)	170
Fit 'N Delicious 12 Inch Chicken Red Onion & Green Pepper	1 slice (3.3 oz)	180
Fit 'N Delicious 12 Inch Diced Red Tomato Mushroom & Jalapeno	1 slice (3.1 oz)	150
Fit 'N Delicious 12 Inch Green Pepper Red Onion & Diced Red Tomato	1 slice (3.1 oz)	150
Fit 'N Delicious 12 Inch Ham Pineapple & Diced Red Tomato	1 slice (2.9 oz)	160
Fit 'N Delicious 12 Inch Ham Red Onion & Mushrooms	1 slice (2.9 oz)	160
Hand Tossed 12 Inch Cheese Only	1 slice (2.9 oz)	220
Hand Tossed 12 Inch Cheese Only Garlic Parmesan	1 slice (3 oz)	220
Hand Tossed 12 Inch Dan's Original	1 slice (3.6 oz)	260
Hand Tossed 12 Inch Ham & Pineapple	1 slice (3.2 oz)	200
Hand Tossed 12 Inch Hawaiian Luau	1 slice (3.5 oz)	240
Hand Tossed 12 Inch Italian Sausage & Red Onion	1 slice (3.5 oz)	240
Hand Tossed 12 Inch Meat Lover's	1 slice (3.7 oz)	300
Hand Tossed 12 Inch Pepperoni	1 slice (2.9 oz)	230
Hand Tossed 12 Inch Pepperoni Lover's	1 slice (3.3 oz)	270
Hand Tossed 12 Inch Pepperoni & Mushroom	1 slice (3.2 oz)	210
Hand Tossed 12 Inch Pepperoni Garlic Parmesan	1 slice (2.9 oz)	230
Hand Tossed 12 Inch Spicy Sicilian	1 slice (3.5 oz)	240
Hand Tossed 12 Inch Supreme	1 slice (3.7 oz)	260
Hand Tossed 12 Inch Triple Meat Italiano	1 slice (3.4 oz)	260
Hand Tossed 12 Inch Ultimate Cheese Lover's	1 slice (2.9 oz)	240
Hand Tossed 12 Inch Veggie Lover's	1 slice (3.6 oz)	200
Pan 12 Inch Cheese Only	1 slice (3.2 oz)	240
Pan 12 Inch Dan's Original	1 slice (3.9 oz)	280
Pan 12 Inch Ham & Pineapple	1 slice (3.4 oz)	230

FOOD	PORTION	CALS
Pan 12 Inch Hawaiian Luau	1 slice (3.6 oz)	260
Pan 12 Inch Italian Sausage & Red Onion	1 slice (3.7 oz)	270
Pan 12 Inch Meat Lover's	1 slice (4 oz)	330
Pan 12 Inch Pepperoni	1 slice (3.2 oz)	250
Pan 12 Inch Pepperoni Lover's	1 slice (3.5 oz)	290
Pan 12 Inch Pepperoni & Mushroom	1 slice (3.4 oz)	240
Pan 12 Inch Spicy Sicilian	1 slice (3.7 oz)	270
Pan 12 Inch Supreme	1 slice (3.9 oz)	290
Pan 12 Inch Triple Meat Italiano	1 slice (3.6 oz)	290
Pan 12 Inch Ultimate Cheese Lover's	1 slice (3.2 oz)	270
Pan 12 Inch Veggie Lover's	1 slice (3.8 oz)	230
PANormous 9 Inch Cheese Only	1 pie (13.4 oz)	1100
PANormous 9 Inch Dan's Original	1 pie (15.9 oz)	1270
PANormous 9 Inch Ham & Pineapple	1 pie (14 oz)	1020
PANormous 9 Inch Hawaiian Luau	1 pie (14.8 oz)	1150
PANormous 9 Inch Italian Sausage & Red Onion	1 pie (15.4 oz)	1210
PANormous 9 Inch Meat Lover's	1 pie (16.3 oz)	1470
PANormous 9 Inch Pepperoni	1 pie (12.9 oz)	1100
PANormous 9 Inch Pepperoni Lover's	1 pie (16 oz)	1290
PANormous 9 Inch Pepperoni & Mushroom	1 pie (13.9 oz)	1050
PANormous 9 Inch Spicy Sicilian	1 pie (15.4 oz)	1220
PANormous 9 Inch Supreme	1 pie (16.2 oz)	1270
PANormous 9 Inch Triple Meat Lover's	1 pie (14.9 oz)	1280
PANormous 9 Inch Veggie Lover's	1 pie (15.4 oz)	1010
Personal Pan 6 Inch Cheese Only	1 (7.2 oz)	590
Personal Pan 6 Inch Dan's Original	1 (8.8 oz)	720
Personal Pan 6 Inch Ham & Pineapple	1 (7.5 oz)	550
Personal Pan 6 Inch Hawaiian Luau	1 (8 oz)	620
Personal Pan 6 Inch Italian Sausage & Red Onion	1 (8.6 oz)	690
Personal Pan 6 Inch Meat Lover's	1 (9.2 oz)	830
Personal Pan 6 Inch Pepperoni	1 (7.1 oz)	610
Personal Pan 6 Inch Pepperoni Lover's	1 (8.1 oz)	720
Personal Pan 6 Inch Pepperoni & Mushroom	1 (7.5 oz)	570
Personal Pan 6 Inch Spicy Sicilian	1 (8.6 oz)	680
Personal Pan 6 Inch Supreme	1 (9 oz)	720
Personal Pan 6 Inch Triple Meat Italiano	1 (8.4 oz)	730
Personal Pan 6 Inch Ultimate Cheese Lover's	1 (7.3 oz)	660
Personal Pan 6 Inch Veggie Lover's	1 (8.2 oz)	550
P'Zone Classic	½ serv (6.1 oz)	470

FOOD	PORTION	CALS
P'Zone Meaty	½ serv (6.6 oz)	550
P'Zone Pepperoni	½ serv (5.5 oz)	450
Stuffed Pizza Rollers	1 (2.7 oz)	220
Thin'N Crispy 12 Inch Cheese Only	1 slice (2.3 oz)	190
Thin'N Crispy 12 Inch Dan's Original	1 slice (3 oz)	240
Thin'N Crispy 12 Inch Ham & Pineapple	1 slice (2.6 oz)	180
Thin'N Crispy 12 Inch Hawaiian Luau	1 slice (2.8 oz)	220
Thin'N Crispy 12 Inch Italian Sausage & Red Onion	1 slice (2.8 oz)	220
Thin'N Crispy 12 Inch Meat Lover's	1 slice (3 oz)	280
Thin'N Crispy 12 Inch Pepperoni	1 slice (2.2 oz)	200
Thin'N Crispy 12 Inch Pepperoni Lover's	1 slice (2.6 oz)	250
Thin'N Crispy 12 Inch Pepperoni & Mushroom	1 slice (2.6 oz)	180
Thin'N Crispy 12 Inch Spicy Sicilian	1 slice (2.8 oz)	220
Thin'N Crispy 12 Inch Supreme	1 slice (3.1 oz)	240
Thin'N Crispy 12 Inch Triple Meat Italiano	1 slice (2.7 oz)	240
Thin'N Crispy 12 Inch Ultimate Cheese Lover's	1 slice (2.3 oz)	220
Thin'N Crispy 12 Inch Veggie Lover's	1 slice (3 oz)	180

PRETZELMAKER
BEVERAGES

FOOD	PORTION	CALS
Breezer Coffee	1 (20 oz)	640
Breezer Mocha	1 (20 oz)	620
Breezer Peach	1 (20 oz)	650
Breezer Raspberry	1 (20 oz)	650
Breezer Strawberry Banana	1 (20 oz)	650
Diet Coke	1 sm (20 oz)	0
Lemonade	1 sm (20 oz)	160

PRETZELS

FOOD	PORTION	CALS
Bites	1 med (7.4 oz)	640
Bites	1 sm (5.3 oz)	450
Bites Cinnamon Sugar	1 serv (5.8 oz)	520
Caramel Nut	1 (4.5 oz)	390
Cinnamon Sugar	1 (4.3 oz)	370
Garlic	1 (4.1 oz)	350
Original	1 (4 oz)	340
Parmesan	1 (4.2 oz)	360
Plain	1 (4 oz)	209
PT Pretzel Dog	1 (6 oz)	440
Ranch	1 (4.1 oz)	240

FOOD	PORTION	CALS
TOPPINGS		
Cream Cheese	1 serv (1.5 oz)	200
Icing Cream Cheese	1 serv (1.5 oz)	180
Ketchup	2 pkg (0.6 oz)	20
Mustard	2 pkg (0.4 oz)	5
Sauce Caramel	1 serv (1.5 oz)	140
Sauce Cheddar Cheese	1 serv (1.5 oz)	70
Sauce Nacho Cheese	1 serv (1.5 oz)	80
Sauce Pizza	1 serv (1.5 oz)	30
QUIZNOS		
SALAD DRESSINGS		
Acai Vinaigrette	1 reg	230
Balsamic Vinaigrette Fat Free	1 reg	130
Blue Cheese	1 reg	345
Honey Dijon	1 reg	450
Peppercorn Caesar	1 reg	480
Ranch	1 reg	350
Tzatziki	1 reg	450
SALADS		
Fresh Farmers Market Caprese Chicken w/o Dressing	1 reg	260
Fresh Farmers Market Chicken Caesar w/o Dressing	1 reg	130
Fresh Farmers Market Cobb w/o Dressing	1 reg	260
Fresh Farmers Market Harvest Chicken w/o Dressing	1 reg	220
Fresh Farmers Market Mediterranean Chicken w/o Dressing	1 reg	180
SANDWICHES		
Classic Sub Classic Club	1 sm	570
Classic Sub Classic Italian	1 sm	520
Classic Sub Honey Bacon Club	1 sm	480
Classic Sub Honey Bourbon Chicken	1 sm	320
Classic Sub Pork Cuban	1 sm	450
Classic Sub The Traditional	1 sm	430
Classic Sub Tuna Melt	1 sm	690
Classic Sub Turkey Bacon Guacamole	1 sm	540
Classic Sub Turkey Ranch & Swiss	1 sm	420
Classic Sub Ultimate Turkey Club	1 sm	560
Classic Sub Veggie	1 sm	510

FOOD	PORTION	CALS
Flatbread Sammies Bistro Steak Melt	1	410
Flatbread Sammies Cantina Chicken	1	280
Flatbread Sammies Chicken Bacon Ranch	1	380
Flatbread Sammies Italiano	1	420
Flatbread Sammies Roadhouse Steak	1	270
Flatbread Sammies Smoky Chipotle Turkey	1	390
Flatbread Sammies Veggie	1	340
Signature Sub Baja Chicken	1 sm	490
Signature Sub Black Angus On Rosemary Parmesan	1 sm	520
Signature Sub Buffalo Chicken	1 sm	470
Signature Sub Chicken Carbonara	1 sm	530
Signature Sub Chicken Bacon Dipper	1 sm	630
Signature Sub Chipotle Prime Rib	1 sm	600
Signature Sub Double Cheese Cheesesteak	1 sm	770
Signature Sub Harvest Chicken	1 sm	370
Signature Sub Honey Mustard Chicken	1 sm	520
Signature Sub Mesquite Chicken	1 sm	500
Signature Sub Peppercorn Steakhouse Dip	1 sm	630
Signature Sub Prime Rib Mushroom & Swiss	1 sm	600
Signature Sub Prime Rib & Peppercorn	1 sm	620
Signature Sub Prime Rib & Blue	1 sm	570
Signature Sub Southern BBQ Pulled Pork	1 sm	520
Toasty Bullets Beef Bacon & Cheddar	1	450
Toasty Bullets Italian	1	500
Toasty Bullets Pesto Turkey	1	380
Toasty Bullets Tuna Melt	1	510
Toasty Bullets Turkey Club	1	460
Toasty Favorites Honey Cured Ham	1 sm	490
Toasty Favorites Meatball	1 sm	450
Toasty Favorites Oven Roasted Turkey	1 sm	500
Toasty Favorites Roast Beef	1 sm	500
Toasty Favorites Turkey & Ham	1 sm	500
Toasty Favorites Veggie Caprese	1 sm	400
Toasty Torpedoes Beef Bacon & Cheddar	1	800
Toasty Torpedoes Italian	1	860
Toasty Torpedoes Pesto Turkey	1	690
Toasty Torpedoes Tuna Melt	1	980
Toasty Torpedoes Turkey Club	1	830

FOOD	PORTION	CALS
RANCH 1		
BEVERAGES		
Barq's Root Beer	1 sm (16 oz)	167
Coca-Cola	1 sm (16 oz)	150
Diet Coke	1 sm (16 oz)	2
Sprite	1 sm (16 oz)	150
CHILDREN'S MENU SELECTIONS		
Kids Meal Chicken Tenders	1 (2 oz)	111
Kids Meal Fries	1 serv (4 oz)	279
Kids Meal Popcorn Chicken	1 (2 oz)	112
MAIN MENU SELECTIONS		
Bowl Chicken Teriyaki	1 (19.3 oz)	504
Chicken Crispy	1 serv (5 oz)	326
Chicken Grilled	1 serv (3.9 oz)	146
Chicken On Mixed Greens	1 serv (21 oz)	340
Chicken Popcorn	1 serv (5.5 oz)	325
Chicken Tenders	1 serv (5.6 oz)	387
Fajita Mix Tomatoes Onion & Carrot	1 serv (3.2 oz)	20
Fajitas Chicken	1 serv (10 oz)	540
Fries	1 med	381
Fries Cheese	1 reg	493
Green Mix For Sandwiches	1 serv (2.5 oz)	31
Peppers & Onions	1 serv (1.6 oz)	27
Platter Chicken Rice	1 (10.9 oz)	273
Popcorn Chicken	1 sm	325
Rice	1 serv (4 oz)	97
Sandwich Chicken & Cheese	1 (11.2 oz)	389
Sandwich Chicken Philly	1 (9.2 oz)	410
Sandwich Crispy Chicken	1 (11.4 oz)	711
Sandwich Crispy Spicy Chicken	1 (11.4 oz)	543
Sandwich Grilled Spicy Chicken	1 (10.3 oz)	363
Sandwich Ranch 1 Classic	1 (9.4 oz)	683
Steamed Vegetables	1 serv (3 oz)	27
Wrap Grilled Chicken Caesar	1 (13.2 oz)	746
SALAD DRESSINGS AND SAUCES		
Dressing Balsamic Vinaigrette	1 oz	71
Dressing Classic Caesar	1 oz	103
Dressing Salad	1 oz	201
Sauce Ancho Chili Pepper	1 oz	134
Sauce BBQ	1 oz	84

FOOD	PORTION	CALS
Sauce Honey Mustard	1 oz	110
Sauce Pepper & Onion Saute	1 oz	143
Sauce Roasted Red Pepper	1 oz	232
Sauce Teriyaki	1 oz	24
SALADS		
Caesar	1 (7 oz)	34
Caesar Grilled Chicken	1 (11.3 oz)	223
Crispy Chicken Club	1 (13.6 oz)	495
Mandarin Chicken	1 (14.5 oz)	553
Mixed Greens w/o Cheese	1 (17 oz)	194
Salad Blend	1 serv (10.3 oz)	45
Southwest Chicken Chop	1 (17.6 oz)	681

RAX

FOOD	PORTION	CALS
BBQ Beef	1	399
BBQ Sandwich	1	716
Cheddar Melt	1	346
Deluxe	1	521
Grilled Chicken	1	526
Jr. Deluxe	1	367
Mushroom Melt	1	599
Philly Melt	1	537
Regular Rax	1	388
Turkey	1	484
Turkey Bacon Club	1	680

RED LOBSTER

BEVERAGES

FOOD	PORTION	CALS
Boston Ice Tea	1 serv	50
Coke	1 serv	100
Diet Coke	1 serv	0
Dr. Pepper	1 serv	150
Harbor Cafe Coffee	1 serv	0
Lemonade Light	1 serv	0
Lemonade Raspberry	1 serv	180
Tea Hot or Cold Unsweetened	1 serv	0
Wine Blush	1 glass	120
Wine Red	1 glass	120
MAIN MENU SELECTIONS		
Artic Char Grilled Broiled or Blackened w/ Broccoli	1 full portion	630

FOOD	PORTION	CALS
Artic Char Grilled Broiled or Blackened w/ Broccoli	1 half portion	340
Barramundi Grilled Broiled or Blackened w/ Broccoli	1 full portion	420
Barramundi Grilled Broiled or Blackened w/ Broccoli	1 half portion	230
Cobia Grilled Broiled or Blackened w/ Broccoli	1 half portion	400
Cobia Grilled Broiled or Blackened w/ Broccoli	1 full portion	760
Cod Grilled Broiled or Blackened w/ Broccoli	1 half portion	170
Cod Grilled Broiled or Blackened w/ Broccoli	1 full portion	300
Corvina Grilled Broiled or Blackened w/ Broccoli	1 full portion	320
Corvina Grilled Broiled or Blackened w/ Broccoli	1 half portion	180
Flounder Grilled Broiled or Blackened w/ Broccoli	1 half portion	200
Flounder Grilled Broiled or Blackened w/ Broccoli	1 full portion	350
Grouper Grilled Broiled or Blackened w/ Broccoli	1 full portion	370
Grouper Grilled Broiled or Blackened w/ Broccoli	1 half portion	210
Haddock Grilled Broiled or Blackened w/ Broccoli	1 half portion	180
Haddock Grilled Broiled or Blackened w/ Broccoli	1 full portion	310
Lake Whitefish Grilled Broiled or Blackened w/ Broccoli	1 full portion	380
Lake Whitefish Grilled Broiled or Blackened w/ Broccoli	1 half portion	210
Mahi Mahi Grilled Broiled or Blackened w/ Broccoli	1 full portion	360
Mahi Mahi Grilled Broiled or Blackened w/ Broccoli	1 half portion	200
Monchong Grilled Broiled or Blackened w/ Broccoli	1 full portion	340
Monchong Grilled Broiled or Blackened w/ Broccoli	1 half portion	190
Opah Grilled Broiled or Blackened w/ Broccoli	1 full portion	510
Opah Grilled Broiled or Blackened w/ Broccoli	1 half portion	280

FOOD	PORTION	CALS
Perch Grilled Broiled or Blackened w/ Broccoli	1 half portion	170
Perch Grilled Broiled or Blackened w/ Broccoli	1 full portion	300
Pompano Grilled Broiled or Blackened w/ Broccoli	1 full portion	430
Pompano Grilled Broiled or Blackened w/ Broccoli	1 half portion	240
Rainbow Trout Grilled Broiled or Blackened w/ Broccoli	1 half portion	220
Red Rockfish Grilled Broiled or Blackened w/ Broccoli	1 full portion	300
Red Rockfish Grilled Broiled or Blackened w/ Broccoli	1 half portion	170
Salmon Grilled Broiled or Blackened w/ Broccoli	1 half portion	270
Salmon Grilled Broiled or Blackened w/ Broccoli	1 full portion	490
Seabass Grilled Broiled or Blackened w/ Broccoli	1 half portion	230
Snapper Grilled Broiled or Blackened w/ Broccoli	1 half portion	210
Sole Grilled Broiled or Blackened w/ Broccoli	1 half portion	140
Tilapia Grilled Broiled or Blackened w/ Broccoli	1 half portion	210
Tuna Grilled Broiled or Blackened w/ Broccoli	1 half portion	200
Wahoo Grilled Broiled or Blackened w/ Broccoli	1 half portion	220
Walleye Grilled Broiled or Blackened w/ Broccoli	1 half portion	170

RED MANGO

FOOD	PORTION	CALS
Blenders Blueberry Moon	1 cup	150
Blenders Captain Berry	1 cup	140
Blenders Green Tea Blueberry	1 cup	130
Blenders Green Tea Honeydew	1 cup	130
Blenders Mango Island	1 cup	150
Blenders Pina Colada	1 cup	160
Blenders Tri-Berry	1 cup	130
Blenders Watermelon Breeze	1 cup	130
Frozen Yogurt All Flavors	½ cup	90

FOOD	PORTION	CALS
ROBEKS		
BAKED SELECTIONS		
Gourmet Pretzels Apple Cinnamon	1	470
Gourmet Pretzels Spinach Feta	1	430
Gourmet Pretzels Tomato Parmesan	1	420
Muffin Banana	1	310
Muffin Blueberry	1	300
Muffin Chocolate	1	320
Power Cookie Breakfast Bar	1	230
Power Cookie Chocolate Chip w/ Walnuts	1	404
Power Cookie Lemon Poppyseed	1	371
Power Cookie Oatmeal Raisin Walnut	1	375
Power Cookie Peanut Butter	1	426
BEVERAGES		
800 Lb Gorilla	1 (12 oz)	434
Freeze Lemon	1 (12 oz)	282
Freeze Orange	1 (12 oz)	290
Fresh Juice ABC	1 (12 oz)	150
Fresh Juice Apple	1 (12 oz)	180
Fresh Juice Carrot	1 (12 oz)	98
Fresh Juice Green-V	1 (12 oz)	96
Fresh Juice G-Snap	1 (12 oz)	120
Fresh Juice Lemonade Raspberry	1 (12 oz)	164
Fresh Juice Monkey C	1 (12 oz)	186
Fresh Juice Orange	1 (12 oz)	168
Naturally Light Banana Mango	1	162
Naturally Light Pineapple Mango	1	172
Naturally Light Raspberry Banana	1	161
Naturally Light Strawberry Pineapple	1	131
Shake Bananasplit	1 (12 oz)	274
Shake P-Nut Power	1 (12 oz)	362
Smoothie Acai Energizer	1 (12 oz)	161
Smoothie Awesome Acai	1 (12 oz)	146
Smoothie Banzai Blueberry	1 (12 oz)	172
Smoothie Berry Brilliance	1 (12 oz)	192
Smoothie Big Wednesday	1 (12 oz)	201
Smoothie Cardio Cooler	1 (12 oz)	244
Smoothie Citrus Stinger	1 (12 oz)	198
Smoothie Cranberry Quest	1 (12 oz)	208
Smoothie Dr. Robeks	1 (12 oz)	186

FOOD	PORTION	CALS
Smoothie Green Tea Sensation	1 (12 oz)	199
Smoothie Guava Lava	1 (12 oz)	206
Smoothie Hummingbird	1 (12 oz)	211
Smoothie Infinite Orange	1 (12 oz)	182
Smoothie Mahalo Mango	1 (12 oz)	201
Smoothie Malibu Peach	1 (12 oz)	181
Smoothie Outrageous Raspberry	1 (12 oz)	182
Smoothie Passionfruit Cove	1 (12 oz)	193
Smoothie Pina Koolada	1 (12 oz)	212
Smoothie Polar Pineapple	1 (12 oz)	183
Smoothie Pomegranate Passion	1 (12 oz)	190
Smoothie Pomegranate Power	1 (12 oz)	217
Smoothie Pro Arobek	1 (12 oz)	260
Smoothie Raspberry Romance	1 (12 oz)	209
Smoothie Robeks Rejuvenator	1 (12 oz)	221
Smoothie South Pacific Squeeze	1 (12 oz)	200
Smoothie Stawnana Berry	1 (12 oz)	188
Smoothie Venice Burner	1 (12 oz)	227
Smoothie Zen Berry	1 (12 oz)	217

SAMURAI SAM'S
BOWLS

FOOD	PORTION	CALS
Low Carb	1 reg	230
Spicy Beef 'N Broccoli	1 reg	620
Spicy Beef 'N Broccoli Brown Rice	1 reg	580
Sumo Brown Rice	1	1022
Sumo White Rice	1	1083
Sweet & Sour Dark Chicken	1 reg	610
Sweet & Sour Dark Chicken Brown Rice	1 reg	570
Sweet & Sour White Chicken	1 reg	580
Sweet & Sour White Chicken Brown Rice	1 reg	540
Teriyaki Dark Chicken	1 reg	540
Teriyaki Dark Chicken Brown Rice	1 reg	500
Teriyaki Dark Chicken & Shrimp	1 reg	492
Teriyaki Dark Chicken & Shrimp Brown Rice	1 reg	451
Teriyaki Dark Chicken & Steak	1 reg	540
Teriyaki Dark Chicken & Steak Brown Rice	1 reg	490
Teriyaki Salmon	1 reg	643
Teriyaki Shrimp Brown Rice	1 reg	407
Teriyaki Steak	1 reg	530

FOOD	PORTION	CALS
Teriyaki Steak Brown Rice	1 reg	490
Teriyaki Steak & Shrimp	1 reg	483
Teriyaki Steak & Shrimp Brown Rice	1 reg	442
Teriyaki Veggie	1 reg	363
Teriyaki Veggie Brown Rice	1 reg	323
Teriyaki White Chicken	1 reg	520
Teriyaki White Chicken Brown Rice	1 reg	470
Teriyaki White Chicken & Shrimp	1 reg	478
Teriyaki White Chicken & Shrimp Brown Rice	1 reg	437
Teriyaki White Chicken & Steak	1 reg	520
Teriyaki White Chicken & Steak Brown Rice	1 reg	480
Yakisoba Dark Chicken	1	842
Yakisoba Dark Chicken & Steak	1	825
Yakisoba Shrimp	1	677
Yakisoba Steak	1	809
Yakisoba Veggie	1	509
Yakisoba White Chicken	1	794
Yakisoba White Chicken & Steak	1	801
SALADS AND SIDES		
Crab Rangoon	1 serv	210
Dressing Chinese	1 serv (3.5 oz)	230
Dressing Chinese Ginger	1 serv (1 oz)	85
Dressing Oriental	1 serv (1 oz)	70
Egg Roll Grilled Chicken	1	150
Salad Oriental Chicken	1 serv	220
Salad Side	1	10
Salad Toss Sesame Chicken	1	490
Soup Asian Noodle	1 serv	89
Teriyaki Sauce	1 serv (1 oz)	40
WRAPS		
Teriyaki Dark Chicken	1	670
Teriyaki Dark Chicken Brown Rice	1	650
Teriyaki Steak	1	650
Teriyaki Steak Brown Rice	1	630
Teriyaki Veggie	1	510
Teriyaki Veggie Brown Rice	1	490
Teriyaki White Chicken	1	640
Teriyaki White Chicken Brown Rice	1	620
Teriyaki White Chicken & Steak	1	649
Teriyaki White Chicken & Steak Brown Rice	1	628

FOOD	PORTION	CALS
SCHLOTZSKY'S DELI		
CHILDREN'S MENU SELECTIONS		
Pizza Cheese	1 serv	479
Pizza Pepperoni	1 serv	523
Sandwich Cheese	1	394
Sandwich Ham & Cheese	1	424
Sandwich Turkey	1	300
DESSERTS		
Carrot Cake	1 serv	717
Cookie Chocolate Chip	1	160
Cookie Fudge Chocolate Chip	1	160
Cookie Oatmeal Raisin	1	150
Cookie	1	160
Cookie White Chocolate Macadamia	1	170
MAIN MENU SELECTIONS		
Salad Caesar	1 serv	103
Salad Garden	1 serv	51
Salad Grilled Chicken Caesar	1 serv	221
Salad Turkey Chef	1 serv	309
Sandwich Angus Roast Beef & Cheese	1 sm	534
Sandwich Chicken Breast	1 sm	342
Sandwich Fresh Veggie	1 sm	342
Sandwich Ham & Cheese	1 sm	508
Sandwich Smoked Turkey Breast	1 sm	353
Sandwich The Original	1 sm	559
Sandwich Turkey	1 sm	602
Sandwich Turkey Bacon Club	1 sm	561
Wraps Asian Chicken	1	537
Wraps Parmesan Chicken Caesar	1	556
SKIPPERS		
CHILDREN'S MENU SELECTIONS		
Kids Catch Chicken Tenderloin + Chips & Kids Side	1 serv	560
Kids Catch Fish Bites + Chips & Kids Side	1 serv	490
Kids Catch Sandwich Grilled Cheese + Chips & Kids Side	1 serv	620
Kids Catch Shrimp + Chips & Kids Side	1 serv	520
MAIN MENU SELECTIONS		
Baked Potato Plain	1	210

FOOD	PORTION	CALS
Basket Chicken & Fish + Chips & Slaw	1 serv	620
Basket Chicken & Shrimp + Chips & Slaw	1 serv	760
Basket Chicken + Chips & Slaw	2 pieces	730
Basket Clam Strips + Chips & Slaw	1 serv	890
Basket Clams & Fish + Chips & Slaw	1 serv	740
Basket Original Recipe Shrimp + Chips & Slaw	1 serv	800
Basket Popcorn Shrimp + Chips & Slaw	1 serv	750
Basket Prawn & Fish + Chips & Slaw	1 serv	730
Basket Prawn Seafood + Chips & Slaw	1 serv	720
Basket Shrimp & Fish + Chips & Slaw	1 serv	650
Basket Shrimp Trio + Chips & Slaw	1 serv	1040
Clam Chowder	1 cup	120
Clam Strips	1 serv	270
Coleslaw	1 sm	170
Fish Bites + Chips & Slaw	6 pieces	490
French Fries	1 reg	180
Grilled Veggies	1 serv	35
Halibut + Chips & Slaw	1 serv	580
Homestyle Chicken Tenderloin	1 piece	190
Hush Puppies	3 pieces	240
Original Fish Fillet	1 piece	80
Original Fish + Chips & Slaw	2 pieces	510
Original Shrimp	9 pieces	220
Sandwich Fish + Chips & Slaw	1 serv	800
Sandwich Fried Chicken + Chips & Slaw	1 serv	1260
Sandwich Grilled Chicken + Chips & Slaw	1 serv	1070
Skippers Platter + Chips & Slaw	1 serv	930
SALADS		
Caesar	1 sm	150
Caesar w/ Chicken	1 sm	340
Caesar w/ Salmon	1 sm	350
Green Salad w/o Dressing	1 sm	25

SMOOTHIE KING

Acai Adventure	1 (20 oz)	435
Angel Food	1 (20 oz)	354
Banana Berry Treat	1 (20 oz)	364
Banana Boat	1 (20 oz)	524
Berry Punch	1 (20 oz)	360
Blackberry Dream	1 (20 oz)	365

FOOD	PORTION	CALS
Blueberry Heaven	1 (20 oz)	325
Caribbean Way	1 (20 oz)	395
Celestial Cherry High	1 (20 oz)	257
Cherry Picket	1 (20 oz)	273
Coconut Surprise	1 (20 oz)	460
Coffee Smoothie Caramel	1 (20 oz)	340
Coffee Smoothie Mocha	1 (20 oz)	260
Coffee Smoothie Vanilla	1 (20 oz)	347
Cranberry Cooler	1 (20 oz)	496
Cranberry Supreme	1 (20 oz)	554
Fruit Fusion	1 (20 oz)	355
Go Goji	1 (20 oz)	433
Grape Expectations	1 (20 oz)	398
Grape Expectations II	1 (20 oz)	548
Green Tea Tango	1 (20 oz)	282
Hearty Apple	1 (20 oz)	405
High Protein Almond Mocha	1 (20 oz)	366
High Protein Banana	1 (20 oz)	322
High Protein Chocolate	1 (20 oz)	366
High Protein Lemon	1 (20 oz)	372
High Protein Pineapple	1 (20 oz)	320
Immune Builder	1 (20 oz)	380
Instant Vigor	1 (20 oz)	366
Island Impact	1 (20 oz)	311
Island Treat	1 (20 oz)	333
Kids' Cup Berry Interesting	1 (12 oz)	277
Kids' Cup Choc-A-Laka	1 (12 oz)	245
Kids' Cup Gimmi-Grape	1 (12 oz)	265
Kids' Cup Smarti Tarti	1 (12 oz)	200
Kids' Kups CW Jr.	1 (12 oz)	270
Kiwi Island Treat	1 (20 oz)	498
Lemon Twist Banana	1 (20 oz)	358
Lemon Twist Strawberry	1 (20 oz)	438
Light & Fluffy	1 (20 oz)	395
Low Carb All Flavors	1 (20 oz)	268
Malts	1 (20 oz)	680
Mangofest	1 (20 oz)	285
Mangosteen Madness	1 (20 oz)	383
Mo'cuccino Caramel	1 (20 oz)	570
Mo'cuccino Mocha	1 (20 oz)	444

FOOD	PORTION	CALS
Mo'cuccino Vanilla	1 (20 oz)	525
Muscle Punch	1 (20 oz)	364
Muscle Punch Plus	1 (20 oz)	366
Orange Ka-Bam	1 (20 oz)	465
Organic Apple Acai	1 (20 oz)	353
Passion Passport	1 (20 oz)	395
Peach Slice	1 (20 oz)	314
Peach Slice Plus	1 (20 oz)	464
Peanut Power	1 (20 oz)	549
Peanut Power Plus Chocolate	1 (20 oz)	717
Peanut Power Plus Grape	1 (20 oz)	749
Peanut Power Plus Strawberry	1 (20 oz)	699
Pep Upper	1 (20 oz)	411
Pina Colada Island	1 (20 oz)	600
Pineapple Pleasure	1 (20 oz)	280
Pineapple Surf	1 (20 oz)	461
Pomegranate Punch	1 (20 oz)	464
Power Punch	1 (20 oz)	428
Power Punch Plus	1 (20 oz)	500
Raspberry Collider	1 (20 oz)	338
Raspberry Sunrise	1 (20 oz)	392
Shakes	1 (20 oz)	670
Slim-N-Trim Chocolate	1 (20 oz)	297
Slim-N-Trim Orange Vanilla	1 (20 oz)	215
Slim-N-Trim Strawberry	1 (20 oz)	375
Slim-N-Trim Vanilla	1 (20 oz)	253
Strawberry Kiwi Breeze	1 (20 oz)	376
Strawberry X-treme	1 (20 oz)	366
Super Punch	1 (20 oz)	395
Super Punch Plus	1 (20 oz)	459
The Activator Chocolate	1 (20 oz)	404
The Activator Strawberry	1 (20 oz)	556
The Activator Vanilla	1 (20 oz)	406
The Hulk Chocolate	1 (20 oz)	876
The Hulk Strawberry	1 (20 oz)	1035
The Hulk Vanilla	1 (20 oz)	872
The Shredder Chocolate	1 (20 oz)	311
The Shredder Strawberry	1 (20 oz)	356
The Shredder Vanilla	1 (20 oz)	283
Yerba Mate Mango	1 (20 oz)	372

FOOD	PORTION	CALS
Yerba Mate Mixed Berry	1 (20 oz)	348
Yerba Mate Pomegranate	1 (20 oz)	372
Yogurt D-Lite	1 (20 oz)	333
Youth Fountain	1 (20 oz)	253

SONIC DRIVE-IN
ADD-ONS

FOOD	PORTION	CALS
Bacon	1 serv (0.5 oz)	70
Cheese	1 serv (0.7 oz)	60
Chili	1 serv (1.2 oz)	50
Green Chilies	1 serv (1 oz)	5
Grilled Onions	1 serv (1 oz)	25
Jalapenos	1 serv (0.7 oz)	5
Slaw	1 serv (1 oz)	45

BEVERAGES

FOOD	PORTION	CALS
Barq's Root Beer	1 sm (14 oz)	160
Coca-Cola	1 sm (14 oz)	140
Cream Pie Shake Banana	1 reg (14 oz)	590
Cream Pie Shake Chocolate	1 reg (14 oz)	660
Cream Pie Shake Coconut Cream	1 reg (14 oz)	580
CreamSlush Blue Coconut	1 reg (14 oz)	430
CreamSlush Cherry	1 reg (14 oz)	440
CreamSlush Grape	1 reg (14 oz)	430
CreamSlush Orange	1 reg (14 oz)	430
CreamSlush Strawberry	1 reg (14 oz)	450
CreamSlush Watermelon	1 reg (14 oz)	440
Diet Coke	1 sm (14 oz)	0
Dr Pepper	1 sm (14 oz)	130
Float Barq's Root Beer	1 reg (14 oz)	300
Float Coca-Cola	1 reg (14 oz)	290
Float Dr Pepper	1 reg (14 oz)	310
Limeade	1 sm (14 oz)	140
Limeade Cherry	1 sm (14 oz)	170
Limeade Strawberry	1 sm (14 oz)	170
Malt Banana	1 reg (14 oz)	490
Malt Caramel	1 reg (14 oz)	550
Malt Chocolate	1 reg (14 oz)	550
Malt Hot Fudge	1 reg (14 oz)	580
Malt Peanut Butter	1 reg (14 oz)	870
Malt Peanut Butter Fudge	1 reg (14 oz)	620

FOOD	PORTION	CALS
Malt Pineapple	1 reg (14 oz)	510
Malt Strawberry	1 reg (14 oz)	520
Malt Vanilla	1 reg (14 oz)	480
Milk 1%	8.5 oz	110
Milk Chocolate 1%	8.5 oz	160
Shake Banana	1 reg (14 oz)	470
Shake Chocolate	1 reg (14 oz)	540
Shake Hot Fudge	1 reg (14 oz)	570
Shake Peanut Butter	1 reg (14 oz)	640
Shake Peanut Butter Fudge	1 reg	610
Shake Pineapple	1 reg (14 oz)	500
Shake Strawberry	1 reg (14 oz)	510
Shake Vanilla	1 reg (14 oz)	470
Sonic Blast Butterfinger	1 reg (14 oz)	580
Sonic Blast M&M's	1 reg (14 oz)	600
Sonic Blast Oreo	1 reg (14 oz)	540
Sonic Blast Reese's Peanut Butter Cup	1 reg (14 oz)	560
Sprite	1 sm (14 oz)	104
Sprite Zero	1 sm (14 oz)	5
BREAKFAST SELECTIONS		
Breakfast Burrito Jr.	1 (4.1 oz)	330
Breakfast Burrito Sausage Egg Cheese	1 (5.9 oz)	480
Breakfast Toaster Bacon Egg Cheese	1 (5.6 oz)	530
Breakfast Toaster Ham Egg Cheese	1 (6.5 oz)	490
Breakfast Toaster Sausage Egg Cheese	1 (6.8 oz)	620
CroisSonic Bacon	1 (5.3 oz)	510
CroisSonic Sausage	1 (6.2 oz)	600
DESSERTS		
Apple Slice w/ Fat Free Caramel Dipping Sauce	1 serv (3.4 oz)	120
Apple Slices	1 serv (2.4 oz)	35
Banana Split	1 (10.8 oz)	420
Cone Vanilla	1 (4.7 oz)	180
Dish Vanilla	1 (6.5 oz)	240
Sundae Chocolate	1 (8.9 oz)	410
Sundae Hot Fudge	1 (8.9 oz)	440
Sundae Pineapple	1 (8.8 oz)	370
Sundae Strawberry	1 (8.8 oz)	380
MAIN MENU SELECTIONS		
California Cheeseburger	1 (9.3 oz)	690
Ched 'R' Bites	12 (3 oz)	280

FOOD	PORTION	CALS
Ched 'R' Peppers	4 (4.2 oz)	330
Chicken Strip Dinner	1 serv (13.5 oz)	930
Chicken Strips	2 (2.5 oz)	200
Chili Cheeseburger	1 (7.9 oz)	660
Coney Extra Long Chili Cheese	1 (9 oz)	660
Coney Regular	1 (5.2 oz)	390
Corn Dog	1 (2.6 oz)	210
Crispy Chicken Bacon Ranch	1 serv (8.9 oz)	610
French Fries	1 sm (2.5 oz)	200
French Fries w/ Cheese	1 sm (3 oz)	270
French Fries w/ Chili & Cheese	1 sm (4.1 oz)	300
Fritos Chili Pie	1 med (4.8 oz)	470
Green Chili Cheeseburger	1 (10 oz)	630
Grilled Chicken Bacon Ranch	1 serv (8.9 oz)	470
Hickory Cheeseburger	1 (8.3 oz)	640
Jalapeno Burger	1 (7.6 oz)	550
Jalapeno Cheeseburger	1 (8.3 oz)	620
Jr. Bacon Cheeseburger	1 (5 oz)	410
Jr. Burger	1 (4.1 oz)	310
Jr. Burger Deluxe	1 (4.7 oz)	350
Jr. Double Cheeseburger	1 (6.7 oz)	570
Jumbo Popcorn Chicken	1 sm (4 oz)	380
Mozzarella Sticks	1 serv (5 oz)	440
Onion Rings	1 med (5.5 oz)	440
Pickle-O's	1 serv (4 oz)	310
Sandwich Breaded Pork Fritter	1 (8.5 oz)	640
Sandwich Crispy Chicken	1 (7.9 oz)	550
Sandwich Fish	1 (8.6 oz)	650
Sandwich Grilled Cheese	1 (3.9 oz)	380
Sandwich Grilled Chicken	1 (7.8 oz)	400
Sonic Bacon Cheeseburger w/ Mayonnaise	1 (9.8 oz)	780
Sonic Burger w/ Ketchup	1 (8.7 oz)	560
Sonic Burger w/ Mayonnaise	1 (8.7 oz)	650
Sonic Burger w/ Mustard	1 (8.5 oz)	560
Sonic Cheeseburger w/ Ketchup	1 (9.3 oz)	630
Sonic Cheeseburger w/ Mayonnaise	1 (9.3 oz)	720
Sonic Cheeseburger w/ Mustard	1 (9.1 oz)	620
SuperSonic Cheeseburger w/ Ketchup	1 (12 oz)	900
SuperSonic Cheeseburger w/ Mayonnaise	1 (12 oz)	980
SuperSonic Cheeseburger w/ Mustard	1 (11.8 oz)	890

FOOD	PORTION	CALS
Thousand Island Burger	1 (8.7 oz)	610
Toaster Sandwich Bacon Cheeseburger	1 (8.5 oz)	670
Toaster Sandwich BLT	1 (5.2 oz)	500
Toaster Sandwich Chicken Club	1 (9 oz)	740
Toaster Sandwich Country Fried Steak	1 (8.5 oz)	670
Tots	1 sm (1.5 oz)	130
Tots w/ Cheese	1 sm (2.2 oz)	190
Tots w/ Chili & Cheese	1 sm (3.2 oz)	220
Wrap Crispy Chicken	1 (8.2 oz)	490
Wrap Fritos Chili Cheese	1 (8.5 oz)	670
Wrap Grilled Chicken	1 (8.8 oz)	390
SALAD DRESSINGS AND SAUCES		
Dressing Honey Mustard	1 serv (1.5 oz)	180
Dressing Italian Fat Free	1 serv (1.5 oz)	40
Dressing Original Ranch	1 serv (1.5 oz)	190
Dressing Original Ranch Light	1 serv (1.5 oz)	110
Dressing Thousand Island	1 serv (1.5 oz)	190
Sauce BBQ	1 serv (1 oz)	45
Sauce Honey Mustard	1 serv (1 oz)	90
Sauce Marinara	1 serv (1 oz)	15
Sauce Ranch	1 serv (1 oz)	140
SALADS		
Crispy Chicken	1 serv (11.4 oz)	340
Grilled Chicken	1 serv (12 oz)	250

SOUPER SALAD
BEVERAGES

Lemonade	1 (24 oz)	190
Lemonade Mango	1 (24 oz)	220
Lemonade Raspberry	1 (24 oz)	220
Lemonade Strawberry	1 (24 oz)	220
Smoothie Mango	1 tall	250
Smoothie Peach	1 tall	230
Smoothie Raspberry	1 tall	230
Smoothie Strawberry	1 tall	230
DESSERTS		
Blueberry Bread	1 piece	150
Brownies	2 pieces	120
Cornbread	1 piece	170
Cottage Cheese	½ cup	90

FOOD	PORTION	CALS
Gingerbread	1 piece	180
Peaches	½ cup	70
Pineapple Tidbits	¼ cup	60
Pudding Banana	½ cup	160
Pudding Chocolate	½ cup	170
Soft Serve Cone Chocolate	1	120
Soft Serve Cone Vanilla	1	120
Sponge Cake	4 pieces	80
Strawberry Parfait	½ cup	100
Vanilla Wafers	4	70
Whipped Topping	½ cup	100
PASTA AND PIZZA		
Chicken Alfredo	1 cup	320
Macaroni & Cheese	1 cup	380
Pizza Slice Cheese	1	70
Pizza Slice Garden	1	80
Pizza Slice Pepperoni	1	90
Pizza Slice Sausage	1	80
Spaghetti & Meatballs	1 cup	280
SALAD DRESSINGS AND SAUCES		
Balsamic Vinegar	1 oz	60
Bleu Cheese	2 oz	220
Caesar	2 oz	280
Chipotle Ranch	2 oz	280
Fat Free French	2 oz	60
Fat Free Italian w/ Cheese	2 oz	30
Green Goddess	2 oz	260
Honey Mustard	2 oz	240
Mayonnaise	2 tbsp	200
Olive Oil	1 oz	240
Peppercorn Ranch	2 oz	220
Pesto Basil	1 tbsp	45
Ranch	2 oz	220
Reduced Calorie Ranch	2 oz	120
Sauce Alfredo	1½ tbsp	45
Sauce Chipotle Pepper	¼ tsp	0
Sauce Cholula Hot	¼ tsp	0
Sauce Jalapeno Cheese	1 serv (2 oz)	35
Sauce Marinara	1½ tbsp	10
Sauce Meaty Marinara	1½ tbsp	40

FOOD	PORTION	CALS
Sauce Sriracha Hot	¼ tsp	0
Sour Cream Light	2 tbsp	40
Tangy Oriental	2 oz	160
Thousand Island	1 oz	300
Vinaigrette Cranberry	2 oz	100
Vinaigrette House	2 oz	220
SALADS		
Apple Walnut	1 cup	130
Asian Chicken	1 cup	80
Asian Shrimp	1 cup	100
Buffalo Chicken	1 cup	70
Caesar Chicken	1 cup	90
Caesar Chicken Salsa	1 cup	80
Caesar Shrimp	1 cup	90
California Chicken Salad	⅓ cup	80
Capri	1 cup	50
Chicago Chopped	1 cup	120
Chickpea	⅓ cup	110
Cobb	1 cup	100
Coleslaw Broccoli	⅓ cup	80
Edamame	⅓ cup	70
Fisherman's Kettle Shrimp & Crab	⅓ cup	120
Gazpacho	⅓ cup	30
Green Goddess Crab	1 cup	70
Italian Antipasto	1 cup	70
Mango Berry	1 cup	110
Marinated Mushrooms	⅓ cup	60
Marinated Oriental Cucumber	⅓ cup	10
Marinated Tomato	1 cup	60
Melon Couscous	⅓ cup	50
Mustard Potato	⅓ cup	80
Paco's Taco	⅓ cup	100
Pasta De Garden	⅓ cup	80
Pasta Fettuccine	⅓ cup	100
Pasta Primavera	⅓ cup	45
Pasta Thai Chicken	⅓ cup	100
Pasta Tuna Skroodle	⅓ cup	130
Red Potato	⅓ cup	50
Rice Florentine	⅓ cup	90

FOOD	PORTION	CALS
Roasted Mushrooms & Artichokes w/ Feta Cheese	⅓ cup	40
Roasted Vegetables	⅓ cup	20
Salad Of The Sea	⅓ cup	50
Salmon Medley	1 cup	70
Santa Fe Corn	⅓ cup	100
Shrimp & Crab Louie	1 cup	130
Southwest Chicken Chipotle	1 cup	90
Sweet Garden Slaw	⅓ cup	35
Tropical Tuxedo	⅓ cup	60
Tuna Fish	⅓ cup	70
SOUPS		
Adobe Rice & Chicken	1 (5 oz)	100
Alaskan Salmon Chowder	1 (5 oz)	70
Beef Mushroom Barley	1 (5 oz)	80
Beef Noodle	1 (5 oz)	80
Beef Shellini	1 (5 oz)	90
Beef Stroganoff	1 (5 oz)	120
Black Bean	1 (5 oz)	80
Broccoli Cheese	1 (5 oz)	70
Cajun Gumbo	1 (5 oz)	110
Cauliflower Cheese	1 (5 oz)	70
Cheddar Chicken Broccoli Stew	1 (5 oz)	140
Cherokee Joe Cornbread	1 (5 oz)	70
Chicken Creole	1 (5 oz)	100
Chicken Enchilada	1 (5 oz)	180
Chicken Gumbo	1 (5 oz)	90
Chicken Mushroom Barley	1 (5 oz)	80
Chicken Noodle	1 (5 oz)	80
Chicken Tetrazini	1 (5 oz)	120
Chicken Tortilla	1 (5 oz)	60
Cream Of Asparagus	1 (5 oz)	140
Cream Of Broccoli	1 (5 oz)	60
Cream Of Cauliflower	1 (5 oz)	60
Cream Of Chicken	1 (5 oz)	100
Cream Of Mushroom	1 (5 oz)	80
Holiday Harvest	1 (5 oz)	90
Vegan Split Pea	1 (5 oz)	90
Vegetable Beef	1 (5 oz)	80
Vegetable Cheese	1 (5 oz)	80

FOOD	PORTION	CALS
Vegetable Lentil	1 (5 oz)	70
Vegetarian Butter Bean	1 (5 oz)	70
Vegetarian Vegetable	1 (5 oz)	50

SOUPLANTATION
BREADS AND MUFFINS
Biscuit Buttermilk	1	190
Cornbread Buttermilk Low Fat	1 piece	140
Focaccia Bruschetta	1 piece	140
Focaccia Honey Wheat Crust BBQ Chicken	1 piece	200
Focaccia Honey Wheat Crust Buffalo Chicken	1 piece	170
Muffin Apple Cinnamon Bran 96% Fat Free	1	130
Muffin Apple Raisin	1	150
Muffin Banana Nut	1	150
Muffin Cappuccino Chip	1	190
Muffin Caribbean Key Lime	1	170
Muffin Carrot Pineapple w/ Oat Bran	1	150
Muffin Cherry Nut	1	150
Muffin Chile Corn Low Fat	1	140
Muffin Chocolate Brownie	1	180
Muffin Chocolate Chip	1	170
Muffin Top Banana Crunch No Sugar Added	1	120
BREAKFAST MENU SELECTIONS
Belgian Waffle	1	90
Biscuit Sweet Cinnamon w/ Frosting	1	270
Biscuit Sweet Maple Buttermilk	1	240
Biscuit Sweet Strawberry Buttermilk	1	250
Breakfast Burrito Country Ham & Egg	1	210
Breakfast Burrito Sweet Pepper Sausage Egg	1	210
Eggs Scrambled	½ cup	135
Focaccia Egg Scramble w/ Bacon	1 piece	180
French Toast	1 slice	150
Oatmeal Plain	¾ cup	110
Potatoes O'Brien	½ cup	140
Sticky Granola Clusters w/ Almonds	¼ cup	270
Sunrise Pasta Mediterranean	1 cup	210
DESSERTS
Apple Medley Fat Free	½ cup	70
Banana Royale Fat Free	½ cup	80
Cake Carrot & Cream Cheese Lava	1 piece	320

FOOD	PORTION	CALS
Cake Chocolate Lava	½ cup	330
Cobbler Apple	½ cup	360
Cobbler Caramel Apple	½ cup	390
Cobbler Cherry Apple	½ cup	330
Cookie Chocolate Chip	1 sm	75
Cookie Bar Chocolate Peanut Butter	1 piece	270
Frozen Yogurt Chocolate Nonfat	½ cup	110
Pudding Banana	½ cup	160
Pudding Butterscotch Low Fat	½ cup	140
Pudding Chocolate Low Fat	½ cup	150
Pudding Chocolate Low Fat No Sugar Added	½ cup	90
MAIN MENU SELECTIONS		
100% Whole Wheat Jalapeno & Salsa Pasta	1 cup	250
Alfredo 4 Cheese	1 cup	390
Alfredo Broccoli w/ Basil	1 cup	380
Alfredo Fettuccine	1 cup	390
Alfredo Fire Roasted Tomato Basil	1 cup	370
Arizona Marinara	1 cup	360
Baked Potato Topper Broccoli Cheese	1 cup	120
Beefy Meatball Stroganoff	1 cup	340
Bruschetta	1 cup	260
Bruschetta Creamy	1 cup	360
Carbonara Pasta w/ Bacon	1 cup	290
Cheesy Scalloped Potatoes w/ Bacon	1 cup	240
Chicken Tetrazzini	1 cup	480
Creamy Cilantro Lime Pesto Hot Pasta	1 cup	360
Creamy Herb Chicken	1 cup	310
Curried Pineapple & Ginger	1 cup	200
Garden Vegetable w/ Italian Sausage	1 cup	300
Pesto Cilantro Lime	1 cup	370
SALAD DRESSINGS		
Avocado Ranch	2 tbsp	150
Bacon	2 tbsp	110
Blue Cheese	1 tbsp	130
Creamy Cucumber Reduced Calorie	2 tbsp	70
Creamy Italian	2 tbsp	120
Creamy Sesame Soy	2 tbsp	170
Green Chili Ranch	2 tbsp	150
Honey Mustard	2 tbsp	150
Honey Mustard Fat Free	2 tbsp	45

FOOD	PORTION	CALS
Italian Fat Free	2 tbsp	25
Vinaigrette Balsamic	2 tbsp	180
Vinaigrette Basil	2 tbsp	160
Vinaigrette Cranberry Orange Low Fat	2 tbsp	80
Vinaigrette Honey Lime Cilantro	2 tbsp	100
Vinaigrette Italian w/ Basil & Romano Cheese	2 tbsp	150
SALADS		
100% Whole Wheat Arugula Citrus	½ cup	210
100% Whole Wheat Creamy Chipotle	½ cup	350
100% Whole Wheat Sicilian Penne w/ Feta & Pepperoni	½ cup	250
100% Whole Wheat Spicy Asian Peanut	½ cup	260
Ambrosia w/ Coconut	½ cup	190
Artichoke Rice	½ cup	190
Aunt Doris' Red Pepper Slaw Fat Free	½ cup	70
Azteca Taco w/ Turkey	1 cup	130
Baja Bean & Cilantro	½ cup	180
Bartlett Pear & Carmelized Walnut	1 cup	180
BBQ Smokehouse w/ Bacon & Peanuts	1 cup	290
Buffalo Chicken	1 cup	180
Caesar Asiago	1 cup	270
California Cobb w/ Bacon	1 cup	190
Cambay Curry w/ Almonds & Coconut	1 cup	220
Carrot Raisin	½ cup	90
Cherry Balsamic Blue Tossed	1 cup	220
Cherry Chipotle Spinach	1 cup	160
Chinese Krab	½ cup	160
Citrus Noodle w/ Snow Peas	½ cup	140
Classic Antipasto	1 cup	280
Classic Greek	1 cup	120
Confetti Avocado Slaw	½ cup	140
Crunchy Island Pineapple	1 cup	160
Curried Rice w/ Mango Chutney	½ cup	170
Field Corn & Very Wild Rice	½ cup	170
Field Greens Citrus Vinaigrette	1 cup	150
Potato BBQ	½ cup	170
Potato Bristo	½ cup	290
Potato Buffalo Blue	½ cup	190
Potato Dijon w/ Garlic Dill Vinaigrette	½ cup	150

FOOD	PORTION	CALS
SOUPS		
8 Vegetable Chicken Stew	1 cup	160
Albondigas Locas Meatball	1 cup	210
Asian Ginger Broth	1 cup	50
Basmati Lentil	1 cup	210
Beef & Barley Stew	1 cup	240
Better Than Mom's Beef Stew	1 cup	270
Big Chunk Chicken Noodle Low Fat	1 cup	170
Border Black Bean & Chorizo	1 cup	240
Broccoli Cheese	1 cup	270
Buffalo Chicken	1 cup	180
Canadian Cheese w/ Smoked Ham	1 cup	350
Cheese Stuffed Cappelletti	1 cup	250
Cheesy Corn Chowder w/ Bacon	1 cup	220
Chesapeake Corn Chowder	1 cup	290
Chicken & Rice	1 cup	160
Chicken Dijon Reduced Sodium	1 cup	210
Chicken Divan	1 cup	240
Chicken Enchilada	1 cup	190
STARBUCKS		
BAKED SELECTIONS		
Apple Fritter	1	480
Bagel French Toast	1	280
Bagel Multigrain	1	280
Bagel Plain	1	280
Bar Cranberry Bliss	1	320
Bar Toffee Almond	1	400
Brownie Espresso	1	340
Cinnamon Roll	1	470
Cocoa Crispy Square	1	420
Cookie Chocolate Chunk	1	420
Cookie Coffee Ginger	1	470
Cookie Penguin	1	370
Cookie Rainbow	1	420
Cookies Mini Black & White	2	240
Croissant Butter	1	370
Doughnut Glazed	1	490
Loaf Banana Nut	1 serv	470
Loaf Iced Lemon	1 serv	500

FOOD	PORTION	CALS
Loaf Marble	1 serv	410
Loaf Pumpkin	1 serv	380
Mallorca Sweet Bread	1	420
Muffin Blueberry	1	310
Muffin Pumpkin Cream Cheese	1	490
Muffin Reduced Fat Chocolate	1	290
Muffin Walnut Bran	1	430
Reduced Fat Coffee Cake Banana Chocolate Chip	1	390
Reduced Fat Coffee Cake Blueberry	1 serv	320
Reduced Fat Coffee Cake Cinnamon Swirl	1 serv	290
Reduced Fat Coffee Cake Pumpkin Chocolate Chip	1	300
Rustic Apple Tart	1	190
Scone Blueberry	1	480
Scone Cran Apple Crumb	1	490
Scone Raspberry	1	470
BEVERAGES		
Apple Juice	1 grande	250
Cafe Americano	1 grande	15
Cafe Au Lait Nonfat Milk	1 grande	70
Caffe Mocha No Whip Nonfat Milk	1 grande	220
Caffe Mocha Whip Nonfat Milk	1 grande	290
Cappuccino Nonfat Milk	1 grande	80
Caramel Apple Cider Whip	1 grande	380
Caramel Apple Spice No Whip	1 grande	310
Caramel Macchiato Nonfat Milk	1 grande	190
Chocolate Milk Nonfat	1 grande	280
Cinnamon Dolce Creme No Whip Nonfat Milk	1 grande	220
Cinnamon Dolce Whip Nonfat Milk	1 grande	290
Coffee Of The Week	1 grande	5
Coffee Of The Week Decafe	1 grande	5
Frappuccino Blended Coffee Cafe Vanilla Whip Nonfat Milk	1 grande	430
Frappuccino Blended Coffee Cafe Vanilla Whip Soy	1 grande	430
Frappuccino Blended Coffee Cafe Vanilla No Whip Soy	1 grande	310
Frappuccino Blended Coffee Caffe Vanilla No Whip Nonfat Milk	1 grande	310

FOOD	PORTION	CALS
Frappuccino Blended Coffee Caramel No Whip Nonfat Milk	1 grande	270
Frappuccino Blended Coffee Caramel No Whip Soy	1 grande	270
Frappuccino Blended Coffee Caramel Whip Soy	1 grande	380
Frappuccino Blended Coffee Cinnamon Dolce No Whip Nonfat Milk	1 grande	260
Frappuccino Blended Coffee Cinnamon Dolce No Whip Soy	1 grande	260
Frappuccino Blended Coffee Cinnamon Dolce Whip Soy	1 grande	370
Frappuccino Blended Coffee Espresso Nonfat Milk	1 grande	190
Frappuccino Blended Coffee Java Chip No Whip Nonfat Milk	1 grande	340
Frappuccino Blended Coffee Java Chip No Whip Soy	1 grande	190
Frappuccino Blended Coffee Java Chip Whip Nonfat Milk	1 grande	460
Frappuccino Blended Coffee Java Chip Whip Soy	1 grande	460
Frappuccino Blended Coffee Mocha No Whip Nonfat Milk	1 grande	260
Frappuccino Blended Coffee Mocha No Whip Soy	1 grande	260
Frappuccino Blended Coffee Mocha Whip Nonfat Milk	1 grande	380
Frappuccino Blended Coffee Pumpkin Spice No Whip Nonfat Milk	1 grande	290
Frappuccino Blended Coffee Pumpkin Spice No Whip Soy	1 grande	290
Frappuccino Blended Coffee Pumpkin Spice Whip Nonfat Milk	1 grande	400
Frappuccino Blended Coffee Pumpkin Spice Whip Soy	1 grande	400
Frappuccino Blended Coffee Whip Nonfat Milk	1 grande	370
Frappuccino Blended Coffee White Chocolate Mocha No Whip Nonfat Milk	1 grande	300

FOOD	PORTION	CALS
Frappuccino Blended Coffee White Chocolate Mocha No Whip Soy	1 grande	300
Frappuccino Blended Coffee White Chocolate Mocha Whip Nonfat Milk	1 grande	410
Frappuccino Blended Coffee White Chocolate Mocha Whip Soy	1 grande	410
Frappuccino Blended Creme Tazo Chai No Whip Nonfat Milk	1 grande	330
Frappuccino Blended Creme Tazo Chai Whip Nonfat Milk	1 grande	570
Frappuccino Blended Creme Vanilla Bean No Whip Nonfat Milk	1 grande	350
Frappuccino Blended Creme Vanilla Bean Whip Nonfat Milk	1 grande	470
Frappuccino Light Blended Coffee Cafe Vanilla Nonfat Milk	1 grande	190
Frappuccino Light Blended Coffee Caramel	1 grande	160
Frappuccino Light Blended Coffee Cinnamon Dolce Nonfat Milk	1 grande	140
Frappuccino Light Blended Coffee Java Chip Nonfat Milk	1 grande	200
Frappuccino Light Blended Coffee Mocha Nonfat Milk	1 grande	140
Frappuccino Light Blended Coffee Nonfat Milk	1 grande	130
Frappuccino Light Blended Coffee Pumpkin Spice Nonfat Milk	1 grande	150
Frappuccino Light Blended Creme Double Chocolaty Chip Whip Nonfat Milk	1 grande	510
Frappuccino Light Blended Creme Pumpkin Spice No Whip Nonfat Milk	1 grande	360
Frappuccino Light Blended Creme Pumpkin Spice Whip Nonfat Milk	1 grande	470
Frappuccino Light Blended Creme Tazo Green Tea No Whip Nonfat Milk	1 grande	380
Frappuccino Light Blended Creme Tazo Green Tea Whip Nonfat Milk	1 grande	490
Frappuccino Light Blended Creme White Chocolate No Whip Nonfat Milk	1 grande	480
Frappuccino Light Blended Creme White Chocolate Whip Nonfat Milk	1 grande	610

FOOD	PORTION	CALS
Frappuccino Light Espresso Nonfat Milk	1 grande	110
Hot Chocolate No Whip Nonfat Milk	1 grande	240
Hot Chocolate Whip Nonfat Milk	1 grande	320
Iced Brewed Coffee	1 grande	90
Iced Cafe Mocha Whip Nonfat Milk	1 grande	290
Iced Caffe Americano	1 grande	15
Iced Caffe Latte Nonfat Milk	1 grande	90
Iced Caffe Mocha No Whip Nonfat Milk	1 grande	170
Iced Caramel Macchiato Nonfat Milk	1 grande	190
Iced Latte Pumpkin Spice No Whip Nonfat Milk	1 grande	220
Iced Latte Pumpkin Spice Whip Nonfat Milk	1 grande	330
Iced Latte Skinny Cinnamon Dolce No Whip Nonfat Milk	1 grande	80
Iced Latte Sugar Free Flavored Syrup Nonfat Milk	1 grande	80
Iced Latte Syrup Flavored Nonfat Milk	1 grande	160
Iced Latte Vanilla Nonfat Milk	1 grande	160
Iced Peppermint White Chocolate Mocha No Whip Nonfat Milk	1 grande	370
Iced Peppermint White Chocolate Mocha Whip Nonfat Milk	1 grande	490
Iced Tazo Latte Black Tea Nonfat Milk	1 grande	170
Iced Tazo Latte Black Tea Soy	1 grande	200
Iced Tazo Latte Chai Nonfat Milk	1 grande	200
Iced Tazo Latte Green Tea Nonfat Milk	1 grande	220
Iced Tazo Latte Green Tea Soy	1 grande	260
Iced Tazo Latte Red Tea	1 grande	200
Iced Tazo Latte Red Tea Nonfat Milk	1 grande	170
Iced White Chocolate Mocha No Whip Nonfat Milk	1 grande	310
Iced White Chocolate Mocha Whip Nonfat Milk	1 grande	430
Latte Caffe Nonfat Milk	1 grande	130
Latte Cinnamon Dolce No Whip Nonfat Milk	1 grande	210
Latte Cinnamon Dolce w/ Sugar Free Syrup Nonfat Milk	1 grande	130
Latte Cinnamon Dolce Whip Nonfat Milk	1 grande	280
Latte Pumpkin Spice No Whip Nonfat Milk	1 grande	260
Latte Pumpkin Spice Whip Nonfat Milk	1 grande	330
Latte Skinny Caramel No Whip Nonfat Milk	1 grande	130

FOOD	PORTION	CALS
Latte Skinny Cinnamon Dolce No Whip Nonfat Milk	1 grande	130
Latte Skinny Hazelnut No Whip Nonfat Milk	1 grande	130
Latte Skinny Vanilla No Whip Nonfat Milk	1 grande	130
Latte Syrup Flavored Nonfat Milk	1 grande	200
Milk Nonfat	1 grande	180
Peppermint White Chocolate Mocha No Whip Nonfat Milk	1 grande	420
Peppermint White Chocolate Mocha Whip Nonfat Milk	1 grande	490
Pumpkin Spice Creme No Whip Nonfat Milk	1 grande	270
Pumpkin Spice Creme Whip Nonfat Milk	1 grande	340
Shaken Black Iced Tea & Lemonade	1 grande	130
Shaken White Iced Tea Blueberry	1 grande	80
Steamed Apple Juice	1 grande	230
Tazo Black Shaken Iced Tea & Lemonade	1 grande	130
Tazo Chai Latte Iced Tea Soy	1 grande	230
Tazo Chai Latte Nonfat Milk	1 grande	200
Tazo Chai Latte Soy	1 grande	230
Tazo Latte Black Tea Nonfat Milk	1 grande	170
Tazo Latte Black Tea Soy	1 grande	190
Tazo Latte Green Tea Nonfat Milk	1 grande	200
Tazo Latte Green Tea Soy	1 grande	220
Tazo Latte Red Tea Nonfat Milk	1 grande	170
Tazo Latte Red Tea Soy	1 grande	190
Tazo Shaken Iced Tea Green	1 grande	80
Tazo Shaken Iced Tea Green & Lemonade	1 grande	130
Tazo Shaken Iced Tea Orange Passion	1 grande	70
Tazo Shaken Iced Tea Passion	1 grande	80
Tazo Shaken Iced Tea Passion & Lemonade	1 grande	130
Tazo Tea	1 grande	0
Vanilla Creme Whip Nonfat Milk	1 grande	270
Vanilla Creme No Whip Nonfat Milk	1 grande	200
Vivanno Blend Banana Chocolate	1 grande (20 oz)	270
Vivanno Blend Orange Mango Banana	1 grande (20 oz)	250
White Chocolate Mocha No Whip Nonfat Milk	1 grande	360
White Chocolate Mocha Whip Nonfat Milk	1 grande	430
SALADS		
Fiesta	1 (9.4 oz)	320

FOOD	PORTION	CALS
Fruit & Cheese Plate	1 (8.6 oz)	400
Vegetable Vinaigrette	1 (10.7 oz)	310
SANDWICHES		
Club Chicken Cheddar Bacon w/ Mayo	1	480
Club Turkey & Avocado	1	390
Egg Salad On Multigrain	1	470
Turkey & Swiss w/ Mayo	1	310
TOPPINGS		
Caramel	1 tbsp	15
Chocolate	1 tsp	5
Flavored Sugar Free Syrup	1 pump	0
Flavored Syrup	1 pump	20
Mocha Syrup	1 pump	25
Sprinkles	1 serv	0

STEAK ESCAPE
BEVERAGES

FOOD	PORTION	CALS
Coca-Cola	16 oz	150
Diet Coke	16 oz	0
Lemonade	16 oz	167
Sprite	16 oz	150
SALADS		
Grilled Side	1 serv (5.9 oz)	40
Grilled w/ Chicken	1 serv (11.1 oz)	177
Grilled w/ Ham	1 serv (10.6 oz)	302
Grilled w/ Steak	1 serv (11.1 oz)	187
Grilled w/ Turkey	1 serv (10.6 oz)	132
SANDWICHES		
7 Inch Cajun Chicken	1 (8.6 oz)	408
7 Inch Capicola Portion	1 serv (1 oz)	31
7 Inch Chicken Portion	1 serv (3.9 oz)	120
7 Inch Classic Italian Sub	1 (8.4 oz)	471
7 Inch Ham Portion	1 serv (3 oz)	75
7 Inch Salami Portion	1 serv (1 oz)	105
7 Inch Steak Portion	1 serv (3.9 oz)	130
7 Inch Turkey Club	1 (7.9 oz)	380
7 Inch Turkey Portion	1 serv (2.9 oz)	75
7 Inch Vegetarian	1 (8.8 oz)	311
7 Inch Wild West BBQ	1 (9.6 oz)	455
Kids Chicken	1 (3.9 oz)	205

FOOD	PORTION	CALS
Kids Ham	1 (3.7 oz)	183
Kids Steak	1 (3.8 oz)	110
Kids Turkey	1 (3.7 oz)	183
SIDES		
Fries	1 cup (32 oz)	996
Fries	1 cup (12 oz)	498
Fries Kids	1 serv (2.9 oz)	249
Fries Loaded Bacon & Cheddar	1 serv (10.8 oz)	905
Fries Loaded Ranch & Bacon	1 serv (10.8 oz)	1044
Kids Chicken Tenders	2 (3.8 oz)	240
Smashed Potatoes Loaded Bacon & Cheddar	1 serv (16.7 oz)	636
Smashed Potatoes Loaded Ranch & Bacon	1 serv (16.7 oz)	692
Smashed Potatoes Plain	1 serv (13.8 oz)	246
Smashed Potatoes w/ Chicken	1 serv (19.9 oz)	383
Smashed Potatoes w/ Ham	1 serv (19.4 oz)	338
Smashed Potatoes w/ Steak	1 serv (19.9 oz)	393
Smashed Potatoes w/ Turkey	1 serv (19.4 oz)	338
TOPPINGS		
BBQ Sauce	1 serv (1 oz)	40
Brown Mustard	1 serv (1 oz)	0
Cheddar	1 serv (1 oz)	116
Dressing Balsamic Vinaigrette	1 serv (1.5 oz)	90
Dressing Bleu Cheese	1 serv (1.5 oz)	184
Dressing Italian	1 serv (0.5 oz)	51
Dressing Ranch	1 serv (0.5 oz)	83
Lettuce	1 serv (1 oz)	2
Margarine	1 serv (1 oz)	203
Mayonnaise	1 serv (1 oz)	101
Parmesan	1 serv (1 oz)	30
Peppers Jalapeno	1 serv (1.5 oz)	11
Peppers Mild	1 serv (1.5 oz)	11
Provolone	1 serv (0.75 oz)	80
Sour Cream	1 serv (1 oz)	61
Tomatoes	1 serv (2 oz)	24
White American	1 serv (1 oz)	101

SUBWAY
ADD-ONS AND SALAD DRESSINGS

American Cheese	1 serv (0.4 oz)	40
Bacon Strips	2	45

FOOD	PORTION	CALS
Banana Pepper Slices	3	0
Cheddar	1 serv (0.5 oz)	60
Fat Free Italian	1 serv (2 oz)	35
Fat Free Red Wine Vinaigrette	1 serv (0.7 oz)	30
Jalapeno Pepper Slices	3	<5
Mayonnaise	1 tbsp	110
Mayonnaise Light	1 tbsp	50
Monterey Cheddar Shredded	1 serv (0.5 oz)	50
Mustard Yellow or Deli	2 tsp	5
Olive Oil Blend	1 tsp	45
Pepperjack Cheese	1 serv (0.5 oz)	50
Provolone	1 serv (0.5 oz)	50
Ranch	1 serv (2 oz)	320
Ranch Lowfat	1.5 tbsp	120
Red Wine Vinaigrette	1 serv (2 oz)	80
Sauce Chipotle Southwest	1.5 tbsp	100
Sauce Fat Free Honey Mustard	1.5 tbsp	30
Sauce Fat Free Sweet Onion	1.5 tbsp	40
Swiss	1 serv (0.5 oz)	50
Vinegar	1 tsp	0
BREADS		
Hearty Italian	6 inch	220
Honey Oat	6 inch	250
Italian	6 inch	200
Italian Herb & Cheese	6 inch	250
Italian White	1 mini	140
Monterey Cheddar	6 inch	240
Parmesan Oregano	6 inch	220
Wheat	6 inch	200
Wheat	1 mini	140
Wrap	1	190
DESSERTS		
Apple Slices	1 pkg	35
Cookie Chocolate Chip	1	210
Cookie Chocolate Chip w/ M&M's	1 (1.6 oz)	210
Cookie Chocolate Chunk	1	220
Cookie Double Chocolate Chip	1 (1.6 oz)	210
Cookie Oatmeal Raisin	1	200
Cookie Peanut Butter	1	220
Cookie Sugar	1	220

FOOD	PORTION	CALS
Cookie White Chip Macadamia Nut	1	220
Raisins	1 pkg	150
SALADS		
Ham w/o Dressing & Croutons	1 serv	120
Oven Roasted Chicken Breast w/o Dressing & Croutons	1 serv	140
Roast Beef w/o Dressing & Croutons	1 serv	120
Subway Club w/o Dressing & Croutons	1 serv	150
Sweet Onion Chicken Teriyaki w/o Dressing & Croutons	1 serv	210
Turkey Breast & Ham w/o Dressing & Croutons	1 serv	120
Veggie Delight w/o Dressing & Croutons	1 serv	60
SANDWICHES		
6 Inch Chicken & Bacon Ranch	1	580
6 Inch Cold Cut Combo	1	410
6 Inch Double Stacked Cold Cut Combo	1	550
6 Inch Double Stacked Italian BMT	1	630
6 Inch Double Stacked Steak & Cheese	1	540
6 Inch Double Stacked Subway Club	1	420
6 Inch Double Stacked Sweet Onion Chicken Teriyaki	1	480
6 Inch Double Stacked Turkey Breast	1	330
6 Inch Ham	1	290
6 Inch Italian BMT	1	450
6 Inch Meatball Marinara	1	560
6 Inch Oven Roasted Chicken Breast	1	310
6 Inch Roast Beef	1	290
6 Inch Spicy Italian	1	480
6 Inch Steak & Cheese	1	400
6 Inch Subway Club	1	320
6 Inch Subway Melt	1	380
6 Inch Sweet Onion Chicken Teriyaki	1	370
6 Inch Tuna	1	530
6 Inch Turkey Breast	1	280
6 Inch Turkey Breast & Ham	1	290
6 Inch Veggie Delite	1	230
Mini Sub Ham	1	180
Mini Sub Roast Beef	1	190
Mini Sub Tuna w/ Cheese	1	320

FOOD	PORTION	CALS
Mini Sub Turkey Breast	1	190
Softwich Santa Fe Turkey	1	520

TACO BELL

FOOD	PORTION	CALS
Border Bowl Southwest Steak	1 serv	600
Border Bowl Zesty Chicken	1 serv	640
Border Bowl Zesty Chicken w/o Dressing	1 serv	440
Burrito 7 Layer	1	490
Burrito Bean	1	350
Burrito Chili Cheese	1	370
Burrito Grilled Stuft Chicken	1	640
Burrito Grilled Stuft Steak	1	630
Burrito Supreme Beef	1	420
Burrito ½ Lb Beef & Potato	1	530
Burrito ½ Lb Combo Beef	1	440
Burrito Fiesta Chicken	1	360
Burrito Fiesta Steak	1	370
Burrito Supreme Chicken	1	400
Burrito Supreme Steak	1	390
Chalupa Baja Beef	1	410
Chalupa Baja Chicken	1	390
Chalupa Baja Steak	1	390
Chalupa Nacho Cheese Beef	1	370
Chalupa Nacho Cheese Chicken	1	360
Chalupa Nacho Cheese Steak	1	340
Chalupa Supreme Beef	1	380
Chalupa Supreme Chicken	1	360
Chalupa Supreme Steak	1	360
Cheesy Fiesta Potatoes	1 serv	290
Cinnamon Twists	1 serv	170
Crunchwrap Supreme	1	560
Crunchwrap Supreme Spicy Chicken	1	540
Crunchy Taco	1	170
Crunchy Taco Supreme	1	210
Empanada Caramel Apple	1	290
Enchirito Beef	1	360
Enchirito Chicken	1	340
Fresco Border Bowl Zesty Chicken w/o Dressing	1 serv	350
Fresco Burrito Bean	1 (7.5 oz)	340

FOOD	PORTION	CALS
Fresco Burrito Fiesta Chicken	1	330
Fresco Burrito Supreme Chicken	1 (8.5 oz)	340
Fresco Burrito Supreme Steak	1 (8.5 oz)	330
Fresco Crunchy Taco	1 (3.2 oz)	150
Fresco Soft Taco Beef	1 (4 oz)	180
Fresco Soft Taco Grilled Steak	1 (4.5 oz)	160
Fresco Soft Taco Ranchero Chicken	1 (4.7 oz)	170
Gordita Baja Beef	1	340
Gordita Baja Chicken	1	320
Gordita Baja Steak	1	320
Gordita Nacho Cheese Beef	1	300
Gordita Nacho Cheese Chicken	1	280
Gordita Nacho Cheese Steak	1	270
Gordita Supreme Beef	1	310
Gordita Supreme Chicken	1	290
Gordita Supreme Steak	1	290
Guacamole Side	1 serv	70
Mexican Pizza	1	530
Mexican Rice	1 serv	180
MexiMelt	1 serv	260
Nacho Supreme	1 serv	440
Nachos	1 serv	330
Nachos Bellgrande	1 serv	770
Pintos 'n Cheese	1 serv	160
Quesadilla Cheese	1	470
Quesadilla Chicken	1	520
Quesadilla Steak	1	520
Salsa Side	1 serv	15
Soft Taco Grande	1	430
Soft Taco Grilled Steak	1	270
Soft Taco Ranchero Chicken	1	270
Soft Taco Supreme Beef	1	250
Sour Cream Side	1 serv	80
Taco Double Decker	1	320
Taco Double Decker Supreme	1	370
Taco Spicy Chicken	1	170
Taco Salad Express	1	610
Taco Salad Fiesta	1	840
Taco Salad Fiesta w/o Shell	1	470
Taco Salad Fiesta Chicken	1	790

FOOD	PORTION	CALS
Taco Salad Fiesta Chicken w/o Shell	1	430
Taquitos Chicken Grilled	1 serv	310
Taquitos Steak Grilled	1 serv	310
Tostada	1	240

TACO BUENO
MAIN MENU SELECTIONS

FOOD	PORTION	CALS
Bueno Chilada Beef	1 (7.9 oz)	523
Bueno Chilada Beef w/o Chili	1 (5.5 oz)	412
Bueno Chilada Beef w/o Queso	1 (5.6 oz)	337
Bueno Chilada Chicken	1 (7.4 oz)	477
Bueno Chilada Chicken w/o Chili	1 (5 oz)	366
Bueno Chilada Chicken w/o Queso	1 (5.1 oz)	290
Burrito Bean	1 (6.4 oz)	490
Burrito Bean w/o Cheddar Cheese	1 (5.9 oz)	412
Burrito Bean w/o Chili	1 (5.2 oz)	434
Burrito Beef	1 (6.9 oz)	510
Burrito Beef Potato	1 (4.8 oz)	350
Burrito Beef Potato w/o Queso	1 (4.1 oz)	305
Burrito Beef Potato w/o Sour Cream	1 (4.3 oz)	330
Burrito Beef w/o Cheddar Cheese	1 (6.4 oz)	432
Burrito Beef w/o Chili	1 (5.7 oz)	455
Burrito Big Ol' Beef	1 (10.6 oz)	772
Burrito Big Ol' Beef w/o Cheddar Cheese	1 (9.6 oz)	615
Burrito Big Ol' Beef w/o Chili	1 (9.4 oz)	716
Burrito Big Ol' Beef w/o Sour Cream	1 (9.6 oz)	715
Burrito Big Ol' Chicken	1 (8.4 oz)	607
Burrito Big Ol' Chicken w/o Cheddar Cheese	1 (7.4 oz)	450
Burrito Big Ol' Chicken w/o Sour Cream	1 (7.4 oz)	551
Burrito Chicken Potato	1 (4.5 oz)	327
Burrito Chicken Potato w/o Queso	1 (3.8 oz)	274
Burrito Chicken Potato w/o Sour Cream	1 (4 oz)	299
Burrito Combination	1 (6.8 oz)	507
Burrito Combination w/o Cheddar Cheese	1 (6.3 oz)	429
Burrito Combination w/o Chili	1 (5.6 oz)	452
Burrito Combination w/o Refried Beans	1 (5.7 oz)	440
Burrito Party	1 (4 oz)	298
Burrito Party w/o Cheddar Cheese	1 (3.8 oz)	259
Chimichanger Cheesecake	1 (2 oz)	210
Cinnamon Chips	1 serv (4.5 oz)	676

FOOD	PORTION	CALS
Corn Tortilla Chips	1 serv (1.5 oz)	219
Guacamole	1 serv (0.9 oz)	55
Jalapenos	1 serv (0.7 oz)	3
Mexican Rice	1 serv (4.2 oz)	469
Muchaco Beef	1 (5.2 oz)	449
Muchaco Beef w/o Cheddar Cheese	1 (4.9 oz)	410
Muchaco Beef w/o Refried Beans	1 (4.2 oz)	392
Muchaco Chicken	1 (4.6 oz)	387
Muchaco Chicken w/o Cheddar Cheese	1 (4.4 oz)	348
Nachos Cheese	1 serv (5.5 oz)	572
Quesadilla Beef Cheese	1 (8.5 oz)	823
Quesadilla	1 (6.5 oz)	709
Quesadilla Chicken	1 (7.9 oz)	761
Quesadilla Kids Cheese	1 (2.2 oz)	219
Quesadilla Mini Cheese	1 (2.7)	274
Refried Beans Powdered	1 serv (6.3 oz)	406
Refried Beans w/o Cheddar Cheese	1 serv (5.8 oz)	327
Refried Beans w/o Chili	1 serv (5.1 oz)	360
Salsa Red	1 serv (2 oz)	14
Soup Tortilla	1 bowl	237
Soup Tortilla w/o Tortilla Strips & Cheese	1 bowl	148
Sour Cream	1 serv (1 oz)	57
Taco Party	1 (1.9 oz)	143
Taco w/o Cheddar Cheese	1 (1.5 oz)	104
Taco Crispy Beef	1 (2.6 oz)	200
Taco Crispy Chicken	1 (1.9 oz)	140
Taco Crispy Chicken w/o Cheddar Cheese	1 (1.7 oz)	100
Taco Crispy w/o Cheddar Cheese	1 (2.4 oz)	161
Taco Soft Beef	1 (3.5 oz)	245
Taco Soft Beef w/o Cheddar Cheese	1 (3.2 oz)	206
Taco Soft Chicken	1 (2.9 oz)	184
Taco Soft Chicken w/o Cheddar Cheese	1 (2.5 oz)	145
Tostada	1 (4.1 oz)	324
Tostada w/o Cheddar Cheese	1 (3.3 oz	207
Tostada w/o Chili	1 (2.9 oz)	269
Tostada w/o Refried Beans	1 (2.5 oz)	234
SALADS		
Nacho Beef	1 (9.3 oz)	759
Nacho Beef w/o Cheddar Cheese	1 (8.8 oz)	681
Nacho Beef w/o Chili	1 (6.9 oz)	648

FOOD	PORTION	CALS
Nacho Chicken	1 (8.9 oz)	713
Nacho Chicken w/o Cheddar Cheese	1 (8.4 oz)	634
Nacho Chicken w/o Chili	1 (6.5 oz)	601
Taco Beef	1 (12.7 oz)	1043
Taco Beef w/o Cheddar Cheese	1 (11.7 oz)	886
Taco Beef w/o Chili	1 (11.5 oz)	987
Taco Beef w/o Guacamole	1 (11.7 oz)	988
Taco Beef w/o Sour Cream	1 (11.7 oz)	986
Taco Beef w/o Tortilla Bowl	1 (9.7 oz)	564
Taco Chicken	1 (9.6 oz)	838
Taco Chicken w/o Cheddar Cheese	1 (8.6 oz)	680
Taco Chicken w/o Guacamole	1 (8.6 oz)	783
Taco Chicken w/o Sour Cream	1 (8.6 oz)	781
Taco Chicken w/o Tortilla Bowl	1 (6.6 oz)	359

TACO CABANA
ADD-ONS

FOOD	PORTION	CALS
Dressing Southwest Ranch	1 serv (1 oz)	112
Guacamole	1 serv (3 oz)	110
Pico De Gallo	1 serv (1 oz)	5
Queso	1 serv (3 oz)	200
Salsa Black Bean & Corn	1 serv (1 oz)	30
Salsa Fuego	1 serv (1 oz)	5
Salsa Pineapple	1 serv (1 oz)	20
Salsa Ranch	1 serv (1 oz)	35
Salsa Roja	1 serv (1 oz)	5
Salsa Verde	1 serv (1 oz)	10
Shredded Cheese	1 serv (1 oz)	110
Sour Cream	1 serv (3 oz)	160

BREAKFAST MENU SELECTIONS

FOOD	PORTION	CALS
Breakfast Burrito Bacon & Egg	1	410
Breakfast Burrito Barbacoa	1	510
Breakfast Burrito Chorizo & Egg	1	400
Breakfast Burrito Potato & Egg	1	440
Breakfast Taco Bacon & Egg	1	230
Breakfast Taco Barbacoa	1	250
Breakfast Taco Chorizo & Egg	1	200
Breakfast Taco Potato & Egg	1	210
Plates Huevos Rancheros	1 serv	770
Plates Steak Fajitas & Scrambled Eggs	1 serv	800
Platter Eggs Mexicana	1 serv	920

FOOD	PORTION	CALS
MAIN MENU SELECTIONS		
Black Beans	1 serv	80
Borracho Beans	1 serv	140
Burrito Bean & Cheese	1	730
Burrito Beef Ground	1	710
Burrito Black Bean	1	450
Burrito Chicken Breast Fajita	1	630
Burrito Chicken Stewed	1	660
Burrito Chicken Ultimo Stewed	1	760
Burrito Steak Fajita	1	650
Burritos Beef Ultimo Ground	1	800
Chips	1 serv (2.5 oz)	180
Fajitas Chicken Personal	1 serv	740
Fajitas Chicken Platter	1 serv	1670
Fajitas Steak Personal	1 serv	760
Flautas Chicken	1	100
Refried Beans	1 serv	250
Taco Beef Ground	1	230
Taco Chicken Breast Fajita	1	190
Taco Steak Fajita	1	200
Taco Crispy Chicken Stewed	1	160
Taco Crispy Ground Beef	1	180
Taco Soft Bean & Cheese	1	300
Taco Soft Black Bean	1	200
Taco Soft Carne Guisada	1	190
Taco Soft Chicken Stewed	1	210
Tortilla Corn	1	70
Tortilla Flour	1	120
TACO JOHN'S		
BREAKFAST SELECTIONS		
Breakfast Burrito Bacon	1 (7.6 oz)	550
Breakfast Burrito Egg	1 (6.6 oz)	420
Breakfast Burrito Egg Bacon	1 (7 oz)	500
Breakfast Burrito Egg Sausage	1 (8.1 oz)	590
Breakfast Burrito Sausage	1 (8.6 oz)	640
Breakfast Taco Bacon	1 (3.7 oz)	270
Breakfast Taco Sausage	1 (4.2 oz)	310
Scrambler Burrito Bacon	1 (8.6 oz)	550
Scrambler Burrito Sausage	1 (9.6 oz)	640

FOOD	PORTION	CALS
Scrambler Potato Ole Bacon	1 sm (9.4 oz)	630
Scrambler Potato Ole Sausage	1 sm (10.5 oz)	720
DESSERTS		
Apple Grande	1 serv (3.4 oz)	270
Choco Taco	1 serv (4 oz)	390
Churro	1 serv (2 oz)	190
Cini-Sopapilla Bites	1 serv (2.6 oz)	210
Giant Goldfish Grahams	1 serv (0.5 oz)	70
MAIN MENU SELECTIONS		
Burrito Bean	1 (6.6 oz)	360
Burrito Beefy	1 (6.6 oz)	440
Burrito Chicken & Potato	1 (8.3 oz)	470
Burrito Chicken Grilled	1 (8.2 oz)	590
Burrito Combination	1 (6.6 oz)	400
Burrito Crunchy Chicken & Potato	1 (8.8 oz)	600
Burrito Grilled Beef	1 (8.2 oz)	600
Burrito Meat & Potato	1 (8.3 oz)	500
Burrito Ranch Beef	1 (7.1 oz)	440
Burrito Ranch Chicken	1 (7 oz)	400
Burrito Smothered	1 (11.3 oz)	510
Burrito Super	1 (8.8 oz)	450
Chili w/o Crackers	1 serv (8 oz)	220
Chili w/o Crackers & Cheese	1 serv (7.5 oz)	160
Chilto	1 serv (4.6 oz)	360
Chips & Queso	1 serv (6.7 oz)	430
Crispy Taco	1 (3.2 oz)	180
Crunchy Chicken w/o Sauce	1 serv (5 oz)	450
Enchiliada Chili	1 serv (7.6 oz)	310
Mexi Rolls w/o Nachos	2 pieces (1.9 oz)	130
Mexican Rice	1 serv (6 oz)	250
Nachos	1 serv (5 oz)	380
Potato Oles	1 sm (5 oz)	430
Potato Oles Chili Cheese	1 serv (10.7 oz)	590
Potato Oles Super	1 serv (9.7 oz)	620
Quesadilla Melt Cheesey	1 (5.6 oz)	440
Quesadilla Melt Fajita Beef	1 serv (8.6 oz)	540
Quesadilla Melt Fajita Chicken	1 (8.6 oz)	510
Refried Beans	1 serv (9.4 oz)	320
Refried Beans w/o Cheese	1 serv (8.9 oz)	260
Sierra Chicken Sandwich	1 (8.2 oz)	350

FOOD	PORTION	CALS
Softshell Taco	1 (4 oz)	220
Super Nachos	1 sm (6.9 oz)	450
Taco Bravo	1 (6.5 oz)	340
Taco Burger	1 (5 oz)	270
Taco Stuffed Grilled	1 (7.4 oz)	560
SALAD DRESSINGS AND TOPPINGS		
Bacon Ranch Dressing	1 serv (1.5 oz)	130
Creamy Italian Dressing	1 serv (1.5 oz)	130
Guacamole	1 serv (2 oz)	90
Hot Sauce	1 serv (1 oz)	10
House Dressing	1 serv (1.5 oz)	70
Mild Sauce	1 serv (1 oz)	10
Nacho Cheese	1 serv (3 oz)	120
Pico De Gallo	1 serv (1 oz)	10
Ranch Dressing	1 serv (1.5 oz)	140
Salsa	1 serv (2 oz)	20
Sour Cream	1 serv (2 oz)	120
Super Hot Sauce	1 serv (1 oz)	10
SALADS		
Softshell Taco Chicken	1 (4 oz)	190
Taco Crunchy Chicken w/o Dressing	1 serv (13.4 oz)	660
Taco w/o Dressing	1 serv (12.7 oz)	520

TACOTIME
DESSERTS

Churro Plain	1 (1.5 oz)	205
Churro w/ Cinnamon & Sugar	1 (2 oz)	245
Crustos	1 serv	294
Empanada Apple	1 (4 oz)	234
Empanada Cherry	1 (4 oz)	240
Empanada Pumpkin	1 (4 oz)	256
MAIN MENU SELECTIONS		
Burrito Big Juan Chicken	1 (13 oz)	594
Burrito Big Juan Seasoned Ground Beef	1 (13 oz)	651
Burrito Big Juan Shredded Beef	1 (13 oz)	633
Burrito Casita Chicken	1 (12 oz)	494
Burrito Casita Seasoned Ground Beef	1 (12 oz)	552
Burrito Casita Shredded Beef	1 (12 oz)	533
Burrito Chicken & Black Bean	1 (10 oz)	478
Burrito Chicken BLT	1 (10 oz)	721

FOOD	PORTION	CALS
Burrito Chicken Ranchero	1 (10.8 oz)	654
Burrito Crisp Chicken	1 (5.5 oz)	336
Burrito Crisp Meat	1 (5.8 oz)	450
Burrito Crisp Pinto Bean	1 (6 oz)	394
Burrito Soft Meat	1 (6.7 oz)	426
Burrito Soft Pinto Bean	1 (6.7 oz)	377
Burrito Veggie	1 (11 oz)	534
Cheddar Fries	1 sm (6 oz)	374
Cheddar Melt	1 (2.8 oz)	250
Mexi-Fries	1 sm (5 oz)	290
Mexi-Rice	1 serv (4 oz)	87
Nachos Grande	1 serv (16.5 oz)	1132
Refritos w/ Chips	1 serv (7 oz)	304
Refritos w/o Chips	1 serv (6.7 oz)	285
Stuffed Fries	1 sm (5 oz)	321
Taco Crisp Seasoned Ground Beef	1 (4.3 oz)	225
Taco Super Soft Chicken	1 (11 oz)	540
Taco Super Soft Seasoned Ground Beef	1 (11 oz)	598
Taco Super Soft Shredded Beef	1 (11 oz)	579
Taco Value Soft	1 (5.3 oz)	314
Taco ½ Lb Shredded Beef	1 (9 oz)	440
Taco ½ Lb Soft Chicken	1 (9 oz)	401
Taco ½ Lb Soft Seasoned Ground Beef	1 (9 oz)	459
Taco Chips	1 serv (2 oz)	150
SALAD DRESSINGS AND TOPPINGS		
Cheddar Cheese	1 serv (2 oz)	223
Dressing Chipotle Ranch	1 serv (1 oz)	165
Dressing Ranch	1 serv (1 oz)	181
Dressing Thousand Island	1 serv (1 oz)	132
Guacamole	1 serv (1 oz)	50
Salsa Nuevo	1 serv (1 oz)	8
Salsa Verde	1 serv (1 oz)	6
Sour Cream	1 serv (1.5 oz)	85
SALADS		
Taco Chicken	1 reg (9.2 oz)	351
Taco Seasoned Ground Beef	1 reg (7.8 oz)	396
Taco Shredded Beef	1 reg (7.8 oz)	377
Tostada Delight Chicken	1 (10.5 oz)	565
Tostada Delight Seasoned Ground Beef	1 (10.5 oz)	623
Tostada Delight Shredded Beef	1 (10.5 oz)	604

FOOD	PORTION	CALS
TCBY		
FROZEN YOGURT AND SORBET		
Hand Scooped Butter Pecan Perfection	½ cup	110
Hand Scooped Chocolate Chocolate Swirl	½ cup	120
Hand Scooped Chocolate Chunk Cookie Dough	½ cup	160
Hand Scooped Cookies & Cream	½ cup	140
Hand Scooped Cotton Candy	½ cup	120
Hand Scooped Mint Chocolate Chunk	½ cup	140
Hand Scooped Mocha Almond	½ cup	150
Hand Scooped No Sugar Added Chocolate Chocolate Swirl	½ cup	90
Hand Scooped No Sugar Added Vanilla	½ cup	80
Hand Scooped No Sugar Added Vanilla Fudge Brownie	½ cup	100
Hand Scooped Pralines & Cream	½ cup	140
Hand Scooped Psychedelic Sorbet	½ cup	290
Hand Scooped Rainbow Cream	½ cup	120
Hand Scooped Rocky Road	½ cup	220
Hand Scooped Strawberries & Cream	½ cup	120
Hand Scooped Vanilla Chocolate Chunk	½ cup	140
Hand Scooped Vanilla Bean	½ cup	120
Soft Serve Frozen Yogurt All Flavors 96% Fat Free	½ cup	140
Soft Serve Frozen Yogurt All Flavors Low Carb	½ cup	110
Soft Serve Frozen Yogurt All Flavors Nonfat	½ cup	110
Soft Serve Frozen Yogurt All Flavors Nonfat No Sugar Added	½ cup	90
Soft Serve Sorbet All Flavors Nonfat Nondairy	½ cup	100
SMOOTHIES		
Berrylicious	1 (16 oz)	290
Black 'N Blueberry	1 (16 oz)	280
Mango Tango	1 (16 oz)	330
Mangolada	1 (16 oz)	340
Mondo Mango	1 (16 oz)	310
Pina Paradise	1 (16 oz)	350
Pink Pineapple	1 (16 oz)	340
Straight Up Strawberry	1 (16 oz)	280
Strawberry Bonanza	1 (16 oz)	320
Strawberry Fling	1 (16 oz)	340

FOOD	PORTION	CALS
TIM HORTONS		
BAKED SELECTIONS		
Bagel Blueberry	1	270
Bagel Cinnamon Raisin	1	270
Bagel Everything	1	280
Bagel Flax Seed	1	290
Bagel Onion	1	260
Bagel Plain	1	260
Bagel Poppy Seed	1	270
Bagel Sesame Seed	1	270
Bagel Sun Dried Tomato	1	310
Bagel Twelve Grain	1	330
Cinnamon Roll Frosted	1	470
Cinnamon Roll Glazed	1	420
Cookie Caramel Chocolate Pecan	1	230
Cookie Chocolate Chip	1	230
Cookie Oatmeal Raisin Spice	1	220
Cookie Peanut Butter Chocolate Chunk	1	260
Cookie Triple Chocolate	1	250
Cookie White Chocolate Macadamia Nut	1	240
Croissant Butter	1	340
Croissant Cheese	1	370
Danish Cherry Cheese	1	330
Danish Chocolate	1	430
Danish Maple Pecan	1	380
Donut Apple Fritter	1	300
Donut Chocolate Dip	1	210
Donut Chocolate Glazed	1	260
Donut Honey Dip	1	210
Donut Maple Dip	1	210
Donut Old Fashion Glazed	1	320
Donut Old Fashion Plain	1	260
Donut Sour Cream Plain	1	270
Donut Walnut Crunch	1	360
Donut Filled Angel Cream	1	310
Donut Filled Blueberry	1	230
Donut Filled Boston Cream	1	250
Donut Filled Canadian Maple	1	260
Donut Filled Strawberry	1	230
Honey Cruller	1	320

FOOD	PORTION	CALS
Muffin Blueberry	1	330
Muffin Blueberry Bran	1	300
Muffin Carrot Wheat	1	400
Muffin Chocolate Chip	1	430
Muffin Cranberry Blueberry Bran	1	290
Muffin Cranberry Fruit	1	350
Muffin Fruit Explosion	1	360
Muffin Raisin Bran	1	360
Muffin Strawberry Sensation	1	350
Muffin Low Fat Blueberry	1	290
Muffin Low Fat Cranberry	1	290
Tea Biscuit Plain	1	250
Tea Biscuit Raisin	1	290
Timbits Apple Fritter	1	50
Timbits Chocolate Glazed	1	70
Timbits Honey Dip	1	60
Timbits Old Fashion Plain	1	70
Timbits Filled Banana Cream	1	60
Timbits Filled Lemon	1	60
Timbits Filled Strawberry	1	60
BEVERAGES		
Cafe Mocha	1 (10 oz)	160
Cappuccino Iced	1 (12 oz)	300
Coffee Decaffeinated Sugar & Cream	1 (10 oz)	75
Coffee Sugar & Cream	1 (10 oz)	75
English Toffee	1 (10 oz)	220
Flavor Shot	1 serv	5
French Vanilla	1 (10 oz)	240
Hot Chocolate	1 (10 oz)	240
Hot Smoothie	1 (10 oz)	260
Iced Cappuccino w/ Milk	1 (12 oz)	180
Tea Sugar & Milk	1 (10 oz)	50
CREAM CHEESE		
Garden Vegetable	1.5 oz	120
Light Plain	1.5 oz	60
Plain	1.5 oz	130
Strawberry	1.5 oz	120
SANDWICHES		
B.L.T.	1	450
Breakfast Bacon Egg Cheese	1	410

FOOD	PORTION	CALS
Breakfast Egg Cheese	1	360
Breakfast Sausage Egg Cheese	1	520
Chicken Salad	1	380
Egg Salad	1	390
Ham & Swiss	1	440
Toasted Chicken Club	1	460
Turkey Breast	1	390
SOUPS		
Beef Stew	1 serv (10 oz)	236
Chicken Noodle	1 serv (10 oz)	120
Chili	1 serv (10 oz)	300
Country Field Mushroom	1 serv (10 oz)	150
Cream Of Broccoli	1 serv (10 oz)	160
Hearty Vegetable	1 serv (10 oz)	70
Minestrone	1 serv (10 oz)	120
Potato Bacon	1 serv (10 oz)	180
Split Pea w/ Ham	1 serv (10 oz)	150
Turkey Rice	1 serv (10 oz)	120
Vegetable Beef Barley	1 serv (10 oz)	110
YOGURT		
Low Fat Creamy Vanilla w/ Berries	1 (6 oz)	160
Low Fat Strawberry w/ Berries	1 (6 oz)	150

T.J. CINNAMONS

FOOD	PORTION	CALS
Chocolate Twist	1	250
Cinnamon Twist	1	280
Mocha Chill w/ Whipped Cream	1 (12.5 oz)	306
Mocha Chill w/o Whipped Cream	1 (12.5 oz)	264
Original Roll w/o Icing	1	507
Pecan Sticky Bun	1	688
TJ Icing	1 serv (1 oz)	117

TOGO'S
SALAD DRESSINGS

FOOD	PORTION	CALS
Asian	1 serv (2.5 oz)	380
Blue Cheese	1 serv (2.5 oz)	260
Buttermilk Ranch	1 serv (2.5 oz)	250
Caesar	1 serv (2.5 oz)	150
Fat Free Serano Grape Vinaigrette	1 serv (2.5 oz)	90
Low Fat Balsamic Vinaigrette	1 serv (2.5 oz)	90

FOOD	PORTION	CALS
SALADS		
Asian Chicken w/o Dressing	1 full serv	200
Chicken Caesar w/o Dressing	1 full serv	210
Cobb w/o Dressing	1 full serv	330
Santa Fe Chicken w/o Dressing	1 full serv	370
Taco w/o Dressing	1 full serv	600
SANDWICHES		
Albacore Tuna	1 reg	660
Avocado & Cucumber	1 reg	560
Black Forest Ham & Cheese	1 reg	670
Capicolla Dry Salami & Provolone	1 reg	1080
Cheese	1 reg	800
Chef's Creations Pacific Cobb	1 reg	710
Chef's Creations Pastrami Reuben	1 reg	990
Chicken Salad	1 reg	650
Egg Salad & Cheese	1 reg	750
Hot BBQ Beef	1 reg	670
Hot Meatball	1 reg	690
Hot Pastrami	1 reg	750
Hot Roast Beef	1 reg	730
Hummus	1 reg	650
Salami & Cheese	1 reg	1100
Turkey & Avocado	1 reg	640
Turkey & Cheese	1 reg	670
Turkey & Cranberry	1 reg	670
Turkey Bacon Club	1 reg	680
Turkey Ham & Cheese	1 reg	690
WHATABURGER		
BEVERAGES		
Barq's Root Beer	1 sm (16 oz)	220
Cherry Coke	1 sm (16 oz)	210
Coca-Cola	1 sm (16 oz)	207
Coffee	1 sm (8 oz)	5
Coffee Decafe	1 sm (8 oz)	5
Diet Coke	1 sm (16 oz)	0
Dr Pepper	1 sm (16 oz)	190
Fanta Orange	1 sm (16 oz)	210
Fanta Strawberry	1 sm (16 oz)	230
Iced Tea Sweetened	1 (34 oz)	430

FOOD	PORTION	CALS
Iced Tea Unsweetened	1 sm (19 oz)	0
Lemonade Hi-C Poppin' Pink	1 sm (16 oz)	200
Malt Chocolate	1 sm (16 oz)	670
Malt Strawberry	1 sm (16 oz)	670
Malt Vanilla	1 sm (16 oz)	600
Milk Reduced Fat	8 oz	120
Orange Juice Tropicana	1 (10 oz)	140
Powerade Fruit Punch	1 sm (16 oz)	130
Shake Chocolate	1 sm (16 oz)	630
Shake Strawberry	1 sm (16 oz)	630
Shake Vanilla	1 sm (16 oz)	560
Sprite	1 sm (16 oz)	200
CHILDREN'S MENU SELECTIONS		
Kid's Meal Chicken Strips	1 serv	770
Kid's Meal Justaburger	1 serv	570
DESSERTS		
Apple Pie A La Mode	1 serv	520
Apple Pie Hot	1	230
Cinnamon Roll	1	400
Cookie Chocolate Chunk	1 (2 oz)	230
Cookie White Chocolate Chunk Macadamia	1 (2 oz)	250
Peach Pie A La Mode	1 serv	570
MAIN MENU SELECTIONS		
Biscuit	1	300
Biscuit Sandwich Bacon Egg & Cheese	1	500
Biscuit Sandwich Egg & Cheese	1	450
Biscuit Sandwich Honey Butter Chicken	1	610
Biscuit Sandwich Sausage Egg & Cheese	1	690
Biscuit w/ Bacon	1	355
Biscuit w/ Gravy	1	530
Biscuit w/ Sausage	1	540
Breakfast Platter w/ Bacon	1 serv	730
Breakfast Platter w/ Sausage	1 serv	930
Breakfast On A Bun w/ Bacon	1	380
Breakfast On A Bun w/ Sausage	1	570
Chicken Strips	1	200
Chicken Strips w/ Gravy	4	840
French Fries	1 sm	260
Gravy White Peppered	1 serv	60
Hashbrown Sticks	4	200

FOOD	PORTION	CALS
Justaburger	1	329
Onion Rings	1 med	420
Pancakes Plain	1 serv	580
Pancakes w/ Bacon	1 serv	630
Pancakes w/ Sausage	1 serv	820
Sandwich Chicken Strip Honey BBQ	1	1110
Sandwich Chicken Strip Junior Honey BBQ	1	720
Sandwich Egg	1	330
Sandwich Grilled Chicken	1	450
Taquito w/ Bacon & Egg	1	370
Taquito w/ Bacon Egg & Cheese	1	420
Taquito w/ Potato & Egg	1	430
Taquito w/ Potato Egg & Cheese	1	470
Taquito w/ Sausage & Egg	1	410
Taquito w/ Sausage Egg & Cheese	1	450
Texas Toast	1 slice	180
Whataburger	1	640
Whataburger Double Meat	1	890
Whataburger Jr.	1	330
Whataburger Triple Meat	1	1140
Whataburger w/ Bacon & Cheese	1	800
Whatacatch	1	480
Whatacatch Dinner	1 serv	1095
Whatachick'n	1	530
SALADS		
Chicken Strips	1 serv	570
Garden Salad	1	60
Grilled Chicken	1 serv	230

WHITE CASTLE
BEVERAGES

Barq's Red Cream Soda	1 sm (21 oz)	260
Barq's Root Beer	1 sm (21 oz)	250
Coca-Cola	1 sm (21 oz)	220
Coffee Black	1 sm (12 oz)	<5
Crave Cooler Coke	1 sm (21 oz)	150
Diet Coke	1 sm (21 oz)	0
Fanta Orange	1 sm (21 oz)	240
Hi-C Flashing Fruit Punch	1 sm (21 oz)	240
Hot Chocolate	1 sm (12 oz)	220

FOOD	PORTION	CALS
Hot Tea	1 sm (12 oz)	0
Iced Tea Sweetened w/ Lemon	1 sm (21 oz)	170
Iced Tea Unsweetened	1 sm (21 oz)	0
Lemonade Raspberry	1 sm (21 oz)	290
Pibb Xtra	1 sm (21 oz)	220
Powerade Mountain Blast	1 sm (21 oz)	140
Sprite	1 sm (21 oz)	220
MAIN MENU SELECTIONS		
Cheeseburger	1	170
Cheeseburger Bacon	1	200
Cheeseburger Bacon Double	1	370
Cheeseburger Double	1	300
Cheeseburger Jalapeno	1	180
Cheeseburger Jalapeno Double	1	320
Chicken Rings	6	210
Clam Strips	1 reg	250
Fish Nibblers	1 reg	280
French Fries	1 reg	310
Mozzarella Cheese Sticks	3	250
Onion Chips	1 reg	480
Sandwich Chicken Breast w/ Cheese	1	200
Sandwich Chicken Ring	1	180
Sandwich Chicken Ring w/ Cheese	1	200
Sandwich Fish w/ Cheese	1	180
White Castle	1	140
White Castle Double	1	250
SAUCES AND SPREADS		
Dressing Ranch	1 serv (1 oz)	150
Ketchup	1 pkg	10
Lemon Juice	1 pkg	0
Mayonnaise	1 pkg	60
Sauce BBQ	1 serv (1 oz)	35
Sauce Fat Free Honey Mustard	1 serv (1 oz)	50
Sauce Hot	1 pkg	0
Sauce Marinara	1 serv (1 oz)	15
Sauce Seafood	1 serv (1 oz)	30
Sauce Tartar	1 pkg	30
Sauce Zesty Zing	1 serv (1 oz)	110

FOOD	PORTION	CALS
WINCHELL'S DONUTS		
Chocolate Bar	1	240
Chocolate Round	1	240
Chocolate Twist	1	240
Croissant	1	260
Glazed Round	1	230
Glazed Twist	1	230
Iced Chocolate	1	230
Traditional	1	215
WORLD WRAPPS		
CHILDREN'S MENU SELECTIONS		
Kid's Bean & Cheese	1	332
Kid's Chicken & Cheese	1	229
Kid's Quesadilla	1	410
Kid's Teriyaki Chicken	1	407
SALADS		
BBQ Ranch Chicken	1 serv	633
Caesar Blackened Salmon	1 serv	612
Caesar Classic	1 serv	417
California Cobb	1 serv	636
Garden Veggie	1 serv	492
Thai Asian Chicken	1 serv	613
SIDES AND SOUPS		
Chips & Mango Salsa	1 serv	224
Chips & Tomato Corn Salsa	1 serv	184
Potstickers	3	170
Soup Thai Lemongrass	1 cup	256
Soup Tortilla	1 cup	191
Yogurt Parfait	1 serv	281
SMOOTHIES		
Black & Blue	1 (16 oz)	319
Blue Mango Boost	1 (16 oz)	295
Caribbean C	1 (16 oz)	276
Georgia Peach	1 (16 oz)	343
Peanut Butter Banana	1 (16 oz)	502
Strawberry Orange Banana	1 (16 oz)	268
Triathlete	1 (16 oz)	341
Tropical Storm	1 (16 oz)	309

FOOD	PORTION	CALS
WRAPS		
Baja Veggie w/ Cheese Sour Cream Avocados	1 sm	541
Barcelona	1 sm	460
Bean & Cheese	1 sm	452
Bombay Curry Veggie	1 sm	495
Buffalo w/ Shrimp	1 sm	422
Burrito w/ Chicken Cheese Sour Cream Avocado	1 sm	576
Burrito w/ Steak Cheese Sour Cream Avocado	1 sm	573
Caribbean Sole	1 sm	523
Chicken Caesar	1 sm	547
Chicken Parmesan	1 sm	495
Portabello & Goat Cheese	1 sm	391
Samurai Salmon	1 sm	543
Spicy Southwest Shrimp	1 sm	460
Tequila Lime Shrimp	1 sm	422
Teriyaki Chicken	1 sm	482
Teriyaki Steak	1 sm	497
Teriyaki Tofu & Mushroom	1 sm	387
Texas Roadhouse BBQ Chicken	1 sm	512
Texas Roadhouse BBQ Steak	1 sm	569
Thai Chicken	1 sm	508
YOGEN FRUZ		
Blend It No Sugar Added Vanilla	1 sm	110
Blend It Probiotic Low Fat Chocolate	1 sm	121
Blend It Probiotic Low Fat Vanilla	1 sm	121
Blend It Probiotic Non Fat Vanilla	1 sm	110
Smoothie Dairy Blueberry Breeze	1 sm	180
Smoothie Dairy Peach Berry Sunset	1 sm	150
Smoothie Dairy Strawberry Banana	1 sm	180
Smoothie Non Dairy Raspberry Blast	1 sm	208
Smoothie Non Dairy Tropical Storm	1 sm	224
Smoothie Non Dairy Very Berry	1 sm	192
Top It Probiotic Soft Serve	1 sm	132
YOGURTLAND		
Arctic Vanilla	½ cup (3 oz)	108
Blueberry Tart	½ cup (3 oz)	127
Cafe Con Leche	½ cup (3 oz)	108
Chocolate Mint	½ cup (3 oz)	100

FOOD	PORTION	CALS
Double Cookies & Cream	½ cup (3 oz)	121
Dutch Chocolate	½ cup (3 oz)	118
French Vanilla No Sugar Added	½ cup (3 oz)	89
Fresh Strawberry	½ cup (3 oz)	108
Green Tea	½ cup (3 oz)	107
Heath Bar	½ cup (3 oz)	132
Mango	½ cup (3 oz)	96
Mango Tart	½ cup (3 oz)	127
NY Cheesecake	½ cup (3 oz)	100
Peach	½ cup (3 oz)	100
Peach Tart	½ cup (3 oz)	127
Peanut Butter	½ cup (3 oz)	119
Pineapple Tart	½ cup (3 oz)	127
Pistachio	½ cup (3 oz)	100
Plain Tart	½ cup (3 oz)	108
Strawberry Tart	½ cup (3 oz)	127
Taro	½ cup (3 oz)	102

ZOUP!
DESSERTS

FOOD	PORTION	CALS
Cookie Chocolate Chunk	1	410
Cookie Peanut Butter	1	420

SANDWICHES

FOOD	PORTION	CALS
Grilled Turkey Club	½	470
Panini Italian Chicken	½	370
Pesto Three Cheese	1	720
Tuna Melt	1	600
Wrap American Farm	½	435
Wrap Asian	½	615
Wrap Chicken Caesar w/o Dressing	½	505
Wrap Greek w/o Dressing	½	485
Wrap Sonoma	½	595
Wrap Tuna	½	365
Zesty Southwest Turkey	½	310

SOUPS

FOOD	PORTION	CALS
Chicken & Dumplings	1 (8 oz)	130
Chicken Potpie	1 (8 oz)	200
Italian Wedding w/ Turkey Meatballs	1 (8 oz)	120
Jamaican Bay Gumbo	1 (8 oz)	140
Lobster Bisque	1 (8 oz)	260

FOOD	PORTION	CALS
Pepper Steak	1 (8 oz)	160
Potato Cheddar	1 (8 oz)	210
Sesame Noodle Bowl	1 (8 oz)	80
Shrimp & Crawfish Etouffee	1 (8 oz)	130
Sicilian Pizza	1 (8 oz)	150
Spicy Crab & Rice	1 (8 oz)	110
Turkey Chili	1 (8 oz)	120
Wild Mushroom Barley	1 (8 oz)	108